SURGICAL attending ROUNDS

SURGICAL attending ROUNDS

Cornelius Mckown Dyke M.D.
Eric J. DeMaria M.D.

third edition

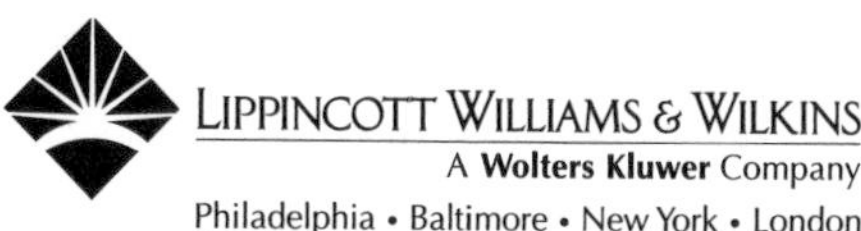

LIPPINCOTT WILLIAMS & WILKINS
A **Wolters Kluwer** Company
Philadelphia • Baltimore • New York • London
Buenos Aires • Hong Kong • Sydney • Tokyo

Acquisitions Editor: Craig Percy
Developmental Editor: Joanne Bersin
Project Manager: Bridgett Dougherty
Manufacturing Manager: Ben Rivera
Marketing Manager: Adam Glazer
Cover Designer: Joseph DePinho
Compositor: TechBooks
Printer: RR Donnelley

530 Walnut Street
Philadelphia, PA 19106 USA
LWW.com

Printed in the USA

Library of Congress Cataloging-in-Publication Data

Surgical attending rounds / [edited by] Cornelius McKown Dyke, Eric J. DeMaria.—3rd ed.
p. ; cm.
Includes bibliographical references and index.
ISBN-13: 978-0-7817-5046-2
ISBN-10: 0-7817-5046-6
1. Surgery—Examinations, questions, etc. I. Dyke, Cornelius M. II. DeMaria, Eric J., 1959-
[DNLM: 1. Surgery—Examination Questions. 2. Surgical Procedures, Operative—Examination Questions. WO 18.2 S9617 2004]
RD37.2.S9745 2004
617′.0076—dc22

2004015710

---

10 9 8 7 6 5 4

CONTRIBUTORS

Michael Aboutanos, M.D., MPH
Assistant Professor of Surgery
Division of Trauma/Critical Care
Department of Surgery
Virginia Commonwealth University Health Systems
Richmond, VA

Robert D. Acton, M.D.
Assistant Professor of Surgery and Pediatrics
Department of Surgery
University of Minnesota
Minneapolis, MN

Gregory K. Albaugh, D.O.
Attending Surgeon
St. Johns Regional Medical Center
Oxnard, CA

Sean Jeffrey Barnett, M.S., M.D.
Surgical Research Fellow
Department of Surgery
University of Minnesota
Minneapolis, MN

J. Christopher Brandys, M.D.
Director of the Cornerstone Wound Healing Center
Department of Surgery
Barrrow Community Hospital
Atlanta, GA

Tim M. Brandys, M.D.
Assistant Professor
Division of Vascular Surgery
Core Program Director
Department of Surgery
University of Ottowa
Ottowa, Canada

Kelli M. Bullard, M.D.
Assistant Professor
Department of Surgery
University of Minnesota
Minneapolis, MN

Attending Surgeon
Department of Surgery
Fairview University Medical Center
Minneapolis, MN

Keith G. Chisholm, M.D.
Adjunct Assistant Professor
Department of Surgery
University of Florida
Gainesville, FL

Attending Surgeon
Department of Surgery
Malcolm Randall VA Medical Center
Gainesville, FL

Nicholas P.W. Coe, M.D.
Professor
Department of Surgery
Tufts University School of Medicine
Springfield, MA

Director, Surgical Education
Department of Surgery
Baystate University Medical Center
Springfield, MA

Eric J. DeMaria, M.D.
Professor
Division of General/Trauma Surgery
Richmond, VA

Director, Center for Minimally Invasive Surgery
General Surgery Division
Virginia Commonwealth University
Richmond, VA

André Duranceau, M.D.
Professor of Surgery
Chief, Division of Thoracic Surgery
Université de Montreal
Montreal, Quebec, Canada

Cornelius McKowan Dyke, M.D.
The Sanger Clinic-Gastonia
Gaston Memorial Hospital
Gastonia, NC

Pasquale Ferraro, M.D.
Division of Thoracic Surgery
Hotel Dieu Hospital
Montreal, Canada

Viriato M. Fiallo, M.D., FACS
Assistant Professor of Surgery
Department of Surgery
Tufts University School of Medicine
Springfield, MA

James S. Gammie, M.D.
Assistant Professor of Surgery
Department of Cardiac Surgery
University of Maryland School of Medicine
Baltimore, MD

D. Lee Gordon, M.D.
Assistant Professor of Surgery
Vanderbilt University Medical Center
Division of Hepatobiliary Surgery and Liver Transplant
Nashville, TN

Dennis C. Gore, M.D.
Associate Professor
Department of Surgery
University of Texas Medical Branch
Galveston, TX

Co-Director, Surgical Intensive Care Unit
Department of Surgery
John Sealy Hospital
Galveston, TX

Jerry Holleman, M.D.
Medical Director, Vascular Center
Vascular Surgery
Carolina Medical Center
1001 Blythe Boulevard
Charlotte, NC

Mohammad K. Jamal, M.D.
Department of Surgery
Division of Minimally Invasive Surgery
Virginia Commonwealth University
Medical College of Virginia
Richmond, VA

Brian J. Kaplan, M.D.
Associate Professor of Surgery
Virginia Commonwealth University
VCU Medical Center
Richmond, VA

General Surgery Program Director
Department of Surgery
Virginia Commonwealth University - MCV Hospital
Richmond, VA

Jeffrey L. Kaufman, M.D.
Surgeon
Department of Surgery
Tufts University School of Medicine
Springfield, MA

Surgeon
Department of Surgery
Baystate Medical Center
Springfield, MA

Nathaniel S. Kreykes, M.D.
Surgery Research Fellow
Department of Surgery
University of Minnesota
Minneapolis, MN

K. Francis Lee, M.D.
Assistant Professor of Medicine
Tufts University School of Medicine
Chief, General and Trauma Surgery
Baystate Medical Center
Springfield, MA

Sophia Lee, M.D.
Resident in Surgery
Virginia Commonwealth University
Richmond, VA

Mark M. Levy, M.D.
Associate Professor of Surgery
Division of Vascular Surgery
Virginia Commonwealth University
Richmond, VA

Chairman, Vascular Surgery
Department of Surgery
VCU Medical Center
Medical College of Virginia
Richmond, VA

D. Scott Lind, M.D.
Associate Professor
Department of Surgery–General
University of Florida College of Medicine
Gainsville, FL

Ronald C. Merrell, M.D.
Professor of Surgery
Virginia Commonwealth University
Richmond, VA

David Page, M.D., FACS
Associate Clinical Professor of Surgery
Department of Surgery
Tufts University School of Medicine
Boston, MA

Director, Undergraduate Student Programs
Department of Surgery
Baystate Medical Center
Springfield, MA

William P. Reed, Jr., M.D.
Department of Surgery
Winthrop University Hospital
Mineola, NY

Professor of Clinical Surgery
State University of New York at Stony Brook
Stony Brook, NY

Daniel A. Saltzman, M.D., Ph.D.
Assistant Professor of Surgery and Pediatrics
Department of Surgery and Pediatrics
University of Minnesota Medical School
Minneapolis, MN

Jeannie F. Savas, M.D.
Program Director of Surgery
Medical College of Virginia
Richmond, VA

Bruce Jay Simon, M.D., FACS
Associate Professor of Surgery
Department of Surgery
State University of New York
Health Sciences Center at Stony Brook
Stony Brook, NY

Director, Trauma and Surgical Critical Care
Department of Surgery
Winthrop University Hospital
Mineola, NY

W. Charles Sternbergh III, M.D.
Program Director
Vascular Surgery
Ochsner Clinic Foundation
New Orleans, LA

Todd M. Tuttle, M.D.
Associate Professor of Surgery
Department of Surgery
University of Minnesota
Minneapolis, MN

Attending Surgeon
Department of Surgery
Fairview University Medical Center
Minneapolis, MN

Ciaran J. Walsh, M.D.
Consultant Surgeon and Coloproctologist
Wirral Hospital
United Kingdom

Jan Wojcik, M.D.
Assistant Professor of Surgery
Tufts University School of Medicine
Chief, Colorectal Surgery
Baystate Medical Center
Springfield, MA

Sharlilne Zacur, M.D.
Resident
Department of Surgery
VCU Medical Center
Richmond, VA

ACKNOWLEDGMENTS

We would like to acknowledge our tremendous authors, who have taken considerable time and effort to help disseminate information. Authorship is frequently relatively thankless, at least compared to the amount of work involved, and the editors of this third edition are grateful.

We would also like to express our gratitude to Joanne Bersin at Lippincott Williams and Wilkins for shepherding this edition to completion. She did so with grace and skill.

Finally, we want to reiterate our communion with our surgical colleagues. The combination of skills necessary to practice surgery is unique within medicine, and the strength of our specialty lies with its practitioners. Although surgery is not the easiest discipline, we believe it is the most fulfilling. This is true today and will be so in the future.

PREFACE

In the 5 years since the publication of the second edition of *Surgical Attending Rounds*, the practice of surgery has changed remarkably. In our minds, the most dramatic changes have revolved around the continued push toward a minimally invasive approach in all fields, from laparoscopic procedures to cardiac surgery. These changes are reflected in this third edition of *Surgical Attending Rounds.* As an example, the recognition of the global epidemic of overweight and obesity has prompted us to include a new chapter on bariatric surgery. Not only has bariatric surgery become an important component of general surgery but also advances in minimally invasive techniques have fueled its expansion and acceptance as an important therapy for a large number of patients.

The successful Socratic question and answer format has been preserved in the third edition. This method of presenting and highlighting information is a demonstrably effective way to retain large amounts of information. Using case scenarios that any student or practitioner of surgery would see in practice engages the reader. For each patient described in the text, critical decision points are emphasized and key data are discussed. First developed by Dr. Francis Lee and Dr. Cornelius Dyke from their own experiences on attending rounds during training, this method of critical examination allows surgeons to review cases and information as they appear on rounds, on exams, and on the wards.

Finally, the editors would like to acknowledge the tremendous contribution of K. Francis Lee to *Surgical Attending Rounds.* Although he was unable to contribute to this third edition as an editor, we are fortunate to have his contribution as an author. Dr. Lee's conviction that surgery is a cognitive discipline permeates this third edition and has influenced all readers of *Surgical Attending Rounds.*

Cornelius McKown Dyke, MD
Gastonia, North Carolina

CONTENTS

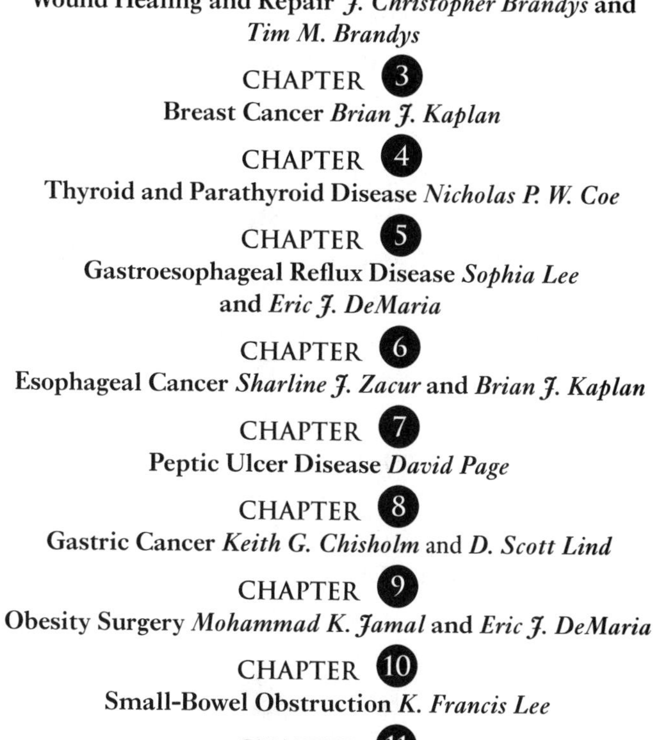

CHAPTER

PREOPERATIVE ANESTHETIC ASSESSMENT OF THE SURGICAL PATIENT

Thomas McNiff and Cornelius Dyke

Mrs. Barr is a 65-year-old woman whom the anesthesiologist is called to see before surgery. She presented to the emergency department with abdominal pain and bilious emesis of 2 days' duration. After evaluation by the general surgery service, she is scheduled for an exploratory laparotomy for a presumed small bowel obstruction. Further medical history reveals hypertension, non-insulin-dependent diabetes mellitus, and severe degenerative joint disease, which limits her ability to walk. She has not seen her primary physician for 2 years. She has a 30-pack-year history of smoking.

Mrs. Barr's surgical history includes an aortofemoral bypass graft 8 years ago and a right femoropopliteal bypass graft 3 years ago. She takes a beta-blocker and a diuretic for hypertension, a nonsteroidal anti-inflammatory for joint pain, and metformin (Glucophage) for diabetes. She has no medical allergies.

Why is an anesthetic assessment needed?

An anesthetic assessment includes taking a pertinent history, performing a physical examination, assigning American Society of Anesthesiologists (ASA) physical status (Table 1.1), and performing appropriate laboratory tests. The anesthetic evaluation is designed to ensure proper preparation of the patient for surgery and to allow risk stratification. Multiple studies and closed claim analyses have indicated that inadequate preoperative planning and errors in patient preparation are the most common causes of anesthetic complications. The Joint Commission on Accreditation of Healthcare Organizations (JCAHO) standards emphasize the importance of the anesthetic assessment by requiring that in any accredited

TABLE 1.1.

AMERICAN SOCIETY OF ANESTHESIOLOGISTS (ASA) STATUS

Classification	Systemic Disease
ASA I	No organic disease
ASA II	Mild or moderate systemic disease without functional impairment
ASA III	Organic disease with definite functional impairment
ASA IV	Severe disease that is life-threatening
ASA V	Moribund patient, not expected to survive
ASA VI	Donor patient for organ harvesting

Note: An "E" classification added to the above denotes an emergency case. (From Ross AF, Tinker JH. Preoperative evaluation of the healthy patient. In: Rogers MC, Tinker JH, Covino BG, et al., eds. Principles and Practice of Anesthesiology. St. Louis, Mo: Mosby–Year Book; 1993:4, with permission.)

facility all patients undergoing sedation or regional or general anesthesia have a standardized preoperative assessment.

What is Mrs. Barr's NPO status?

NPO (nil per os; nothing by mouth) status is used to assess the patient's likelihood of having a full stomach and thus having increased risk of aspiration. Patients with normal gastric motility require more than 4 hours to empty the stomach of solid matter (1). However, patients with decreased gastric motility are always considered to have full stomachs and to be at increased risk for aspiration. Decreased motility can occur in patients with intestinal obstruction, trauma patients, obese patients, gravid women, and patients with diabetes mellitus.

What is rapid-sequence intubation?

Rapid-sequence intubation is a technique used for patients at risk for aspiration. The patient is preoxygenated with 100% oxygen and an intravenous (IV) anesthetic agent is administered, followed rapidly by IV succinylcholine. Cricoid pressure is applied to occlude the esophagus in the event of passive regurgitation (Fig. 1.1) and is maintained until tracheal intubation is confirmed by measuring end-tidal carbon dioxide, documenting bilateral breath sounds, and noting inflation of the endotracheal tube cuff has occluded the trachea.

Mrs. Barr has been NPO for 2 days. What else does this imply?

Any NPO period creates a fluid deficit. Fluid deficits contribute to hemodynamic instability and risk of cardiac and renal complications. Correction of fluid deficit is based on calculation of maintenance fluid and third-space volume requirements.

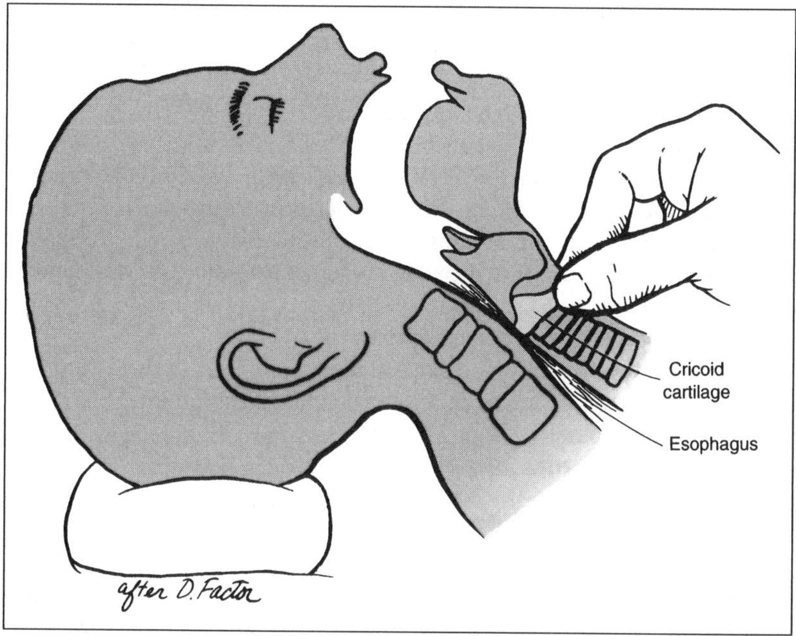

Figure 1.1. Use of the Sellick maneuver. Pressure is applied to the cricoid cartilage to occlude the esophagus. Cricoid pressure prevents aspiration of gastric contents during the administration of anesthesia. (From Stehling LC. Management of the airway. In: Barash PG, Cullen BF, Stoelting RK, eds. Clinical Anesthesia. Philadelphia, Pa: JB Lippincott Co; 1992:695, with permission.)

Maintenance IV fluids are calculated according to body weight for both children and adults. The initial 10 kg of a person's body weight is allotted at 4 mL per kg; the second 10 kg is allotted at 2 mL per kg; and any remaining weight is allotted at 1 mL per kg.

Calculation of the patient's fluid deficit is based on maintenance volume and the number of hours he or she has been NPO. Half of this fluid is replaced during the first hour of surgery, and 25% of the volume is replaced during each of the subsequent 2 hours.

Additional intraoperative fluid requirements are calculated according to third-space fluid losses anticipated in the operating room, which are also based on the patient's weight. Operations without much fluid loss, such as eye surgery, have third-space losses of 2 mL per kg per hour. Operations with moderate fluid losses, such as ventral hernia repair, are replaced at 6 mL per kg per hour. Large operations with much exposed viscera, such as abdominal aorta resection or exploratory laparotomy, have large fluid shifts and patients are given an additional

10 to 15 mL per kg per hour. The overall determinant of adequate fluid resuscitation is urine output, which should be at least 0.5 mL per kg per hour.

Why is a patient's anesthetic history important?

History repeats. If old charts are available, review them to determine ease of laryngoscopy and intubation, type of anesthetic used, and any complications associated with anesthesia. If old charts are not available, ask the patient what types of anesthetics he or she has had (e.g., regional versus general). Seek details of the previous anesthetics: ask the patient whether he or she has ever been told that the anesthesiologist had difficulty placing a breathing tube, and ask whether he or she required prolonged postoperative ventilation.

Why is a family history of problems with anesthetics important?

A family history of problems with anesthetics may indicate inherited risks (e.g., malignant hyperthermia). Many patients have not had prior surgery, but the family history might help the anesthesiologist become aware of inherited conditions that may threaten life.

Mrs. Barr states that she had general anesthesia for her aortobifemoral bypass graft and had no problems. However, her sister almost died of an intraoperative "fever."

What is malignant hyperthermia?

Malignant hyperthermia is an autosomal dominant trait that causes severe fevers and massive catabolism. It is triggered by administration of some anesthetic agents. Initially, it manifests as tachycardia and cardiac dysrhythmia, which can result in complete cardiac collapse. Malignant hyperthermia may not manifest until 24 hours after exposure. The physiologic mechanism is believed to be an excessive release of calcium from the sarcoplasmic reticulum in skeletal muscle, which results in severe muscle contractures. Anesthetic agents known to trigger malignant hyperthermia are the volatile anesthetics (e.g., halothane, desflurane, isoflurane), succinylcholine, and decamethonium (2). Total IV anesthesia and regional anesthesia are generally considered safe for these patients. Malignant hyperthermia is associated with other disorders, such as Duchenne's muscular dystrophy and King-Denborough syndrome (3).

After obtaining a complete history, perform a thorough physical examination, paying particular attention to the airway and cardiovascular, pulmonary, and neurologic systems. Also assess other pertinent organ systems.

Why is an examination of the airway important?

Examination of the airway allows the anesthesiologist to assess how easy it will be to intubate the patient and to anticipate any difficulty with the airway.

Considerations during examination include the Mallampati classification, extent of mouth opening, hyomental distance, and neck range of motion.

What is the Mallampati classification?

The Mallampati classification system assesses the size of the tongue relative to the oropharyngeal cavity (Fig. 1.2). It is performed with the patient sitting upright and the head in a neutral position. The patient maximally opens his

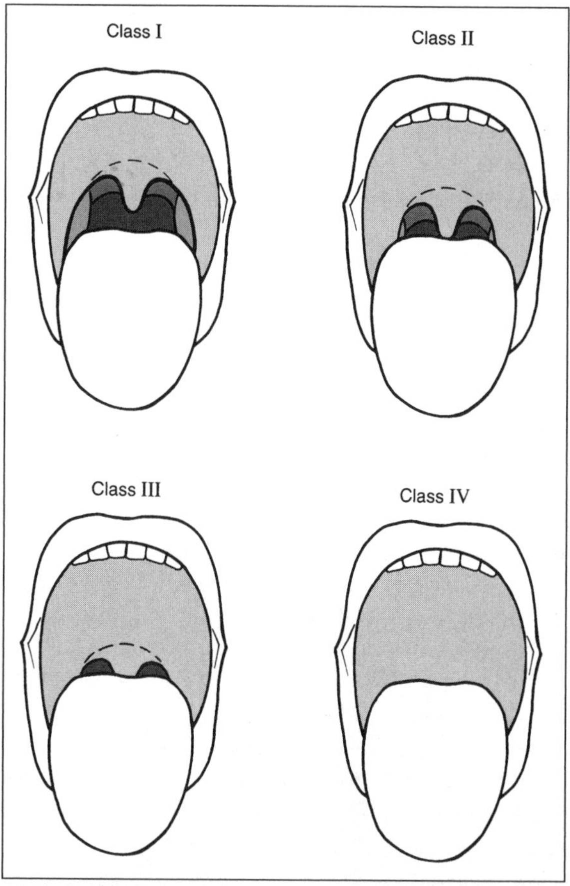

Figure 1.2. Mallampati classification system. Difficulty of intubation increases from Class I to Class IV. (From Cooper SD, Benumof JL, Reisner LS. The difficult airway: risk, prophylaxis, and management. In: Chestnut DH, ed. Obstetric Anesthesia. St. Louis, Mo: Mosby–Year Book; 1994:581, with permission.)

or her mouth and maximally protrudes his or her tongue. The patient should not phonate because this falsely raises the soft palate and gives an erroneous classification. The airway is classified by what structures are visualized:

- *Class I:* the soft palate, fauces, uvula, and anterior and posterior tonsillar pillars
- *Class II:* the soft palate, fauces, and uvula
- *Class III:* the soft palate and base of the uvula
- *Class IV:* the soft palate not visible

There is a correlation between Mallampati class and ease of laryngoscopy. Class I patients are expected to be relatively easy to intubate, whereas class IV patients are expected to be difficult to intubate. This score combined with range of motion of cervical vertebrae and presence or absence of dentition allows relatively accurate prediction as to the difficulty of intubation.

Why does the anesthesiologist want to know the patient's height and weight?

The dosage of most drugs used in the operating room is determined by body weight (milligrams per kilogram). Spinal and epidural anesthesia dosing is based on height. Also, in the event that a pulmonary artery catheter is placed, body surface area (BSA) is used for such calculations as cardiac index and systemic vascular resistance index.

How is BSA calculated?

$$\text{BSA} = \sqrt{[\text{height (cm)} \times \text{weight (kg)}]/3600}$$

Units are in meters squared.

Mrs. Barr is unable to provide information about exercise tolerance because degenerative joint disease limits her mobility.

Why is exercise status important?

Exercise status is used in the risk stratification of patients at risk for cardiovascular complications (Table 1.2). Mrs. Barr has multiple risk factors for coronary artery disease, including advanced age, hypertension, peripheral vascular disease, obesity, diabetes mellitus, and a history of smoking.

Cardiovascular complications account for 25% to 50% of all deaths following noncardiac surgery. These complications include myocardial infarction (MI), congestive heart failure (CHF), and thromboembolism. Mortality rates for perioperative MI are reported in several series as greater than 50%. The American College of Cardiology/American Heart Association (ACC/AHA) has published guidelines on perioperative cardiovascular evaluation for noncardiac surgery. The ACC/AHA guidelines include exercise ability as part of an eight-step algorithm

TABLE 1.2.

INDICATORS OF HIGH-RISK PATIENTS WHO NEED A THOROUGH EVALUATION

Cardiovascular	Pulmonary	Neurologic
Third heart sound gallop	Chronic lung disease	Central nervous system injury
Jugular venous distention	FEV_1 >2.0 L	Carotid bruit
MI within 6 months	Obesity	
Dysrhythmias	Hypercapnia at rest	
Age >70 years	Age >70 years	
Emergency operation	Site of operation	
Important aortic stenosis	Smoking history	
Poor general health		

FEV_1, forced expiratory volume in 1 second; MI, myocardial infarction. (From Roberts SL, Tinker JH. Perioperative myocardial infarction. In: Gravenstein N, Kirby RR, eds. Complications in Anesthesiology. Philadelphia, Pa: Lippincott–Raven Publishers; 1996:339, with permission.)

for preoperative work up. The first three steps of the guideline consider the urgency of the operation and the recentness of any cardiac evaluation or intervention. Steps four through seven consider exercise ability, surgical risk, and clinical predictors. (See Algorithm 1.1)

What effect does beta-blockade have on surgical risk?

The preoperative use of beta-blocking drugs has been shown to decrease the incidence of postoperative adverse cardiac events. Starting beta-blockers preoperatively in the patient undergoing major noncardiac surgery decreases cardiac complications and improves short- and long-term survival (4).

Mrs. Barr takes metformin. How should this be addressed preoperatively?

Have the patient discontinue metformin 12 to 24 hours before surgery because it increases the patient's risk of developing lactic acidosis. The patient should not resume metformin until stable hemodynamics and baseline renal function occur.

How should diabetes mellitus be treated perioperatively?

The goal of glucose control is to maintain glucose levels between 80 and 150 mg/dL. The dangers of hypoglycemia and resultant neurologic injury have long been recognized. More recently, hyperglycemia in the perioperative setting has been shown to impair wound healing and increase the incidence of wound infections. In patients who are treated with oral agents, withhold these agents the day of surgery. Check glucose levels and treat with short-acting insulin. In patients who are treated with insulin, withhold their short-acting insulin on the day of surgery. Administer intermediate-acting formulations at half the baseline dose. The recent advent of more complex regimes for tight glucose control, including insulin pumps and multiple types of insulin, have increased the complexity of perioperative insulin management. Endocrinology consultation may be particularly helpful.

What are this patient's options for postoperative pain control?

The three most commonly employed techniques for control of pain after abdominal surgery are intermittent IV opioid administration, IV patient-controlled analgesia (PCA), and analgesics administered in the epidural space.

What is IV PCA?

PCA is a device attached to the patient's maintenance IV line that allows administration of opioids to be programmed. A baseline infusion of opioids is ordered, and the patient controls how often additional boluses are given. PCA devices have a lockout period that prevents overdosing. Most hospitals have printed PCA order forms. A typical order includes a loading dose, a maintenance dose with lockout interval, and a 4-hour maximum dose limit. Antiemetics and antipruritics should be routinely ordered because the most common side effects of PCA are pruritus and nausea or emesis.

What is epidural anesthesia?

An epidural catheter is placed, usually preoperatively, into the epidural space. The level of required anesthesia helps to determine the spinal level at which the catheter is placed. The catheter is attached to an infusion pump that can continuously infuse a local anesthetic or opioid. Epidural PCA operates along the same principles as IV PCA. Contraindications to epidural catheter placement include refusal by the patient, uncorrected coagulopathy, local infection at the sight of the puncture, uncorrected hypovolemia, and anticipated major blood loss (5). The main risks associated with epidural catheter placement include blood vessel puncture, dural puncture, backache, and severe hypotension. Spinal headache is caused by inadvertent entry into the cerebrospinal fluid (dural puncture). The risks caused by epidural placement range from blood vessel puncture (2.8%) to permanent paralysis (0.02%) (6).

After the epidural anesthetic is placed but before the procedure, the anesthesiologist notes that the patient is very lethargic and has facial twitching.

Why should the anesthesiologist be concerned?

Although it is very unlikely with spinal anesthesia, the anesthesiologist must be concerned about a toxic local reaction to the anesthetic. These reactions may also occur when the surgeon uses concurrent local anesthesia or when a large dose of local anesthetic is inadvertently given in the vascular system instead of the subcutaneous tissue.

What is the maximum amount of lidocaine or bupivacaine that should be administered to a patient?

In average-sized adults, the maximum dose of lidocaine is approximately 500 mg, and the maximum dose of bupivacaine (Marcaine) is about 200 mg. The route of administration affects the rate of uptake. Intercostal blocks result in the highest plasma levels of local anesthetics, followed by brachial plexus blocks. Spinal anesthesia results in extremely low levels of anesthetic in the plasma.

How are lidocaine and bupivacaine toxicity manifested?

Local anesthesia toxicity manifests primarily through the cardiac and central nervous systems, with bupivacaine having more cardiac disturbances than lidocaine. The patient may exhibit tinnitus, perioral dysesthesias, seizures, or unconsciousness. Hypercarbia decreases the seizure threshold significantly; therefore, opioids must be used with caution. Cardiac manifestations of bupivacaine are primarily conduction abnormalities, dysrhythmia, and cardiac arrest (7).

Mr. Jackson, an 80-year-old man, presents for a transurethral resection of the prostate (TURP) for a slowly bleeding prostate tumor. His hematocrit is 39%. His medical history is significant for rheumatoid arthritis and a few episodes of CHF. Further questioning reveals that the patient's father had to be on a ventilator after general anesthesia for a small inguinal hernia repair because he "could not breathe."

What is pseudocholinesterase deficiency?

Pseudocholinesterase, or plasma cholinesterase, deficiency is an inherited disorder that results in varying levels of plasma cholinesterase. Plasma cholinesterase is the enzyme responsible for the metabolism of succinylcholine, mivacurium (a nondepolarizing neuromuscular relaxant), and ester anesthetics (e.g., cocaine, procaine, chloroprocaine, tetracaine). Patients with this disorder are typically asymptomatic; however, they may exhibit prolonged apnea after administration of succinylcholine or mivacurium. This condition may be exacerbated by echothiophate eye drops or by severe liver dysfunction. Neuromuscular blockade may last 120 to 300 minutes or longer (8).

Mr. Jackson's physical examination is remarkable for decreased neck extension, a short hyoid mental distance, and a Mallampati III airway. The patient is alert and well oriented.

What is the optimal type of anesthesia for this patient?

Two major factors specifically make spinal anesthesia the optimal choice for this patient: his cardiac status and the type of surgery he is having. His family history of presumed pseudocholinesterase deficiency and his difficult airway preclude the use of succinylcholine or mivacurium for rapid-sequence intubation, and his airway makes the use of longer-acting muscle relaxants undesirable. An awake intubation with general anesthesia is another option for this patient, and it may be considered ideal by some anesthesiologists because it allows the airway to be secured early.

What is TURP syndrome?

TURP syndrome occurs when the patient undergoing transurethral resection of the prostate absorbs large quantities of hypotonic irrigation solution used during surgery, resulting in volume overload and hyponatremia. Symptoms include altered mental status, cyanosis, pulmonary edema, and eventual cardiac collapse from CHF. Glycine toxicity also manifests as altered mental status due to hyperammonemia. TURP syndrome is related to the length of surgery, the irrigating pressure of solution, and the extent of resection (9). Spinal anesthesia allows continual assessment of the patient's mental status and pulmonary status.

What is spinal anesthesia?

Also known as subarachnoid block, spinal anesthesia is local anesthesia delivered directly into the subarachnoid space. Any of several types of local anesthetic can be used depending on the anticipated duration of the surgery. The most commonly used anesthetics are lidocaine, bupivacaine, and tetracaine. The subarachnoid entry for TURP is usually performed at the L4–5 or L3–4 interspace. The level, or height, of anesthesia depends primarily on the volume instilled.

What are the risks of spinal anesthesia?

The main risks of spinal anesthesia are pruritus, urinary retention, bleeding, infection, spinal headache, intravascular absorption of medication, and a "high spinal." Pruritus is common after intrathecal (spinal) opioid administration. Bleeding abnormalities must be ruled out by a thorough history before subarachnoid anesthesia is attempted because a hematoma may have permanent neurologic sequelae. Infection is rare but can result in meningitis. If there is evidence of infection where the block is to be placed, never perform subarachnoid block, and use strict sterile technique. Spinal, or postdural puncture, headache is more common with subarachnoid blocks than with epidural catheter placement, occurring in approximately 11% of patients undergoing spinal anesthesia. Factors associated with a high incidence of postdural puncture headache are female gender, pregnancy, young age, large needle size, needle orientation, and multiple attempts (10). Postdural puncture headache is usually treated conservatively with IV fluid hydration and analgesics.

What is a high spinal?

When the level of anesthesia is too high on the spinal cord, higher cord function may be impaired (most serious being the inhibition of respiration). As the level of anesthesia rises cephalad above T2, the patient subjectively feels dyspneic, with upper limb paresthesias and weakness. The patient has difficulty speaking because of the inability to exchange air. In extreme cases, loss of consciousness occurs. The treatment for a high spinal is early recognition and prompt institution of mechanical ventilation until the spinal anesthesia regresses (11).

Mr. Jackson is a good candidate for a subarachnoid block, so the surgical team must be prepared for a difficult airway in the event that the block fails or results in a high spinal. Preparations for a difficult airway (e.g., laryngeal mask airway, lighted stylet, fiberoptic laryngoscope) should be available in case of a complication, such as a failed subarachnoid anesthesia, a toxic reaction, or a high subarachnoid anesthesia.

A 40-year-old man, Mr. McMahon, presents for thoracotomy and left pneumonectomy for cancer. He has an extensive smoking history (75 pack-years) and easily becomes dyspneic. He is 6′2″ tall and weighs 80 kg. The remainder of his medical and surgical history is unremarkable. Physical examination is unremarkable except for bilateral distant breath sounds with wheezing throughout.

What preoperative studies are necessary for this patient?

Basic laboratory work for Mr. McMahon includes a complete blood count with quantitative platelet count, blood type, crossmatch for 2 units of packed red blood cells, basic chemistry, liver function testing, chest radiograph, and electrocardiogram.

What information can an arterial blood gas measurement provide?

A preoperative measurement of arterial blood gas on room air provides the physician with the baseline values for this patient. It allows assessment of the extent of any hypoxemia and hypercarbia. Patients with baseline compensated respiratory acidosis (i.e., $Pa{CO_2}$ above 45 mm Hg) are at particular risk (12).

What are the types of acid-base abnormalities, and what can be expected with each?

There are four basic types of abnormalities: respiratory acidosis, respiratory alkalosis, metabolic acidosis, and metabolic alkalosis. They are commonly found in combination, and the combinations are usually compensatory (13).

To simplify the assessment of arterial blood gases, check pH first. Normal pH is 7.35 to 7.45; a pH below 7.35 is considered acidotic, and a pH above 7.45 is considered alkalotic. A normal pH implies either no abnormality (if the carbon dioxide and bicarbonate levels are normal) or a compensated disorder. The pH is never overcompensated; that is, in the presence of respiratory acidosis, the bicarbonate level never overcompensates to make the pH alkalotic. Metabolic compensation occurs at a much slower rate (over many hours to days) than does respiratory compensation. The four possible acid-base abnormalities are summarized here and in Table 1.3.

TABLE 1.3.

DETERMINING ACID–BASE ABNORMALITY THROUGH pH AND ARTERIAL BLOOD GASES

Abnormality	pH	Carbon Dioxide (CO_2)	Bicarbonate Acid–Base (HCO_3^-)
Acute respiratory acidosis	↓	↑	–
Chronic respiratory acidosis	↓/–	↑	↑ (compensated)
Acute respiratory alkalosis?	↑	↓	–
Chronic respiratory alkalosis	↑/–	↓	↓ (compensated)
Acute metabolic alkalosis	↑	–/↑	–
Chronic metabolic alkalosis	↑/–	↑	↑ (compensated)
Acute metabolic acidosis	↓	–/↓	–
Chronic metabolic acidosis	↓/–	↓	↓ (compensated)

1. The patient who is acidotic or has a carbon dioxide level greater than 45 (normal carbon dioxide level is 35 to 45 mm Hg) has *respiratory acidosis.* If the bicarbonate level is high (normal bicarbonate level is 22 to 26 mmol per L), one can expect that the acidosis is compensated. If the bicarbonate level is low, one can assume that the patient has a mixed primary respiratory and metabolic acidosis.
2. The patient who is alkalotic with a low carbon dioxide level has *respiratory alkalosis.* If the bicarbonate level is low, it is compensated; if it is high, the patient can be assumed to have mixed primary respiratory and metabolic alkalosis.
3. The patient who is alkalotic with a high bicarbonate level has *metabolic alkalosis.* If the carbon dioxide level is high, it is compensated; if it is low, it is a *mixed primary metabolic and respiratory alkalosis.*
4. The patient who is acidotic with a low bicarbonate level has *metabolic acidosis.* If the carbon dioxide level is low, it is compensated; if it is high, it is a *mixed primary metabolic and respiratory acidosis.*

What is anion gap acidosis and what are its major causes?

Anion gap acidosis cannot be accounted for by the major cations and anions in the body (i.e., sodium, chloride, bicarbonate) (13). It primarily arises from an excess of minor anions (e.g., lactate, ketones, organic acids). The human body normally has an anion gap of less than 12, which is typically calculated by subtracting the major plasma anions from the major plasma cations $(Na^+) - [(Cl^-) + (HCO_3^-)]$. Common causes of metabolic acidosis with an anion gap include diabetic ketoacidosis, lactic acidosis, aspirin toxicity, methanol ingestion, uremia, and ethylene glycol ingestion.

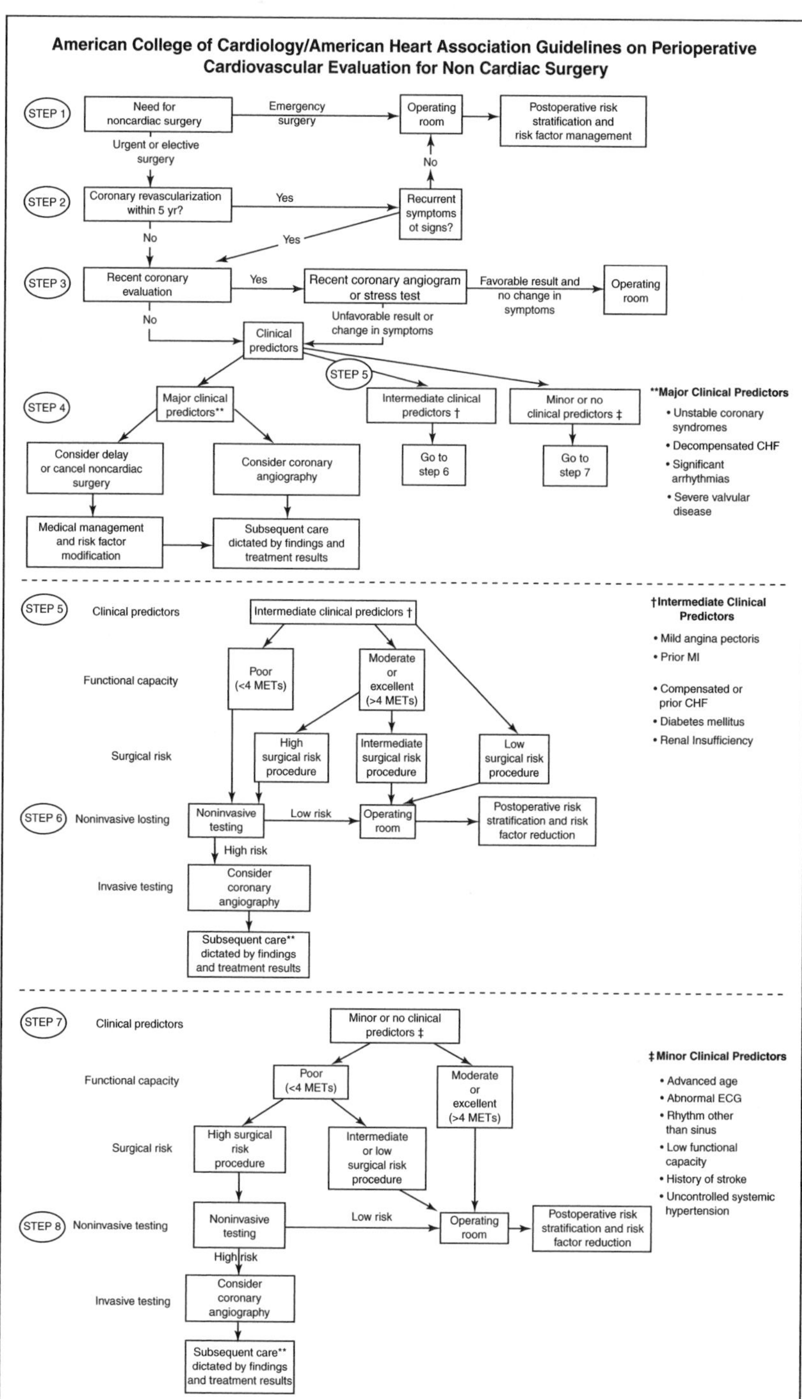

Algorithm 1.1.

REFERENCES

1. James CF. Pulmonary aspiration of gastric contents. In: Gravenstein N, Kirby RR, eds. Complications in Anesthesiology. Philadelphia, Pa: Lippincott–Raven Publishers; 1996:176.
2. Malignant hyperthermia. In: Gravenstein N, Kirby RR, eds. Complications in Anesthesiology. Philadelphia, Pa: Lippincott–Raven Publishers; 1996:149.
3. Brownell AKW. Malignant hyperthermia: relationship to other diseases. Br J Anaesth. 1988;60:303.
4. Mangano DT, Layug EL, Wallace A, et al. Effect of atenolol on mortality and cardiovascular morbidity after noncardiac surgery. Multicenter study of Perioperative Ischemia Research Group. N Engl J Med. 1996;335:1713–1720.
5. Covino BG, Lambert DH. Epidural and spinal anesthesia. In: Barash PG, Cullen BF, Stoelting RK, eds. Clinical Anesthesia. Philadelphia, Pa: JB Lippincott Co; 1992:815.
6. Dawkins CLM. Anatomy of the complications of extradural and caudal block. Anaesthesia. 1969;24:554.
7. Covino BG. Pharmacology of local anesthetic agents. In: Rogers MC, Tinker JH, Covino BG, et al., eds. Principles and Practice of Anesthesiology. St. Louis, Mo: Mosby–Year Book; 1993:1247–1249.
8. Rosenberg H, Fletcher J, Seitman D. Pharmacogenetics. In: Barash PG, Cullen BF, Stoelting RK, eds. Clinical Anesthesia. Philadelphia, Pa: JB Lippincott Co; 1992: 603–605.
9. Mazze RI, Fujinaga M, Wharton RS. Fluid and electrolyte problems. In: Gravenstein N, Kirby RR, eds. Complications in Anesthesiology. Philadelphia, Pa: Lippincott–Raven Publishers; 1996:470.
10. Brown DL. Spinal, epidural, and caudal anesthesia. In: Miller RD, ed. Anesthesia. New York, NY: Churchill Livingstone; 1994:1521.
11. Vandam LD. Complications of spinal and epidural anesthesia. In: Gravenstein N, Kirby RR, eds. Complications in Anesthesiology. Philadelphia, Pa: Lippincott–Raven Publishers; 1996:567.
12. Benumof JL, Alfrey DD. Anesthesia for thoracic surgery. In: Miller RD, ed. Anesthesia. New York, NY: Churchill Livingstone; 1994:1666–1667.
13. Shapiro BA, Peruzzi WT. Interpretation of blood gases. In: Ayres SM, Grenvik A, Holbrook PR, et al., eds. Textbook of Critical Care. Philadelphia, Pa: WB Saunders; 1995:279.

CHAPTER

2

WOUND HEALING AND REPAIR

J. Christopher Brandys and Tim M. Brandys

A 17-year-old man is brought to the emergency room directly from the local high school track and field meet. While running in the 100-yard hurdles, he was injured on the last hurdle, sustaining a 15 by 3-cm laceration down the medial aspect of his right thigh. You are consulted regarding the best management of the local track star's injury.

What are the key features of your initial assessment?

Proper initial management of the wound promotes healing, reduces infection, and prevents complications. Critical considerations include identification of factors that potentiate infection, such as the elapsed time from injury, the degree of contamination, the depth of injury, and the presence of devitalized tissue or foreign material in the wound. Injuries by animal or human bite also need accurate and prompt identification. The patient's ability to respond to potential infection is also important. Significant medical problems that affect wound healing include diabetes, cardiovascular disease, immunocompromised states, and medications that suppress the immune system. Tetanus status and nutritional status are also critical. Important features on examination of the wound include neurovascular compromise, function distal to the injury, the depth of wound and any involved structures (e.g., compound fracture, tendon injury), and the presence of devitalized tissue or foreign material.

What is the best method to close the wound?

There are three options for wound closure: primary (immediate suture closure), secondary (healing by secondary intention), or tertiary closure (delayed primary closure). When deciding, significant factors include the potential for wound infection, the condition of the soft tissues and the tension required to approximate them, and the need for hemostasis. Most wounds that are less than 6 hours old are in "the golden period" and contain less than 10^5 colonies of organisms per gram of tissue and can be closed primarily (1). Acute wounds can also be classified into four categories: clean, clean-contaminated, contaminated, and dirty and infected (2). Do not close puncture wounds, human bites, wounds with inadequate hemostasis, and wounds under excessive tension. Devitalized tissues and foreign bodies must be removed before primary closure. Diabetics and immunocompromised patients will have a higher risk of infection and subsequent dehiscence.

Does this patient require tetanus prophylaxis?

The risk of tetanus is increased if the wound is more than 6 hours old, is deeper than 1 cm, or is contaminated. Crush or missile injuries and bite wounds also require a tetanus shot (3). Assess the patient's tetanus immune status and give appropriate tetanus toxoid with or without immunoglobulin as indicated.

Does this patient require prophylactic antibiotics?

Prophylactic antibiotics are indicated for contaminated wounds in patients who are immunocompromised, are diabetic, or have indwelling prosthetic devices such as heart valves or joint prostheses. Bite wounds, necrotic wounds, and wounds contaminated with gastrointestinal or urologic organisms also should receive prophylactic antibiotics (4).

What are the four phases of wound healing?

The four phases that acute and chronic wounds must pass through are hemostasis, inflammation, proliferation, and remodeling (Table 2.1).

The platelet is the most important component of the hemostasis phase. Not only does it help to form the wound clot (or temporary matrix) but also its alpha granules release growth factors, which play a critical role in accelerating wound healing.

Neutrophils, monocytes, and macrophages direct the inflammatory phase by removing devitalized tissue and destroying bacteria. They phagocytose bacteria and release proteases (matrix metalloproteinases [MMPs]).

The fibroblast and myofibroblast produce collagen during the proliferative phase and initiate wound contraction. By 6 weeks, collagen synthesis has peaked and the wound has achieved approximately 75% of its eventual tensile strength (5). Keratinocytes re-epithelialize the wound.

Fibroblasts then regulate remodeling as immature collagen (type 3) is broken down and mature collagen (type 1) is synthesized and re-aligned to increase the tensile strength of the wound.

In the wound center, you are asked to assess a 25-year-old man from a long-term care facility who has a chronic wound on his right ischial

TABLE 2.1.

PHASES OF WOUND HEALING

Phase	Duration	Appearance	Principal Cell Type	Function
1 Hemostasis	Immediate	Fibrin clot	Platelet	Formation of wound clot, release of cytokines
2 Inflammatory	Day 1–5	Edema, exudate, erythema	Neutrophil, macrophage	Phagocytosis, release of MMPs
3 Proliferation	Day 5–21	Red granulation tissue	Fibroblast, myofibroblast, keratinocyte	Collagen synthesis, wound contraction, epithelialization
4 Remodeling	Week 3–52	Scar	Fibroblast	Collagen turnover, realignment, cross-linking

MMP, matrix metalloproteinases.

region. He has a history of spinal cord injury from a motor vehicle accident 5 years earlier. The majority of his day is spent in a wheelchair. On examination, he has a dry eschar with surrounding erythema over the right ischial tuberosity and redness over the left ischial tuberosity.

What are the underlying etiologic factors of this wound?

This patient's functional status clearly plays a large role in his predisposition to ulcer formation. Decubitus ulcers (from the Latin *decumbere-* "to lie down") result from pressure, shear, friction, and moisture. Tissue necrosis can result when interface pressure on soft tissues between a bony prominence and support surface exceeds 32 mm Hg (6), the pressure at which tissue capillaries collapse. Other factors to consider include the patient's nutritional and immune status.

What stage are these wounds?

Staging of decubitus ulcers is critical to allow for effective communication between members of the health care team and to document progress of the wound as it heals. The right ischial wound cannot be staged until it is débrided to healthy tissue. The left ischium has a stage I wound. The National Pressure Ulcer Advisory Panel (NPUAP) classification is useful:

Stage I: redness of the skin
Stage II: ulceration of the epidermis with or without dermis

Stage III: ulceration into the subcutaneous tissue
Stage IV: ulceration to bone, tendon, or fascia

Why has this chronic wound failed to heal?

Chronic wounds are defined as wounds that have been present more than 12 weeks and are not progressing through the four phases of wound healing. Most chronic wounds are stuck in phase 2, the inflammatory phase.

The prolonged inflammatory phase appears to be triggered by the presence of necrotic debris, bacterial infection (or bioburden), cellular debris (senescent cells) (7), and decreased levels of cytokines and growth factors (8). These stimuli result in an exaggeration and prolonged release of proteases (including MMPs), which degrade the extracellular matrix faster than it can take hold in the wound bed. Wound exudate analysis has shown the level of MMPs to be up to 116 times normal compared to the acute healing wound (9). These proteases include collagenases (MMP1, MMP8, MMP13), gelatinases (MMP2, MMP9), and stromelysins (MMP3, MMP10, MMP11). The activity of these enzymes appears to be regulated by several tissue inhibitors of metalloproteinases (TIMP), which are decreased in the chronic wound (10).

What is the role of debridement?

Frequent debridement of the chronic wound bed has been shown to accelerate wound healing (11). Debridement is intended to remove necrotic debris, the cellular burden (senescent cells), and the biofilm of contaminated or infected matrix from the wound bed (12). In doing so the stimulus for white cell migration and the inflammatory process within the wound is removed (13). Debridement can be performed by surgical debridement, mechanical debridement (whirlpool, pulsed lavage), enzymatic means (papain-urea or collagenase), or autolytic means.

How is the bioburden managed?

Quantitative tissue cultures reveal whether the wound is contaminated or infected (more than 10^5 colonies per g of tissue) (14). Specific organisms can be addressed with topical agents such as ionic silver or cadexomer iodine. Agents such as povidone iodine (Betadine), 3% hydrogen peroxide, and 0.5% sodium hypochlorite (Dakin solution) kill fibroblasts and keratinocytes (15) and should be avoided. Systemic antibiotics may be required if extensive soft tissue, bone, or systemic infection is present.

What are the essentials of treatment of the chronic wound?

A multidisciplinary approach involving initial débridement of the wound, staging of the wound, treatment of underlying infection including osteomyelitis, offloading with appropriate support surfaces, assessment and supplementation of nutrition, possible coverage with myocutaneous or fasciocutaneous flap, and postoperative rehabilitation and physical therapy are all critical.

During the initial débridement, you notice that the patient has a stage IV ischial ulcer with exposed bone.

How do you determine the presence of osteomyelitis? What dressings should you use?

Twenty-five percent of non-healing pressure ulcers have underlying osteomyelitis (16). Osteomyelitis can be diagnosed most definitely by bone biopsy and culture (17). Triple-phase bone scan or magnetic resonance imaging may help to assess the extent of infected bone.

Following débridement, aim initial dressings at maintaining a moist wound environment, managing exudate, and reducing bioburden in the wound. There have been dramatic and significant advances in the array of dressings available (Table 2.2). With the development of these sophisticated new dressings, wet-to-dry gauze as primary dressings have become obsolete. It is critical to realize that no one dressing is appropriate for all classifications of wounds and no one dressing is best for all four phases of wound healing. Excellent wound care requires regular reassessment of the wound.

You are asked to assess a 50-year-old woman in the wound center. She has a large ulcer just above the medial malleolus on her left ankle, which has been present intermittently for 3 years. She is currently using wet-to-dry gauze dressings twice daily, wrapping the dressing with an Ace bandage, and cleansing the wound with hydrogen peroxide.

On obtaining the history, you note the patient had a deep venous thrombosis (DVT) in this leg 3 years ago following a brief hospitalization. Physical examination reveals significant pitting edema in the left leg. The ulcer measures 4- by 5-cm and is shallow in depth with irregular edges, and there is greenish drainage from a pale wound bed. The surrounding skin is hyperpigmented and indurated with areas of light discoloration and darkly stained tissues.

What are the possible causes of this ulcer?

The key to managing leg ulcers is first to determine their underlying etiology. The initial history and physical should allow classification of the wound. Ninety percent of leg ulcers fall into one of four categories: venous, arterial, diabetic, or decubitus (Table 2.3), although overlap can occur.

What is the etiology of this wound?

This patient has a venous ulcer secondary to chronic venous hypertension. Patients with an ambulatory venous pressure of 80 mm Hg or greater at the ankle

TABLE 2.2.

BASIC WOUND DRESSINGS

Dressing Class	Clinical Example Brand	Phase of Wound Healing: Indication	Performance	Dressing Interval
Non-adherents	Mepitel, Adaptic, Xeroform	Phase I, II: Interface to cover skin grafts, viscera, and so on	Non-adherence	q1–4 days
Films	Op-Site, Tegaderm	Phase II–III: Clean superficial and deep wounds	Trap moisture, protect wound from soiling	q1–5 days
Hydrogels	Intrasite, Curasol	Phase I–III: Superficial and deep wounds	Provide moisture, promote autolysis	q1 day
Hydrocolloids	Duoderm, Replicare	Phase II–III: Clean, superficial wounds	Protective, mildly absorbtive, maintain moisture	q1–3 days
Enzymes	Santyl, Accuzyme	Phase II–III: Wounds with necrosis, maintenance débridement	Digest proteins, collagen	q1 day
Topical antimicrobials	Cadexomer iodine, silver	Phase II–III: Iodosorb, acticoat, silvasorb, arglaes	Inhibit MRSA pseudomonas, virus	q1–7 days
Collagen	Oasis	Phase III: To enhance matrix formation	Promote granulation and epithelialization; absorbs MMPs	q4–7 days
	Promogran	Phase II: Wounds with matrix destruction		q1–7 days
Foams	Allevyn, Lyofoam	Phase II: Superficial, deep wounds	Absorbs exudate	q1–2 days
Algimates	Sorbsan, Kaltostat	Phase II: Cavity wounds, sinus tracts	Absorbs exudate	q1 day
Hydrofiber	Aquacel	Phase II:		q1 day
Growth factors	Regranex platelet gel	Phase II: Accelerate wound healing	Promote granulation and epithelialization	q1 day q7 days
Tissue substitutes	Apligraf, Dermagraft	Phase III: Venous, diabetic wounds, accelerate wound healing	Promote granulation and epithelialization	q7 days
Negative pressure wound therapy	Wound vac.	Phase II–III: Cavity wounds, high exudates, skin grafts, burns, wound dehiscence	Absorbs exudates, increases perfusion to wound bed, protective	q1–3 days

will have a greater than 80% incidence of ulceration (18). Prolonged venous hypertension results in leaky capillaries with red blood cells and macromolecules entering the interstitial space. Hemosiderin is deposited and stains the tissues, resulting in discoloration of the skin. An inflammatory response recruits leukocytes to the interstitium with ensuing release of proteases. MMP2 activity degrades the epidermal basement membrane leading to ulceration (19).

What is the initial treatment?

Initial treatment of this chronic venous ulcer includes débridement if necessary, culture for bacterial infection, topical dressings to manage exudate and bioburden, and elevation and compression to reduce interstitial edema and venous hypertension.

How is compression best applied?

Typically, compression is applied using a multilayer system such as Profore, developed at Charing Cross Hospital. Assess potential peripheral arterial disease; the ankle-brachial index (ABI) should be greater than 0.7 before applying compression.

The four-layer system applies 40 mm Hg compression at the ankle, thus improving tissue capillary PO_2 levels in the wound bed (20) and increasing the hydrostatic force in the interstitium, driving protein and fluid back into the capillary space. The four-layer wrap can be left in place up to 1 week, depending on the amount of bioburden in the wound, and effectively maintains compression throughout (unlike Unna's boot). Once the ulcer is healed, the patient can be fitted for long-term compression stockings to prevent recurrence.

Is there a role for surgical correction of venous insufficiency?

Up to 40% of patients are candidates for surgical procedures aimed at reducing ulcer recurrence, including sclerotherapy; saphenous vein ligation, stripping, or ablation; perforator vein ligation; or venous bypass. Surgical intervention and compression therapy can reduce 4-year recurrence rates to approximately 25% versus 67% for compression alone (21).

What is the SEPS (Subfascial Endoscopic Perforator Surgery) procedure?

This is a minimally invasive technique replacing the open Linton procedure for ulcers secondary to incompetent perforators from the deep to superficial venous system. The perforating veins can be clipped or ablated using incisions remote from the ulcer with a subfascial endoscopic approach.

A 70-year-old woman is referred to the wound center with a painful ulceration on the dorsum of her left forefoot. Her history is significant for claudication, a past history of myocardial infarction, and 50 pack-years of smoking. On examination, the foot is shiny and pale. It becomes red

TABLE 2.3.

LOWER EXTREMITY ULCERS

Type	Location	Appearance of Leg	Perfusion	Appearance of Wound	Symptoms
Arterial	Distal extremity, sites of trauma	Shiny, hairless, dependent rubor	Nonpalpable pulse, $TcPo_2$ <30 ABI <0.5	Pale, deep, punched out, dry or wet gangrene	Pain, claudication, rest pain
Venous	Gaiter distribution	Edema, hyper pigmentation, lipodermatosclero-sis, stasis dermatitis	Palpable pulse, normal ABI, $TcPo_2$ normal or decreased	Superficial, broad, irregular margins	Mild to moderate pain
Diabetic	Site of bony deformities	Dry, hammer toes, Charcot deformity	Pulse may be palpable, decreased $TcPo_2$	Deep, circular wounds with surrounding callus	Insensate
Pressure	Over bony prominences		Palpable pulse	Stage I-IV	

ABI, ankle-brachial index; $TcPo_2$, Transcutaneous Po_2 measurement.

when dependent. No pulse can be palpated below the femoral position in either extremity. The wound has a black dry eschar with surrounding erythema but is cool to the touch.

What class of wound is this? What tests are useful to assess the degree of arterial insufficiency and the healing potential for this chronic wound?

This is an arterial ulcer. The healing potential of wounds in the ischemic lower extremity may be predicted with non-invasive evaluation, including the ABI, Doppler waveform analysis, toe pressures in the diabetic patient, and transcutaneous PO_2 measurement (Table 2.4). Laser Doppler is also useful when available. If the healing potential is low and the patient is a candidate for revascularization, consider angiography followed by endovascular or conventional surgical revascularization. If the patient is not a surgical candidate or has anatomy precluding revascularization then basic wound care plus cilostazol (Pletal), growth factors, hyperbaric evaluation with oxygen challenge, and arterial compression boots (Art Assist, Circulator Boot) may be of some use. Primary amputation may also have to be considered.

A 50-year-old man presents with a chronic ulcer on the weight-bearing surface of his right forefoot over the first metatarsal head. He has a 10-year history of type I diabetes. On examination, he has a 2+ dorsalis pedis pulse and hammer toe deformities of his right foot. He is unable to sense the 5.07 per 10 g monofilament on the Semmes-Weinstein Test. The wound has significant callus around it, is circular in shape, and has a greenish exudate. On probing, the wound is deep and leads to bone.

What type of wound is this and what are the etiologic factors?

This is a diabetic foot ulcer; 15% of diabetics will develop a lower extremity ulcer in their lifetime. The peripheral neuropathy of diabetes affects the autonomic,

TABLE 2.4.

HEALING POTENTIAL IN THE ISCHEMIC LOWER EXTREMITY

	Healing Potential		
Non-Invasive Study	High	Medium	Low
ABI	>0.8	0.5–0.8	<0.5
Wave forms	Triphasic	Monophasic	Absent
Toe pressure	>50 mm Hg	30–50 mm Hg	<30 mm Hg
$TcPO_2$	>40 mm Hg	30–40 mm Hg	<30 mm Hg
Laser Doppler	>30 mm		<30 mm

Courtesy of Bill Marston, The Wound Course 2003.

ABI, ankle-brachial index; $TcPO_2$, .

motor, and sensory systems with resulting dry skin, intrinsic muscle loss with foot deformity, and loss of protective sensation. Vascular impairment and a propensity for infection potentiate the development of wounds and complicate their healing. Diabetics have a five times greater chance of infection occurring in wounds (22). Diabetes also results in glycosylation of connective tissue and impairs wound healing.

What is the initial management?

With a palpable pulse, this patient appears to have adequate arterial perfusion. Tissue capillary PO_2 evaluation or toe pressures may confirm this. Treatment includes débridement with removal of callus and devitalized tissue, tissue cultures with treatment of soft tissue infection, and assessment for osteomyelitis. Structural changes to the foot from diabetic neuropathy result in a shift of normal weight bearing to unprotected easily traumatized areas. This makes pressure-offloading devices such as accommodative footwear (molded insoles, custom made orthoses, depth footwear, ankle-foot orthoses) critical to promote healing. In more extreme cases, local surgical procedures are necessary to produce pressure relief including Achilles tendon lengthening and metatarsal head excision.

Can anything be done to accelerate wound healing?

Four advanced wound care technologies accelerate the proliferative phase of wound healing: negative pressure wound therapy, growth factors, hyperbaric oxygen therapy, and tissue substitutes containing living, cultured cells.

Negative pressure wound therapy (or vacuum-assisted closure) provides an infinitely absorbent system to manage exudates and increases perfusion to the wound by opening the capillary bed and removing surrounding interstitial edema, resulting in accelerated wound healing rates (23).

Growth factors can be applied topically to the proliferative wound bed in the form of platelet-derived growth factor (PDGF) becaplermin (Regranex) (24) or as platelet gels containing multiple PDGFs: epidermal growth factor (EGF), transforming growth factor (TGF-B), vascular endothelial growth factor (VEGF), fibroblast growth factor (FGF), keratinocyte growth factor (KGF), and others.

Tissue substitutes such as Apligraf and Dermagraft contain living cultured fibroblasts with or without keratinocytes. They deliver growth factors to the wound bed as well as a biologic matrix and do not have the morbidity of a donor graft. They appear to be especially useful in venous and diabetic foot ulcers.

Hyperbaric oxygen therapy requires the patient to breathe 100% O_2 while at greater than atmospheric pressure. It is indicated in chronic wounds that are demonstrated to be hypoxic by $TcPO_2$ evaluation and respond to oxygen dosing. Approved indications by the Undersea and Hyperbaric Medical Society include gas gangrene, crush injury, necrotizing soft tissue infections, refractory osteomyelitis, acute ischemia, and diabetic wounds of the lower extremity.

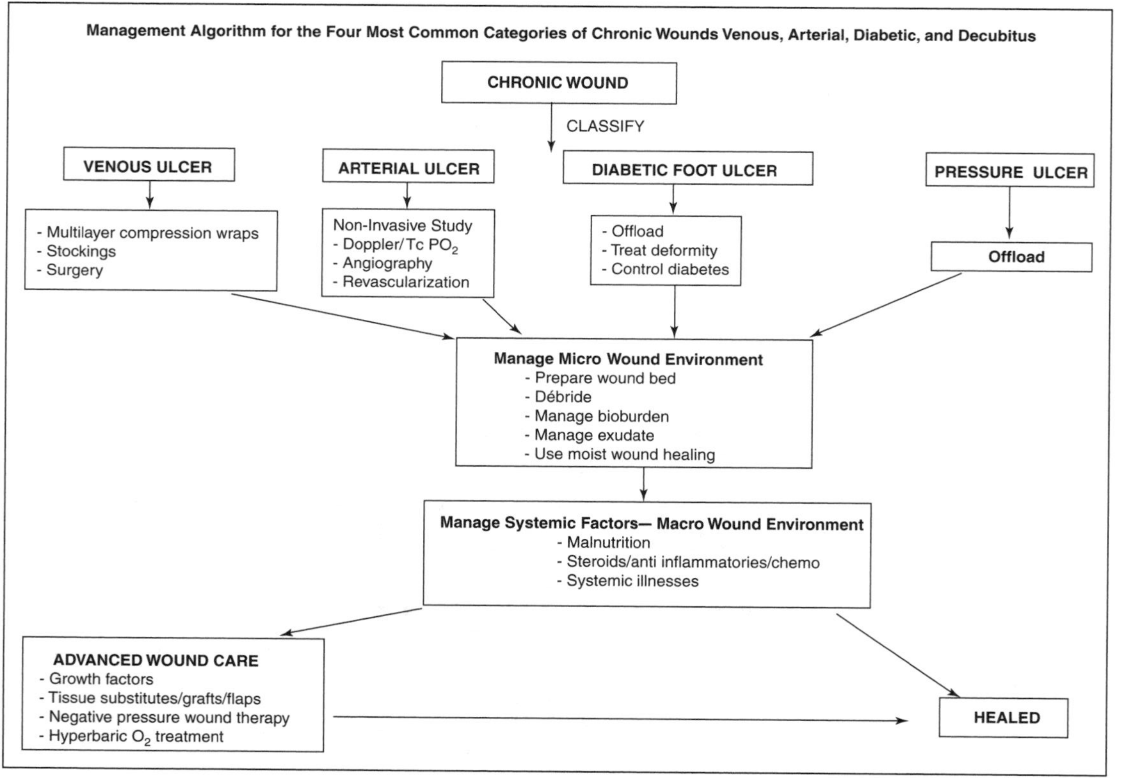

Algorithm 2.1.

REFERENCES

1. Robson MC, Duke WF, Krizek TJ. Rapid bacterial screening in the treatment of civilian wounds. J Surg Res. 1973;14:426–430.
2. Altemeir, WA. Manual on control of infection in surgical patients. American College of Surgeons Committee on Control of Surgical Infections of the Committee on Pre- and Postoperative Care. Philadelphia: JB Lippincott, 1976;280.
3. American College of Surgeons, Committee on Trauma. A Guide to Prophylaxis against Tetanus in Wound Management, 1984 Revision. Chicago, Ill: The American College of Surgeons; 1984.
4. Edlich RF, Rodeheaver GT, Morgan RF, et al. Principles of emergency wound management. Ann Emerg Med. 1988;17:1284–1302.
5. Lawrence WT, Bevin AG, Sheldon GF. Acute wound care: approach to acute wound management. In: Wilmore DW, Cheng LY, Harken AH, et al. ed. American College of Surgeons. Scientific American Surgery. Vol 1. New York, NY: WebMD Corporation; 2000:3–21.
6. Landis DM. Studies of capillary blood pressure in human skin. Heart. 1930;15:209.
7. Mendez MV, Raffetto JD, Phillips T, et al. The proliferative capacity of neonatal skin fibroblasts is reduced after exposure to venous ulcer wound fluid: a potential mechanism for senescence in venous ulcers. J Vasc Surg. 1999;30:734–742.
8. Yager DR, Nwomeh BC. The proteolytic environment of chronic wounds. Wound Repair Regen. 1999;7:433–441.
9. Tarnuzzer RW, Schultz GS. Biochemical analysis of acute and chronic wound environments. Wound Repair Regen. 1996;4:321.
10. Bullen EC, Longaker MT, Updike DL, et al. Tissue inhibitor of metalloproteinases-1 is decreased and activated gelatinases are increased in chronic wounds. J Invest Dermatol. 1995;104:236–240.
11. Steed DL, Donohoe D, Webster MW, et al. Effect of extensive débridement and treatment on the healing of diabetic foot ulcers. Diabetic Ulcer Study Group. J Am Coll Surg. 1996;183:61–64.
12. Falanga V. Wound bed preparation and the role of enzymes: a case for multiple actions of therapeutic agents. Wounds. 2002;14:47–57.
13. Mulder GD, Vandeberg JS. Cellular senescence and matrix metalloproteinase activity in chronic wounds. Relevance to débridement and new technologies. J Am Podiatr Med Assoc. 2002;92:34–37.
14. Heggers JP, Robson MC, Ristroph JD. A rapid method of performing quantitative wound cultures. Mil Med. 1969;134:666–667.
15. Lineaweaver W, Howard R, Soucy D, et al. Topical antimicrobial toxicity. Arch Surg. 1985;120:267–270.
16. Sugarman B. Pressure sores and underlying bone infection. Arch Intern Med. 1987;147:553–555.
17. Deloach ED, Christy R, Check WE, et al. Osteomyelitis underlying severe pressure sores. Contemp Surg. 1992;40:25–32.
18. Nicolaides AN, Hussein MK, Szendro G, et al. The relation of venous ulceration with ambulatory venous pressure measurements. J Vasc Surg. 1993;17:414–419.

19. Saito S, Trovato MJ, You R, et al. Role of matrix mettalloproteinases-1, 2, and 9 and tissue inhibitor of matrix mettalloproteinase-1 in chronic venous insufficiency. J Vasc Surg. 2001;34:930–938.
20. Roberts G. Some effects of sustained compression on ulcerated tissues. Angiology. 2002;53:451–456.
21. McDaniel HB, Marston WA, Farber MA, et al. Recurrence of chronic venous ulcers on the basis of clinical, etiologic, anatomic, and pathophysiologic criteria and air plethysmography. J Vasc Surg. 2002;35:723–728.
22. Cruse PJ, Foord R. A 5 year prospective study of 23, 649 surgical wounds. Arch Surg. 1973;107:206–210.
23. Argenta LC, Monykwas MJ. Vacuum-assisted closure: a new method for wound control and treatment: clinical experience. Ann Plast Surg. 1997;38:563–576.
24. Kallianimen LK, Hirschberg J, Marchant B, et al. Role of platelet derived growth factor as an adjunct to surgery in the management of pressure ulcers. Plastic Reconstr Surg. 2000;106:1243–1248.

CHAPTER 3

BREAST CANCER

Brian J. Kaplan

Mrs. Murphy is a healthy 55-year-old woman who has a new cluster of microcalcifications on her annual screening mammogram. She is advised to have a biopsy. Mrs. Murphy has no previous breast problems. She is past menopause and has no breast symptoms. On physical examination there is no lymphadenopathy, and her breasts are normal.

What are the mammographic signs of malignancy?

Mammographic signs of malignancy include stellate or dominant masses, architectural distortion, and skin or nipple thickening or retraction. Some types of microcalcifications are also associated with malignancy. The size, shape, number, density, and extent of microcalcifications help to determine the risk of a malignancy being present. Comparison to previous mammograms is essential. Additional coned or compression mammograms may be needed to define the calcifications.

It also is very important to discuss the findings with the radiologist. The American College of Radiology has proposed a classification system to help management decisions. Not all radiologists use this system, but consulting with the radiologist should help to classify the risk. If there is any doubt, obtain the opinion of a second radiologist (1).

After review of the mammograms, the radiologist believes Mrs. Murphy's abnormality is new and moderately suspicious.

What is the best way to sample this lesion for biopsy?

One option is a needle localized breast biopsy (NLB). The radiologist places a long wire through the skin to the microcalcifications, using stereotactic guidance. During surgery, the wire is followed to the lesion; then a wide excision is done around the tip of the wire. To ensure that the microcalcifications are in the specimen, a radiograph of the specimen is taken. The procedure is complete only after the calcifications in the specimen are seen to be the same as those in the mammogram (2).

Sterotactic core biopsy (SCB) is quickly replacing NLB as the initial diagnostic modality for nonpalpable breast lesions. Stereotactic guidance is used to take tissue samples with large-gauge needles. Long-term follow-up of SCB shows that sensitivity and specificity is greater than 90% (3).

SCB has several advantages over NLB. It is less costly, allows for better cosmesis, is associated with a shorter recovery time, and, if the biopsy is positive, allows for optimal preparation of the patient and surgeon and a lower incidence of positive margins (4). Results from SCB must be concordant. In addition, some lesions such as atypical ductal hyperplasia and radial scar warrant NLB because there is an incidence of carcinoma in these patients that is not found due to the small sample size taken in SCB.

Mrs. Murphy undergoes a stereotactic core biopsy. The pathologist confirms the presence of the microcalcifications in the specimen and makes a diagnosis of ductal carcinoma in situ (DCIS).

What is DCIS?

Almost 30% of breast neoplasms diagnosed by mammography are DCIS, a precancerous lesion characterized by malignant cells in the ducts but showing no evidence of invasion through the basement membrane. However, these lesions may progress to invade the basement membrane. It is thought that if untreated, 20% to 30% of these patients develop invasive ductal carcinoma. This is a demanding diagnosis for the pathologist. As high as 10% of these lesions may be reclassified as benign or malignant on review by a second pathologist (5).

What are Mrs. Murphy's options?

The patient has two options: total mastectomy (removal of the breast with preservation of underlying musculature) or lumpectomy with radiation. Total mastectomy is associated with a cure rate of approximately 98% to 99%. Lumpectomy with clear margins and adjuvant radiotherapy has shown to have approximately 5% to 8% recurrence rate. The National Surgical Adjuvant Breast and Bowel Project (NSABP) B-17 randomized women to radiation or observation only after lumpectomy (6). There was no difference in survival between the two groups. Addition of radiation resulted in a statistically significant difference in local recurrence. Generally, adjuvant radiotherapy is recommended for all patients after lumpectomy.

Mrs. Murphy undergoes a lumpectomy. Pathology shows a small focus of DCIS with negative margins. She is referred to a radiation oncologist.

Is there any other therapy that should be considered? Does she need an axillary node dissection?

Without further treatment, 2.6% of cases of DCIS recur per year; 50% of these recurrences are invasive. Death among patients with recurrent DCIS is very unusual. As for the role of axillary node dissection, less than 1% of axillary node dissections performed for DCIS show metastatic disease. Obviously, in these cases, an area of invasion was not seen by the pathologist. Axillary node dissection is not recommended for the treatment of patients with DCIS. Counsel the patient about the use of tamoxifen. NSABP B-24 showed that the addition of tamoxifen to women treated with lumpectomy and radiation reduced breast cancer events at 5 years (8.2% vs. 13.4%) (7).

Mrs. Gaudet is a 60-year-old woman with a 4-month history of a left breast mass that is asymptomatic. During this time, the mass has enlarged. She is otherwise healthy, and a review of systems does not reveal any concerns. She has never had a mammogram. On examination, there is no supraclavicular or infraclavicular lymphadenopathy. With the patient sitting with her hands above her head, a skin retraction at the upper outer quadrant is clearly visible. Palpation of the left breast reveals a 2-cm irregular, partially mobile mass in the same quadrant. There also are several enlarged nodes in the left axilla.

What is the differential diagnosis of this lump?

Breast cancer is a disease of aging. The risk of developing breast cancer between the ages of 20 and 30 years is 0.04%. The risk of developing breast cancer between the ages of 65 and 75 years is 3.2%. A woman who lives 110 years has a 10% risk of developing breast cancer. Therefore, as a woman ages, the likelihood of a new breast mass being cancer increases. This means that the differential diagnosis varies among age groups. For women older than 50 years, this mass should be considered a malignancy until proven otherwise. It also may be fibrocystic change (especially if she is taking hormone replacement therapy) or fat necrosis (8).

How should the physician proceed to a diagnosis?

A diagnostic mammogram would be useful. This provides more information about the characteristics of the mass and any other suspicious lesions, and it allows evaluation of the contralateral breast.

What should be done if the mammogram does not show a mass?

"A suspicious lump is a suspicious lump" until there is a histologic diagnosis. Mammograms miss 10% to 15% of cancers. Options for obtaining tissue for diagnosis are a fine-needle aspiration biopsy (FNAB), a core biopsy, and an open biopsy. FNAB is an excellent first test. Interpreting the result requires a pathologist skilled in cytology. The final pathology should provide a reasonable explanation for the mass and be concordant with the mammogram and clinical examination.

Mrs. Gaudet undergoes FNAB, and the cytologist reports finding atypical cells suspicious for malignancy.

How should Mrs. Gaudet now be treated?

At this point there still is no diagnosis. It is now time to perform a core or open biopsy. I prefer a core biopsy in this clinical scenario because the level of suspicion is high. Core biopsy can be done in the office, and it allows for further decision making to be done when the pathology is available. This reduces cost, reduces time, and most importantly allows the patient to adequately prepare. In addition, potentially there may be one operation instead of two or more.

Mrs. Gaudet undergoes a core biopsy. The finding is invasive ductal cancer.

What treatment is now necessary?

There are two main issues in the treatment of breast cancer: local control and treatment of systemic disease. Local recurrence rates after lumpectomy alone approach 30%. The best local control of this cancer is obtained by the addition of radiotherapy to the affected breast or by a mastectomy. The mortality related to breast cancer is the same after either of these options; deaths occur because of metastatic disease. Therefore, physicians must try to determine who is at greatest risk for developing or harboring metastasis, which is called *staging the disease* (9).

How should the axilla be staged?

Axillary staging is performed to provide the clinician with prognostic information and for local control. The role of formal axillary dissection has come into question since the late 1990s. The reasons are multifactorial. Chemotherapy is offered to many patients, regardless of nodal status. Unless high-dose chemotherapy is better for high-risk patients, the number of positive nodes is not important. Increased use of mammography has resulted in finding more lymph node–negative cancers and in sentinel node mapping and biopsy. In addition, there is a small but real morbidity associated with axillary dissection including lymphedema, loss of range of motion, seroma, and nerve damage.

The sentinel lymph node (SLN) concept initially was used widely for melanoma (10). The technology has been subsequently applied to breast cancer (11). The SLN is the first node to receive lymphatic drainage from a primary tumor. Thus, it is the first node to which a tumor will metastasize. If the SLN is negative for metastatic disease, the remaining nodes in the lymphatic basin are also likely to be negative. The ability to detect a SLN is greater than 90% (12) in experienced hands. The false-negative rate is variable but has been reported to be from 5% to

15%. A study by Guiliano (11) showed no axillary recurrences in patients with early breast cancer. There are two large multicenter trials led by the American College of Surgeons Oncology Group and NSABP that will help substantiate other single institution studies in the literature and provide long-term follow-up.

How is a sentinel node biopsy performed?

One millicurie of technetium sulfur colloid, in 4 to 8 mL, is injected around the tumor. Another option is to inject intradermally above the tumor. In the operating room, 1 to 24 hours after radiotracer injection, 3 to 5 mL of isosulfan blue is injected either around the tumor or in the subareolar region. A handheld gamma probe is used with visual identification of blue lymphatics to identify the SLN. All of the hot or blue nodes (usually 1 to 3) are removed until axillary bed counts approach background counts. I routinely send the SLN for imprint cytology. If this is positive, I perform a completion axillary dissection.

So what exactly are the options available to Mrs. Gaudet?

Mrs. Gaudet has two choices: total mastectomy and SLN biopsy or a lumpectomy and SLN biopsy.

Mrs. Gaudet chooses to have a total mastectomy and SLN biopsy.

What are the anatomic landmarks used in a mastectomy?

The breast sits on the anterior chest wall lateral to the sternum and extending to the mid-axillary line. The tail of Spence is an extension of the breast to the axilla. In the vertical axis, the breast extends from the second to the sixth ribs.

Intraoperative frozen section reveals that the SLN is positive for carcinoma.

What are the levels of the axilla and the important structures?

The axilla is the site of the main lymph node basin draining the breast. The status of the lymph nodes is one of the principle factors of staging patients with breast cancer. At least 10 lymph nodes are needed to make sure nodal metastases are not missed. The axilla has level I, level II, and level III nodes that are lateral to, under, and medial to the pectoralis minor muscle, respectively.

The standard operation is dissection and removal of level I and II lymph nodes. The operation entails dissection and identification of the axillary vein, which may sustain damage. The major risk is to adjacent nerves. The intercostal brachial nerve is a sensory nerve to the posteromedial aspect of the upper arm. It is frequently damaged, and patients may have postoperative pain or numbness. The long thoracic nerve lies on the chest wall and innervates the serratus anterior muscle. Damage to this nerve results in a winged scapula. Finally, the thoracodorsal nerve can be damaged, resulting in weakness in the latissimus dorsi muscle.

Mrs. Gaudet undergoes an uneventful operation. The final pathology shows a 2-cm infiltrating ductal carcinoma. Of 20 lymph nodes, 3 are positive for metastasis. The pathologist also determines that the tumor is estrogen receptor positive.

Should Mrs. Gaudet receive adjuvant chemotherapy?

Mrs. Gaudet is postmenopausal and has an estrogen receptor–positive tumor and node–positive disease. Therefore, she has a 50% to 60% chance of developing metastatic disease. The recommendation is that she begin a 5-year course of tamoxifen, an antiestrogen drug, and to consider chemotherapy.

If Mrs. Gaudet were still menstruating, what would be her adjuvant therapy?

The recommendations for adjuvant chemotherapy depend on menopausal status and the patient's risk of recurrence (13). The risk of recurrence is categorized as low, intermediate, or high according to the size and grade of the tumor, the presence or absence of estrogen receptors, and any lymphatic or vascular invasion. Decisions regarding chemotherapy are made on an individual basis and include an assessment of performance status. If Mrs. Gaudet were premenopausal she would be offered multiagent chemotherapy. There are two recommended regimens: either six cycles of cyclophosphamide, methotrexate, and 5-fluorouracil (CMF) or four cycles of doxorubicin (Adriamycin) and cyclophosphamide (AC).

Mrs. Gaudet's 35-year-old daughter, Ms. Gaudet, attends your clinic. She is worried about her risk of developing breast cancer. Findings of a complete history and physical examination are normal. A thorough review of the family history determines that Mrs. Gaudet's sister was diagnosed with breast cancer at age 45 years, and Mrs. Gaudet's mother died of breast cancer at age 40 years.

What percentage of breast cancers is inherited?

As much as 5% to 10% of breast cancers may be inherited. Breast cancer may be divided into three categories:

1. *Sporadic:* no relatives with breast cancer for two generations
2. *Familial:* breast cancer in one or more first- or second-degree relatives
3. *Hereditary:* the same as familial but the cancers occur at a younger age, are frequently bilateral, are associated with other primary tumors, and appear to be inherited in an autosomal dominant pattern

What hereditary syndromes are associated with an increased risk of breast cancer?

The BRAC1 gene, or hereditary breast-ovary cancer syndrome, may account for 40% to 50% of hereditary breast cancer. As much as 80% of women who inherit this gene develop breast cancer, and 40% develop ovarian cancer. The

BRAC2 gene has also been identified with an increased risk of breast cancer. Other less common syndromes include Li-Fraumeni syndrome, ataxia, telangiectasia, Cowden's disease, and Bloom's syndrome.

How should the physician deal with Ms. Gaudet's problem?

Ms. Gaudet should be offered genetic testing. Testing for BRAC1 and BRAC2 is commercially available. Genetic counseling before and after such testing is required.

Ms. Gaudet goes for genetic counseling and testing and is found to be positive for the BRAC1 gene. She returns to discuss a management plan.

What options are available to Ms. Gaudet?

Intense follow-up and prophylactic mastectomy are the two choices. Follow-up entails biannual physical examinations and annual mammograms beginning immediately for Ms. Gaudet, who is 35 years old (annual mammograms start at age 20 years for BRAC1-positive women). Also, because of the risk of ovarian cancer, screening pelvic and transvaginal ultrasounds are used. There is no evidence that this protocol reduces cancer deaths in this group of patients. Studies are needed to determine the best method of follow-up.

In patients who are BRAC1 positive, prophylactic mastectomy does not eliminate the risk but has been shown to reduce risk and extend life expectancy (14). The best management plan has not yet been determined, but careful communication with geneticists and early involvement of a plastic surgeon is advisable (15).

Ms. Cromwell is a 25-year-old woman with painful breasts. She is a jogger, and it has become difficult for her to run. On examination, both breasts are found to be tender, particularly in the upper outer quadrants. Both breasts are nodular and firm. There is no lymphadenopathy.

What is fibrocystic change of the breast?

Fibrocystic change is a benign process that is present to some degree in all women. It is usually asymptomatic, but women may notice breast nodules or have mastalgia or nipple discharge. Biopsies may show cysts, fibrosis, sclerosing adenosis, or epithelial hyperplasia (Table 3.1).

What other information is needed to manage Ms. Cromwell's case?

More information about the characteristics of the pain is needed. For example, is the pain related to her menstrual cycle, or is it cyclic? Elicit any history of trauma and identify aggravating and relieving factors, such as movement.

Ms. Cromwell describes the pain as a dull, achy pain that is at its worst 7 to 10 days before menses. At that time, the pain radiates into her

TABLE 3.1.

DIFFERENTIAL DIAGNOSIS OF BREAST PAIN

True breast pain	
	Cyclical
	Noncyclical trigger spot
Musculoskeletal	
	Tietze's syndrome
	Cervical root syndrome
	Rib injury
	Thoracic spine osteoarthritis
Inflammatory	
	Breast abscess
	Mammary duct octasia
Miscellaneous	
	Pregnancy
	Mondor's syndrome
	Trauma
	Psychologic
	Psychosexual
Breast cancer	
	5% have pain
	0.5% of patients with breast pain have cancer

axilla. There is no history of trauma. Anything that causes pressure or movement of her breasts is uncomfortable.

How should you proceed?

It is important to determine why Ms. Cromwell has now sought medical attention. Many patients worry that pain is a sign of cancer. Although 5% to 10% of patients with cancer have breast pain, only 0.5% of patients with reported breast pain have cancer. In women older than 35 years, a mammogram may be suggested to rule out a mass. There is spontaneous resolution of the pain in 20% to 50% of patients; and 10% to 20% of women seek further help (16).

What is the treatment of this pain?

For the majority of women, simple reassurance is all that is needed. First-line treatment is analgesics and heat. Reduction in caffeine intake and dietary fat may be beneficial. Evening primrose oil is a dietary supplement that has been found to be effective. Hormone agonists (e.g., danazol) and antagonists (e.g., tamoxifen) are effective but have a significant number of side effects. These agents should be reserved for unresponsive patients and those with severe pain.

Is mastectomy an option for patients with intractable pain?

Surgery does not guarantee relief of pain. Many patients continue to have pain; painful scars may develop; and the end result may be dissatisfying. Surgery is not recommended as a treatment for mastalgia.

Mrs. Gomez is a 30-year-old mother of a 5-year-old boy. She has a 2-month history of bloody discharge from her right nipple. She notices some blood on her nightgown every morning and is able to express a small amount of blood. She does monthly breast examinations and has not noticed any masses. There is no family history of breast cancer. Physical examination reveals no masses, and the physician cannot express any blood from the nipple.

How can the diagnosis be confirmed?

The first step is to ask Mrs. Gomez to try to express blood. If she is unable to do so, she should be asked not to examine herself for a few days, and a return appointment should be arranged. The hope is that sufficient blood will accumulate to demonstrate the problem.

Mrs. Gomez returns a week later, and the physician is able to express blood from a duct at the 2-o'clock position on the right breast.

What investigations are indicated?

The obvious concern is that there is cancer. Other causes of bloody discharge include ductal papilloma, Paget's disease of the nipple, and fibrocystic change (Table 3.2). Mammography may identify an occult mass and therefore is the best first test. A galactogram may identify a lesion in the duct. This is done by cannulation of the affected duct and injection of a contrast medium.

Mrs. Gomez has a normal mammogram, but a galactogram reveals a small growth consistent with a duct papilloma.

What is a papilloma?

A papilloma is a benign lesion; however, the problem is that 0.5% of these lesions are papillary cancers. The association of a breast mass and calcifications constitute a stronger indication of cancer. Excisional biopsy of the affected duct with wire localization is the next best investigation and is also the treatment for this problem in the majority of women.

Mrs. Smith is a 52-year-old woman who is referred to surgery because of a breast abscess. Mrs. Smith has noticed that her left breast gradually has enlarged and become uncomfortable during the past month. The breast became red and mildly tender 2 weeks ago. She sought medical attention and was prescribed antibiotics. Despite this treatment, the problem has become worse.

TABLE 3.2.

CAUSES OF NIPPLE DISCHARGE

Bloodstained
- Duct papilloma
- Intraduct cancer (30%)
- Paget's disease of nipple
- Fibrocystic change

Serous
- Duct hyperplasia
- Cancer
- Pregnancy

Greenish-brown
- Mammary duct ectasia
- Fibrocystic change

Purulent
- Breast abscess

Creamy
- Duct ectasia

Milky
- Postlactation
- Drug induced (OCP)
- Prolactinoma

During examination, the patient is afebrile. Her left breast is obviously very much enlarged. The skin over the breast is red, tense, and dimpled. No discrete mass can be identified. There is no lymphadenopathy.

Why have the antibiotics not worked?

The bacteria associated with breast abscesses in Mrs. Smith's age group differ from those associated with lactation, and they may be caused by gram-negative anaerobes. Therefore, it is possible that the wrong antibiotics were chosen. It also is possible that the abscess will need surgical drainage. The diagnosis also may be wrong. Mrs. Smith has the classic features of an inflammatory carcinoma of the breast.

How can a diagnosis be determined for Mrs. Smith?

Mrs. Smith should have an immediate breast ultrasound to look for an abscess.

An ultrasound is done, and no abscess is seen.

Should the antibiotics be changed?

No. Mrs. Smith should have a mammogram.

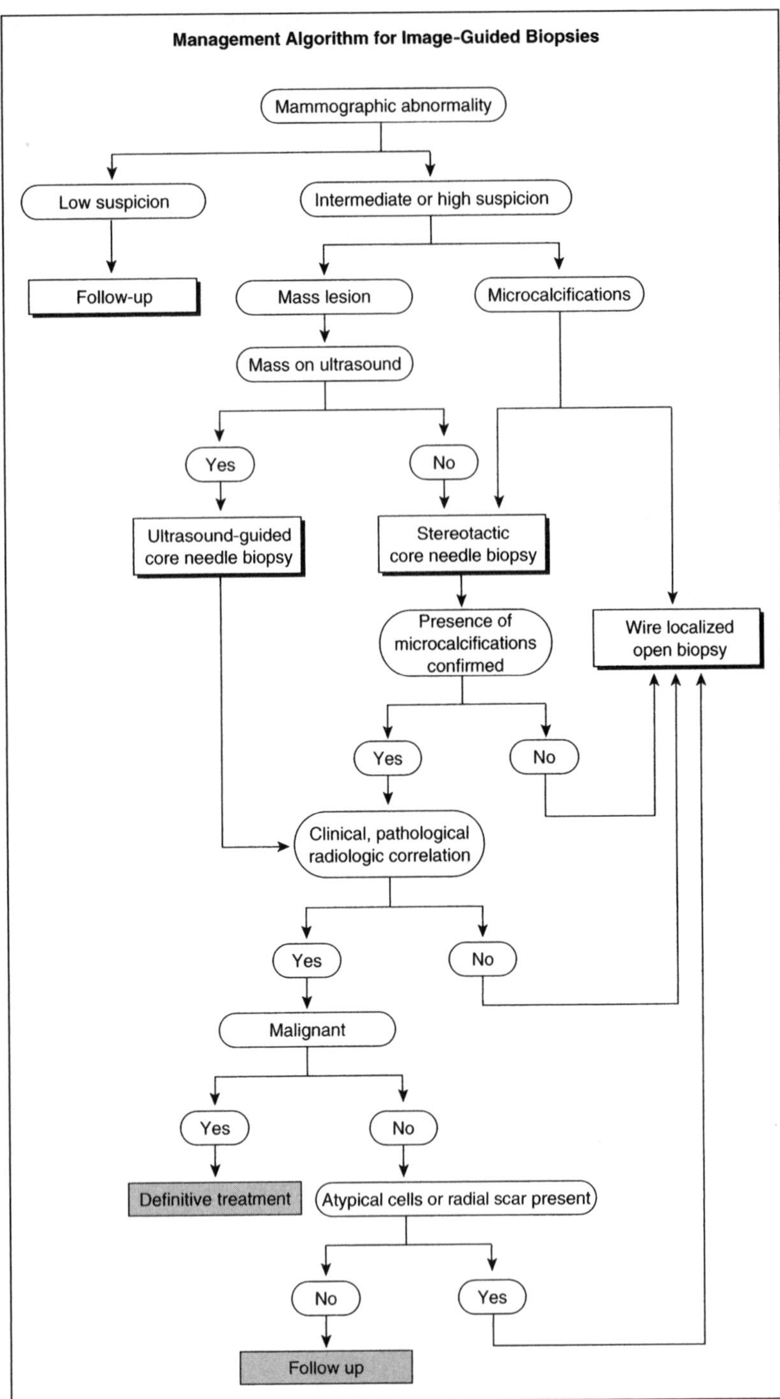

Algorithm 3.1.

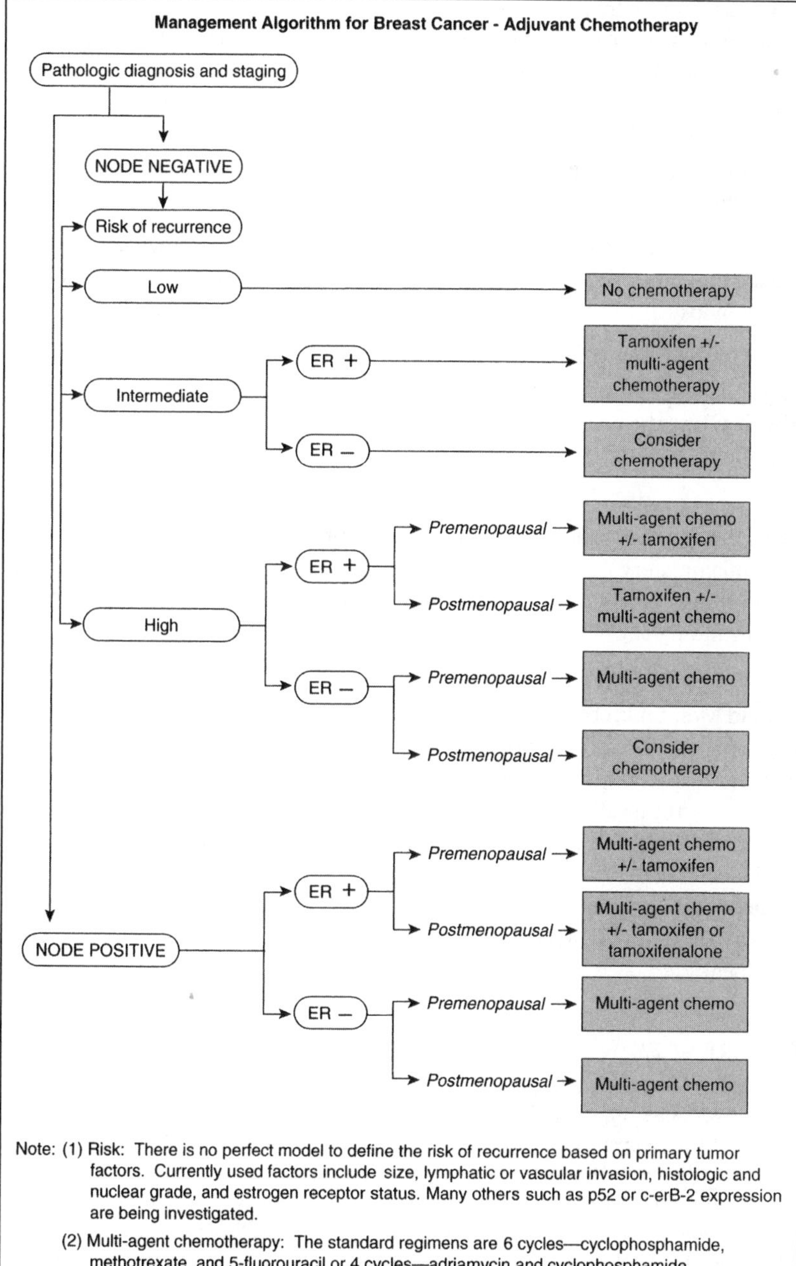

Note: (1) Risk: There is no perfect model to define the risk of recurrence based on primary tumor factors. Currently used factors include size, lymphatic or vascular invasion, histologic and nuclear grade, and estrogen receptor status. Many others such as p52 or c-erB-2 expression are being investigated.

(2) Multi-agent chemotherapy: The standard regimens are 6 cycles—cyclophosphamide, methotrexate, and 5-fluorouracil or 4 cycles—adriamycin and cyclophosphamide.

Algorithm 3.2.

What is inflammatory cancer of the breast?

Inflammatory cancer of the breast is the most aggressive form of breast cancer. It accounts for 1% to 3% of breast cancers. The classic presentation is an enlarging breast, erythema, and skin edema resulting in characteristic dimpling of the skin resembling the skin of an orange (*peau d'orange*). In most cases, the cancer is widely infiltrating, so that no mass is palpable. Invasion of the dermal lymphatics is common.

It is very important to make a quick diagnosis and not delay treatment any further. A mammogram may show a mass or demonstrate the extent of infiltration. A punch biopsy of affected skin and a core biopsy of the breast should be sufficient for diagnosis, but if there is any doubt, perform an incisional biopsy.

Mrs. Smith's skin biopsy does not show invasion of the dermal lymphatics, but the core biopsy of the breast reveals a poorly differentiated adenocarcinoma.

Does the negative skin biopsy mean this is not an inflammatory carcinoma?

No. Inflammatory carcinoma is a constellation of clinical signs associated with an aggressive breast cancer. Mrs. Smith has those clinical signs and now has a biopsy finding of cancer.

Should Mrs. Smith be scheduled for surgery?

Inflammatory carcinoma of the breast is not treated with surgery, at least not at first. Historically, when surgery or radiation therapy or both were the primary treatments, the local recurrence rates were 50% to 80%, and metastasis occurred in more than 90% of patients. Multiagent chemotherapy is now the first treatment of choice, followed by radiation and surgery. This change in management has reduced local recurrence rates to 10% to 20% and has improved 5-year survival from 5% to 50% (17). Mrs. Smith should be sent to a medical oncologist to begin treatment.

REFERENCES

1. Clinical practice guidelines for the care and treatment of breast cancer. CMAJ. 1998;158:S9–14(3 Suppl)
2. D'Orsi C, Kopans DB. Mammography interpretation: the BI-RADS method. Am Fam Physician. 1997;55:1548–1552.
3. Nguyen M, McCombs MM, Ghandehari S, et al. An update of core needle biopsy for radiologically detected breast lesions. Cancer. 1996;78:2340–2345.
4. Lind DS, Minterr, Steinbach B. Stereotactic core biopsy reduces the reexcision rate and cost of mammographically detected cancer. J Surg Res. 1998;78:23–26.
5. Eusebi V, Feudale E, Foschini M, et al. Long-term follow-up of in situ carcinoma of the breast. Semin Diagn Pathol. 1994;11:223.

6. Fisher B, Costantino J, Redmond C, et al. Lumpectomy and radiation for treatment of intraductal breast cancer: findings from the National Surgical Adjuvant Breast and Bowel Project B-17. N Engl J Med. 1993;328:1581–1586.
7. Fisher B, Dingman J, Wolmark N, et al. Tamoxifen in the treatment of intraductal breast cancer: National Surgical Adjuvant Breast and Bowel Project B-24 randomised controlled trial. Lancet. 1999;353:1993–2000.
8. Henderson IC. Risk factors for breast cancer development. Cancer. 1993;71(Suppl):2127.
9. Fisher B, Anderson S, Redmond CK, et al. Reanalysis and results after 12 years of follow-up in a randomized clinical trial comparing total mastectomy with lumpectomy with or without irradiation in the treatment of breast cancer. N Engl J Med. 1995;333:1456.
10. Morton DL, Wen D, Wong JH, et al. Technical details of intraoperative lymphatic mapping for early stage melanoma. Arch Surg. 1992;127:392–399.
11. Guiliano AE, Kirgan DM, Guenther JM, et al. Lymphatic mapping and sentinel lymphadenectomy for breast cancer. Ann Surg. 1994;2:335–340.
12. Harlow SP, Krag DN. Sentinel lymph node—why study it: implications of the B-32 study. Semin Surg Oncol. 2001;20:224–229.
13. Early Breast Cancer Trialists Collaborative Group. Systemic treatment of early breast cancer by hormonal, cytotoxic, or immune therapy: 133 randomized trials involving 31,000 recurrences and 24,000 deaths among 75,000 women. Lancet. 1992;339:1–15.
14. Schrag D, Kuntz KM, Garber JE, et al. Decision analysis—effects of prophylactic mastectomy and oophorectomy on life expectancy among women with BRCA1 or BRCA2 mutations. N Engl J Med. 1997;336:1465–1471.
15. Lynch HT, Lynch JF. Breast cancer genetics: family history, heterogeneity, molecular genetic diagnosis and genetic counseling. Curr Probl Cancer. 1996;20:329–365.
16. Klimberg VS. Etiology and management of breast pain. In: Harris JR, ed. Diseases of the Breast. Philadelphia, Pa: Lippincott-Raven Publishers; 1996:99–106.
17. Buzdar AU, Singletary E, Booser DJ, et al. Combined modality treatment of stage III and inflammatory breast cancer. Surg Oncol Clin N Am. 1995;4:715–734.

CHAPTER

THYROID AND PARATHYROID DISEASE

Nicholas P.W. Coe

THYROID DISEASE

Patricia Arnold is a 35-year-old woman with an asymptomatic neck mass, which she first noticed 3 weeks ago. Her history is unremarkable except for childhood tonsillectomy and adenoidectomy. She is taking birth control pills and has no known drug allergies. A family history reveals that a maternal aunt had Graves' disease; no other members had thyroid disease. The patient has a 20-pack-year smoking history and has one to two alcoholic drinks per week. A review of various other systems does not reveal any significant findings.

The physical examination reveals a healthy-looking woman in no acute distress. Her vital signs are normal: temperature, 36.5° C; blood pressure, 135/70 mm Hg, pulse rate 80 beats per minute; and respiratory rate, 18 breaths per minute. The head and neck examination reveals no exophthalmos, lid lag, or intraoral lesions; the neck mass is not associated with any cervical adenopathy. The lungs are clear to auscultation; the heart rate and rhythm are regular and without murmurs; and the abdominal examination is normal. Neurologic function is intact, and findings are nonfocal.

What is the differential diagnosis for a neck mass?

Approximately 50% of neck masses that persist beyond 3 to 4 weeks originate from the thyroid gland. Inflammatory lesions, nonthyroidal malignant lesions, and congenital lesions account for the remaining 50%. Malignant lesions, such as lymphoma, carcinoma of the thyroid, and metastatic tumor from another head and neck site, are most common in adults, whereas inflammatory lesions are most common in children. Congenital lesions, such as thyroglossal duct and branchial cleft cysts, are also very common in children.

The 3-cm mass, which appears to be originating from the right thyroid lobe, is firm and not tender. There is no associated fever, chills, pressure, or symptoms of thyrotoxicity.

What are the symptoms of thyrotoxicity?

Heat intolerance, weight loss with increased appetite, tachycardia (sleeping pulse rate faster than 80 beats per minute), atrial arrhythmias, congestive heart failure (especially in the elderly), hyperkinetic behavior, emotional instability, insomnia, fatigue, muscle weakness, amenorrhea, and diarrhea are all symptoms of thyrotoxicity.

What does *thyroid* mean and where is the thyroid gland?

The word *thyroid* is derived from the Greek *thyreos,* or shield. The thyroid gland originates from two sites. The tuberculum impar at the base of the vallate papillae of the tongue forms the foramen cecum. The thyroid tissue descends into the neck along the line of the thyroglossal duct. The lateral component, which contributes the calcitonin-producing C cells, is derived from the fourth pharyngeal pouch.

The mature thyroid gland, which weighs about 20 g, drapes over the anterolateral aspect of the upper trachea just below the cricoid cartilage. The two lobes, connected by the isthmus, lie along the sides of the larynx and trachea, extending up to the level of the middle of the thyroid cartilage. The pyramidal lobe is a diverticulum extending upward from the isthmus. These lobes are between the trachea medially and the carotid sheaths and sternocleidomastoid muscles laterally; the strap muscles lie anterior to the thyroid lobes. The parathyroid glands and the recurrent laryngeal nerves are on the posterior surface of the lateral lobes of the thyroid gland. The nerves are typically found in the tracheoesophageal groove. A thin, fibrous capsule surrounds the thyroid gland.

What are the risk factors for thyroid malignancy?

A careful personal and family history helps determine whether a patient has any special risk factors for thyroid malignancy. Low-dose radiation exposure (300 to 1000 cGy) is associated with well-differentiated thyroid cancer (1). More than 90% of thyroid carcinomas in patients with a history of irradiation are papillary. Low doses of radiation were commonly used between 1945 and 1955 to treat an enlarged thymus. Radiation was also used from the 1930s to the 1960s to treat diseases such as ringworm, keloids, capillary hemangiomata, and tubercular lymphadenopathy. In more recent times, exposure to radiation from the Chernobyl nuclear accident in April 1986 placed residents of the Ukraine, the Gomel region of Belorussia, and possibly other widespread areas of central Europe at high risk for developing thyroid malignancy. Immigrants from these areas now live in many parts of the Unites States.

A higher incidence of malignancy is also found in patients with a thyroid mass who are younger than 20 years, patients older than 60 years, and men than in the general population. A family history of thyroid disease is often present, especially in female relatives; this has little bearing on the treatment of the patient, but the possibility of the familial form of thyroid carcinoma should always be kept in mind.

Significant findings on physical examination include a hard mass with poorly defined borders, cervical adenopathy adjacent to the thyroid or in the posterior triangle, fixation of the gland, and vocal cord paralysis.

How should a thyroid mass be evaluated?

The main features that have to be determined are (a) whether the mass is malignant and (b) whether it is hyperfunctioning. The patient should also be questioned about symptoms of compression such as difficulty swallowing or a choking sensation.

If a patient has no symptoms or signs of thyrotoxicosis, the simplest and most economical way to begin the workup is to determine the thyroid-stimulating hormone (TSH) level and obtain a fine-needle aspirate (FNA) of the thyroid with a 21- to 25-gauge needle. If the TSH level is normal, the patient is not likely to be thyrotoxic; if there is any doubt, determine thyroxine (T_4) and triiodothyronine (T_3) levels. Ultrasonography may be helpful in a patient whose neck is difficult to examine, but ultrasonography has largely been superseded by FNA for distinguishing between cystic and solid lesions. Radioactive scanning with iodine 123 (^{123}I) or technetium 99m (^{99m}Tc)-labeled compounds can differentiate among cold lesions (those with low or no radioisotope uptake), warm lesions (those that take up the radioisotope but show no evidence of thyrotoxicosis), and hot lesions (those that concentrate the isotope to a greater degree than the remaining thyroid). Cold lesions raise suspicion of malignancy and are always evaluated with FNA. Warm and hot lesions are only rarely malignant and do not require FNA.

What are the advantages and disadvantages of needle biopsy in the evaluation of a thyroid nodule?

FNA biopsy is safe, fast, sensitive, and cost effective, and it can be performed on an outpatient basis. Papillary, medullary, and anaplastic carcinomas can be diagnosed with this method. Certain elements, such as atypia and a microfollicular pattern, suggest malignancy, whereas a macrofollicular pattern or abundant colloid is more consistent with a benign lesion. However, this technique does not allow differentiation between malignant and benign follicular tumors because that distinction is made on the basis of vascular and/or capsular invasion, features that cannot be determined from an FNA.

What is the therapeutic approach if the FNA indicates that the lesion is benign?

If an experienced thyroid cytopathologist considers the aspirate to be benign, the patient is offered the option of treatment with suppressive doses of L-thyroxine, and the biopsy is repeated in 3 to 6 months.

What is the mechanism of thyroxine suppression?

The activity of the thyroid gland is regulated by the central nervous system (CNS) and by the serum level of iodine. The hypothalamus secretes thyrotropin-releasing hormone, which stimulates the anterior pituitary gland to release TSH. TSH stimulates the production and release of thyroid hormone and induces hyperplasia (TSH is also known as thyrotropin) and vascularity of the thyroid gland.

Secretion of TSH is inhibited by the negative feedback effect of endogenous or exogenous thyroid hormone. Thyroid suppression may be given in doses of L-thyroxine sufficient to suppress TSH to barely detectable levels. This decrease in TSH may shrink the lesion by inhibiting the hyperplastic effect of TSH. There is, however, a significant association with increased osteoporosis and the onset of atrial fibrillation in these patients. Some endocrinologists will use exogenous thyroid hormone to suppress TSH only to low levels of normal or just below normal because of this major concern. The thyroid tumors do not usually shrink but the patient should be given the option to try this treatment modality.

How is thyroid hormone formed?

The principal function of the thyroid gland is to produce thyroid hormone, which regulates cellular metabolism. The production of thyroid hormone depends on dietary iodine, which is actively transported from the plasma into the thyroid where it is oxidized and rapidly incorporated into a macromolecule, thyroglobulin. Tyrosine molecules are iodinated at one (monoiodotyrosine) or two (diiodotyrosine) sites, and these are subsequently coupled to form T_3 and T_4.

Hydrolysis of thyroglobulin releases T_3 and T_4 into the circulation, but thyroglobulin is not released except in disease states (Fig. 4.1). The active thyroid hormones attach to a plasma protein, thyroxine-binding globulin. In the plasma, the T_4-T_3 ratio ranges from 10:1 to 20:1. In the periphery, T_4 is converted to T_3, which enters the tissues quickly because of its lower affinity for protein and is three to four times as active as T_4. The half-life of T_4 (7 to 8 days) is longer than that of T_3 (3 days). The metabolic functions of thyroid hormone include increased calorigenesis, increased protein synthesis, and altered carbohydrate and lipid metabolism.

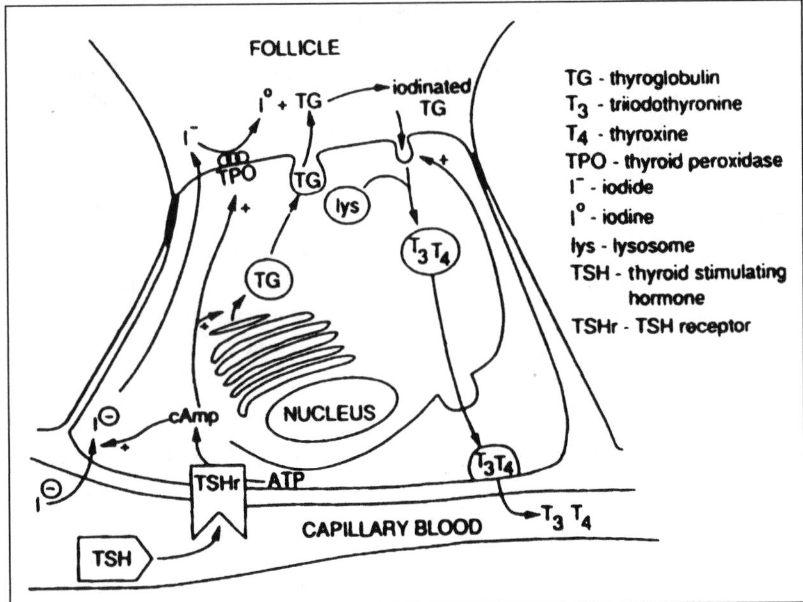

Figure 4.1. Iodinated thyroglobulin stored as thyroid hormones in the follicle. (From Lawrence PF, Bell RM, Dayton MT, eds. Essentials of General Surgery. 2nd ed. Baltimore: Williams & Wilkins, 1992:294, with permission.)

What are the indications for surgery in thyroid disease?

Surgical treatment of thyroid disease should be considered for the following conditions:

Malignancy

- Carcinoma proved with FNA
- A lesion suspicious for carcinoma on FNA
- As prophylaxis for patients with familial thyroid cancer

Nonmalignant thyroid mass

- Toxic multinodular goiter
- Solitary toxic nodule
- Graves' disease

Compression symptoms from a thyroid mass

Ms. Arnold's ultrasound examination reveals a solid nodule. A ^{123}I scan reveals a cold nodule, and FNA reveals cells suggestive of papillary carcinoma.

What are the pathologic types of thyroid cancers?

Four main types of thyroid cancers can be distinguished according to their pathology: papillary, follicular, medullary, and anaplastic. More than 90% of all thyroid cancers are papillary and follicular (well-differentiated) carcinomas.

Papillary carcinomas are well-differentiated lesions. The peak incidence is in the third to fourth decades, and women are affected three times as often as men. Papillary carcinomas contain concentric layers of calcium called *psammoma bodies.* Papillary cancers are the slowest-growing thyroid cancers, and they spread through the lymphatic system. When thyroid tissue is found in the posterior triangle of the neck, the condition has been referred to as *lateral aberrant thyroid.* This actually represents a papillary cancer that has metastasized to a lymph node. Accessory thyroid tissue, separate from the thyroid, can be found in the central compartment of the neck. Usually this does not represent metastatic thyroid cancer but rather an embryonic rest of thyroid tissue. The multicentricity rate of papillary thyroid cancer is 80% on microscopic examination, but probably less than 5% have a clinical effect. Papillary metastases usually concentrate iodine and can be treated with radioiodine. Some papillary thyroid cancers show features of follicular cancer and are known as follicular variants of papillary cancer. They behave in the same way as papillary cancers.

Follicular carcinomas are generally also well-differentiated tumors. Pure follicular cancers, as distinct from follicular variants of papillary cancer, differ from papillary tumors in that they exhibit less multicentricity and are more likely to spread hematogenously to bone, lung, and liver. Follicular metastases may concentrate iodine, but to a lesser degree than papillary lesions. When iodine uptake is demonstrated, they can be treated with radioiodine.

Medullary carcinomas are less common tumors, comprising 3% to 5% of thyroid cancers. They are calcitonin-producing tumors that originate from the C cells; amyloid deposits in the stroma of the tumor are diagnostic. Bilateral multicentricity is more commonly found in familial cases but is still common in the sporadic variety. Medullary cancers occur in families as components of both multiple endocrine neoplasia (MEN) type II and the familial medullary carcinoma syndrome (see Chapter 23). MEN type IIA, or Sipple's syndrome, also includes pheochromocytomas and hyperparathyroidism (HPT). MEN type IIB is a less common form that includes mucosal neuromas, ganglioneuroma of the bowel, and a marfanoid appearance; HPT is rare. An elevated serum calcitonin level is diagnostic of medullary carcinoma and is also a useful screening tool for familial transmission and to monitor recurrence. Evaluation of point mutations in the *Ret* protooncogene is part of the workup of these patients and their families (2).

Anaplastic carcinomas account for less than 5% of thyroid cancers and occur later in life than the other types. These cancers are characterized by extremely rapid and widespread growth. Patients present with a sometimes painful and enlarged thyroid gland. These tumors are highly aggressive and are associated with a very short life expectancy.

What is the treatment for a patient with a presentation such as Ms. Arnold's if the FNA indicates papillary carcinoma?

The lesion must be excised, but the extent of resection—thyroid lobectomy alone versus total thyroidectomy (Fig 4.2)—has been debated extensively (3,4).

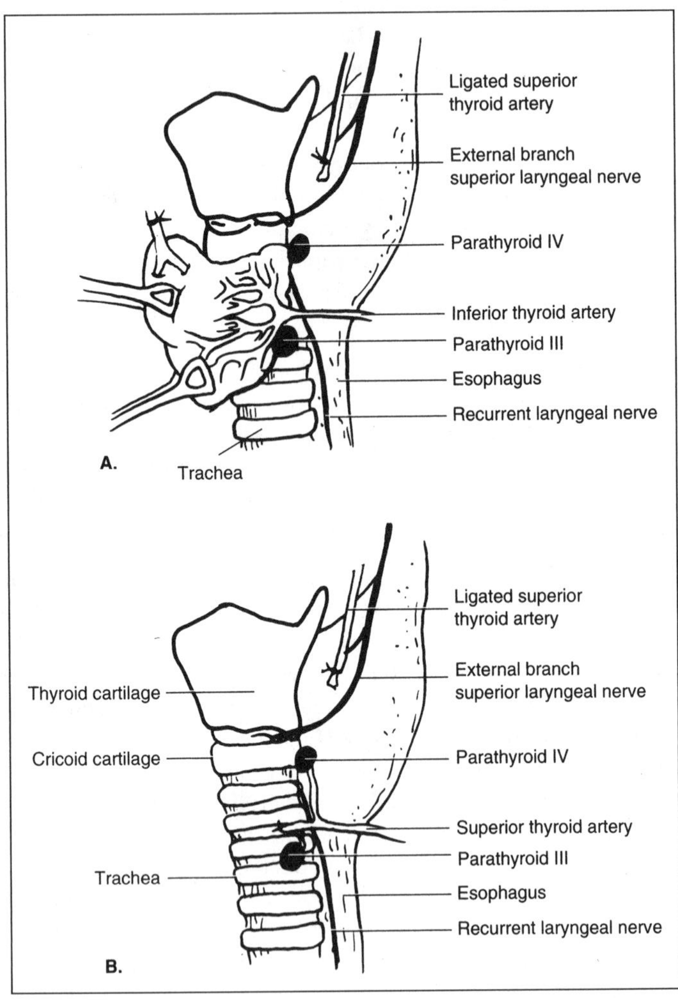

Figure 4.2. **A.** Anteromedial reflection of thyroid gland. **B.** Anatomy after total thyroidectomy. (Adapted from Doherty GM, Norton JA. Thyroid and parathyroid. In: Lawrence PF, ed. Essentials of General Surgery. 2nd ed. Baltimore: Williams & Wilkins, 1992:298, with permission.)

Lobectomy is advocated by some because it minimizes the operative risks of nerve and parathyroid injury; multicentric disease rarely becomes a clinical problem; and thyroid cancers in general are not very aggressive. More extensive surgical ablation (total thyroidectomy) is promoted because it allows postoperative scanning with ^{131}I for metastatic disease because no normal thyroid tissue (which concentrates iodine more vigorously than papillary or follicular metastases) remains in the neck; it facilitates follow-up with thyroglobulin levels; and it eliminates recurrence caused by multicentricity. One large study has shown a survival benefit for total thyroidectomy over lobectomy (5). A majority of endocrine surgeons favor total thyroidectomy for lesions larger than 2 to 3 cm.

After total thyroidectomy, L-thyroxine is given for life in doses sufficient to maintain normal levels of TSH. Radioiodine is used to ablate any residual functional thyroid tissue in the neck after thyroidectomy and to destroy widespread metastases. Improved survival was demonstrated after treatment with total thyroidectomy, radioiodine ablation, and TSH suppression for life in a study of 1355 patients who were followed for 40 years (5,6).

What is the treatment if the FNA shows atypical follicular cells?

The treatment decision in this instance continues to be difficult. The question is whether this tumor is a follicular adenoma, follicular hyperplasia, follicular carcinoma, or a follicular variant of papillary carcinoma. In addition, malignancy cannot be determined from intraoperative frozen sections (7), which adds to the uncertainty of the diagnosis. When the pathologic interpretation is that the lesion is a follicular carcinoma, the debate over the extent of operative resection is similar to that for papillary carcinoma. Advocates of total thyroidectomy for well-differentiated thyroid carcinoma recommend this procedure for lesions that cytology suggests are malignant and for lesions larger than 3 cm. If the cytology is indeterminate, generally a lobectomy is performed followed later by completion thyroidectomy if the permanent sections show malignancy. The surgeon and patient must balance the risk of a total thyroidectomy for possibly benign disease against the risk of further anesthesia and another procedure.

What are Hürthle cell carcinomas?

Hürthle cell carcinomas are aggressive variants of follicular cell origin. As with follicular carcinomas, capsular or vascular invasion by the tumor indicates malignancy, but some Hürthle cell tumors behave in a malignant fashion even without these pathologic features. Size appears to be an important criterion. As a general rule, lesions less than 3 cm in diameter behave benignly, whereas those larger than 6 cm have tendency to behave as a malignancy (8).

How are medullary carcinomas treated?

Medullary carcinomas are aggressive lesions that are markedly multicentric and that commonly metastasize to the lymph nodes. Total thyroidectomy with a central node dissection is performed for disease limited to the thyroid (9). A unilateral or bilateral modified radical neck dissection is indicated when metastatic disease is suspected because of elevated calcitonin levels and nodes that are either palpable or demonstrated by ultrasound and FNA studies to contain metastatic disease. Development of medullary thyroid cancer in patients with MEN II is virtually 100% and prophylactic total thyroidectomy at an early age is recommended in all these patients.

How are anaplastic carcinomas treated?

Anaplastic carcinomas are characterized by extremely rapid growth and a very poor prognosis. Thyroidectomy does not improve the prognosis and is performed only to prevent airway compression. Chemotherapy and radiation therapy may offer some benefit as palliation (10).

Ms. Arnold is scheduled for neck exploration and thyroid resection for a papillary carcinoma.

What are the main steps in a thyroidectomy?

General endotracheal anesthesia is induced, and the neck is extended. A curvilinear transverse incision is made in the line of a natural skin crease just below the cricoid cartilage over the thyroid isthmus. The incision is carried through the skin, subcutaneous tissue, platysma (innervated by the facial nerve), and cervical fascia overlying the pretracheal muscles and anterior jugular veins. After the subplatysmal flaps are developed, the cervical fascia is opened in the midline. The strap muscles (sternohyoid and sternothyroid) are separated. They are only divided for very large lesions. If the tumor infiltrates the sternothyroid muscle, the muscle should be resected en bloc with the thyroid (Fig. 4.3).

What are the characteristics of the blood supply to the thyroid gland?

The thyroid has an abundant arterial blood supply from the superior thyroid arteries, which arise as the first branch of the external carotid arteries, and the inferior thyroid arteries, which arise from the thyrocervical trunks of the subclavian artery. There is no middle thyroid artery. Although the thyroid ima, an inferior artery that is said to arise from the arch of the aorta, is mentioned in many texts, it is rarely if ever found. The venous drainage consists of paired superior, inferior, and middle thyroid veins (Fig. 4.2).

The patient undergoes total thyroidectomy for treatment of a papillary carcinoma.

What are the complications of thyroidectomy?

The most serious injury is to the recurrent laryngeal nerve.

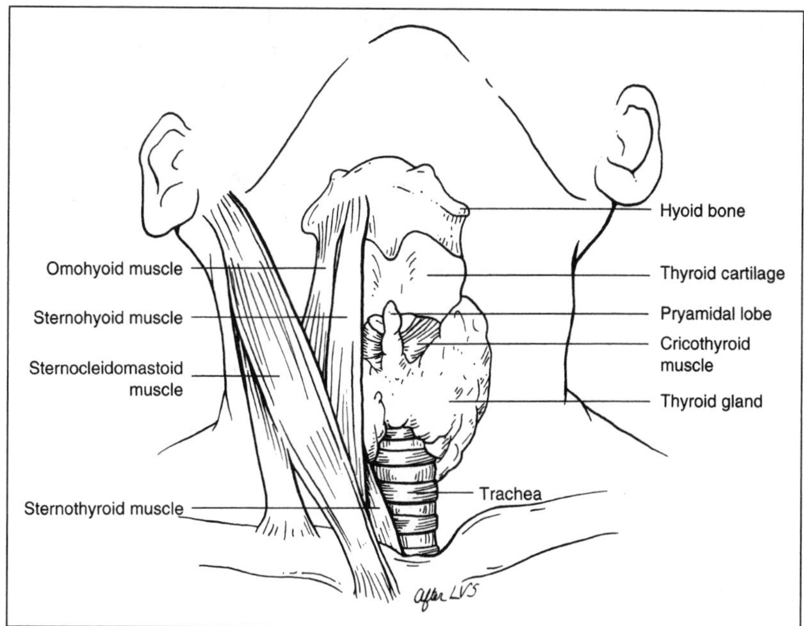

Figure 4.3. Gross anatomy of the neck and thyroid gland. (Adapted from Greenspan FS, ed. Basic and Clinical Endocrinology. 3rd ed. Norwalk, Conn: Appleton & Lange; 1991:189, with permission.)

How can that happen?

With an experienced thyroid surgeon and the use of magnification (loupes), this complication is infrequent. The nerve is most vulnerable at the level of the two upper tracheal rings, where the middle portion of the thyroid lobe is attached to the tracheal cartilage by the suspensory ligament of Berry. The nerve is usually posterior to this ligament; however, variations in position occur and the nerve may be displaced by the thyroid mass.

What happens if the recurrent laryngeal nerve is injured?

The recurrent laryngeal nerve is motor to all the muscles of the larynx except the cricothyroid. Therefore, injury results in vocal cord paralysis, and the affected vocal cord assumes a paramedian position. In most cases, nerve injury is an indirect result of adjacent dissection leading to neuropraxia or axonotmesis and function returns within a few days to 3 months. Division of the nerve (neurotmesis) results in permanent loss of function and repair attempts have a very poor track record. Unilateral injury causes various levels of hoarseness. Bilateral nerve injury may lead to the inability to protect the airway and usually the need for a tracheostomy.

What other nerves may be injured during thyroidectomy?

The external branch of the superior laryngeal nerve may be damaged during the mobilization of the superior pole of the thyroid. This is the motor nerve of the inferior pharyngeal constrictor and cricothyroid muscles, and injury is manifested by limitation of the force of voice projection and lowering of the pitch. This function usually improves during the first 3 months after thyroidectomy but may persist if the nerve is divided.

What other complications may occur?

Hypoparathyroidism and hemorrhage.

What are the signs and symptoms of hypoparathyroidism, and how would you treat it?

The parathyroids are very delicate and despite meticulous dissection, clinically significant hypoparathyroidism after thyroid resection is usually a temporary problem. The signs and symptoms of hypoparathyroidism occur within the first few days after surgery. The early symptoms are perioral numbness, tingling of the fingers, and in extreme cases, carpopedal spasm. The threshold of muscular excitability is lowered, and involuntary spasms occur. The following are classic signs of hypo-parathyroidism:

- *Chvostek's sign:* ipsilateral facial muscles contract when the facial nerve is tapped against the bone just anterior to the ear.
- *Trousseau's sign:* carpal spasm occurs after the brachial artery is occluded for 3 minutes with an inflated sphygmomanometer cuff.
- *Spontaneous carpopedal spasm:* hands and feet contract spontaneously. This is called *tetany.*

The calcium level is measured postoperatively in any patient undergoing total thyroidectomy. It is probably unnecessary to perform this study when only one side has been explored. If the patient is symptomatic or if the calcium level falls to less than 7.5 to 8 mg/dL, oral calcium replacements are given (500 mg of elemental calcium in the form of 1250 mg of calcium carbonate (Os-Cal) or 600 mg. of calcium as 1500 mg. of calcium citrate (Caltrate) every 6 hours). Most postoperative hypoparathyroidism resolves over the first few days or weeks. If the hypocalcemia is unresponsive to oral calcium supplementation, oral vitamin D (calcitriol 0.25 to 0.5 μg daily) may be given.

How is postoperative hemorrhage managed?

This potentially serious complication is fortunately uncommon. Accumulation of blood or formation of a clot in the closed space around the trachea can lead to airway constriction. The treatment is to open the wound and evacuate the clot at the bedside and obtain hemostasis in the operating room. Tracheostomy is contraindicated if the clot is evacuated. If airway control is needed, the patient can be intubated orally.

After the thyroidectomy, Ms. Arnold's voice appears to be unchanged from the preoperative period, and she has no complications. She is discharged from the hospital.

What is the prognosis for the different types of thyroid cancers?

Several prognostic scoring systems have been developed for well-differentiated thyroid cancer. Two such systems are the AGES system (*a*ge of patient; *g*rade, *e*xtent, and *s*ize of tumor) (11) and the AMES system (*a*ge, *m*etastatic disease, and *e*xtent and *s*ize of tumor) (12). Papillary carcinoma has the most favorable prognosis, with approximately 95% survival at 10 and 20 years. The prognosis for follicular and medullary carcinomas is less favorable, with 80% of patients surviving at 10 years and 71% at 20 years (13). Anaplastic carcinomas have a poor prognosis: fewer than 10% of patients survive 1 year (14).

What is the recommended follow-up for the different types of carcinomas?

The follow-up for well-differentiated carcinomas consists of physical examination, thyroglobulin measurements, ultrasonography, chest radiography, and ^{131}I nuclear scanning. For patients with medullary carcinoma, the follow-up is similar, but it also includes calcitonin measurement and molecular analysis of the *Ret* protooncogene. This is important for family members for evaluation of familial carcinoma.

Ms. Arnold is prescribed L-thyroxine supplements. At the first postoperative clinic visit, her wound appears to be well healed, and she reports feeling well.

Barbara Morin has had a thyroid nodule for a few years and has been referred by her primary care physician. She has been told that the nodule is not cancer.

What are the common causes of thyroid nodules besides carcinoma?

Other causes are multinodular goiter or follicular hyperplasia, Hashimoto's disease (lymphocytic thyroiditis), and follicular adenoma.

What does *goiter* mean, and what causes it?

Goiter is benign enlargement of the thyroid gland. The term is derived from the Latin *guttur*, which means throat. The pathogenesis of multinodular goiter in most cases is unknown; the involvement of growth factors is being investigated (15). TSH clearly plays a role in iodine deficiency states, but iodine deficiency is rare in the United States today.

What are the clinicopathologic manifestations of goiter, and what is the recommended therapy?

The thyroid gland may have nodules of variable size and number or be smooth and diffusely enlarged. Patients with goiter may be asymptomatic, although they more commonly complain of a neck mass or an increase in neck size, sometimes with pressure symptoms. On physical examination there will usually be a palpable mass that moves on swallowing. If the goiter extends retrosternally, the patient's face becomes suffused with blood when the arms are raised above the head because the goitrous mass obstructs venous return from the head (Pemberton's sign). Thyrotoxicosis can also develop in patients with a long-standing history of multinodular goiter (toxic multinodular goiter).

A multinodular goiter that produces no symptoms may not require treatment. Indications for surgery are pressure, cosmetic deformity, persistent growth of the goiter, and a nodule suspicious for cancer.

What is Hashimoto's thyroiditis?

Hashimoto's thyroiditis, or chronic lymphocytic thyroiditis, is the most common form of chronic thyroiditis. It is an autoimmune disease in which antibodies to thyroglobulin are formed. The thyroid may be diffusely enlarged and firm or it may be reduced in size or even difficult to palpate at all. The presence of nodules may cause this condition to be confused with a multinodular goiter or carcinoma. Hashimoto's thyroiditis is seen predominantly in women, with a mean age of 50 years. Common complaints are neck enlargement and associated pain and tenderness. Most patients are euthyroid or, most commonly, hypothyroid. Occasionally, Hashimoto's thyroiditis can result in hyperthyroidism.

A high serum titer of thyroid antibodies is diagnostic of this disease. Needle aspiration and cytologic examination may be indicated to rule out carcinoma.

The treatment of Hashimoto's disease depends on severity. In some patients, no therapy is indicated, whereas other patients require thyroid replacement therapy to relieve hypothyroidism. Surgery is indicated for pressure, for suspected carcinoma, and for cosmetic reasons. After surgery, most patients will need to take replacement doses of thyroid hormone.

What are the other types of thyroiditis and how do they differ from Hashimoto's disease?

Following are the other types of thyroiditis.

Acute suppurative thyroiditis, the rarest form of thyroiditis, usually occurs after an acute upper respiratory tract infection. Clinical manifestations include sudden severe pain around the thyroid gland, dysphagia, fever, and chills. Treatment includes antibiotics and drainage of the abscess.

de Quervain's disease (subacute thyroiditis) is not thought to be autoimmune. Sudden onset of thyroid pain and swelling is a common presenting feature. The erythrocyte sedimentation rate is elevated. A brief course of steroids may relieve symptoms, and spontaneous recovery is common. Surgery is not indicated.

Riedel's struma (chronic thyroiditis) is a rare condition in which patients have profound hypothyroidism that is usually irreversible. The thyroid gland is so hard that an open biopsy must be performed to distinguish this lesion from thyroid carcinoma. Patients with chronic thyroiditis have lower titers of circulating autoantibodies than those with Hashimoto's disease. Thyroid hormone replacement therapy relieves the hypothyroidism but does not affect the disease.

What is toxic multinodular goiter and how does it differ from Graves' disease or a solitary toxic nodule?

Patients with long-standing nontoxic multinodular goiter may develop hyperthyroidism because one or more of the nodules develop autonomous hyperfunction. This form of hyperthyroidism, known as Plummer's disease, is usually not as severe as Graves' disease. Antithyroid drugs offer no long-term benefit because the disease is relatively resistant to these drugs. Similarly, radioiodine ablation is inefficient in destroying hyperactive thyroid tissue, and recurrence is more common than with Graves' disease because of the intrinsic autonomy of the thyroid tissue (16,17). Many patients have prominent thyroid masses and resulting compression; therefore, the preferred treatment for patients who are otherwise well is total or subtotal thyroidectomy after the patient has been rendered euthyroid with propylthiouracil or methimazole.

What is Graves' disease and how is it treated?

Graves' disease, or toxic diffuse goiter, is a systemic autoimmune disease caused by immunoglobulin (IgG) antibodies to the TSH receptor. These antibodies bind the hormone receptor and stimulate the thyroid gland. Graves' disease affects women six to seven times as commonly as men. Both Graves' disease and Hashimoto's thyroiditis have a high familial incidence. The thyroid gland in these patients is symmetrically and diffusely enlarged. The cardinal signs of Graves' disease are thyroid enlargement, exophthalmos, tachycardia, and tremor. Common symptoms include heat intolerance and weight loss. Eye signs, mild in most patients, include (a) upper lid spasm with retraction, (b) external ophthalmoplegia, (c) exophthalmos with proptosis, (d) supraorbital and infraorbital edema, and (e) conjunctive congestion and edema.

Treatment options include antithyroid drugs, radioactive iodine, or thyroid resection. Commonly used drugs include methimazole and propylthiouracil. These drugs block synthesis of thyroid hormone by inhibiting iodide organification and iodotyrosine coupling (Fig. 4.1). In addition, propylthiouracil inhibits peripheral conversion of T_4 to T_3 by blocking the action of the 5′ deiodinase enzyme. The normal metabolic rate is restored within 6 weeks of treatment. After drug withdrawal, hyperthyroidism recurs in about 25% to 40% of patients. The advantages of radioactive iodine therapy are that remission occurs in 80% to 98% of patients, surgery with its potential for complications is avoided, and costs are reduced. Its disadvantages are that it takes longer to control the disease and the incidence of permanent hypothyroidism is high, up to 90% at 10 years. Radioiodine therapy is contraindicated in pregnant or lactating women.

When is surgical treatment indicated for Graves' disease?

Subtotal or total thyroidectomy is indicated in young adults with severe disease and large goiters, in patients who are refractory to medical therapy or whose symptoms recur, in patients who desire a rapid response, in patients who do not wish the radiation exposure risks (e.g., patients who have frequent contact with young children), and in patients for whom radioiodine is contraindicated. The thyrotoxic state is corrected in more than 95% of patients. Total thyroidectomy has been advocated by some surgeons because (a) it is safe when performed by an experienced surgeon, (b) there is almost no recurrence of hyperthyroidism, and (c) the exophthalmos and other eye signs resolve more completely. Pretibial myxedema, which is seen in a few patients, also responds best to total surgical thyroid ablation (18).

What is the preoperative treatment?

Patients with active Graves' disease and those with toxic multinodular goiter require preoperative treatment to avoid thyroid storm (discussed next) and to shrink the thyroid gland. Antithyroid drugs establish a euthyroid state. Iodine is administered 8 to 10 days before surgery to decrease the vascularity of the thyroid gland. These large doses of iodine cause a dramatic but short-lived decrease in iodine organification (the Wolff-Chaikoff effect). Administering beta-adrenergic blockers adds to the safety of this procedure. Propranolol decreases the pulse rate of patients with thyrotoxicosis. Many patients are treated preoperatively with a combination of propylthiouracil, iodine, and propranolol.

What is thyroid storm?

Thyroid storm is an acute adrenergic outburst that is augmented by the presence of thyroid hormone and that manifests clinically as hyperthermia, tachycardia, hypertension, and eventual hypotension and death. Thyroid storm was a frequent and life-threatening condition before preoperative control of thyrotoxicosis was possible. Today, thyroid storm is rare, but it still occurs spontaneously in patients with unrecognized hyperthyroidism. Treatment is directed at inhibiting the production of thyroid hormone and at antagonizing its effects. Large doses of propranolol are beneficial in reducing the tachycardia. Intravenous (IV) iodine is given in addition to steroids because of the danger of adrenal insufficiency. Oxygen and IV glucose should be given to treat the hypermetabolic state, and a hypothermia blanket may be used. This complication has a 10% mortality rate.

What is the management of a patient with a thyroid nodule who complains of heat intolerance and tremor?

Heat intolerance and tremor suggest that the patient may be thyrotoxic with an autonomous nodule. Under these circumstances, FNA should not be performed until thyroid function is studied. Determine T_3, T_4, and TSH levels, and perform a thyroid scan. Although the nodule is the most likely source of hyperfunction, it is essential to rule out a cold nodule in an otherwise hyperfunctioning gland. Such a nodule is suspect for malignancy, whereas hot nodules are rarely malignant.

Ms. Morin's laboratory report indicates that she has elevated T_3 and T_4 levels and a low TSH level. A ^{99m}Tc scan shows a single hyperfunctioning nodule.

What is the recommended treatment?

There are two steps to management. The first is to achieve a euthyroid state with methimazole or propylthiouracil. After the patient is euthyroid, either a thyroid lobectomy or radioiodine ablation can be performed. Generally, surgical resection is preferred because many nodules persist after radioiodine ablation (17).

PARATHYROID DISEASE

Mary Knowles is a 55-year-old woman with a long history of hypertension and recurrent nephrolithiasis who has had progressive fatigue and muscular weakness over the past 3 months. She is otherwise in good health and does not have weight loss, night sweats, or other constitutional complaints. She is taking clonidine for hypertension. The family history and physical examination are unremarkable, and she has no history of neck irradiation. She is afebrile and her vital signs are stable. The results of the blood chemistry screen are within normal limits except that the serum calcium level is 12.8 mg per dL and the serum phosphate level is 2.2 mg per dL.

What is the differential diagnosis for hypercalcemia in this patient?

The most common causes of hypercalcemia are primary HPT and malignancy, which account for more than 90% of cases. Medications, most commonly thiazides, lithium, excess intake of vitamin D, or vitamin A intoxication may cause hypercalcemia. Endogenous causes such as granulomatous disorders (sarcoidosis, berylliosis, tuberculosis, coccidioidomycosis, and histoplasmosis) and endocrine disorders (hyperthyroidism, adrenal insufficiency, and familial hypocalciuric hypercalcemia), immobilization, and Paget's disease may also lead to hypercalcemia (19,20).

Which tests help develop the diagnosis?

If exogenous causes are excluded, primary HPT is the most likely diagnosis because of the patient's history of symptomatic hypercalcemia in the absence of weight loss or other systemic symptoms that suggest malignancy. Confirm hypercalcemia first. In sick patients, it is important to correct serum calcium values for variations in serum albumin:

$$\text{Adjusted } Ca^{2+} = (\text{serum } Ca^{2+}) + 0.8 \times [4 - (\text{serum albumin})]$$

However, in most patients it is unnecessary to measure the serum albumin. The level of ionized calcium can clarify any ambiguity. The serum phosphate level, which is less than 3 mg per dL in primary HPT, should also be determined. In a hypertensive patient, urinary catecholamine metabolites must be evaluated to rule out pheochromocytoma. Other laboratory findings include a serum chloride level less than 102 mEq per L, serum chloride-phosphate ratio less than 33, elevated serum alkaline phosphatase, elevated urinary calcium, and elevated urinary cyclic adenosine monophosphate.

The next step is to obtain an intact parathyroid hormone (PTH) assay and a 24-hour urinary calcium measurement. An understanding of PTH physiology and the availability of the intact assay have made much of the extensive workup performed in the past unnecessary.

What is the function of PTH, and how does its measurement help diagnosis?

PTH is an 84–amino acid peptide secreted only by the parathyroid glands. In the circulation, the intact hormone (half-life, less than 3 minutes) is rapidly cleaved into the active aminoterminal fragment containing amino acids 1 to 34 (short half-life) and an inactive carboxyterminal fragment (long half-life, about 20 hours) and cleared by the liver. Assays for the carboxyterminal, midregion, and aminoterminal fragments are available, but the assay for intact hormone (also known as the sandwich or two-site assay) is superior (21). This assay uses antibodies to PTH fragments 1 to 34 and 39 to 84. An elevated serum calcium level, together with increased intact PTH level and elevated 24-hour urinary calcium excretion, is diagnostic of primary HPT. The assay for intact PTH does not cross-react with PTH-related protein and thus effectively rules out malignancy as a cause of hypercalcemia.

Why is it important to measure 24-hour urinary calcium excretion?

It is important to measure urinary calcium excretion to rule out familial hypercalcemic hypocalciuria (FHH) (22). FHH is an autosomal dominant disease characterized by mildly elevated serum calcium, but unlike primary HPT, it is associated with decreased urinary calcium excretion. It is generally considered a disease not of the parathyroids but of renal calcium excretion. PTH levels may be low, normal, or high in FHH; when the value is high, an erroneous diagnosis of HPT may be suggested. The ratio of calcium clearance to creatinine clearance is less than 0.01.

What are the normal physiologic mechanisms for calcium and phosphate homeostasis?

PTH and vitamin D are the primary factors that regulate serum calcium and phosphate concentrations (23). PTH stimulates osteoclastic bone resorption, increases tubular reabsorption of calcium, retards renal tubular reabsorption of phosphate, and indirectly increases intestinal absorption of calcium by inducing renal hydroxylation of vitamin D. The action of PTH on the kidney occurs within seconds to minutes, whereas its effects on bone and gut take hours to days. PTH is synthesized in the chief cells of the parathyroid gland, and its release is controlled in a negative feedback loop by the calcium concentration.

Vitamin D is synthesized in the skin in response to sunlight and is also a dietary component. Two hydroxylations convert it to its active form. The first hydroxylation, in the liver, converts it to 25-hydroxyvitamin D. The second hydroxylation, which occurs in the kidney, produces the active form, 1,25-dihydroxyvitamin D, and it is directly stimulated by PTH and low calcium or phosphate concentrations. This active form increases intestinal absorption of calcium and phosphate, promotes mineralization of bone by calcium and phosphate, and enhances PTH-mediated mobilization of calcium and phosphate from bone. Along with its primary effect of increasing serum calcium levels, 1,25-dihydroxyvitamin D inhibits PTH secretion (24). Increased serum calcium or phosphate levels inhibit the renal hydroxylating enzyme.

What is the role of calcitonin in serum calcium homeostasis?

Calcitonin plays an important role in the maintenance of skeletal mass during periods of calcium stress such as growth spurts, pregnancy, and lactation. The increased demands for calcium during these periods may cause calcium to be depleted from the bony skeleton by osteoclastic bone resorption. Calcitonin inhibits this effect (25).

What is the pathophysiology of hypercalcemia associated with malignancy?

Hypercalcemia secondary to an underlying malignancy occurs (a) through bone resorption by primary or metastatic tumor cells in direct contact with bone (breast cancer, multiple myeloma, and other hematologic cancers) or (b) through osteoclastic activity of a circulating humoral factor secreted by tumors such as breast, renal, and ovarian cancers and squamous cell carcinoma of the lung. This factor, characterized in the late 1980s, is known as PTH-related protein (PTHrP) (26). PTHrP has extensive homology with the N-terminal portion of PTH, which accounts for the similarity of its action in producing humoral hypercalcemia of malignancy (HHM). The C-terminals of PTH and PTHrP differ considerably, however, so the assay for intact PTH does not detect PTHrP. In the past, serum assays of C-terminal PTH were unreliable in differentiating primary HPT from

HHM, necessitating an extensive workup. With the intact assay, patients with HHM are shown to have suppressed levels of PTH.

How is primary HPT differentiated from sarcoidosis and other causes of hypercalcemia?

Hypercalcemia in sarcoidosis is believed to result from increased production of vitamin D secondary to enhanced extrarenal production of 1,25-dihydroxy vitamin D in granulomata (27). Intact PTH levels are low in sarcoidosis as well as in other causes of hypercalcemia, such as Paget's disease, immobilization, excessive calcium intake, vitamin D intoxication, and thyrotoxicosis. Thiazides increase renal tubular absorption of calcium, and their use may be associated with increased levels of PTH. The diagnosis of primary HPT cannot therefore be made until thiazide treatment has been stopped and the patient has been restudied.

What is the relationship between symptomatic disease and serum calcium levels in patients with hypercalcemia?

Symptoms of hypercalcemia are related to the degree and duration of the hypercalcemia. With regard to symptoms caused by hypercalcemia alone, patients with serum calcium levels less than 11.5 mg per dL are rarely symptomatic, whereas patients with levels between 11.5 and 13 mg per dL may or may not display symptoms. Severe hypercalcemia (calcium level higher than 13 mg per dL) is almost always associated with symptoms, and the risk of severe organ damage is significant.

Appropriate laboratory tests, including the PTH level, are performed on Ms. Knowles, and the diagnosis of primary HPT is confirmed.

What are the principal symptoms of primary HPT?

More than half of patients diagnosed with primary HPT after routine serum chemistry screening are asymptomatic, in comparison with 18% of patients before the introduction of routine screening in the 1970s. Symptoms include nephrolithiasis; bone pain or fractures; gastrointestinal distress such as peptic ulcer, pancreatitis, or constipation; muscle pain, lethargy, or weakness; and delirium, depression, coma, or exacerbation of preexisting psychiatric disease (hence the mnemonic; "stones, bones, moans, groans and psych overtones").

What are typical radiologic findings in primary HPT?

Standard radiography of the middle and distal phalanges of the hand to show subperiosteal bone resorption and skull radiography to demonstrate the moth-eaten appearance of HPT are rarely done today because overt clinical bony disease is present in only about 10% of patients. Osteitis fibrosa cystica, which is characterized by resorption of bone, focal eroded areas, reactive fibrosis, cyst formation, and brown tumors, was once the major clinical manifestation of primary HPT but is now also uncommon. Bone densitometry, which is a much more sensitive indicator of bone disease such as osteoporosis, can guide decisions to operate on otherwise asymptomatic patients, especially women who are in or past menopause (28).

Ms. Knowles's radiologic workup is negative. She returns to the clinic for a discussion of possible surgery for primary HPT.

What are the indications for surgery in primary HPT?

Surgical intervention is indicated in all cases of symptomatic disease, except in patients for whom the operative risk is prohibitive. Indications include radiographic evidence of bone disease (including bone resorption, cysts, pathologic fractures, or osteoporosis demonstrated by bone densitometry), nephrolithiasis, decreased renal function, gastrointestinal complications (peptic ulcer disease or pancreatitis), neuromuscular disease, and acute hypercalcemic symptoms.

Should asymptomatic patients undergo surgery?

This is a hotly debated, highly controversial topic. Those who advocate surgery for cases of asymptomatic primary HPT recommend this course because (a) there are no defined criteria for early identification of patients whose disease will eventually become symptomatic, (b) patients often resist the prolonged and rather intensive follow-up required for nonoperative management, and (c) the cost of nonoperative monitoring is often higher than the cost of operation. In addition, some authors believe that if an appropriate history has been obtained, only 10% of patients are found to be truly asymptomatic (29). Surgery can be delayed in asymptomatic patients who express interest in nonoperative management and are willing to undergo the prolonged, regular follow-up to evaluate progress of the disease. The most persuasive argument for recommending surgery in this group of patients is that the risks and cost of long-term nonoperative therapy exceed the cost and potential morbidity of parathyroidectomy. The incidence of complications (e.g., hypertension, nephrolithiasis, impaired renal function, nephrocalcinosis) arising from nonoperative disease within 5 years of follow-up is considerably higher than the 25% originally reported (30). This debate continues unabated.

What are the embryologic and anatomic features of the parathyroid glands?

The upper parathyroid glands develop from the fourth branchial pouch and descend into the neck with the thyroid, remaining in close association with the upper portion of the thyroid lobes. Their blood supply is from either the superior or inferior thyroid artery depending on their location. The lower parathyroid glands arise from the third branchial pouch along with the thymus, and they descend with the thymus, usually coming to rest in the neck but on occasion continuing into the mediastinum. This long migration in embryologic life appears to account for the variable location of these glands. In approximately 50% of persons, these glands are found on the lateral or posterior surface of the lower pole of the thyroid gland. The inferior thyroid artery supplies blood. Ordinarily, there are four parathyroid glands that weigh, on average, 30 to 35 mg.

What are common ectopic locations of the parathyroid glands?

Parathyroid glands have been found as high as the carotid artery bifurcation and as low as the pericardium. The superior glands have the most constant position, behind the upper thyroid lobe or at the cricothyroid junction posteriorly in nearly 80% of cases. Most ectopic superior glands are within the surgical capsule of the upper pole of the thyroid. Roughly 1% of superior glands are in the retropharyngeal or retroesophageal region. Superior parathyroid adenomas have a tendency to migrate from the normal position into the posterior superior mediastinum.

The inferior parathyroid glands are more widely distributed than the superior glands. The most common location for these glands is the anterolateral or posterolateral surface of the lower thyroid gland (in 40% to 50% of cases). The majority of ectopic glands are found within the thymus, either in the lower neck within the thymic tongue or inside the mediastinal thymus (in 1% to 2% of cases). Approximately 15% of inferior glands reportedly lie lateral to the thyrothymic tract and the lower thyroid pole, and an additional 5% are intrathyroidal. In rare instances, the lower parathyroid gland is high in the neck lateral to the upper thyroid lobes or in proximity to the carotid sheath because of early developmental arrest. These glands are typically associated with a thymic remnant (Fig. 4.4).

What causes primary HPT, and what are its pathologic characteristics?

Single adenomas cause disease in approximately 80% to 85% of patients; 10% to 15% have multiglandular disease, either double adenomas or diffuse hyperplasia; and fewer than 1% have cancer. In most cases of primary HPT, the cause is unknown. A protooncogene and chromosomal mutations have been described in small subsets of patients, generally those who have inherited parathyroid abnormalities (31). As with hyperthyroidism, there is an association between irradiation of the head and neck and HPT. Patients who have been exposed to low-level radiation either for medical treatment or after a nuclear accident (e.g., the Chernobyl incident) are at increased risk.

What role do localization studies have in the preoperative assessment for parathyroid disease?

The localization techniques include scanning with ^{99m}Tc sestamibi or sestamibi alone. These agents are taken up rapidly by actively metabolizing mitochondria in both the thyroid and the parathyroid glands but are washed out more quickly from the thyroid. Ultrasonography may also be used, but studies such as computed

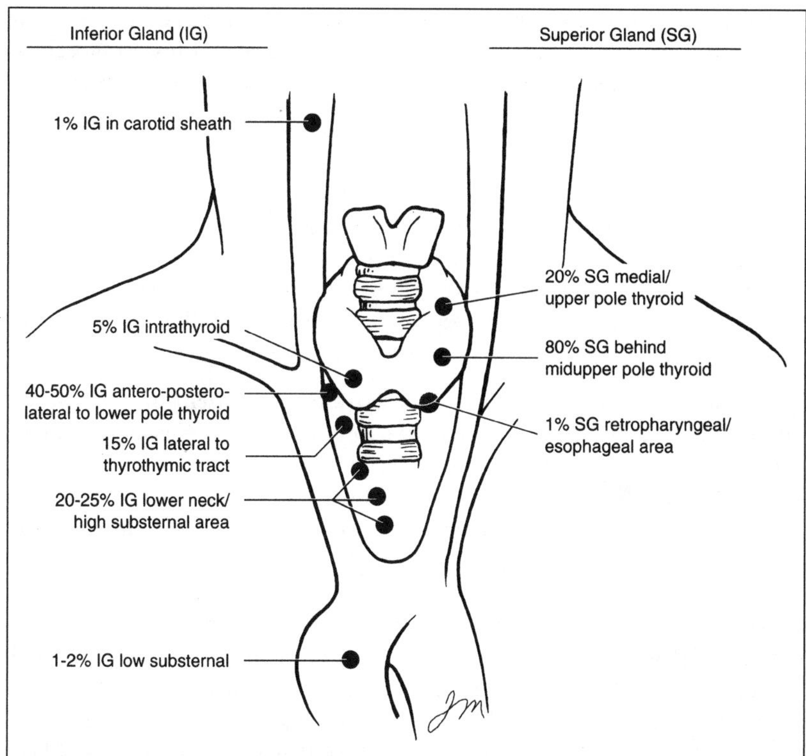

Figure 4.4. Possible locations and frequencies of the parathyroid gland.

tomography (CT), magnetic resonance imaging (MRI), and selective venous sampling for PTH are generally reserved for cases of recurrent or persistent HPT.

The need for preoperative localization studies has been questioned. Most surgeons believe that exploration of the neck by an experienced parathyroid surgeon (one who performs more than 12 parathyroid operations a year) can achieve a cure rate greater than 90%, which is better than the sensitivity of localization studies, and they therefore do not recommend preoperative localization (32). The arguments in favor of preoperative localization are that (a) a positive sestamibi scan in the neck virtually eliminates the possibility of an ectopic location for the parathyroid tissue and (b) the use of rapid intraoperative PTH assays (33) allows a limited exploration, which saves time and discomfort (34).

There is agreement, however, that preoperative localization studies should be performed in patients with persistent or recurrent HPT that has prompted reexploration. In these patients, an intensive effort is made to localize the glands because of the high incidence of ectopic tumors and because the increased scarring and loss of tissue planes from previous surgery make extensive dissection difficult. With preoperative localization, unnecessary dissection can be avoided, complications can be reduced, and surgical results can be improved.

The rapid intraoperative PTH assay is a chemoluminescent assay that takes 7 minutes to incubate. This technique requires preoperative localization. A PTH level is drawn preoperatively. Then, under local or general anesthesia, a 2- to 3-cm incision is made and the enlarged gland is identified and excised. A second PTH level is drawn 10 minutes after excision (five times the half-life of PTH, which is 2 minutes). If the PTH level falls by 50% and below 50 pg per mL (i.e., below normal levels), no further exploration is performed. The drop in PTH indicates excision of hyperplastic parathyroid tissue.

Ms. Knowles requires parathyroidectomy for treatment of her disease and gives her consent to proceed. Two operative strategies are possible: (a) the limited, minimally invasive exploration using the rapid intraoperative PTH assay or (b) exploration of both sides of the neck to identify all parathyroid glands before any resection is done. The right superior parathyroid gland is enlarged.

What is the appropriate treatment in patients with such findings?

Enlargement of only one gland with the others being normal is an indication of adenoma, which must be removed. Evaluation of the other glands will depend on the PTH assay. If the level falls appropriately, then no further exploration is necessary. If the level does not fall, the other three glands must be identified. Magnification allows confirmation of the normal glands and biopsy is not required (35). This reduces the rate of postoperative hypoparathyroidism. However, if the normalcy of the glands is in doubt, biopsy is essential. Sporadic cases, in which two glands are enlarged and the others appear normal, should be treated with removal of the enlarged glands and biopsy of the normal glands. Enlargement of four glands constitutes hyperplasia, and treatment consists of removing three glands and part of a fourth (subtotal parathyroidectomy); a well-vascularized remnant of roughly 50 mg of tissue should be retained. This remnant gland is pared to size before all remaining glands are excised to ensure that the remnant is not ischemic.

How is the distinction between parathyroid adenoma and hyperplasia made intraoperatively?

This differentiation, which is made by the surgeon, requires bilateral exploration and identification of all parathyroid glands under magnification. An effective procedure is to resect abnormal glands on the basis of macroscopic criteria, such as any gland that weighs more than 70 mg, which are considered the upper normal limit. Histologic examination is generally unreliable for differentiating parathyroid adenoma from hyperplasia or abnormal from normal parathyroid tissue. Pathologic examination is important for identifying parathyroid tissue and distinguishing it from thyroid or lymph node.

How are parathyroid glands that are in unusual locations identified?
A helpful procedure to localize parathyroid glands during a neck exploration is to locate the junction of the inferior thyroid artery and the recurrent laryngeal nerve. Most inferior parathyroid glands lie anterior and caudal to this point; most superior glands lie posterior and cephalad to it (Fig. 4.4).

When glands are not found in the usual sites, attention must be directed to known ectopic sites. If a lower parathyroid gland is missing, the ipsilateral thymus should be surgically delivered into the field, removed, and examined for the missing gland. Failure to identify the missing gland in the thymus should prompt exploration of the ipsilateral carotid sheath. If this, too, is negative, thyroid lobectomy is indicated on the side of the missing gland. The rationale for this is that 2% to 5% of inferior parathyroid glands lie in the lower third of the ipsilateral thyroid lobe.

If an upper gland is missing, the retroesophageal, retrocarotid, carotid sheath, and posterior mediastinal regions should be explored. It is important that the upper pole of the thyroid be fully mobilized; division of the superior thyroid vessels must be included if necessary because the upper parathyroids are frequently tucked behind the superior pole. If fewer than two superior glands are identified at this point, a posterolateral thyroidotomy or a partial or total thyroid lobectomy is indicated (36,37). Intraoperative ultrasonography may be used to determine whether an intrathyroidal nodule is a parathyroid gland.

What is the procedure if four normal glands are identified on exploration for primary HPT?
If four normal glands and no parathyroid tumor are found, the normal-appearing glands are biopsied and confirmed to be normal parathyroid glands. Their positions are marked with surgical clips. Although the supernumerary gland is usually in the mediastinum, explore all possible ectopic sites accessible through the neck. If a tumor still remains unidentified, it is unlikely to be in the neck, and the neck is closed.

Why is mediastinal exploration not the initial neck exploration if no abnormal parathyroid glands have been found in the neck?
There are several reasons to delay mediastinal exploration in this situation: (a) the neck dissection may have interrupted the blood supply of an ectopic parathyroid adenoma, rendering the patient normocalcemic; (b) a correctly performed neck exploration that shows negative results raises concern about the diagnosis and indicates the need for additional studies; (c) the actual site of an ectopic gland may not have been determined, and localization studies may be needed to

distinguish between a parathyroid gland high in the neck and a mediastinal gland; and (d) if the lesion is in the thorax, careful planning and use of minimally invasive technology may avoid a formal median sternotomy.

What is the incidence of normocalcemia after surgery for primary HPT?

The incidence of normocalcemia after an initial neck exploration performed by an experienced parathyroid surgeon is greater than 95%.

What are the major complications of surgery?

Major complications include hypoparathyroidism, recurrent laryngeal nerve injury, and persistent or recurrent HPT. Postoperative hemorrhage is rare (see How is postoperative hemorrhage managed?, earlier).

Ms. Knowles's single enlarged gland, an adenoma, is removed. Her immediate postoperative period is unremarkable. During morning rounds the next day, Ms. Knowles complains of numbness around her mouth and is found to have a positive Chvostek's sign.

What are Chvostek's and Trousseau's signs?

Chvostek's sign, an indicator of hypocalcemia, is a contraction of the facial muscles in response to tapping the facial nerve trunk in front of the ear. This sign results from the increased neuromuscular irritability induced by hypocalcemia. Chvostek's sign may be found in up to 10% of the normal population.

Another useful sign of hypocalcemia is *Trousseau's sign,* in which carpal spasm, an indication of latent tetany, is induced by occluding the brachial artery for 3 minutes with a blood pressure cuff. Trousseau's sign is caused by increased tetanic activity resulting from ischemia in patients with hypocalcemia.

What are the symptoms of hypocalcemia, and when are they likely to occur?

Circumoral numbness, apprehension with or without dyspnea, weakness, headaches, extremity paresthesia (tingling of the fingertips), muscle cramps, laryngeal stridor, and convulsions may occur in hypocalcemia. The drop in calcium level is variable. Although the lowest serum calcium levels are usually seen 24 to 48 hours after surgery, symptomatic hypocalcemia is fairly common within the first 12 to 18 hours.

What are the most common causes of hypocalcemia after surgery for parathyroid disease?

Hypocalcemia after surgery is usually caused by hungry bone syndrome or hypoparathyroidism resulting from operative trauma or underactivity of the suppressed remaining glands; it has a reported incidence of 13% to 30%. Other causes include hypomagnesemia, which may exaggerate hypocalcemia through impairment of PTH secretion and action on target tissues, and alkalosis, which can produce tetany even in the presence of a normal total blood calcium level by lowering the ionized calcium level.

What is hungry bone syndrome and how is it treated?

Hungry bone syndrome develops after parathyroidectomy as a result of extensive remineralization of the skeleton. It should be suspected in patients with known osteopenia on bone densitometry, in women who are in or past menopause, and in patients with long-standing disease (38). Postoperatively, as normal parathyroid function resumes, the calcium level should fall, and the phosphate level should increase. Hungry bone syndrome is suspected when the phosphate level fails to increase or falls even further. In addition, calcium levels in hungry bone syndrome tend to decrease faster and more dramatically. Calcium and phosphate levels are monitored closely beginning the evening of surgery, and calcium replacement is given as oral calcium supplements (500 mg of elemental calcium in the form of 1250 mg of calcium carbonate or 600 mg of calcium as 1500 mg of calcium citrate every 6 hours). IV calcium and vitamin D (given orally as calcitriol 0.25 μg daily) are not commonly required. Because most patients are discharged the day of or the day after surgery, outpatient follow-up must include close monitoring of calcium levels. In patients at risk, calcium replacement begins immediately after the operation without a wait for a decline in serum calcium levels.

What are other possible causes of hypoparathyroidism in the postoperative period?

Hypoparathyroidism can be caused by direct operative trauma, removal of all parathyroid tissue, transient vascular compromise of the remaining parathyroid tissue, or reduced secretion of PTH from atrophic parathyroid tissue (a result of long-term hypercalcemic suppression).

What is the treatment for hypoparathyroidism?

Hypoparathyroidism is treated if there are symptoms or signs of neuromuscular irritability (e.g., positive Chvostek's or Trousseau's signs) together with hypocalcemia; hypocalcemia alone is not treated unless the calcium level decreases to less than 8 mg per dL. The treatment is similar to that for hungry bone syndrome.

Ms. Knowles is found to have postoperative hypocalcemia, which is treated with oral calcium. With the increase of her serum calcium level, her perioral symptoms resolve. She is discharged home in satisfactory condition and scheduled for follow-up in the clinic a week later.

Do other features of HPT, such as kidney stones, high blood pressure, and neuromuscular symptoms, persist after surgery?

After surgery and normalization of urinary calcium excretion, formation of urinary calculi ceases in 91% of patients; however, deterioration of renal function and hypertension may persist. Psychiatric disturbances and neuromuscular problems caused by primary HPT are usually reversed. Parathyroidectomy does not reverse the diffuse osteopenia, but the rate of skeletal deterioration should be slowed or halted. Patients with osteopenia receive calcium replacements for life.

What is the role of medical therapy in primary HPT?

Although surgery is the mainstay of treatment in primary HPT, medical therapy is used in cases of life-threatening hypercalcemia (acute primary HPT) and in patients for whom surgery is unacceptably risky.

Management of acute primary hyperparathyroidism. Acute life-threatening hypercalcemia is a rare manifestation of HPT. Typical features include serum calcium levels higher than 14 mg/dL and CNS disorders (confusion, disorientation, coma), gastrointestinal problems (abdominal pain, anorexia, nausea, weight loss), and neuromuscular dysfunction (fatigue, muscle weakness). The precipitating cause is usually volume depletion or stress. Two thirds of these patients have diagnostic features of HPT (history of hypercalcemia, presence of nephrolithiasis or nephrocalcinosis, radiographically demonstrated bone disease) (39). Emergency treatment consists of volume repletion with IV saline followed by furosemide to promote a sodium, hence calcium, diuresis. Mithramycin, through its inhibition of osteoclastic activity, can often prevent further accelerated bone resorption. The large amounts of potassium and magnesium lost during HPT crisis must be replaced. Parathyroidectomy is typically performed after the patient has improved and the diagnosis is confirmed; however, urgent operative intervention is advocated by many surgeons in the absence of a prompt response to medical therapy by the patient (39).

Management of patients for whom surgery is unacceptably risky. The medical treatment of chronic hypercalcemia caused by primary HPT is much less effective than parathyroidectomy. Management includes walking to decrease mobilization of calcium from bone and judicious use of diuretics, as these may worsen a negative calcium balance. Other agents that inhibit or counteract the actions of PTH on bone or intestine include oral phosphate, estrogens for postmenopausal women, and selective estrogen receptor modulators (e.g., Evista) and bisphosphonates (e.g., Fosamax), which impair the function of osteoclasts. These treatments are sometimes used for patients with mild asymptomatic hypercalcemia and those with persistent or recurrent disease. To date, there is no effective long-term medical management of primary HPT. A new class of agents that affects the extracellular calcium-sensing receptor function of the parathyroid cells is being studied (40).

What preoperative findings suggest parathyroid carcinoma?

Parathyroid carcinomas are rare (incidence less than 0.5%), but any of these preoperative findings suggest that diagnosis: severe hypercalcemia (greater than 13 mg per dL), a markedly elevated PTH level (above 1000 pg per mL), a palpable cervical mass in a hypercalcemic patient (adenomas are almost never palpable), hypercalcemia associated with an unexplained unilateral vocal cord paralysis, or HPT recurring several months after an apparently successful parathyroidectomy.

What findings at surgery confirm this diagnosis?

The tumors are hard and surrounded by dense fibrous tissue, giving them a whitish appearance that is in marked contrast to the reddish-brown color of hyperactive glands in benign disease. A histologic diagnosis of parathyroid carcinoma is difficult, especially from a frozen section. The only findings diagnostic of malignancy are invasion of surrounding structures and lymph node metastases.

How does a diagnosis of malignancy alter surgical management?

En bloc resection is performed, with care being taken to maintain capsular integrity. Cure rates have been reported in more than 50% of patients with this technique. Penetration of the tumor capsule disseminates cancer cells and is likely to result in local implantation in the operative site. Radical neck dissection is performed only if clinically involved lymph nodes are present. Excision of recurrent or metastatic disease is attempted and is certainly indicated for control of severe hypercalcemia.

What are the most likely diagnoses in a young woman who has persistent asymptomatic hypercalcemia a year after subtotal parathyroidectomy and who has a family history of hypercalcemia?

After a diagnosis of FHH has been ruled out by repeat urine studies, the diagnoses of familial HPT and MEN syndromes are considered. Familial HPT is a rare disorder that appears to be autosomal dominant with incomplete penetrance (41). Unlike the MEN syndromes, this is a single disease without associated abnormalities. The clinical and laboratory presentations are identical to those of nonfamilial primary HPT. The incidence of multiglandular disease with chief cell hyperplasia is high.

What is the incidence of HPT in the MEN syndromes?

HPT is a significant element of the MEN-I and MEN-IIA syndromes, both of which are autosomal dominant disorders. The genetic abnormality in MEN-I is a tumor suppressor gene that encodes the protein menin and is located on the long arm of chromosome 11. The genetic abnormality responsible for MEN-IIA is located in the pericentromeric region of chromosome 10 and is known as the RET protooncogene. RET mutations enhance cellular growth. The MEN-I syndrome consists of HPT in 90% to 97% of those affected, pancreatic tumors in 30% to 80%, and pituitary tumors in 15% to 50%. The MEN-IIA syndrome consists of pheochromocytomas (commonly bilateral) or bilateral adrenal medullary hyperplasia in 50%, HPT in 10% to 25%, and medullary carcinoma of the thyroid or C-cell hyperplasia in 100%. HPT is rare in the MEN-IIB syndrome, which consists of medullary carcinoma, pheochromocytomas, marfanoid habitus, neuromas of the tongue or conjunctiva, and ganglioneuromas of the plexuses of Meissner and Auerbach. The HPT in these syndromes is typically caused by chief cell hyperplasia (42,43).

What are the appropriate screening tests for family members?

Initial screening for MEN-I includes measurement of serum calcium, whereas screening for MEN-II entails basal and stimulated calcitonin assays. Screening for MEN-II is particularly important because it allows diagnosis of medullary carcinoma at an early stage, when it is still curable.

How does a diagnosis of MEN syndrome affect treatment?

For treatment of the parathyroid component of these syndromes, a diagnosis of MEN-I alerts the surgeon to perform an adequate parathyroid resection when hyperplasia is present because of the increased risk (as high as 50%) of recurrent disease postoperatively. Some surgeons continue to perform subtotal parathyroidectomy in these patients; others recommend total parathyroidectomy with autotransplantation of the parathyroid remnant into the forearm. If graft-dependent hypercalcemia occurs, the transplanted tissue can be resected easily. In patients with MEN-IIA, attention is first directed to treatment of pheochromocytoma or adrenal hyperplasia and then to thyroidectomy. All four parathyroid glands are identified and samples taken for biopsy, with subsequent resection of enlarged glands only. When this principle is followed, recurrent disease is rare.

What leads to an unsuccessful initial parathyroid resection?

Some 2% to 5% of patients undergoing parathyroid explorations subsequently require reexploration for persistent HPT. The factors implicated include inexperience of the surgeon leading to inadequate exploration of the neck and superior mediastinum, abnormal parathyroid gland location, and underestimation of multiglandular disease.

What is the preoperative evaluation in patients being considered for parathyroid reoperation?

The preoperative evaluation should include reconfirmation of the biochemical diagnosis of HPT, exclusion of FHH and MEN as possible diagnoses, careful review of previous operative notes and pathologic specimens, and localization studies.

How are abnormal glands localized in patients with recurrent or persistent HPT?

Noninvasive studies include CT, ultrasonography, ^{99m}Tc sestamibi scintigraphy, and MRI. Although CT and MRI are best for imaging the mediastinum, ultrasonography is sensitive to lesions in the neck and is much cheaper. If noninvasive imaging is inadequate, invasive studies, such as intraarterial digital subtraction angiography, conventional selective angiography, parathyroid venous sampling, and intraoperative ultrasonography are conducted. These procedures have allowed localization in up to 95% of cases.

Are there alternatives to surgical reexploration in patients with recurrent or persistent HPT in whom a mediastinal adenoma has been localized by angiography?

An alternative to surgical reexploration is angiographic ablation of the adenoma with ionic contrast material. Ablation is feasible in approximately 70% of patients with mediastinal adenomas. Even if it is unsuccessful, this procedure does not preclude surgical resection (44).

What is the operative strategy for parathyroid reoperation?

Disease will be found on neck reexploration in 60% to 70% of patients. Thus, the neck is usually explored first at reoperation unless a mediastinal adenoma has been found preoperatively. In the latter instance, either a partial or a complete sternotomy is performed, and attention is first directed to the thymus and then to posterior dissection of the mediastinum. More recently, the exploration has been performed using thorascopic techniques. The same surgical procedures recommended for a thorough neck exploration at initial operation apply on reexploration with regard to locating ectopic adenomas or parathyroid tissue in the neck. When HPT recurs in patients who were thought to have had adequate resection after initial neck exploration, the parathyroid disease is treated as hyperplasia; subtotal parathyroidectomy or total parathyroidectomy with autotransplantation is performed. During reexploration of patients in whom only biopsy-proven normal glands were detected at initial operation, identification and removal of the abnormal gland without further attempts to identify normal glands is usually successful.

What is secondary HPT?

Secondary HPT, or reactive HPT of renal disease, a compensatory response to lowered serum calcium levels by the parathyroid glands, is the result of progressive loss of nephrons. Several interrelated factors promote it. Renal disease suppresses the addition of the second hydroxyl group to form active 1,25-dihydroxyvitamin D; it also leads to decreased phosphate excretion and hyperphosphatemia. As a result, calcium absorption from the gut is decreased and ionized calcium levels are lowered, which enhances production of PTH. This in turn leads to hyperplasia of parathyroid chief cells. The hypocalcemia is also fueled by a skeletal resistance to the action of PTH (45).

What are the major clinical manifestations of this disorder?

Clinical manifestations include bone pain and tenderness, especially in the pelvic girdle; pathologic fractures; proximal muscle weakness; severe pruritus;

gastrointestinal problems, including peptic ulcer disease, nausea, and vomiting; painful extraskeletal calcifications, especially in periarticular sites; and ischemic necrosis of various tissues caused by progressive vascular calcification (46).

What is the recommended treatment?

The initial goals of therapy are to prevent parathyroid hyperplasia and secondary HPT by controlling hyperphosphatemia and negative calcium balance. Hyperphosphatemia is treated by lowering phosphate intake and administering aluminum hydroxide or carbonate to minimize intestinal absorption of phosphorus. Calcium levels are enhanced by oral calcium supplements and calcitriol and by dialysis with solutions containing high concentrations of ionized calcium (3 to 3.5 mEq per L).

What are the indications for parathyroidectomy in secondary HPT?

Indications for parathyroidectomy include hypercalcemia, either spontaneous or appearing during treatment with small doses of vitamin D; progressive increase in serum PTH to more than 20 times normal levels; bone pain; skeletal complications; pruritus; and soft tissue calcifications. For maximum benefit, parathyroidectomy should be performed before renal osteodystrophy leads to extensive bone involvement. Four hyperplastic glands are usually found at surgery, and a total parathyroidectomy with autotransplantation of parathyroid tissue is recommended (47). However, some surgeons recommend total parathyroidectomy without transplantation, relying on the presence and function of additional parathyroid rests and oral calcium supplementation to control calcium levels (48).

What is the significance of aluminum intoxication in patients with chronic renal failure, and how is it treated?

Aluminum accumulation in patients with chronic renal failure impedes bone mineralization, with resultant osteomalacia, which may occur with bone pain, fractures, and proximal muscle weakness. This condition is easily confused with renal osteodystrophy from secondary HPT and should be ruled out before surgery. Desferrioxamine, an aluminum chelator, is used to treat aluminum intoxication.

What are the effects of renal transplantation on secondary HPT?

Hypercalcemia and the skeletal effects of secondary HPT may be diminished or even cured by renal transplantation.

What is tertiary HPT, and how is it treated?

Tertiary HPT is secondary HPT in which PTH secretion has become autonomous. Hypertrophied parathyroid tissue continues to secrete increased quantities of PTH despite hypercalcemia. The diagnosis is established by an elevated serum calcium level in a previously hypocalcemic patient with chronic renal failure and secondary HPT. The most pertinent example is persistent HPT after successful renal transplantation.

Management is conservative, and adequate time must be allowed for PTH levels to return to normal. Parathyroidectomy is reserved for patients with symptomatic disease and for those in whom severe asymptomatic hypercalcemia (serum calcium level higher than 12.5 mg per dL) persists for more than a year after the transplant (49). The workup and operative strategies are similar to primary hyperparathyroidism, although multigland disease is more common.

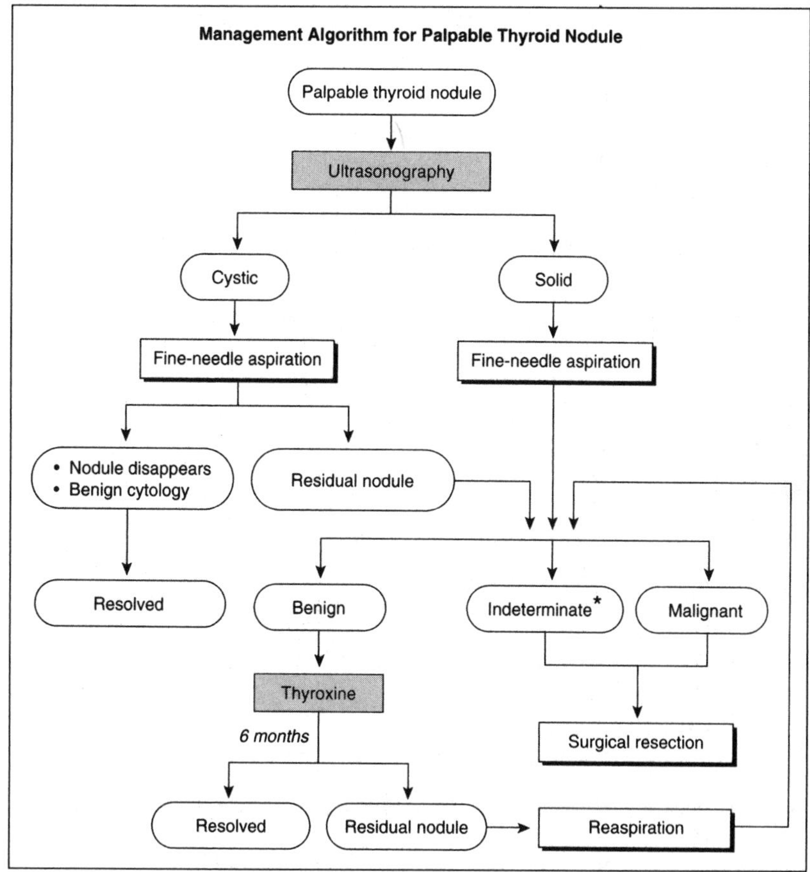

Algorithm 4.1. (Adapted from Doherty GM, Norton JA. Thyroid and parathyroid. In: Lawrence PF, ed. Essentials of General Surgery. 2nd ed. Baltimore, Md: Williams & Wilkins; 1992:299, with permission.)

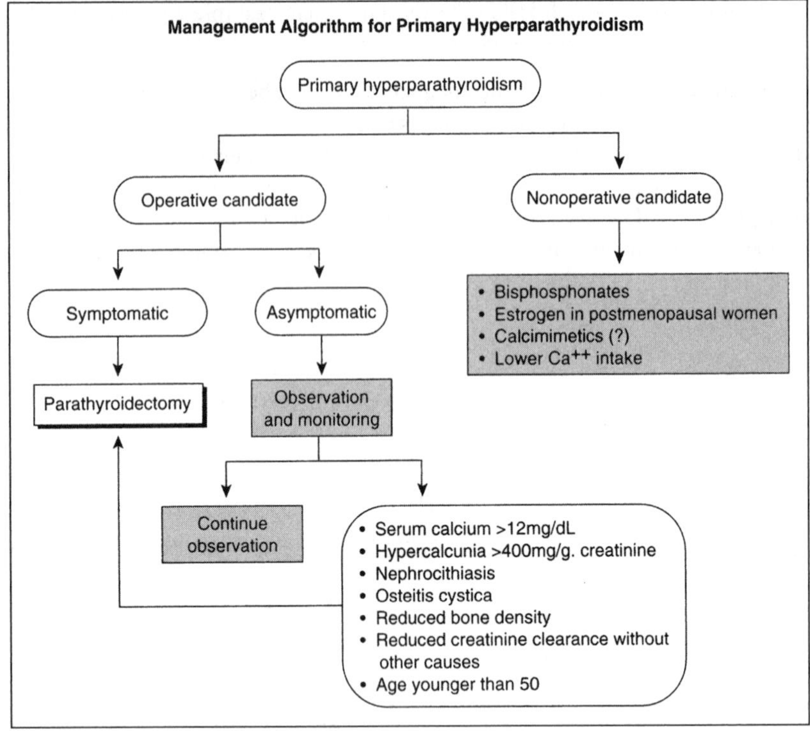

Algorithm 4.2.

REFERENCES

1. Frank R, Vander Velde TL, Doherty GM. Management of nodular thyroid disease and thyroid cancer associated with neck irradiation. Probl Gen Surg. 1997;14:27–33.
2. Gagel RF, Goepfert H, Callender DL, et al. Changing concepts in the pathogenesis and management of thyroid carcinoma. CA Cancer J Clin. 1996;46:261–283.
3. Cady B. Arguments against total thyroidectomy. Probl Gen Surg. 1997;14:44–51.
4. Clark OH, Levin K, Zeng QH, et al. Thyroid cancer: the case for total thyroidectomy. Eur J Cancer. 1988;24:305–313.
5. Mazzaferri EL, Jhiang SM. Long term impact of initial surgical and medical therapy on papillary and follicular thyroid cancer. Am J Med. 1994;97:418–428.
6. Schlumberger MJ. Papillary and follicular thyroid carcinoma. N Engl J Med. 1998;338:297–306.
7. Chen H, Nicol TL, Udelsman R. Follicular lesions of the thyroid: does frozen section alter operative management? Ann Surg. 1995;222:101–106.
8. Chen H, Nicol TL, Zeiger MA, et al. Hürthle cell neoplasms of the thyroid: are there factors predictive of malignancy? Ann Surg. 1998;27:542–546.

9. Soybel DI, Wells SA. Medullary thyroid carcinoma. In: Cady B, Rossi R, eds. Surgery of the Thyroid Glands. 3rd ed. Philadelphia, Pa: WB Saunders; 1991:152–178.
10. Clark OH, Duh QY. Thyroid cancer. In: Greer MA, ed. The Thyroid Gland. New York, NY: Raven Press; 1990:537–572.
11. Hay ID, Grant CS, Taylor WF, et al. Ipsilateral lobectomy versus bilateral lobar resection in papillary thyroid carcinoma: a retrospective analysis of surgical outcome using a novel prognostic system. Surgery. 1987;102:1088–1095.
12. Cady B, Rossi R. An expanded view of risk-group definition in differentiated thyroid carcinoma. Surgery. 1988;104:947–953.
13. Grant CS, Hay ID. Staging and prognosis in differentiated thyroid carcinoma. Probl Gen Surg. 1997;14:34–43.
14. Lee HK, Graham ML. Anaplastic thyroid cancer: diagnosis, prognosis and treatment. Probl Gen Surg. 1997;14:124–131.
15. Studer H, Gerber H. Non-toxic goiter. In: Greer MA, ed. The Thyroid Gland. New York, NY: Raven Press; 1990:391–404.
16. Orgiazzi JJ, Mornex R. In: Greer MA, ed. The Thyroid Gland. New York, NY: Raven Press; 1990:405–495.
17. Soh EY, Duh QY. Diagnosis and management of hot nodules (Plummer's disease). Probl Gen Surg. 1997;14:165–173.
18. Winsa B, Rastad J, Larrson E, et al. Total thyroidectomy in therapy-resistant Graves' disease. Surgery. 1994;116:1068–1075.
19. Bilezikian JP. Etiologies and therapy of hypercalcemia. Endocrinol Metab Clin North Am. 1989;18:389–413.
20. Chan FKW, Koberle LMC, Thys-Jacobs S, et al. Differential diagnosis, causes, and management of hypercalcemia. Curr Probl Surg. 1997;34:456–461.
21. Nussbaum SR, Potts JT. Advances in immunoassays for parathyroid hormone: clinical applications to skeletal disorders of bone and mineral metabolism. In: Bilezikian JP, Marcus R, Levine MA, eds. The Parathyroids. New York, NY: Raven Press; 1994:157–169.
22. Heath H III. Familial benign (hypocalciuric) hypercalcemia: a troublesome mimic of mild primary hyperparathyroidism. Endocrinol Metab Clin North Am. 1989;18:723–740.
23. Brown EM. Homeostatic mechanisms regulating extracellular and intracellular calcium metabolism. In: Bilezikian JP, Marcus R, Levine MA, eds. The Parathyroids. New York, NY: Raven Press; 1994:15–54.
24. Mallette LE. Regulation of blood calcium in humans. Endocrinol Metab Clin North Am. 1989;18:601–610.
25. Brunt LM, Halverson JD. The endocrine system. In: O'Leary JP, Capote LR, eds. The Physiologic Basis of Surgery. 2nd ed. Baltimore, MD: Williams & Wilkins; 1996:388.
26. Broadus AE, Mangin M, Ikeda K, et al. Humoral hypercalcemia of cancer: identification of a novel parathyroid hormone-like peptide. N Engl J Med. 1988;319:556.
27. Chan FKW, Koberle LMC, Thys-Jacobs S, et al. Differential diagnosis, causes, and management of hypercalcemia. Curr Probl Surg. 1997;34:489–492.

28. Silverberg SJ, Gartenberg F, Jacobs TP, et al. Longitudinal measurements of bone density and biochemical indices in untreated primary hyperparathyroidism. J Clin Endocrinol Metab. 1995;80:723–728.
29. Thomas JM, Cranston D, Knox AJ. Hyperparathyroidism: patterns of presentation, symptoms and response to operation. Ann R Coll Surg Engl. 1985;67:79–82.
30. Mowschenson PM, Silen W. Developments in hyperparathyroidism. Curr Opin Oncol. 1990;2:95–100.
31. Chan FKW, Koberle LMC, Thys-Jacobs S, et al. Differential diagnosis, causes, and management of hypercalcemia. Curr Probl Surg. 1997;34:462–464.
32. Kaplan EL, Yoshiro T, Salti G. Primary hyperparathyroidism in the 1990's. Ann Surg. 1992;215:300–317.
33. Irvin GL, Prudhomme DL, Deriso GT. A new, practical intraoperative parathyroid hormone assay. Am J Surg. 1994;219:574–581.
34. Sfakianakis GN, Irvin GL, Foss WM, et al. Efficient parathyroidectomy guided by SPECT-MIBI and hormonal measurements. J Nucl Med. 1996;37:798–804.
35. Oertli D, Richter M, Kraenzlin M, et al. Parathyroidectomy in primary hyperparathyroidism: preoperative localization and routine biopsy of unaltered glands are not necessary. Surgery. 1995;117:392–396.
36. Levin KE. The reasons for failure in parathyroid operations. Arch Surg. 1989;124:911–915.
37. Rossi RL, Cady B. Surgery of the parathyroid glands. In: Cady B, Rossi RL, eds. Surgery of the Thyroid and Parathyroid Glands. 3rd ed. Philadelphia: WB Saunders. 1991:283–294.
38. Brasier AR, Nussbaum SR. Hungry bone syndrome: clinical and biochemical predictors of its occurrence after parathyroid surgery. Am J Med. 1988;84: 654–660.
39. Fitzpatrick LA, Bilezikian JP. Acute primary hyperparathyroidism. Am J Med 1987;82:275–282.
40. Chan FKW, Koberle LMC, Thys-Jacobs S, et al. Differential diagnosis, causes, and management of hypercalcemia. Curr Probl Surg. 1997;34:477.
41. Goldsmith RE, Sizemore GW, Chen I, et al. Familial hyperparathyroidism: description of a large kindred with physiologic observations and a review of the literature. Ann Intern Med. 1976;84:36–43.
42. Metz DC, Jensen RT, Bale AE, et al. Multiple endocrine neoplasia type I. In: Bilezikian JP, Marcus R, Levine MA, eds. The Parathyroids. New York, NY: Raven Press; 1994:591–646.
43. Gagel R. Multiple endocrine neoplasia type II. In: Bilezikian JP, Marcus R, Levine MA, eds. The Parathyroids. New York, NY: Raven Press; 1994:681–698.
44. Miller DL, Doppmann JL, Chang R. Angiographic ablation of parathyroid adenomas: lessons from a 10-year experience. Radiology. 1987;165:601–607.
45. Martin KJ, Slatopolsky E. The parathyroids in renal disease. In: Bilezikian JP, Marcus R, Levine MA, eds. The Parathyroids. New York, NY: Raven Press; 1994:711–745.
46. Sitges-Serra A, Caralps-Riera A. Hyperparathyroidism associated with renal disease. Surg Clin North Am. 1987;67:359–377.

47. Romanus ME, Farndon R, Wells SA. Transplantation of the parathyroid glands. In: Johnston IDA, Thompson NW, eds. Endocrine Surgery. Stoneham, Mass: Butterworth; 1983:25–40.
48. Kaye M, D'Amour P, Henderson J. Elective total parathyroidectomy without autotransplant in end-stage renal disease. Kidney Int. 1989;35:1390–1399.
49. D'Alessandro AM, Melcer JS, Pirsch JD. Tertiary hyperparathyroidism after renal transplantation: operative indications. Surgery. 1989;106:1049–1056.

CHAPTER

GASTROESOPHAGEAL REFLUX DISEASE

Sophia Lee and Eric J. DeMaria

Andrew Grant is a 45-year-old man who has a 3-year history of heartburn that is particularly bothersome at night when he is in bed. The heartburn worsens when he bends over; antacids provide relief. Occasionally, he wakes up at night coughing and choking.

Mr. Grant's medical history is significant for hypertension and bronchial asthma, for which he takes calcium channel blockers and albuterol by inhaler, respectively. He smokes a pack of cigarettes and drinks 10 cups of coffee daily. He also admits to significant intermittent consumption of alcohol.

The physical examination reveals no problems; Mr. Grant is well developed and well nourished, his vital signs are within normal limits, and his chest, cardiovascular system, and abdomen appear to be normal. The rectal examination is normal and the stool is guaiac negative. The physician makes a provisional diagnosis of gastroesophageal reflux disease (GERD) on the basis of the history.

What is the prevalence of GERD in the United States?

GERD is a chronic illness that affects approximately 7% of the adult population daily in the United States. Although about 38% of the population has heartburn, only those with severe symptoms (approximately 10% of this group) seek the advice of their physician (1).

What are the clinical features of GERD?

The typical symptoms of GERD are heartburn and regurgitation. However, the absence of these symptoms does not exclude GERD. Conversely, only about a third of patients with typical symptoms have endoscopic evidence of GERD.

Atypical symptoms of GERD include substernal chest pain (approximately 50% of patients with noncardiac chest pain have reflux disease), hoarseness caused by reflux laryngitis, hiccups, asthma (34% to 89% of asthmatics have GERD) (2,3), ear pain, loss of dental enamel, night sweats, chronic coughing, globus sensation, hypersalivation, heartburn during intercourse (reflux dyspareunia), and dysphagia secondary to stricture.

What is the pathophysiology of GERD?

Gastroesophageal reflux to a certain extent is a normal continual phenomenon. Prolonged contact of the esophageal mucosa with gastric juice leads to pathologic conditions such as esophagitis and subsequently to stricture and metaplasia (Barrett's esophagus). Innate mechanisms protect the esophagus from abnormal reflux (4), and when these fail, signs and symptoms of GERD appear. These protective mechanisms can be described as esophageal, gastric, and duodenal.

Esophageal Factors

Lower esophageal sphincter mechanism. Dysfunction of the lower esophageal sphincter (LES) is the most important esophageal factor in the pathophysiology of reflux. Once the high-pressure zone of the lower esophageal sphincter is lost, reflux of gastric contents occurs. Many factors affect the LES and can precipitate reflux symptoms. The anatomic factors that are believed to contribute to the LES are mentioned later in this chapter.

Peristalsis. Another important factor is esophageal peristalsis. Primary peristalsis results from a swallowing reflex that propels the bolus of food down the esophagus and lowers the LES to allow the bolus passage into the stomach. Secondary peristaltic waves are initiated in the esophagus. These so-called stripping waves clear any refluxed material from the esophagus into the stomach.

Salivary bicarbonate. Swallowed salivary bicarbonate neutralizes gastric acid in the esophagus and thus protects the esophageal lining.

Esophageal mucosa. The esophageal mucosa has inherent defense mechanisms against the noxious gastric secretions. Bicarbonate in the unstirred water layer adjacent to the mucosa protects the mucosa from H^+ and pepsin. This mechanism is believed to play only a minor role in humans. Other protective mechanisms of the esophageal mucosa are intercellular tight junctions, epithelial transport (Na^+–H^+ exchange), epithelial buffers, and the lipid bilayer of the stratum corneum (3). Along with these factors, an adequate esophageal blood supply helps in cell replication, regeneration, and repair and in adequate nutrition of the epithelium.

Gastric Factors

Gastric distention. Gastric distention reduces the LES pressure and promotes reflux. Patients with Zollinger-Ellison syndrome are prone to reflux disease because of the increased gastric volume secondary to gastric hypersecretion.

Increased intraabdominal pressure. Obese patients and pregnant women have increased intraabdominal pressure, which raises the pressure gradient across the LES, causing reflux of gastric contents.

Duodenal Factors

Alkaline reflux. The alkaline reflux of biliary and pancreatic juices can injure the esophagus (4), a well-documented occurrence after resection of the LES following total gastrectomy.

A possible role for *Helicobacter pylori* in the pathogenesis of GERD has been suggested in number of studies. However, the link between GERD and *H. pylori* is complex and poorly defined.

What are the differential diagnoses?

GERD needs to be distinguished from gastritis, infectious esophagitis, pill esophagitis, peptic ulcer disease, non-ulcer dyspepsia, biliary tract disease, coronary artery disease, and esophageal motor disorders.

What investigations aid in the diagnosis of GERD?

The initial diagnosis is based largely on the history. Several tests can help in diagnosis and management of the disease.

Tests for Mucosal Injury

Esophagogastroduodenoscopy. Esophagogastroduodenoscopy (EGD) is usually the first test to be performed. It is useful for the detection of mucosal injury and for the surveillance of Barrett's metaplasia. Endoscopic appearance can be misleading, as biopsy of a "normal" mucosa may reveal florid inflammatory changes. Histology helps make the diagnosis of esophagitis and Barrett's metaplasia.

Barium esophagram. Reflux may be demonstrated with a barium esophagram even in normal persons. Reflux becomes pathologic when it is excessive, frequent, and associated with symptoms and signs of reflux disease. A barium esophagram reveals mucosal abnormalities, strictures, motility dysfunction, and a short esophagus. This allows surgery to be customized to the patient's needs.

Tests for Abnormal Reflux

The 24-hour pH monitor. One of the most specific and sensitive tests for GERD, pH monitoring quantifies the actual periods when acid is in contact with the esophageal mucosa. The pH electrode is positioned 5 cm above the manometrically defined upper limit of the LES. It allows the correlation of these exposures with the subjective feeling of heartburn. A normal 24-hour pH study virtually rules out reflux disease. Some new probes (e.g., Bilitec) also monitor any biliary contents in the esophagus.

Barium study. A barium study of the upper gastrointestinal (GI) tract can demonstrate reflux and the presence of hiatal hernia. Reflux itself is not considered pathologic because some degree of reflux is normal, as mentioned earlier. A barium study may also show evidence of mucosal injury, abnormalities of esophageal motility, and gastroparesis.

Test for Gastric Emptying

Gastroesophageal scintiscan. Delayed gastric emptying can be detected with this scan, in which a technetium 99 (^{99}Tc) sulfur colloid–labeled diet is used. About 5% of patients with reflux disease have poor gastric emptying. If these patients undergo antireflux surgery, the steep increase in intragastric pressure postoperatively can cause wrap disruption or gastric perforation. To prevent these complications, a pyloroplasty may be added to the fundoplication.

Test for Esophageal Motility

Esophageal manometry. This test is helpful in individualizing the surgery and to exclude major motor disorders. The LES pressure in patients with reflux disease is usually 6 mm Hg or less. Most patients, therefore, require a 360° wrap. A partial wrap is indicated if the LES pressure is high or if the esophageal motility is poor. Patients with a high LES pressure may still have abnormal reflux, and patients with a low LES pressure may have a normal esophagus.

Other Test

Bernstein's test. This test is useful to determine symptom correlation with esophageal acidification in patients without endoscopic evidence of esophagitis. Saline or 0.1N HCl at a rate of 6 to 8 mL per min is infused via a nasogastric tube into midesophagus.

What are the recommended changes to Mr. Grant's lifestyle?
The first step in the treatment of reflux disease is a change in lifestyle.

Diet. A diet low in fat, mint, chocolates, coffee, and alcohol improves the LES pressure and reduces reflux. Also avoid foods known to cause symptoms. Many beverages have a very acidic pH and can exacerbate symptoms, including colas, red wine, and orange juice (pH 2.5 to 3.5). Obese patients who lose weight by dieting may have less heartburn as a result of both better diet and decreased intraabdominal pressure.

Sleeping position and time. Patients are advised to raise the head end of the bed and sleep on their left side. Head of bed elevation is important for individuals with nocturnal or laryngeal symptoms. Gravity helps to clear the esophagus of the gastric refluxate and to decrease the symptoms of reflux. Patients are also advised to delay going to bed until 3 to 4 hours after the last meal to allow the stomach to empty.

Smoking. Smoking worsens reflux disease by decreasing the LES pressure and increasing the time taken for esophageal clearance.

Medications. Medications that decrease the LES (e.g., calcium channel blockers in the case of Mr. Grant) should be changed. Medications that worsen reflux are listed in Table 5.1.

Other factors. Tight clothes and exercise can aggravate the symptoms of reflux. Although stress does not directly cause GERD, it makes the patient more sensitive

TABLE 5.1.

FACTORS THAT AFFECT LES PRESSURE

Factors That Increase LES Pressure

Diet: Protein, coffee
Drugs: Cisapride, metoclopramide, bethanechol, norepinephrine, phenylephrine
Hormones: Gastrin, bombesin, motilin, substance P, L-encephalin
Other: Antireflux surgery, gastric alkalization

Factors That Decrease LES Pressure

Diet and lifestyle: Fatty diet, old age, exercise, chocolate, mint, alcohol, cigarettes
Drugs: Atropine, epinephrine, theophylline, nitroglycerin, prostaglandin F_2, oral contraceptives, diazepam, dopamine, meperidine, calcium channel blockers, barbiturates, prostaglandins E_1 and E_2
Hormones: Secretin, cholecystokinin, glucagon, somatostatin, neuropeptide Y, vasoactive intestinal peptide, and calcitonin gene–related peptide
Medical conditions: Diabetes, pregnancy, hiatal hernia, gastric acidification, hypothyroidism, amyloidosis, gastrectomy, placement of nasogastric tube

LES, lower esophageal sphincter.

to the symptoms of reflux and has therefore been historically associated with GERD. Promotion of salivation with either chewing gum or oral lozenges may help relieve mild heartburn because salivation neutralizes refluxed acid.

Mr. Grant tries conservative measures for a few months, but his symptoms do not improve.

Which single test is appropriate at this stage?

Upper GI endoscopy (or esophagogastroduodenoscopy [EGD]) is the initial test usually recommended for diagnosing the extent and severity of the disease. EGD also allows for concurrent biopsy and dilation (5).

EGD on Mr. Grant reveals inflammation in the lower portion of the esophagus and a small sliding hiatal hernia. No other abnormalities are noted. A biopsy is performed on the distal esophagus.

What are the histologic features of GERD?

Some 94% of the patients with significant GERD have histologic abnormalities; in 40% to 65% of patients, abnormalities are visible during endoscopy. The histologic features that correlate with reflux are the subject of considerable debate. Findings, even in carefully controlled experiments on animals, are inconsistent. These features are common in GERD:

1. Segmented leukocytes (neutrophils and eosinophils) infiltrating the mucosa
2. *Balloon cells:* enlarged, round squamous cells with a pale-staining cytoplasm and a degenerative nucleus caused by the pathologic swelling of the cell
3. *Epithelial hyperplasia:* basal cell zone thickness of the mucosa
4. *Papillomatosis:* elongated papillae of lamina propria extending to within a few epithelial cell layers of the mucosal surface
5. *Erosions:* denudation of the superficial layers of the mucosa
6. *Ulcers:* full-thickness destruction of the mucosa and muscularis mucosae
7. Distention and congestion of the microvasculature in the papilla of the lamina propria
8. Barrett's esophagus

What is a hiatal hernia, and what is its association with GERD?

Hiatal hernia is herniation of the stomach through the esophageal hiatus. There are three types of hiatal hernia:

Sliding hernia. The phrenoesophageal membrane becomes lax; the LES is pulled up in the thorax along with a portion of the stomach.

Paraesophageal hernia. The stomach herniates into the thorax, but the LES remains in its intraabdominal location.

Mixed hernia. The hiatal hernia is a combination of the sliding and para-esophageal types.

GERD and hiatal hernia are common conditions that may coexist in a patient. No evidence supports a cause-and-effect theory. Hiatal hernia can exacerbate reflux disease by two mechanisms. With the sliding hernia, the LES gets pulled up in the thorax; the LES pressure is thereby reduced and reflux increases. A hiatal hernia may also trap the gastric secretions that have refluxed into the esophagus and hinder their clearance, prolonging exposure to acid juices and worsening the esophageal injury.

Where is the esophagogastric junction?

The precise location of the esophagogastric junction is a matter of controversy. There are three opinions:

1. It is the junction of the squamous and columnar epithelium (Z line, or ora serrata). This opinion is not accepted by many because the last few centimeters of the esophagus may be normally lined with columnar epithelium.
2. It is the junction of the esophageal circular muscle layer and the oblique muscle fibers of the stomach known as the collar of Helvetius.
3. It is the site at which the tubular esophagus joins the gastric pouch.

What is the normal resting pressure of the LES? What anatomic features contribute to the sphincter mechanism?

The LES is more a physiologic than an anatomic entity. It is the name given to the distal 1 to 5 cm of the esophagus that acts as a high-pressure zone. The resting pressure of the LES is normally 10 to 20 mm Hg. In GERD, the resting pressure is usually less than 6 mm Hg.

Various anatomic factors may contribute to the sphincter mechanism of the LES:

1. Reflection of the phrenoesophageal membrane from the muscular margins of the diaphragmatic hiatus to the esophagus. This tethers the LES in the intraabdominal position.
2. Intraabdominal position of the LES. The transmission of positive intraabdominal pressure to the distal esophagus increases the LES pressure above the negative pressure of the intrathoracic esophagus.
3. The right crus of the diaphragm encircles the esophagus and on contraction may act as a pinchcock, closing the esophagus.
4. The acute angle of insertion of the esophagus into the stomach (angle of His) helps prevent reflux.
5. The oblique sling fibers of the muscle layer of the stomach at the gastroesophageal junction.
6. The rosette-like configuration of the gastric mucosa at the gastroesophageal junction helps prevent reflux.

What factors affect LES pressure?

The factors that affect LES pressure are listed in Table 5.1.

How is GERD managed medically?

GERD is a chronic disease, and most patients' symptoms can be controlled with medications. The objectives of treatment are relief of symptoms, avoidance of complications, healing of esophagitis, and ideally, healing of any mucosal metaplasia. However, the natural history of the disease does not change with medications, and symptoms recur after therapy is stopped. The following therapies may be used.

Lifestyle changes. These have been discussed in a previous section.

Antacid therapy. Antacids may provide short-term systematic relief, but they are ineffective for long-term therapy of GERD. Ingestion of large quantities of calcium-containing antacids may result in serum electrolyte abnormalities, such as the milk-alkali syndrome.

H_2 receptor blockers. When changes in lifestyle and antacid therapy are ineffective, H_2 receptor blockers are used. The H_2 receptor blockers offer a therapeutic gain of 10% to 24% relative to placebo for healing esophagitis (6). The commonly used ones are ranitidine (Zantac), cimetidine (Tagamet), nizatidine (Axid), and famotidine (Pepcid); famotidine is the most potent.

Proton pump inhibitors (H^+,K^+-ATPase inhibitors). These drugs are much more powerful than H_2 blockers with a therapeutic gain of 57% to 74% relative to placebo (6). One dose of inhibitor reduces gastric acid secretion by 90% in a normal person. Proton inhibitors lead to more rapid healing and symptom relief than H_2 receptor blockers. When H_2 blockers fail, omeprazole (Prilosec) is the drug most commonly used. Other proton pump inhibitors are lansoprazole (Prevacid) and pantoprazole.

Prokinetic agents. Other medications, such as prokinetic agents and sucralfate, may be added as adjunctive therapy to control GERD symptoms. Sucralfate provides a protective lining for the mucosa in an acid environment. It is used in the treatment of peptic ulcer disease and to prevent stress gastritis; however, its role in GERD is small. Cisapride (Propulsid) is available only on a severely restricted basis in the United States because of concerns related to cardiac arrhythmia (7). Others include metoclopramide (Reglan), domperidone (Motilium), bethanechol (Urecholine), and erythromycin.

The drugs may be combined for synergistic effect. When standard doses are ineffective, higher doses of these medications may be used. It is fairly common for patients with severe reflux symptoms to be treated with twice the normal doses of omeprazole, ranitidine, and sucralfate.

What are the side effects of H_2 blockers and H^+,K^+-ATPase inhibitors?

H_2 blockers are fairly safe. Common side effects include diarrhea, headache, fatigue, muscular pains, drowsiness, and constipation. Cimetidine and to a lesser extent ranitidine reversibly bind to oxidases of the cytochrome P450 system and inhibit hepatic metabolism of drugs such as phenytoin, warfarin, and theophylline, which raises the serum level of these medications. Other effects may include gynecomastia resulting from elevated serum prolactin levels and a reduction in procainamide secretion by the renal tubules, leading to higher serum levels.

Proton pump inhibitors are similarly well tolerated; common GI side effects are dyspepsia, nausea, vomiting, flatulence, and diarrhea. Headaches are less common, as is inhibition of P450 system of liver enzymes and attendant drug interactions. Reduction of acid secretion causes hypergastrinemia, atrophic gastritis, nitrosamine production, bacterial overgrowth, and enteric infections such as *Campylobacter* gastroenteritis, all of which may lead to gastric malignancy. Long-term administration of high doses of omeprazole to rats causes gastric carcinoid tumors; however, this has not been observed in humans. Long-term therapy with omeprazole has been associated with vitamin B_{12} malabsorption (8).

Mr. Grant is prescribed a 3-month course of high-dose omeprazole and metoclopramide. However, his symptoms persist after therapy, and he still wakes up with a choking sensation at night and has coughing spells. He now complains of dysphagia with solid food. Endoscopy is repeated; it reveals esophagitis and a stricture in the lower esophagus. The latter problem is corrected successfully by endoscopic dilation.

What is the pathophysiology of peptic stricture?

Strictures are a result of the healing process of ulcerative esophagitis. Collagen is deposited and, with time, the collagen fibers contract narrowing the esophageal lumen. The strictures are usually short in length and contiguous with the gastroesophageal junction.

What are the different types of esophageal dilators and what are their respective advantages and disadvantages?

Three types of esophageal dilators are commonly used:

Mercury-filled rubber bougie. Examples are the Hurst (round tip) and Maloney (tapered tip) types. These are easy to use but require repeated blind passages. The operator has a good feel for the resistance. These dilators are not useful in very tight or irregular strictures.

Guided, fixed-size dilator. Examples are Eder Puestow metal olives and Celestin, Savary Gilliard, Buess, and Keymed advanced dilators. They are passed over a guidewire and because of their relative stiffness they can negotiate tight and irregular strictures. The disadvantages include pharyngeal and dental injury; also, the operator does not have a good feel for resistance.

Balloon dilator. Various types of balloon dilators can traverse irregular strictures. They have the advantage of not causing any shearing damage because the force applied is radial, but the balloons are fragile and easily displaced.

Surgery is recommended to Mr. Grant at this stage.

What are the indications for surgery in GERD?
The indications for surgery are as follows:

- Failed medical therapy with persistent esophagitis or persistent symptoms
- Complications of GERD, such as Barrett's esophagus, stricture refractory to medical treatment, or bleeding from refractory esophagitis
- Healthy young patient who prefers surgery to lifelong medication
- Extraesophageal symptoms from reflux that are refractory to medical treatment

What are some antireflux procedures?
Antireflux procedures can be divided into these groups (9):

Partial Fundoplication

- *Belsey Mark IV:* thoracic approach, anterior 270° wrap, crural repair
- *Toupet:* abdominal approach, posterior 270° wrap, crural repair
- *D'or:* abdominal approach, anterior 270° wrap, crural repair
- *Hill:* abdominal approach, posterior wrap, anchor gastroesophageal junction to the median arcuate ligament

Total Fundoplication

- *Floppy Nissen:* abdominal approach, 360° wrap, crural repair
- *Rosetti Nissen:* same as floppy Nissen but no division of short gastric arteries

Antireflux Prosthesis

- *Angelchik prosthesis:* discredited because of problems of slippage, perforation, and stricture

Experimental Procedures

- Endoscopic injection of biopolymer in LES (e.g., Enteryx)
- Endoscopic injection of sodium morrhuate into gastric cardia

- Endoscopic gastroplasty/plication (e.g., Bard EndoCinch, Wilson-Cook endoscopic suturing device)
- *Stretta procedure:* radiofrequency treatment
- *Narbona sling procedure:* abdominal approach, mobilization of hepatic ligamentum teres, and formation of a sling around the gastroesophageal junction onto the anterior stomach

Common laparoscopic procedures used for reflux disease are the floppy Nissen and Toupet fundoplications with 85% to 95% success rate in relieving symptoms and healing esophagitis. Partial fundoplication is recommended in patients with poor esophageal motility.

What are the goals of surgery for reflux disease?

The primary goal of surgery is to reestablish the competency of the LES. These are the technical goals:

1. To place an adequate length (1.5 to 2 cm) of the distal esophagus in the positive pressure environment of the abdomen
2. To maintain or restore overall LES pressure to twice the resting gastric pressure (e.g., 12 mm Hg for a gastric pressure of 6 mm Hg)
3. To avoid too competent an LES by use of a 60-French bougie in the esophagus before wrap placement and use of a wrap no longer than 1.5 cm
4. To perform crural repair

A floppy Nissen procedure is performed laparoscopically on Mr. Grant. He is discharged home the day after surgery. Initially, he notices some dysphagia and inability to belch, but these problems improve with time. Heartburn and regurgitation decrease, and he does not have choking spells at night.

What are some complications of antireflux surgery?

The mortality from antireflux surgery is approximately 1%, and the morbidity after surgery approaches 10%.

Specific complications of antireflux surgery can be operative or postoperative. Operative complications specific to reflux surgery include splenic trauma leading to splenectomy and its attendant problems, perforated esophagus, and inadvertent vagotomy. The usual postoperative complications specific to reflux surgery are gas bloat syndrome, inability to vomit or belch, and dysphagia.

General complications of any surgery include atelectasis, pleural effusion, bleeding, wound infection, deep venous thrombosis, and pulmonary embolism.

Most of these complications specific to antireflux surgery are self-limited and diminish with time. Good results are evident in more than 90% of patients 10 years after a Nissen procedure (10).

What are some technical reasons for a failed surgical repair?

The following are some common reasons for surgical failure:

1. Partial or complete breakdown of the repair
2. Placement of the wrap around the stomach instead of around the esophagus
3. Overtight wrap (fails to mobilize the short gastric vessels) or overlong wrap
4. Herniation of the wrap into the chest
5. Necrosis or fistula in the lower esophagus
6. Inadvertent division of the vagus nerve

What are the complications of GERD?

Severe GERD can cause erosions, ulcerations, stricture, and metaplasia. The difference between an erosion and an ulcer is that an erosion is only a mucosal injury, whereas an ulcer is deeper. Ulcers can bleed, perforate, or cause strictures. Metaplasia (Barrett's esophagus) can lead to dysplasia and malignancy.

Other complications attributed to GERD are laryngitis, hoarseness, cough, bronchitis, asthma, pneumonitis, and hemoptysis. Apnea and sudden infant death syndrome have been associated with reflux disease in children.

What is the stepwise progression for diagnosis and management of GERD?

See Algorithm 5.1 for management of GERD.

What is Barrett's esophagus and why is it important? What are the usual histologic features?

Barrett's esophagus was first described in 1950 by Sir Norman Barrett of England. His initial hypothesis that this was a congenital condition with columnar cells lining the distal esophagus has largely been discarded. It is now considered to be acquired from long-standing reflux disease. Repeated and prolonged peptic acid and alkaline reflux damage the esophageal mucosa, which undergoes repair and regeneration. Barrett's esophagus is essentially a metaplasia of the damaged squamous epithelium of the esophagus to the columnar type, which has a propensity for dysplasia and neoplasia. Approximately 10% of patients with severe GERD have Barrett's disease (1), and 0.5% to 10% of patients with Barrett's esophagus eventually develop carcinoma. Even patients with easily controlled symptoms of reflux disease may have severe dysplasia accompanying Barrett's esophagus. Patients with Barrett's disease have a risk of malignancy that is 40 times higher than the general population. This translates into a sevenfold lifelong risk of developing adenocarcinoma. The risk is the same as that of a 55-year-old smoker developing lung cancer (6). The histologic features of Barrett's disease are usually subdivided into three distinct patterns:

1. *Specialized, or intestinal, type:* the most common variety, it is characterized by villous architecture, mucous glands, and goblet cells, features that are normally seen in the small bowel.

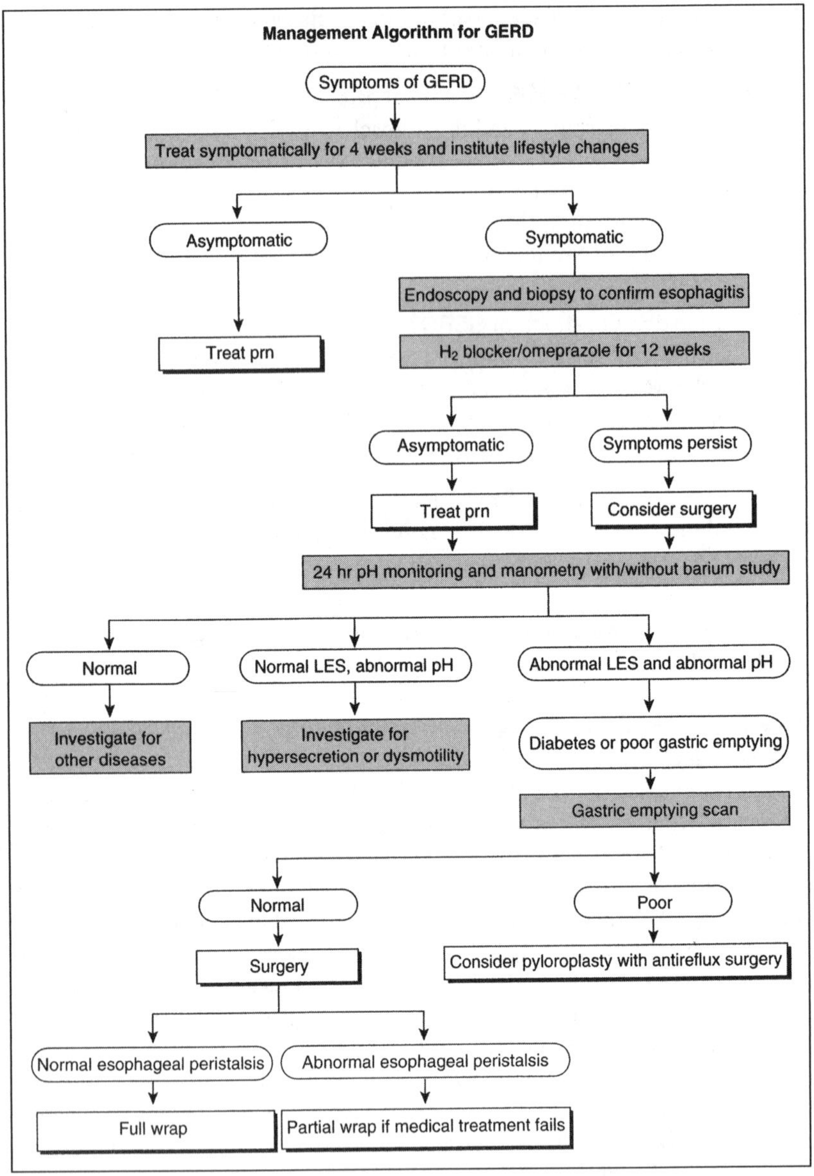

Management Algorithm for GERD

Symptoms of GERD
→ Treat symptomatically for 4 weeks and institute lifestyle changes
- Asymptomatic → Treat prn
- Symptomatic → Endoscopy and biopsy to confirm esophagitis → H_2 blocker/omeprazole for 12 weeks
  - Asymptomatic → Treat prn
  - Symptoms persist → Consider surgery

(Both) → 24 hr pH monitoring and manometry with/without barium study
- Normal → Investigate for other diseases
- Normal LES, abnormal pH → Investigate for hypersecretion or dysmotility
- Abnormal LES and abnormal pH → Diabetes or poor gastric emptying → Gastric emptying scan
  - Normal → Surgery
    - Normal esophageal peristalsis → Full wrap
    - Abnormal esophageal peristalsis → Partial wrap if medical treatment fails
  - Poor → Consider pyloroplasty with antireflux surgery

Algorithm 5.1.

2. *Junctional type:* this type has mucosa resembling the cardia of the stomach.
3. *Fundic type:* this type, in which the mucosa resembles the gastric fundus with parietal and chief cells, is the type associated with malignancy.

Coexistence of different types is usual.

How is Barrett's disease treated, and what are the results of surgery?

The treatment of Barrett's disease is controversial. Algorithm 5.2 shows management strategies. It is not clear whether nonoperative treatment prevents dysplasia or reduces the degree of dysplasia that may already be present. Similarly, although some literature suggests that surgery may cure a few patients with dysplastic Barrett's disease, the consensus is that antireflux surgery does not cure the condition, although it may delay or prevent the development of dysplasia.

How are esophageal motility disorders classified?

Esophageal motility disorders can be primary or secondary.

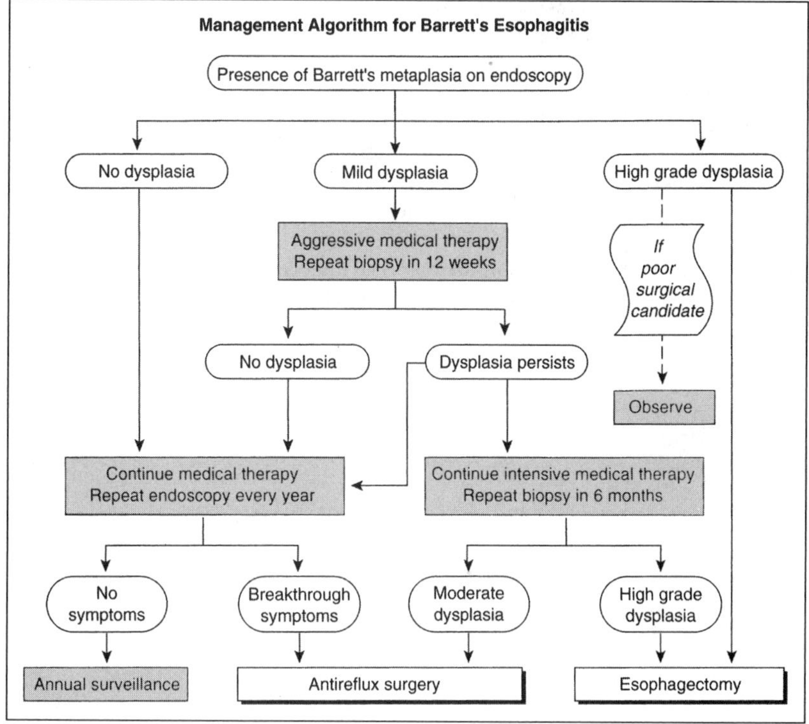

Algorithm 5.2.

Primary disorders include achalasia, diffuse and segmental esophageal spasm, nutcracker esophagus, hypertensive lower esophageal sphincter, and other nonspecific disorders.

Secondary disorders, which include systemic sclerosis, polymyositis, dermatomyositis, systemic lupus erythematosus, and mixed connective tissue disease, chronic idiopathic intestinal pseudo-obstruction, neuromuscular disorders, endocrine disorders, and metastatic disorders, are secondary to collagen disorders.

REFERENCES

1. Nebel OT, Fornes MF, Castell DO. Symptomatic gastro-esophageal reflux: incidence and precipitating factors. Am J Dig Dis. 1976;21:953–956.
2. Sontag SJ, O'Connell S, Khandelwal S. Most asthmatics have gastroesophageal reflux with or without bronchodilator therapy. Gastroenterology. 1990;99:613.
3. Harding SM, Richter JE, Guzzo MR. Asthma and gastroesophageal reflux: acid suppressive therapy improves asthma outcomes. Am J Med. 1996;100:395.
4. Cohen S. The pathogenesis of gastro-esophageal reflux disease: a challenge in clinical physiology. Ann Intern Med. 1992;117:1051–1052.
5. Orlando RC. Esophageal epithelial defenses against acid injury. Am J Gastroenterol. 1994;89:S48–S52.
6. Sontag SJ. The medical management of reflux esophagitis. Role of antacids and acid inhibition. Gastroenterol Clin North Am. 1990;19:683.
7. Wysowski DK, Bacsanyi J. Cisapride and fatal arrhythmia. N Engl J Med. 1996;149:2486.
8. Marcuard SP, Albernax L, Khazanie PG. Omeprazole therapy causes malabsorption of cyanocobalamin. Ann Intern Med. 1994;120:211.
9. Lillemoe KD, Johnson LF, Harmon JW. Alkaline esophagitis: a comparison of the ability of components of gastroduodenal contents to injure the rabbit esophagus. Gastroenterology. 1983;85:621–628.
10. Weinberg DS, Kadish SL. The diagnosis and management of gastroesophageal reflux disease. Med Clin North Am. 1996;80:411–429.

CHAPTER

6

ESOPHAGEAL CANCER

Sharline J. Zacur and Brian J. Kaplan

Mr. Gill is a 61-year-old African American man who was in good health until 3 months ago when he began experiencing difficulty swallowing. Initially, his dysphagia was limited to solid foods when he felt a piece of steak get stuck in his throat. During the past two weeks he has had progressive dysphagia to include difficulty swallowing liquids. Mr. Gill has no history of vomiting, odynophagia, cough, or hemoptysis, but he does report a 20-pound weight loss since the beginning of his symptoms. His past medical history includes poorly controlled hypertension and coronary artery disease. His surgical history is significant for a right inguinal hernia repair. His current medications include hydrochlorothiazide, aspirin, and enalapril. He has a 45-pack-year smoking history and currently smokes a pack a day. He reports social alcohol use.

On physical examination, his vital signs are as follows: pulse 86 beats per minute, blood pressure 152/80 mm Hg, respirations 14 breaths per minute, and temperature 98.3°F. Head and neck examination reveals poor dentition and no lymphadenopathy. He is anicteric and no carotid bruits are heard. His cardiovascular and respiratory examinations are unremarkable. Mr. Gill has normal bowel sounds with no abdominal tenderness or masses. Rectal examination is normal with negative occult blood in the stool. His neurologic examination is normal.

What is the differential diagnosis of dysphagia?

Dysphagia due to luminal narrowing may be a result of esophagitis, Schatzki ring, benign strictures, benign tumors, or malignant tumors. Patients with Plummer-Vinson syndrome have cervical dysphagia, secondary to a cervical esophageal web, and iron deficiency. Extrinsic compression of the esophagus may be caused by a Zenker's diverticulum, mediastinal masses, an enlarged thyroid, vertebral osteophytes, an aberrant right subclavian artery, a left atrial enlargement, an aortic aneurysm, or a right-sided aorta. Dysphagia resulting from esophageal dysmotility may be caused by muscle weakness, achalasia, diffuse esophageal spasm, or scleroderma.

What is the difference between mechanical and motor dysphagia?

Mechanical dysphagia may result from a large food bolus, intrinsic luminal narrowing, or extrinsic compression. *Motor dysphagia* occurs because of difficulty initiating swallowing, abnormal peristalsis, or disorders of the smooth and striated esophageal muscles.

What are the early and late manifestations of esophageal cancer?

The most common symptoms of esophageal cancer are dysphagia and weight loss.

Dysphagia with solid foods often progresses to include liquids, which indicates a luminal compromise of 60%. Dysphagia may be associated with odynophagia, emesis, aspiration pneumonia, malnutrition, and weight loss. Body weight loss of greater than 2% has been reported to have a significant decrease on 5-year survival (1). Advanced disease may manifest with tracheoesophageal fistulas, vocal cord paralysis secondary to recurrent laryngeal nerve involvement, and severe pain.

Mr. Gill was seen by his family physician, and the following laboratory tests were obtained: hemoglobin 13.2 g per dL (normal 12 to 15 g per dL), white blood count 8.4 (normal 4.3 to 10), sodium 138 mEq per L (normal 135 to 145 mEq per L), potassium 4.5 mEq per L (normal 3.5 to 5.0 per L), aspartate aminotransferase 10μ (normal 10 to 40μ), alanine aminotransferase 16μ (normal 10 to 40μ), alkaline phosphatase 37 IU (normal 21 to 91 IU), bilirubin 0.8 mg per dL (normal 0.3 to 1.0 mg per dL), and albumin 3.5 g per dL (normal 3.5 to 5.5 g per dL). A barium contrast examination revealed a mucosal irregularity with an annular lumen narrowing at the midesophageal level (Fig. 6.1).

What is the diagnostic evaluation of a patient suspected to have esophageal cancer?

The patient must undergo esophagoscopy with biopsy of the suspected tumor to confirm the diagnosis of esophageal carcinoma. Direct visualization can also determine location and length of the involved segment. Bronchoscopy can evaluate tracheobronchial invasion in a patient with a history suggestive of advanced disease. The patient may present with progressive pneumonia, chocking, coughing with feedings, or aspiration of bile-stained mucus from the airway. Nishimura et al. determined that the accuracy rate of diagnosing tracheobronchial invasion based on bronchoscopy was 78%; this rate was greater than

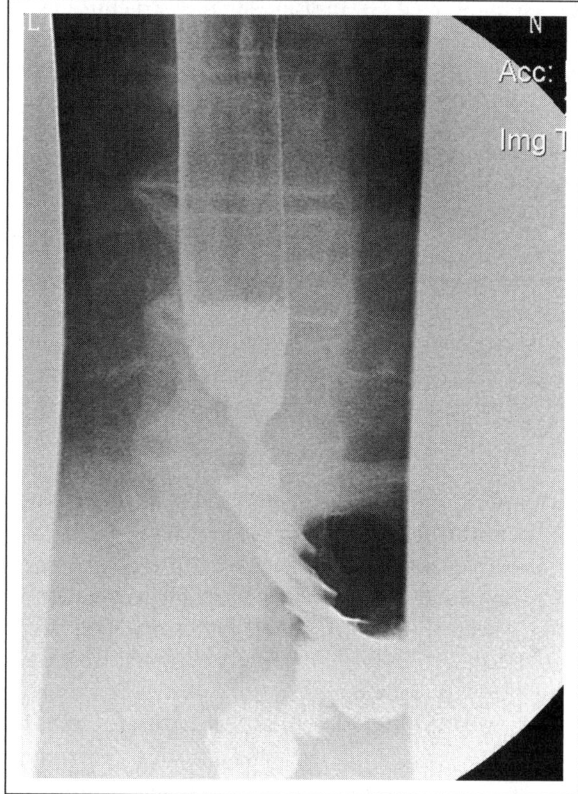

Figure 6.1. Esophagogram showing a distal esophageal carcinoma presenting as a luminal narrowing.

computed tomography (CT) (58%) but less than bronchoscopic ultrasound (91%) (2).

Mr. Gill was referred to a gastroenterologist who performed an esophagoscopy and biopsy of a nearly obstructing mass seen at 27 cm from the incisors. Pathology of the biopsy specimen revealed squamous cell carcinoma of the esophagus.

Once diagnosed with esophageal cancer, what examinations should be used to stage him?

CT is an essential study to evaluate patient anatomy, confirm the presence of distant metastasis, and assess lymph node involvement. CT scan cannot, however, precisely determine the stage of cancer. A CT scan with contrast has a sensitivity of 70% to 80% in detecting hepatic metastasis larger than 2 cm, but smaller liver metastasis may go undetected (3). Invasion of other structures may be difficult to detect on CT and has high interobserver variability. Accuracy rates range from 59% to 82% (4). Furthermore, CT has a sensitivity of 34% to 61% for mediastinal and 50% to 76% for abdominal lymphadenopathy (3).

Esophageal ultrasound (EUS) is capable of showing individual layers of the esophagus by combining endoscopy and high frequency ultrasound. It can identify the extent of tumor wall invasion and especially locate involved lymph nodes that might otherwise be missed by CT scan. Accuracy of EUS in T staging is 84%, and it increases in T3 to T4 carcinomas and with operator experience (3). Fine-needle aspiration biopsy of lymph nodes can be achieved under EUS guidance, providing greater staging information. Positron emission tomography (PET) cannot demonstrate tumor invasion as well as EUS; however, PET can locate distant metastasis undetected by CT scan. The role of PET has yet to be elucidated.

Is there a role for minimally invasive surgery in esophageal tumor staging?

Comparable to the use of mediastinoscopy in lung cancer staging, there has been an increase in using mediastinoscopy, thoracoscopy, and laparoscopy to search for and biopsy lymph nodes undetectable by imaging techniques. Laparoscopy is also useful for detecting liver metastasis and omental implants. A review of the literature by Reed and Eloubeidi reported that thoracoscopic accuracy was 93% and laparoscopic accuracy was 94% (3). Luketich et al. reported 32% of patients who underwent CT and EUS had a T stage change after thoracoscopy and laparoscopy (5). Nguyen et al. had similar results, reporting a change in treatment plan for 36% of patients staged with minimally invasive techniques. The specificity of detecting occult metastatic disease was 100% (6). This staging benefit must be compared to the risks of an additional invasive procedure.

Mr. Gill had an EUS, which revealed invasion of the muscularis propria. There were no lymph nodes seen. Thus, his stage is T2, N0. His CT scans of the chest, abdomen, and pelvis showed that they were free of metastasis.

What is the length of the esophagus?

The esophagus measures an estimated 25 cm in length, and it begins at the inferior edge of C6, connecting the pharynx to the cardia of the stomach. The cervical portion of the esophagus begins below the cricopharyngeus muscle and spans about 5 cm until T2 or the suprasternal notch. The thoracic esophagus then begins at the thoracic inlet, measures roughly 20 cm, and is further divided into upper, middle, and lower segments. These thoracic portions are located as follows: upper third, T2–5 (suprasternal notch to carina); middle third, T5–8 (carina to inferior pulmonary vein); lower third, T8–12 (inferior pulmonary vein to gastroesophageal junction). Endoscopic examinations report measurements beginning at the incisor teeth and ending about 5 cm beneath the diaphragm.

Typically, this measurement is 38 to 40 cm in men and can vary according to height.

What are the layers of the esophagus?

The esophagus is only composed of an epithelial layer and a muscular layer. Unlike other gastrointestinal organs, there is no serosa. Squamous epithelium lines the mucosa, and the musculature of the esophagus consists of an outer longitudinal and an inner circular layer. The upper third of the esophagus is composed of striated muscle that allows voluntary movements, such as swallowing; however, the distal two thirds is made up of smooth muscle, which permits involuntary movement.

What is the blood supply to the esophagus?

The arterial blood supply is segmental and results in an extensive intramural vascular plexus. The cervical esophagus receives its supply from the inferior thyroid artery. The thoracic esophageal portion is supplied by blood from thoracic branches, some directly off of the aorta. As for the abdominal esophageal segment, the inflow is from both the left gastric and inferior phrenic arteries. Venous drainage parallels the arterial network. The cervical esophagus drains into the inferior thyroid vein, whereas the thoracic region is drained by the bronchial, azygos, or hemiazygos veins. The distal esophagus has venous drainage into the left gastric (coronary) vein.

What is the lymphatic drainage of the esophagus?

The lymphatic plexus, located in the submucosa of the esophagus, mainly spreads in a longitudinal fashion. The cervical esophagus drains cephalad into the internal jugular, paratracheal, and deep cervical lymph nodes. However, the middle and lower thoracic segments of the esophagus drain caudad to the subcarinal/ pulmonary hilar nodes and to the paraesophageal/celiac nodes, respectively.

Are most esophageal tumors benign or malignant?

Most esophageal tumors are malignant because only 0.5% of total esophageal masses are benign. Benign tumors are classified by their location, mucosal or intramural, and consist of leiomyomas, benign polyps, hemangiomas, lipomas, and esophageal duplication cysts. Leiomyomas, as the most common, represent 60% of benign neoplasms. Squamous cell carcinoma accounts for the most common malignant tumor worldwide; however, there is an increase in adenocarcinoma incidences, especially in the United States and Western Europe.

Where are most esophageal malignancies located?

Only 15% of esophageal cancers occur in the upper portion of the esophagus compared with 50% in the middle and 35% in the lower segments. The higher percentages seen in the lower segments compared to the upper are, in majority, related to Barrett's esophagus.

What risk factors does our patient have?

In Western countries, esophageal cancer tends to be most common in African American men older than age 50. There is an association between squamous cell carcinoma and tobacco and alcohol usage. An extremely high prevalence of esophageal cancer is also seen in China and Iran. In China, environmental factors such as nitrosamines in the soil and contamination of food by fungi and yeast were found to be carcinogenic. In Iran, the pyrrolysates found in opium and the ingestion of extremely hot teas are thought to contribute to an increase in the incidence of esophageal cancer. Nutritional factors such as malnutrition, vitamin deficiencies, poor dentition, and anemia are also linked to increasing the risk of esophageal cancer. Other risk factors include Plummer-Vinson syndrome, achalasia, lye strictures, irradiation esophagitis, and *tylosis* (familial keratosis palmaris and plantaris). Gastroesophageal reflux disease (GERD) and Barrett's esophagus are risk factors for adenocarcinoma of the esophagus, which is more common in whites than African Americans.

What is the 2002 American Joint Committee for Cancer Staging system for esophageal cancer?

Esophageal cancer is based on the tumor, node, metastasis (TNM) system (Tables 6.1 and 6.2) (7).

What are the available treatment modalities?

Surgery, radiation, and chemotherapy are the available treatments.

TABLE 6.1.

ESOPHAGEAL CANCER TNM CLASSIFICATION

Tumor (T) Classification

T_{is} = high grade dysplasia
T_1 = tumor invasion of the lamina propria or submucosa
T_2 = tumor invasion of the muscularis propria
T_3 = tumor invasion of adventitia
T_4 = tumor invasion of adjacent structures

Nodal (N) Classification

N_0 = no lymph node metastasis
N_1 = regional lymph node metastasis

Metastasis (M) Classification

M_0 = no distal metastasis
M_{1a} = upper thoracic tumors metastatic to cervical; nodes lower thoracic tumors metastatic to celiac nodes
M_{1b} = other nonregional lymph node metastases or distant metastases

TABLE 6.2.

ESOPHAGEAL CANCER STAGING

Stage	T	N	M
0	T_{is}	N_0	M_0
I	T_1	N_0	M_0
IIa	T_2	N_0	M_0
	T_3	N_0	M_0
IIb	T_1	N_1	M_0
	T_2	N_1	M_0
III	T_3	N_1	M_0
	T_4	any N	M_0
IVa	any T	any N	M_{1a}
IVb	any T	any N	M_{1b}

Mr. Gill is referred to a surgeon, who admits him to the hospital for an esophagectomy.

What examinations should be ordered for Mr. Gill's preoperative assessment?

Standard preoperative workup includes a chest radiograph, electrocardiogram, and current blood laboratories, especially coagulation studies and blood type and screen. Serum electrolyte abnormalities must be corrected. Abnormal findings on the chest radiograph, such as abnormal mediastinal soft tissues, dilation of the esophagus, pulmonary metastasis, and air–fluid levels in obstruction, may be seen; however, a normal chest radiograph is common, even in advanced stages of esophageal cancer. Pulmonary function can be improved by ceasing cigarette smoking 2 weeks before surgery and starting incentive spirometry or chest physiotherapy. Unable to maintain a normal diet, poor nutritional status is often seen. Avoid gastrostomy tubes because the stomach is often used as an esophageal replacement.

What is the surgical treatment of esophageal cancer?

Esophagectomy is the standard treatment for surgical candidates with localized esophageal cancer. The three surgical approaches one may perform are the Ivor-Lewis esophagectomy, which combines a right thoracotomy and a laparotomy, the transthoracic or thoracoabdominal approach through a left thoracotomy, and the transhiatal esophagectomy, which combines left cervical and abdominal incisions. The advantages of the transhiatal approach include avoiding a thoracotomy and its associated postoperative pain and avoiding a mediastinal anastomosis and its risk of an intrathoracic leak. However, the transhiatal approach precludes an extended lymph node dissection. Goldminc et al. reported no difference in postoperative morbidity or long-term survival between patients having transhiatal and transthoracic esophagectomies when compared in a prospective randomized trial (8). Wu and Posner concluded that both procedures are equal and that surgical experience determines the morbidity of either one (9).

Debate continues regarding standard lymphadenectomy (limited to paraesophageal and lesser curve nodes) and extended en bloc three-field lymphadenectomy (cervical, mediastinal, and celiac axis nodes). Extended lymph node dissection involves longer operative times and greater blood loss. However, one must recall the prognostic implications with discovery of lymph node involvement. Altorki et al. reported a prospective observational study in which three-field lymphadenectomy revealed positive cervical lymph nodes in 36% of patients (despite tumor location and type) and upstaged 30% of patients (10).

Is there a role for minimally invasive surgery in the treatment of esophageal cancer?

Minimally invasive esophagectomy (MIE) was developed due to the high morbidity and mortality associated with conventional open esophagectomy. Techniques vary; they may be totally laparoscopic, combined thoracoscopic and laparoscopic, or hand-assisted laparoscopic.

Patient selection is an important consideration. Stage IV patients requiring palliation would greatly benefit from a minimally invasive resection. Proponents of laparoscopic esophagectomy also state that patients with T2 or T3 disease would profit because laparoscopic lymph node resections would be done under magnification and immunosuppression associated with an open procedure would be decreased (11). An experienced laparoscopic surgeon can potentially reduce the length of procedure and hospital stay. Advantages include less surgical morbidity and increased number of lymph nodes resected. However, there are risks of conversion to an open procedure (0 to 29%) and port site recurrence, in addition to other complications associated with esophagectomy (12). One study compared MIE to transthoracic and transhiatal esophagectomy. The authors reported shorter operative times, less blood loss, decreased length of intensive care unit and hospital stay with MIE. Neither group had a significantly greater incidence of anastomotic leak or pulmonary complications (13).

What is used to replace the esophagus during esophagectomy?

The stomach is the most common gastric replacement. Stomach reconstruction includes preserving the right gastroepiploic artery and occasionally performing a pyloroplasty to prevent postvagotomy gastric outlet obstruction. If the stomach is unable to be used as the esophageal replacement, a previous gastric resection has been performed, or total gastrectomy is planned, a colonic conduit may be constructed. Davis et al. reported significantly longer operative time, blood loss, anastomotic leakage, and intraabdominal sepsis in patients with colonic interposition grafts. However, both gastric and colonic replacement groups had equal overall mortality and survival (14).

The most common segment used is the left colon. It is smaller, less likely to dilate, and successful at propelling a food bolus. The blood supply is consistent and the length is adequate for any reconstruction. The disadvantage of a left colon graft is that it requires an extensive procedure. The right colon or a loop of jejunum may also be used. The right colon is not used often because it is thin-walled and has a short pedicle. A jejunal graft can be placed as a Roux-en-Y loop or interpositioned conduit for patients who plan on total gastrectomy as part of their procedure. Free jejunal grafts, using microvascular anastomosis, can be employed for failed bowel interpositions as a salvage procedure (15).

What is the operative mortality of an esophagectomy?
The operative mortality rate can vary from zero to 5% (9).

What are the possible causes of morbidity after esophageal resection?
Possible causes of morbidity include anastomotic leak and stricture, wound infection and dehiscence, subphrenic abscess, delay in gastric emptying, pneumonia, pleural effusion, hemorrhage, splenic injury, recurrent laryngeal nerve damage, and ischemia of the conduit.

What is the role of adjuvant therapy?
Adjuvant therapy is given to treat systemic disease, which is otherwise incurable by surgical resection. In one study, survival significantly increased from 8.6 months to greater than 20 months in patients who received both neoadjuvant and adjuvant chemotherapy compared with surgery alone (16).

What is the role of neoadjuvant therapy?
The role of neoadjuvant (preoperative) therapy is to combat disseminated systemic disease and facilitate surgical resection by decreasing bulky tumor size. Risks include increased postoperative morbidity, such as anastomotic leaks, and possible generation of chemoresistant tumor cells. Several studies have documented an increase in survival with chemoradiation before esophagectomy, which remains a vital part of treatment (17). Walsh et al. randomized esophageal adenocarcinoma patients into preoperative chemoradiation and surgery alone groups, and they demonstrated a significant increase in survival in the multimodality group (32% vs. 6% 3-year survival) (18).

Other studies show no advantage to neoadjuvant treatment. A multi-institutional randomized trial showed no difference in survival of patients who received 5-fluorouracil /cisplatin before their surgeries to those who did not, regardless of cancer type (19). Kim and Bains reported several studies showing increased survival in chemotherapy responders compared to nonresponders, which may be important in tailoring patient treatment (20).

What is the role of radiation or chemoradiation as primary treatment?

Chemoradiation, without surgical resection, has been shown to be more effective as primary treatment when compared with radiation alone. Five-year survival was 26% in the chemoradiation group in contrast to 0% in the radiation alone group for patients with locally advanced disease in a randomized controlled trial by Cooper et al. (21). In addition to improved survival, another phase III trial reported better control of local disease and distant metastasis when using chemoradiation compared with radiation alone (17). The complete role of primary chemoradiation alone has yet to be determined but may play a role in poor operative risk patients.

If a patient is not a candidate for curative resection, how can dysphagia be palliated?

Palliation may be performed by esophagectomy and cervical esophagogastrostomy in safe surgical candidates. Intubation of the esophagus with a prosthetic tube is another option. Recently, dilation and esophageal stenting has been shown to increase luminal diameter, but offers no survival advantage over tube intubation (22). Laser ablation and electrical coagulation are other potential palliative treatments. Palliative radiation may be an option but it is not long-lasting.

Mr. Gill underwent a transhiatal esophagectomy and esophagogastrostomy. His postoperative course was uncomplicated. There was no tumor invasion of adjacent structures. The pathology report revealed squamous cell carcinoma of the esophagus invading the muscular wall and involving unilateral lymph nodes.

What are Mr. Gill's chances of a 5-year survival?

Ellis et al. reported a 5-year survival in patients with stage I as 50.3%; stage IIA 22.5%; stage IIB 22.5%; stage III 10.7%; stage IV 0% (23). Overall, 5-year survival was 24.7%. Mr. Gill has stage III disease, and his chance of 5-year survival is 10.7%.

The diagnosis of Barrett's esophagus could have been higher on the differential if Mr. Gill presented as a white man with a prolonged history of GERD.

What is Barrett's esophagus?

Barrett's esophagus is an intestinal metaplasia of columnar epithelium lining the esophagus identified by endoscopic biopsy. Chronic GERD has been identified as a major risk factor.

What is the relationship between Barrett's esophagus and adenocarcinoma of the esophagus?

Theoretically, chronic GERD causes esophagitis, which in turn leads to dysplasia. Dysplastic cells acquire genetic alterations, which may cause progression to invasive carcinoma. Spechler reported that 0.5% of patients with Barrett's esophagus develop adenocarcinoma each year (24). Progression from high-grade dysplasia to adenocarcinoma ranges from 10% to 59% within 5 years.

What is the treatment for Barrett's esophagus?

The cause of Barrett's esophagus is GERD; therefore, the treatment begins by decreasing reflux with proton pump inhibitors or H_2-receptor antagonists. Also, fundoplication may be performed to prevent gastric acid from reaching the esophagus.

A meta-analysis performed by Corey at al. concluded that an anti-reflux procedure does not significantly decrease the risk of adenocarcinoma development in patients with Barrett's esophagus. Therefore, fundoplication should not be recommended as a preventative technique against adenocarcinoma development (25). Patients must continue to have routine endoscopy and biopsy sampling every 2 to 3 years in search of dysplasia.

What would Mr. Gill's treatment be if he presented with dysplastic Barrett's esophagus, and would the treatment differ from that of adenocarcinoma?

Low-grade dysplasia may be followed closely by endoscopy and biopsy sampling every 6 to 12 months in addition to antireflux measures. However, the treatment for high-grade dysplasia in surgical candidates is an esophagectomy. This procedure, in theory, can prevent the progression from dysplasia to neoplasm. Other options include endoscopic ablative therapy and intense surveillance. Similarly, invasion or adenocarcinoma is treated by esophagectomy.

SUMMARY

Although squamous cell carcinoma is the most common malignant tumor of the esophagus, the incidence of adenocarcinoma is increasing. Progressive dysphagia and weight loss are typically the presenting symptoms. The diagnostic evaluation of suspected esophageal cancer includes esophagoscopy with biopsy, EUS, and CT of the chest. The surgical treatment for esophageal cancer is esophagectomy with esophagogastrostomy. The role of minimally invasive techniques has yet to be determined as technology advances. Chemoradiation, as a primary treatment alone, is promising, but further studies are being performed. Adenocarcinoma can arise from Barrett's esophagus; therefore, esophagectomy is the recommended treatment when patients develop high-grade dysplasia.

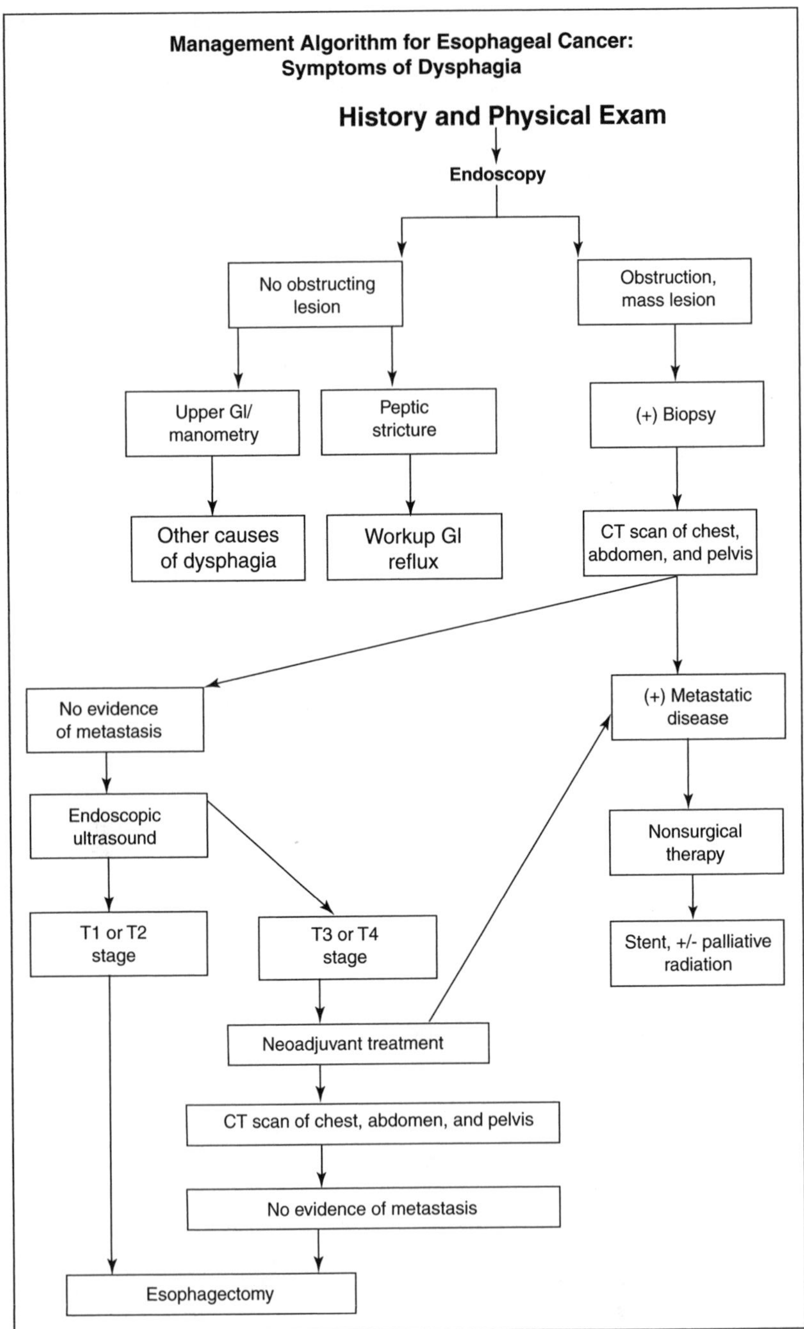

Algorithm 6.1.

REFERENCES

1. Ikeda M, Natsugoe S, Ueno S, et al. Significant host- and tumor-related factors for predicting prognosis in patients with esophageal carcinoma. Ann Surg. 2003;238:197–202.
2. Nishimura Y, Osugi H, Inoue K, et al. Bronchoscopic ultrasonography in the diagnosis of tracheobronchial invasion of esophageal cancer. J Ultrasound Med. 2002;21:49–58.
3. Reed C, Eloubeidi M. New techniques for staging esophageal cancer. Surg Clin North Am. 2002;82:697–710.
4. Iyer RB, Silverman EP, Dunnington JS, et al. Diagnosing, staging and follow-up of esophageal cancer. AJR Am J Roentgenol. 2003;181:785–793.
5. Luketich JD, Meehan M, Schauer PR, et al. Minimally invasive surgical staging for esophageal cancer. Surg Endosc. 2000;14:700–702.
6. Nguyen NT, Roberts PF, Follette DM, et al. Evaluation of minimally invasive surgical staging for esophageal cancer. Am J Surg. 2001;182:702–706.
7. Rice T, Blackstone E, Rybicki L, et al. Refining esophageal cancer staging. J Thorac Cardiovasc Surg. 2003;125:1103–1113.
8. Golminc M, Maddern G, Le Prise E, et al. Oesophagectomy by a transhiatal approach or a thoracotomy: a prospective randomized trail. Br J Surg. 1993;80:367–370.
9. Wu P, Posner M. The role of surgery in the management of oesophageal cancer. Lancet. 2003;4:481–488.
10. Altorki N, Kent M, Ferrara C, et al. Three-field lymph node dissection for squamous cell and adenocarcinoma of the esophagus. Ann Surg. 2002;236: 177–183.
11. Swanstrom LL. Minimally invasive surgical approaches to esophageal cancer. J Gastrointest Surg. 2002;6:522–526.
12. Litle V, Buenaventura P, Luketich J. Minimally invasive resection for esophageal cancer. Surg Clin North Am. 2002;82:711–728.
13. Nguyen NT, Follette DM, Wolfe BM, et al. Comparison of minimally invasive esophagectomy with transthoracic and transhiatal esophagectomy. Arch Surg. 2000;135:920–925.
14. Davis PA, Wong S, Law J. Colonic interposition after esophagectomy for cancer. Arch Surg. 2003;138:303–308.
15. Mansour KA, Bryan FC, Carlson GW. Bowel interposition for esophageal replacement: twenty-five year experience. Ann Thorac Surg. 1997;64:752–756.
16. Roth JA, Pass HI, Flanagan MM, et al. Randomized clinical trial of preoperative and postoperative adjuvant chemotherapy with cisplatin, vincristine, and bleomycin for carcinoma of the esophagus. J Cardiovasc Surg. 1988;96:242–248.
17. Kaplan B, Posner M. Neoadjuvant therapy of esophageal carcinoma. Surg Oncol. 2002;501–511.
18. Walsh TN, Noonan N, Hollywood D, et al. A comparison of multimodal therapy and surgery for esophageal adenocarcinoma. N Engl J Med. 1996;335:462–467.
19. Kelsen DP, Ginsberg R, Pajak TF, et al. Chemotherapy followed by surgery compared with surgery alone for localized esophageal cancer. N Engl J Med. 1998;339:1979–1984.

20. Kim HJ, Bains MS. Randomized clinical trials in esophageal cancer. Surg Oncol. Clin N Am 2002;11:89–109.
21. Cooper JS, Guo MD, Herskovic A, et al. Chemoradiotherapy of locally advanced esophageal cancer: long-term follow up of a prospective randomized trial. JAMA. 1999;281:1623–1627.
22. Boyce H. Stents for palliation of dysphagia due to esophageal cancer. N Engl J Med. 1993;329:1345–1346.
23. Ellis F, Heatly G, Balogh K. Proposal for improved staging criteria for carcinoma of the esophagus and cardia. Eur J Cardiothorac Surg. 1997;12:361–364.
24. Spechler S. Barrett's esophagus. N Engl J Med. 2002;346:836–842.
25. Corey KE, Schmitz SM, Shaheen NJ. Does a surgical antireflux procedure decrease the incidence of esophageal adenocarcinoma in Barrett's esophagus? A meta-analysis. Am J Gastroenterol. 2003;98:2390–2394.

CHAPTER

PEPTIC ULCER DISEASE

David Page

Robbie Steele is a 49-year-old insurance agent with epigastric pain. For approximately 6 months, Mr. Steele has had vague abdominal distress after meals and at night, and he now uses antacids on a regular basis. However, the antacids are no longer effective. Although he admits to one instance of blood in his stool and occasional nausea, he denies repeated melena, change in bowel habits, or weight loss. He smokes a pack of cigarettes a day, uses aspirin sparingly, and drinks socially. The remainder of his history is negative.

What other important information should be obtained?

The following information should be elicited:

- When antacid use was started
- Use of other over-the-counter antacids or histamine receptor antagonists
- Any vomiting of blood
- Diminished ability to eat a whole meal
- Heartburn

Mr. Steele has used antacids for 1 to 2 years for epigastric pain as well as for heartburn. He vomited blood once 6 months ago, but his appetite has not been impaired. His weight dropped 10 pounds during the past year. Mr. Steele has an average build with normal vital signs, and other than being nervous, he is not in acute distress. The findings of the head, neck, and chest examinations are normal. The abdominal examination reveals epigastric tenderness with deep palpation. There is no guarding or rebound tenderness, and bowel sounds are present. No mass or groin hernia is present. Findings of rectal examination and hemoccult tests are negative.

What is the first step in assessing a new patient with symptoms such as Mr. Steele's?

The clinician must determine how sick the patient is. Factors that must be considered include severity of pain and associated symptoms, hemodynamic status, and any indications for immediate surgery. The need for urgent workup for acute symptoms must be determined, and a plan for resuscitation, if needed, must be made.

What is the differential diagnosis for epigastric pain?

Diagnoses include but are not limited to peptic ulcer disease, gastritis, pancreatitis, pancreatic cancer, biliary tract disease, abdominal aortic aneurysm, early appendicitis, gastroenteritis, and ischemic heart disease.

Why is acute myocardial infarction (MI) included in the differential diagnosis of epigastric pain?

Pain from the inferior wall of the left ventricle may be referred to the epigastrium and can be associated with nausea, vomiting, and diaphoresis.

Mr. Steele's laboratory tests show the following: hemoglobin level, 14.2 g per dL; hematocrit, 41%; white blood cell count, 12,800 per mL; normal blood urea nitrogen, creatinine, amylase, and lipase levels. Liver function is normal. An electrocardiogram (ECG) shows normal sinus rhythm at 82 per minute with no acute changes.

What is the most likely diagnosis according to the laboratory results?

The normal ECG eliminates acute MI. Normal liver function studies suggest there is probably no acute biliary tract disease, although an ultrasound examination is needed if cholecystitis is suspected. Normal amylase and lipase levels rule out pancreatitis and, along with a normal hemoglobin, reduce the likelihood of pancreatic carcinoma. Gastritis, gastroenteritis, and early appendicitis are unlikely but possible according to his history and presentation. The absence of a palpable pulsatile mass on initial examination reduces the possibility of abdominal aortic aneurysm. Peptic ulcer disease is the most likely diagnosis.

How is peptic ulcer disease confirmed?

Upper endoscopy (esophagogastroduodenoscopy) is the next step toward confirming the diagnosis and defining the extent of the disease. This test not only allows ulcers to be seen but also helps rule out other diagnoses such as reflux esophagitis, Barrett's esophagus, and gastritis. All gastric ulcers must be sampled for biopsy (four-quadrant specimens must be obtained), and if the ulcers appear suspect for malignancy, gastric washings must be obtained for cytologic examination. Gastric ulcers that have not healed as determined by endoscopy after several weeks of treatment must also be aggressively assessed with repeat biopsies. Although cancer of the duodenum is unusual, biopsy of anomalous, nonhealing duodenal ulcers is necessary. Experience in Japan has demonstrated that early diagnosis and treatment of gastric cancer improve survival (1).

What is the incidence of peptic ulcer disease?

Approximately 5 million Americans have peptic ulcer disease (2). Ulcers occur most commonly in men aged 45 to 55 years, although they also occur in the elderly and occasionally in children and adolescents.

What causes peptic ulcer disease?

Historically, excess gastric acid was believed to be the single cause of peptic ulcer disease. It is now estimated, however, that 90% of duodenal ulcers and 80% of gastric ulcers are associated with *Helicobacter pylori,* the putative causative agent (3). This organism is found in the gastric mucous layer or on the gastric mucosa. Other factors associated with peptic ulcers are cigarette smoking, high alcohol intake, nonsteroidal antiinflammatory drug use, and a stressful lifestyle. Excess gastric acid production continues to accompany peptic ulceration.

Mucosal injury of the stomach (gastric ulceration or stress gastritis) is associated with specific stressors such as major body surface burns (Curling's ulcer), multiple organ failure, multiple trauma, and head injuries (Cushing's ulcer) (4).

What is *H. pylori* and how is *H. pylori* infection diagnosed?

H. pylori is a spiral flagellated organism found worldwide. In countries such as China, where *H. pylori* infects more than half the population during early childhood, the rate of gastric cancer, also associated with this organism, is high. *H. pylori* infection is linked to both duodenal and gastric ulcers and to the lymphoid type of mucosal lymphoma. Approximately two thirds of the world population is infected with *H. pylori.* In the United States, the organism is most often seen in African Americans, Hispanics, the elderly, and the poor (5). Three tests diagnose *H. pylori* infection: rapid urease test, serologic antibody measurement, and urea breath test. The organism may also be seen on endoscopic biopsy.

What is the treatment for peptic ulcer disease?

Uncomplicated peptic ulcer disease is treated medically with a number of agents. Triple therapy based on proton pump inhibitors is the most common treatment aimed at eliminating *H. pylori* (6). Surgical intervention is reserved for recalcitrant cases that progress to complications such as bleeding, obstruction, perforation, and intractability. Before the role of *H. pylori* in peptic ulcer disease was discovered, primary treatment centered on histamine receptor antagonists such as cimetidine, ranitidine, and famotidine. Proton pump inhibitors have proven to be more potent acid suppression agents than H_2 antagonists but are not used for long-term treatment. Five proton pump inhibitors are available:

three older drugs—omeprazole, lansoprazole and pantoprazole—and two newer drugs—rabeprazole and esomeprazole. The latter two newer proton pump inhibitors offer more consistent acid inhibition, especially in the elderly patient (7). Sucralfate, an aluminum salt of sulfated sucrose that binds to the ulcer base and promotes healing, is used to treat acute duodenal ulcers. Pain resolution with sucralfate is less prompt than with H_2 blockers.

The standard treatment for peptic ulcer disease focuses on treatment of *H. pylori* infection, as well as acid suppression, with any of several drug combinations. The original 14-day course of triple treatment consisting of bismuth, metronidazole, and either tetracycline or amoxicillin is often replaced by combinations of new drugs. Other choices include regimens combining (a) omeprazole and clarithromycin; (b) ranitidine, bismuth citrate, and clarithromycin; and (c) lansoprazole and either amoxicillin alone or amoxicillin with clarithromycin (8–10). Also, treatment with esomeprazole, amoxicillin, and clarithromycin is effective (11). The choice of treatment is up to the individual physician.

What are the goals of peptic ulcer treatment and how is therapy assessed?
The goals of treatment are to provide rapid relief of symptoms, promote permanent healing of the ulcer, avoid recurrence, reduce ulcer-related complications, and control treatment costs (12). After treatment, the eradication of *H. pylori* must be confirmed by either endoscopic biopsy or a urea breath test. If the results are negative, no further medical treatment is needed.

How successful is treatment with triple or alternative therapy for *H. pylori*?
The rates of recurrence of gastric and duodenal ulcers are 4% and 6%, respectively, after successful eradication of *H. pylori,* compared with 59% and 67%, respectively, if the organism persists (13). Failure to eradicate *H. pylori* varies between 10% and 20% of treated patients (14).

Mr. Steele completes a course of triple therapy consisting of esomeprazole, amoxicillin, and clarithromycin, and his symptoms resolve. He returns to his investment job with his usual enthusiasm and resumes smoking. About 2 months later, he goes to the emergency department because of gnawing epigastric pain. Endoscopy, performed within the next 2 weeks, reveals a recurrent duodenal ulcer. He is reluctant to undergo further medical treatment and requests a more permanent alternative.

What are the alternatives to medical treatment for gastric ulcer disease?
Laparoscopic (minimally invasive) surgery has influenced the surgical management of peptic ulcers (15). Enthusiasm for surgical therapy has been renewed because of shorter hospital stays, acceptable recurrence rates after proximal gastric vagotomy, and a probable overall reduction in cost as compared with long-term pharmacologic management. Surgical treatment is mandatory if medical therapy

fails and symptoms become intractable. Surgery is indicated if gastric outlet obstruction, significant bleeding, or perforation occurs. However, a patient should undergo more than one course of conservative, nonsurgical treatment before a surgeon is consulted. This may be in the form of a second proton pump inhibitor/antibiotic regimen or re-endoscopy and heater probe or injection therapy for acute hemorrhage.

Mr. Steele ignores his doctor's advice to undergo another course of medical treatment and refuses surgery. About 4 months later he arrives in the emergency room vomiting bright red blood. His blood pressure is 80/60 mm Hg, his pulse is 110 beats per minute, and he is diaphoretic.

What is the first step in managing a patient in a condition such as Mr. Steele's?

Mr. Steele is in hemorrhagic shock and must be resuscitated immediately. Oxygen must be given, normal saline or lactated Ringers solution must be administered via one or two large-bore intravenous lines, and blood must be drawn for typing, cross-matching, and routine laboratory tests. A Foley catheter and a nasogastric tube must also be inserted and the fluid balance monitored. Preparations must be made for emergency upper endoscopy.

What is the differential diagnosis for upper gastrointestinal hemorrhage?

Possible diagnoses include but are not limited to reflux esophagitis, esophageal cancer, esophageal varices, gastritis, gastric cancer, foreign body trauma to the esophagus or stomach, Dieulafoy's ulcer, gastric and duodenal ulcers, and swallowed blood from an upper aerodigestive lesion.

What endoscopic findings suggest ongoing bleeding or rebleeding from a peptic ulcer?

Endoscopic assessment of upper gastrointestinal bleeding identifies patients at high risk for rebleeding. These individuals may require prolonged hospitalization and repeat assessment. Patients who have ulcers with a clean base or with small, flat blood spots do not require endoscopic treatment and may be sent home with appropriate medications (16). Those with active arterial bleeding or with a visible nonhemorrhaging vessel should be treated endoscopically with a heat probe or, rarely, injection therapy.

An emergency upper endoscopic examination of Mr. Steele reveals a pyloric channel ulcer that has a clot at the base. The endoscopist elects not to disturb the clot and terminates the procedure.

What are the indications for surgical treatment of bleeding peptic ulcers?

Emergency surgery for hemorrhage must be performed for the following three conditions:

1. The patient continues to hemorrhage and remains in shock despite maximum resuscitation; surgery is usually contemplated if the patient does not respond to administration of 6 to 8 units of blood.
2. The patient stops bleeding clinically and rebleeds as proven endoscopically; if a patient rebleeds massively, surgery is indicated without repeat endoscopy; if stable, the patient may undergo a second attempt at endoscopic control of the bleeding.
3. The patient bleeds slowly but persistently and requires 2 or 3 units of blood per day for several consecutive days.
4. The patient fails endoscopic treatment.

Relative indications for a more aggressive surgical approach to the bleeding ulcer patient include profound shock on presentation where surgery becomes part of the act of resuscitation. Other factors include severe or multiple comorbid conditions, advanced age, rare blood type, and refusal to accept blood transfusions. A special subset in need of immediate surgical intervention is the elderly patient with a rebleed, a large ulcer, and several comorbid illnesses.

What is the recommended surgical procedure for a hemorrhagic ulcer?

Three standard procedures may be considered in this setting:

1. Oversewing of the bleeding ulcer with highly selective (proximal gastric) vagotomy may be performed open or laparoscopically. In the urgent setting with massive bleeding, the open approach is expedient and stops the hemorrhage more quickly. The recurrence rate is 10% to 15%, but few postoperative complications occur.
2. Oversewing of bleeding ulcer with truncal vagotomy and pyloroplasty is probably the most often used procedure and is performed open. Complete division of the vagus nerve requires a drainage procedure, such as pyloroplasty, to avoid gastric stasis.
3. Oversewing of ulcer with antrectomy (hemigastrectomy) and truncal vagotomy has the lowest recurrence rate (2% to 3%) but is associated with more postoperative complications than the other procedures.

What are other indications for surgery in peptic ulcer disease?

In addition to massive bleeding, other indications for surgery in patients with peptic ulcer disease are perforation, obstruction, and intractability. Studies of the cost of peptic ulcer disease suggest that earlier surgery may be a less expensive alternative to lifelong pharmacologic therapy (13).

What is the recommended surgical procedure in a patient with a perforated ulcer?

Operative options for a patient with a perforated peptic ulcer are similar to those for bleeding. In an emergency, the surgeon uses an omental patch (called a *Graham patch*) to close the perforation rather than oversewing as with a bleeding point. The rigidity of the surrounding tissue makes oversewing a perforation risky or impossible. However, primary excision of the ulcer with a tensionless closure is sometimes possible.

How is gastric outlet obstruction (acquired pyloric obstruction) treated?

Both nonsurgical and surgical procedures are effective, depending on the degree of scarring and stenosis. Balloon dilation via endoscopy is preferred for lesser degrees of obstruction and may be repeated as needed. For severe pyloric stenosis not remediable by dilation, operative intervention becomes necessary.

Which operation is indicated for gastric outlet obstruction secondary to peptic ulcer disease?

Truncal vagotomy with pyloroplasty or truncal vagotomy with antrectomy are both useful for patients with symptoms and radiologic or endoscopic proof of gastric outlet obstruction. After gastric resection, reconstruction of the stomach may be with either a Billroth I (gastroduodenostomy) or a Billroth II (gastrojejunostomy) anastomosis (Fig. 7.1). Truncal vagotomy with gastroenterostomy or a Roux-en-Y anastomosis are less desirable options.

Which surgical procedures are used for intractability?

The same procedures as for gastric obstruction are used. Laparoscopic proximal (parietal cell) gastric vagotomy is least invasive; open gastric resection with truncal vagotomy is most aggressive and has the highest complication rate. However, results with laparoscopic surgery should be assessed and compared with the time-tested open procedures before laparoscopic surgery is accepted as the standard (15).

Over time, Mr. Steele takes his medication less consistently, and his ulcer symptoms worsen. Eventually, he develops intractable pain and some gastric outlet obstruction. He is counseled about options and agrees to undergo elective antrectomy and truncal vagotomy.

What are the short-term complications and long-term problems of gastric resection and vagotomy?

Postgastrectomy complications are related to anatomic changes (absence of pyloric meter), the influence of vagotomy, and include several nutritional factors. Although many patients have these symptoms to a lesser degree immediately after peptic ulcer surgery, only 1% to 2% develop truly debilitating symptoms. Short-term problems include the following:

- Early and late dumping syndromes are thought to result from the absence of the pylorus and the presentation of a high osmolar fluid load to the small bowel in a bolus. This causes epigastric pain, nausea, light-headedness,

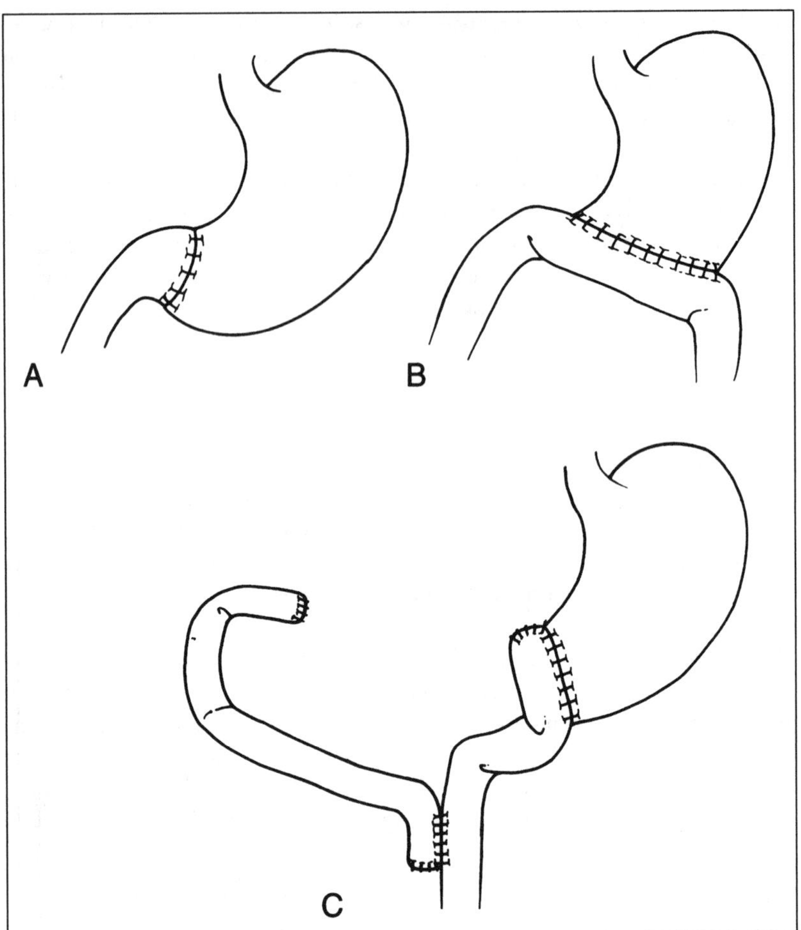

Figure 7.1. A: Billroth I (gastroduodenostomy) anastomosis. **B:** Billroth II (gastrojejunostomy) anastomosis. **C:** Billroth II with Roux-en-Y anastomosis.

and possibly syncope. Early dumping symptoms occur within minutes of eating; similar distress characterizes late dumping, which occurs an hour or more after a meal and which may be associated with reactive hypoglycemia.

- Alkaline reflux gastritis occurs when alkaline bile is refluxed into the stomach in the absence of a pyloric barrier and patients have postprandial epigastric discomfort, nausea, and occasionally vomiting. These persons have endoscopic evidence of bile in the stomach, as well as biopsy-proven gastritis. Treatment includes H_2-receptor antagonists, changes in diet, and bile-binding drugs. A Roux-en-Y gastrojejunostomy is the surgical treatment for recalcitrant cases.

- Postvagotomy diarrhea occurs in a small proportion of patients undergoing truncal vagotomy. Its prevention is one of the primary rationales for parietal cell vagotomy.
- Nutritional deficiencies include iron-deficiency anemia, vitamin B_{12} anemia (loss of intrinsic factor), and protein-calorie deficits.
- Cancer in the gastric remnant may occur 15 to 20 years after surgery. Long-term endoscopic follow-up is important (4).

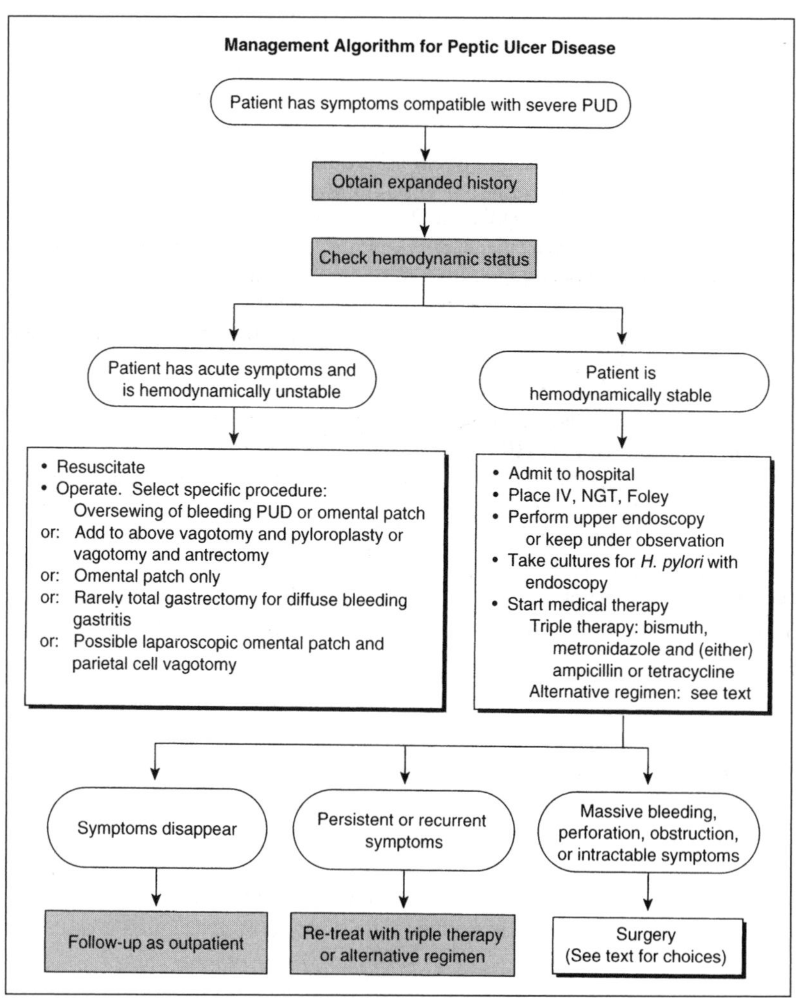

Algorithm 7.1.

REFERENCES

1. Fielding JWL. Gastric cancer: different diseases. Br J Surg. 1989;76:1227.
2. Vakil N, Fennerty B. The economics of eradicating *Helicobacter pylori* infection in duodenal ulcer disease. Am J Med. 1996;100:60S–63S.
3. NIH Consensus Development. *Helicobacter pylori* in peptic ulcer disease. JAMA. 1994;272:65–69.
4. Mulholland MW. Stomach and duodenum. In: Greenfield LJ, Mulholland MW, Oldham KT, et al., eds. Surgery: Scientific Principles and Practice. Philadelphia, Pa: JB Lippincott Co; 1993:661–702.
5. Hunt RH. Eradication of *Helicobacter pylori* infection [review]. Am J Med. 1996;100:42S–51S.
6. Laine L. Review article: esomeprazole in the treatment of *Helicobacter pylori* [review article]. Aliment Pharmacol Ther. 2002;16(4 Suppl):115–118.
7. Thjodleifsson B. Treatment of acid-related diseases in the elderly with emphasis on the use of proton pump inhibitors. Drugs Aging. 2002;19:911–927.
8. Hunt RH. Peptic ulcer disease: defining the treatment strategies in the era of *Helicobacter pylori.* Am J Gastroenterol. 1992;92(4 Suppl):36S–43S.
9. Walsh JH, Peterson WL. The treatment of *Helicobacter pylori* infection in the management of peptic ulcer disease. N Engl J Med. 1995;333:984–991.
10. Howden CW. Optimizing the pharmacology of acid control in the acid-related disorders. Am J Gastroenterol. 1997;92(4 Suppl):17S–21S.
11. Johnson TJ, Hedge DD. Esomeprazole: a clinical review. 2002;59(14):1333–9.
12. Hunt RH et al. Optimizing acid suppression for treatment of acid-related diseases. Dig Dis Sci. 1995;40(2 Suppl):24S–49S.
13. Hopkins RJ, Girardi LS, Turney EA. Relation between *Helicobacter pylori* eradication and reduced duodenal and gastric ulcer recurrence: a review. Gastroenterology. 1996;110:1244–1252.
14. Casas AT, Gadacz TR. Laparoscopic management of peptic ulcer disease. Surg Clin North Am. 1996;76:515–522.
15. Villanueva C, Balanzo J. A practical guide to the management of bleeding ulcers. Drugs. 1997;53:389–403.
16. Jiranek GC, Kozarek RA. A cost-effective approach to the patient with peptic ulcer bleeding. Surg Clin North Am. 1996;76:83–103.

CHAPTER

8

GASTRIC CANCER

Keith G. Chisholm and D. Scott Lind

David Lee is a 68-year-old man who has been having progressive anorexia, postprandial fullness, and vague abdominal discomfort for the past 3 months. He has lost 20 pounds over this period. He denies dysphagia, vomiting, or bright red blood per rectum. His medical history is unremarkable with the exception of hypertension that is well controlled with an angiotensin-converting enzyme (ACE) inhibitor.

Mr. Lee's physical examination is also unremarkable, other than mild midepigastric tenderness to deep palpation. Rectal examination reveals no masses, but his stool is guaiac positive. Laboratory values reveal a hemoglobin count of 9.2 g/dL, which indicates a mild anemia. Levels of serum electrolytes, transaminases, and alkaline phosphatase are within normal limits, and serum albumin is normal.

What is the differential diagnosis for this patient?

Considering the patient's symptoms, both benign and neoplastic disease processes are part of the differential diagnosis. Given Mr. Lee's age, however, malignancy is a prime concern. A cancer of the gastrointestinal (GI) tract must be high on the list, given the patient's symptoms: anorexia, weight loss, anemia, and guaiac-positive rectal examination.

In the United States, colorectal cancer is the most common GI cancer, with an estimated 147,500 new cases diagnosed in 2003. Gastric cancer (estimated 22,400 new cases in 2003) and esophageal cancer (estimated 13,900 new cases in 2003) are the third and fifth most common GI malignancies in the United States (1). However, worldwide, gastric cancer is the second largest cause of cancer-related deaths (2). Peptic ulcer disease may present with similar symptoms of anorexia, anemia, and hemoccult-positive stools. Weight loss may also be present. In this situation, it is paramount for the clinician to eliminate the diagnosis of malignancy.

What are some of the early symptoms of gastric cancer?

Some of the initial symptoms of gastric cancer include weight loss, abdominal pain, nausea, and anorexia. These symptoms are nonspecific and are often overlooked by both the patient and the physician; as a result, the disease is often advanced when it is diagnosed. Currently, as with colorectal cancer, there are no screening recommendations for gastric cancer. Therefore, investigation is usually prompted by symptoms; however, symptoms are usually harbingers of advanced cancers. Proximal gastric cancer (i.e., cancer of the esophagogastric junction) causes dysphagia, and distal gastric cancer (i.e., prepyloric cancer) results in gastric outlet obstruction. GI hemorrhage resulting from gastric cancer is usually occult. Rarely is bleeding severe enough to result in gross hematochezia.

What is an acceptable initial diagnostic or therapeutic step for this patient?

Empiric therapy with H_2 blockers or proton pump inhibitors (PPIs) for presumed peptic ulcer disease is probably inappropriate considering Mr. Lee's age along with his symptoms. An acceptable initial diagnostic test is an upper GI (UGI) radiographic study. A UGI study is an appropriate screening test for suspected peptic ulcer disease or gastric malignancy. The accuracy of this study is increased with double contrasted technique to approximately 90% for diagnosing gastric cancer (3). However, do not allow normal results to preclude further evaluation of the patient's symptoms.

Computed tomography (CT) scans are popular because they are relatively benign procedures and are fairly comprehensive imaging studies. For these reasons, a patient with similar symptoms may get referred to you having already undergone a CT scan, which is an inappropriate initial diagnostic test in this case. CT scans have nearly 100% sensitivity for detecting malignant or potentially malignant gastric lesions when the gastric wall thickness is 1 cm or greater. However, specificity is unacceptably low, at less than 50% (4).

An alternative initial study is an esophagogastroduodenoscopy (EGD) with a flexible fiberoptic endoscope. EGD is often combined with colonoscopy, using a separate, larger flexible fiberoptic endoscope. This double approach is sometimes useful when the symptoms are not specifically related to the upper or lower parts of the GI tract but when guaiac positive stools and anemia are thought to be caused by blood loss within the GI tract.

Endoscopy and contrast studies of the UGI tract are complementary in their diagnostic capabilities. In other words, endoscopy may provide information that was missed by UGI radiography and vice versa. If the surgeon does not perform endoscopy as part of his or her practice, UGI radiography provides a road map for any surgery that is contemplated. The advantage of endoscopy as a diagnostic test is that it permits biopsy of lesions that are visualized.

A UGI radiographic study reveals a 4-cm ulcer on the greater curve of the distal stomach.

What is the next step in the continuing evaluation of this patient?

Endoscopy is the next step for diagnostic workup for suspected gastric cancer. Unlike ulcers associated with peptic disease, ulcers located in the stomach deserve interrogation by biopsy because there is a higher incidence of malignancy with gastric ulcers. Endoscopy allows the physician to obtain a tissue sample for histologic diagnosis (i.e., to distinguish between benign and malignant ulcers) and to define the extent of the lesion. Because a single endoscopic biopsy sample does not have much diagnostic value, take multiple samples from various parts of the ulcer (e.g., the base, slope, and rim). Combine histologic analyses of these biopsy specimens with brush cytology to increase diagnostic accuracy. Occasionally, endoscopy fails to detect a gastric malignancy. In addition, false-negative results are obtained with endoscopic biopsies from patients with gastric lymphoma because this malignancy is submucosal.

Pathology results of the endoscopic biopsy and brushing specimens from Mr. Lee's EGD reveal poorly differentiated adenocarcinoma.

What are the histologic types of gastric malignancies, and what is the relative incidence of each type?

Approximately 95% of malignant neoplasms of the stomach are adenocarcinomas. Several methods of classifying gastric cancer have been developed. In 1926, Borrmann classified gastric cancer into four types: *I*, polypoid; *II*, ulcerated; *III*, ulcerated and infiltrating; and *IV*, infiltrating. In 1965, Lauren reclassified gastric cancer into intestinal and diffuse types. The *intestinal type* includes polypoid and superficial spreading cancers and the *diffuse type* includes linitis plastica (5). This classification is not part of the formal staging of gastric cancer. Prognosis remains more dependent on depth of invasion and nodal status rather than the histologic classification.

The intestinal type is more common in populations in which gastric cancer is highly prevalent. It develops mostly in the distal one third of the stomach. Patients with intestinal type gastric cancer have a better prognosis. The diffuse type, on the other hand, is more common in populations at low risk. It arises more commonly on the proximal stomach and gastroesophageal junction. A separate, distinct entity called *early gastric cancer* (EGC) is defined as gastric cancer confined to the mucosa or submucosa, regardless of size, histologic type, or lymph node status.

There are other types of gastric malignancy. GI stromal tumors (GISTs); primary gastric lymphoma (the most common extranodal lymphoma); and adenosquamous, squamous, and carcinoid neoplasms occur in the stomach relatively rarely.

What is linitis plastica?

Linitis plastica literally means leather bottle. It is a morphologic variant of gastric adenocarcinoma characterized by a diffusely infiltrating tumor that incites a desmoplastic response, which results in a rigid, nondistensible stomach with no discernable intraluminal mass. Patients with linitis plastica have a dismal prognosis.

What additional tests can help determine the extent of disease and why is this important?

In addition to a chest radiograph to detect pulmonary metastasis, radiographic studies should include CT of the abdomen and pelvis. CT yields information about possible liver metastases, invasion of adjacent organs, and lymph node involvement. CT is not, however, sensitive for peritoneal carcinomatosis and it cannot reliably establish unresectability of a tumor.

Endoscopic ultrasonography (EUS) is used to assess the depth of penetration of the lesion into the gastric wall as well as localized lymph node involvement. These findings usually correlate well with the operative findings. EUS and CT findings allow more accurate preoperative staging and thus help identify patients who may benefit from neoadjuvant (preoperative) therapy.

What is the anatomic distribution of adenocarcinoma of the stomach and its pattern of spread?

Approximately half of all gastric cancers arise in the gastric antrum, and about one-fourth arise in the body of the stomach. Recently, there has been an increase in cancer of the proximal stomach and gastroesophageal junction, particularly in young white men. The incidence of distal cancers has decreased (2). A thorough understanding of the patterns of spread of the disease is necessary to plan rational therapy. The patterns of extension of gastric carcinoma are as follows:

1. Direct spread within the wall of the stomach, either proximally to involve the esophagus or, less commonly, distally to involve the pylorus and duodenum
2. Direct extension to involve contiguous organs, such as the spleen, pancreas, colon, and left lobe of the liver
3. Peritoneal dissemination as a result of serosal penetration by the tumor
4. Lymphatic spread to involve local or distant lymph nodes
5. Bloodborne metastases, particularly to the liver

Virchow's node, Irish's node, Sister Mary Joseph's node, Krukenberg's tumor, and Blumer's shelf are all eponyms that may be associated with gastric cancer. How is each defined?

1. **Virchow's node** is a palpable left supraclavicular lymph node that is often associated with an advanced GI malignancy.
2. **Irish's node** denotes a palpable left axillary lymph node.

3. **Sister Mary Joseph's node** is a palpable periumbilical lymph node.
4. **Krukenberg's tumor** is a malignant tumor of the ovary that arises from a GI malignancy because of either peritoneal or hematogenous metastases.
5. **Blumer's shelf** is an extraluminal mass that is palpable during a rectal or pelvic examination; it is the result of peritoneal metastases from a GI malignancy to the pelvic cul-de-sac.

Is the incidence of gastric cancer increasing or decreasing worldwide?

Over the past 70 years, the incidence of gastric cancer has declined dramatically in the United States. In 1930, gastric cancer was the most frequent cancer in adults, with an incidence of 38 per 100,000 individuals. The incidence decreased to 8 per 100,000 in 1980 and leveled off in the mid-1980s (6). With approximately 25,000 new cases being reported per year and with about 15,000 deaths per year, gastric cancer remains a significant national health problem.

In addition, gastric cancer is an enormous health problem worldwide. The incidence of gastric cancer in Japan is 10 times higher than in the United States. In Japan, gastric cancer screening programs have greatly improved the detection of early lesions. In Western countries, screening is not economically justified except in high-risk patients.

What are some risk factors for gastric cancers?

1. **Gastric polyps** occur in two histologic types: hyperplastic and adenomatous. Hyperplastic polyps are not considered premalignant: however, patients with adenomatous polyps of the stomach are at increased risk for gastric cancer. The incidence of malignancy in patients with adenomatous gastric polyps correlates with the size and number of polyps (7).
2. **Chronic atrophic gastritis** and intestinal metaplasia are both associated with an increased risk of gastric cancer. In fact, some physicians have proposed a pathway of disease progression from chronic atrophic gastritis (with intestinal metaplasia as a maladaptive response) to dysplasia, then to carcinoma in situ, and finally to invasive carcinoma (8).
3. **Pernicious anemia** is not precisely defined as a risk factor for gastric cancer, but the risk is established. Patients may benefit from periodic endoscopic surveillance.
4. **Ménétrier's disease**, or giant hyperplasia of the gastric mucosal folds, is a rare protein-losing enteropathy associated with a slightly increased incidence of gastric cancer.
5. **Gastric remnant carcinoma** arises in the part of the stomach that remains after a previous gastric resection, usually done for previous benign disease. It is more common after Billroth II reconstruction than Billroth I. Despite the decreasing incidence of primary gastric cancer, the incidence of gastric remnant cancer is rising, probably due to the high frequency of gastric resections

performed in the 1950s and 1960s. One proposed theory is that the high pH in the gastric remnant permits the overgrowth of bacteria that convert dietary nitrates and nitrites into carcinogenic compounds. In addition, bile reflux may also promote gastric cancer. These cancers develop many years after gastric resection; therefore, some physicians advocate endoscopic screening of patients beginning 10 to 20 years after surgery. On one hand, existing data do not justify endoscopic screening of asymptomatic patients. On the other hand, asymptomatic patients who have undergone a gastric resection merit intensive investigation, including endoscopy. Gastric remnant cancer was first described by Balfour in 1922 (9).

6. **Gastric ulcers** are rarely associated with cancer. However, in any gastric ulcer, malignancy must be ruled out. Nonhealing gastric ulcers especially should raise suspicion of malignancy because such ulcers are probably malignant from the outset.
7. ***Helicobacter pylori* infection** has been strongly implicated in the pathogenesis of adenocarcinoma of the stomach. Because almost all patients with gastric cancer are infected with this gram-negative bacillus, it is postulated that the presence of longstanding, untreated *H. pylori* modifies the exposure of other risk factors, such as deficiency in dietary antioxidants, tobacco smoking, or alcohol consumption. This leads to chronic gastritis that slowly progresses to cancer. In addition, certain strains of *H. pylori* may be more carcinogenic than others (e.g., cagA+) (10). Whether adequate antibiotic treatment of *H. pylori* reduces the risk of gastric adenocarcinoma remains to be determined. There is also an association between *H. pylori* and low-grade B cell lymphoma of the stomach. These lesions usually regress with eradication of *H. pylori*, and patients have a good prognosis (11). Although the oncogenic potential of viruses has long been known, the association between *H. pylori* and gastric malignancy suggests that bacteria may also play a role in cancer.

What are some of the molecular mechanisms of gastric cancer?

Our understanding of the molecular biology of gastric cancer is still in its infancy, but some important advances have been made. Several abnormalities in oncogenes, tumor suppressor genes, and growth factor expression have been identified in gastric cancer. The tumor suppressor gene p53 on the short arm of chromosome 17 plays a key role in regulating the cell cycle. Advanced gastric cancers have a higher rate of p53 tumor suppressor gene mutation than do early cancers, suggesting that p53 suppression may have prognostic significance. Overexpression of the *ras* protein p21 has also been found in gastric cancer. In addition, the bcl-2 protooncogene, which plays a critical role in programmed cell death (apoptosis), is associated with gastric cancer.

Abnormalities of several growth factors and growth factor receptors have also been found in gastric cancer, including fibroblast growth factor, transforming growth factor, and epidermal growth factor receptor. Overexpression of epidermal growth factor receptor is associated with aneuploidy, proliferation, and lymph node involvement in gastric cancer. *H. pylori* may help facilitate carcinogenesis. In a single-family cluster of gastric cancer, eradication of *H. pylori* eliminated DNA aneuploidy, p53 expression, and c-myc expression (12). Understanding the molecular basis of gastric cancer will lead to more effective methods of primary prevention, secondary prevention (early diagnosis), and treatment.

If Mr. Lee is of Japanese descent, is he at any greater or lesser risk for having an aggressive gastric cancer?

Although population studies demonstrate a nearly 10-fold incidence of gastric cancer in Japan (75 to 150 per 100,000) compared to the United States (8 to 15 per 100,000), migration studies have failed to show a continued increased incidence when persons move from areas of high incidence to areas of low incidence. In fact, the incidence decreases as new generations assimilate into new environments. However, stage for stage, Japanese–American patients show a better survival than other American patients (13).

What is early gastric cancer?

Early gastric cancer is confined to the mucosa and submucosa and does not penetrate the muscularis. Patients have an excellent prognosis when treated with adequate surgery, with more than 90% of patients surviving at 5 years. As a result of aggressive endoscopic screening, early gastric cancer makes up a larger percentage of gastric cancer in Japan than it does in the United States. In part, this accounts for the better survival of patients with gastric cancer in Japan.

Mr. Lee undergoes EUS, which reveals that the lesion has penetrated the serosa; however, no nodal enlargement is detected. CT scan fails to delineate any adenopathy or contiguous organ involvement, and his liver appears to be free of metastases. His chest radiograph is unremarkable.

Does laparoscopy have a role in the management of gastric cancer?

Imaging studies are somewhat insensitive for detecting peritoneal spread of cancer; therefore, laparoscopy has been used increasingly to stage gastric cancer patients with greater accuracy. Laparoscopy may identify occult peritoneal metastasis, avoiding unnecessary laparotomy in patients with advanced disease (14). Laparoscopy may even be helpful in surgical assessment after completion of neoadjuvant treatment.

Laparoscopic ultrasound may be helpful in evaluating the liver for occult metastases as well. Additionally, a jejunostomy tube can be placed under laparoscopic guidance to provide enteral support for the patient undergoing neoadjuvant therapy. Further improvements in laparoscopic instruments will probably broaden the role for laparoscopy in the management of gastric cancer.

What is neoadjuvant therapy and what is its role in the management of gastric cancer?

Neoadjuvant therapy is the planned use of chemotherapy or radiation therapy or a combination of both before surgery. The good response rates achieved with neoadjuvant therapy for esophageal cancer, combined with the disappointing results achieved with postoperative adjuvant therapy for gastric cancer, have prompted investigators to evaluate neoadjuvant therapy for gastric cancer (15). Possible advantages of delivering chemotherapy or radiation therapy preoperatively are listed.

1. Because surgery produces scarring and ischemia, there is comparatively greater blood flow to the tumor before surgery. This preoperative undisturbed blood flow facilitates the delivery of chemotherapeutic agents and improves the effectiveness of radiation therapy.
2. Resection may stimulate the growth of remaining tumor cells and cause the proliferation of tumor cell clones that are resistant to chemotherapy and radiation therapy.
3. Postoperative complications may delay the initiation of adjuvant therapy and thereby limit its effectiveness.
4. Because most patients with gastric cancer present with advanced disease, either locally or regionally, neoadjuvant therapy may downstage unresectable tumors to resectable lesions.
5. Neoadjuvant therapy serves as an in vivo assay of the tumor's sensitivity to chemotherapy or radiation therapy and therefore more readily predicts which patients will benefit from these therapies after surgery.

What are some disadvantages of neoadjuvant therapy for gastric cancer?

Disadvantages of neoadjuvant therapy for gastric cancer are listed.

1. Chemotherapy or radiation therapy may show toxicity.
2. If neoadjuvant therapy is ineffective, the delay of definitive surgical therapy may result in tumor growth.
3. Increased surgical morbidity and mortality are associated with preoperative chemotherapy or radiation therapy.

Whether chemotherapy or radiation can convert unresectable tumors to resectable ones is an intriguing concept. Whether these response rates translate into disease-free or improved overall survival has not been proved. Furthermore, caution must be used when interpreting data from neoadjuvant trials because of variation in techniques used for pre-therapy staging (e.g., CT and laparoscopy or laparotomy), lack of standardized surgical techniques and histopathologic evaluation, and relatively short median duration of follow-up. At present, neoadjuvant treatment cannot be routinely recommended other than during clinical trials. Further data from well-designed prospective, randomized trials are needed.

What is the treatment of choice for Mr. Lee in the absence of any neoadjuvant protocol?

Resection offers the only chance for cure. Surgery, be it resection or bypass, can also provide effective palliation. Because most patients with gastric cancer have locally advanced or metastatic disease at presentation and because recurrent disease is seen in nearly one half of patients treated with curative resection, other modes of treatment have been intensely investigated.

Preoperatively, perform comprehensive blood work, obtain an electrocardiogram, and adequately hydrate the patient. In addition, direct attention to full bowel preparation and nutritional support.

Bowel preparation. Although CT may not detect adjacent organ involvement, gastric cancer can invade either the colon or the transverse mesocolon (i.e., the blood supply to the transverse colon) directly, necessitating concomitant partial colectomy. Bowel preparation reduces the septic complications of colon surgery and allows the surgeon to perform a primary colonic anastomosis rather than a colostomy. A standard mechanical prep can be given the day before the procedure. In addition, the patient is given nonabsorbable oral antibiotics (i.e., erythromycin base and neomycin) in a timed manner with the oral purgative. Also, because of the achlorhydria in the stomach, some surgeons advocate intraoperative gastric lavage with antibiotics (delivered through a nasogastric tube) to reduce the likelihood of postoperative infectious complications.

Nutritional support. In patients such as Mr. Lee, who have significant weight loss and low serum albumin levels, some surgeons advocate intensive preoperative nutritional support via a nasoenteral feeding tube or with total parenteral nutrition provided through a central venous catheter. However, in the absence of profound malnutrition or the need for a prolonged preoperative evaluation, advocacy for preoperative total parenteral nutrition is limited, and this approach may simply prolong the hospital course and predispose the patient to infection of the central venous catheter.

After giving Mr. Lee a detailed description of the operative procedure and its risks and benefits, he gives informed consent. During exploratory laparotomy, bimanual palpation reveals that the liver is grossly free of tumor and there are no peritoneal implants or palpable adenopathy. The tumor itself is located in the antrum, on the greater curvature of the stomach, and it grossly penetrates the serosa.

How is the appropriate surgical procedure for patients with gastric cancer selected?

The surgical approach for gastric resection of gastric cancer depends primarily on the location of the lesion. Potential approaches include a transabdominal incision, an abdominal incision combined with a right thoracotomy, or a left thoracoabdominal incision.

Proximal Gastric Cancer

Proximal gastric cancer is probably best treated by radical total gastrectomy. This procedure entails en bloc removal of the omentum, the stomach, the first portion of the duodenum, and the surrounding lymph nodes. Microscopic spread of proximal gastric cancer frequently occurs beyond the gross extent of the tumor and may involve a significant portion of the distal esophagus.

Although radical total gastrectomy can be performed solely via the transabdominal route, the surgeon may have to enter the chest to obtain a sufficient esophageal margin. One option is to use a right subcostal incision that extends across the midline with extension through the eighth intercostal space into the left side of the chest. The disadvantage of this approach is that if a high esophageal transection is required, the beating heart and aortic arch severely limit the exposure and make the anastomosis technically demanding.

An alternative is to perform a midline abdominal incision with a separate right thoracotomy, the so-called Ivor-Lewis technique. This affords excellent exposure for an esophageal anastomosis. The extent of lymph node dissection with radical total gastrectomy is controversial, and this issue is addressed later in this chapter. Radical proximal gastrectomy, in which part of the distal stomach is left intact and anastomosed to the esophagus, results in severe alkaline (bile) reflux gastritis and should be avoided.

Distal Gastric Cancer

Distal gastric cancer is best treated by radical distal subtotal gastrectomy. This procedure consists of en bloc removal of the omentum, 80% to 85% of the stomach, and the first portion of the duodenum, at least 3 cm distal to the pylorus and a 6-cm proximal margin. The lymph node dissection is the same as for a radical total gastrectomy.

Metastatic Gastric Cancer

Metastatic gastric cancer is a spectrum of disease from small peritoneal implants to multiple large liver lesions to ascites with contiguous organ involvement and carcinomatosis. In the past, palliative bypass (i.e., gastrojejunostomy) has been the treatment for symptomatic stage IV gastric cancer patients. Recent data suggest that palliative gastrectomy better treats the potential complications of gastric obstruction, perforation, and bleeding. If technically feasible, in a good operative candidate, a subtotal gastrectomy should be performed.

Palliative gastric resection has not been associated with increased incidence of morbidity and mortality compared to bypass procedures in multiple studies. Additionally, it provides a modest improvement in median survival, on average doubling survival to nearly a year. Contraindications include advanced age, significant comorbidities, inability to resect the primary tumor, hepatic or distant nodal tumor burden that will result in short survival, and large (>2.5 cm) peritoneal implants (15).

Who performed the first successful gastrectomy?

Historically, Theodore Billroth carried out the first successful gastrectomy on January 29, 1881, for an obstructing adenocarcinoma of the pylorus. Unfortunately, the patient died of recurrent disease about 14 months later (5).

To what extent should lymphadenectomy be performed for gastric cancer?

The extent of lymphadenectomy necessary for gastric cancer is controversial in the United States. In Japan, an aggressive approach has been adopted, and extended lymphadenectomy during gastric resection has been championed. The routes of lymphatic spread have been precisely mapped, and extended lymphadenectomy is performed to remove not only all lymph nodes at risk but also nodes that are one level beyond those predicted to contain microscopic disease. The Japanese Gastric Cancer Association's staging system categorizes the lymph nodes into 16 regional nodal stations (16):

1. Right cardial
2. Left cardial
3. Lesser curvature
4. Greater curvature
5. Suprapyloric
6. Infrapyloric
7. Along the left gastric artery
8. Along the common hepatic
9. Celiac axis
10. Splenic hilum
11. Splenic artery
12. Hepatoduodenal ligament
13. Retropancreatic
14. Root of the mesentery
15. Transverse mesocolon
16. Para-aortic

Accordingly, the more extensive the lymphadenectomy, the higher the D value of the dissection. A D1 dissection includes stations 1 through 6. A D2 dissection includes stations 1 through 11; D3 includes stations 1 through 14; and D4 includes stations 1 through 16. The Japanese champion D2 dissections. Japanese data indicate an acceptable safety profile and superior outcomes (17).

Large-scale European data have failed to reproduce similar outcomes. In fact, the Dutch Gastric Cancer Group showed 33% and 35% 5-year survival rates for

D2 and D1 dissections respectively. More importantly, there was 28% morbidity and 6.5% mortality for D1 procedures compared with 46% morbidity and 13% mortality for D2 procedures (18). The British Medical Research Council Trial showed similar results. Based on available data, it is recommended that Western countries perform a D1 dissection with retrieval of 20 to 25 lymph nodes (19).

What variations of the blood supply to the stomach should surgeons be aware of?

The stomach has a rich blood supply. The lesser curvature of the stomach is supplied with blood by the left gastric artery, which arises from the celiac axis, and by the right gastric artery, which arises from the hepatic artery. The lesser curvature of the stomach, in turn, branches off the celiac axis. The greater curvature is supplied by the right gastroepiploic artery, a branch of the gastroduodenal artery, and by the left gastroepiploic artery, a branch of the splenic artery.

In addition, the splenic artery sends numerous short branches, the vasa brevia, or short gastric arteries, to the upper portion of the greater curve. There is an anatomic variation in the blood supply that the surgeon must know about when performing a gastrectomy. Occasionally, the left hepatic artery arises from the left gastric artery, and if the surgeon is not aware of this aberrant vessel, ligation of the left gastric artery can result in ischemia of the left lobe of the liver.

Does radical total or subtotal gastrectomy require splenectomy?

The lymphatic tissue along the splenic vessels is a route of spread of gastric cancer and theoretically should be included in any potential curvature en bloc resection. Nevertheless, retrospective data suggest that prophylactic splenectomy offers no benefit and may increase morbidity and mortality (20). However, direct adherence of a gastric tumor to the distal pancreas of spleen must not preclude en bloc resection of these organs.

How is GI continuity restored after resection of the tumor?

After radical total gastrectomy, reconstruction is usually accomplished by a Roux-en-Y esophagojejunostomy. The small bowel is transected at a convenient point distal to the ligament of Treitz. The distal limb of the small intestine is then anastomosed to the esophagus by connecting the end of the esophagus to the side of the jejunum.

The esophagojejunostomy can be hand sewn, but because of limited exposure in this area, an end-to-end anastomosis (EEA) stapler may better facilitate construction of the anastomosis. To restore GI continuity, the transected end of the proximal small bowel is anastomosed to the side of the Roux limb. To minimize bile reflux, this anastomosis is constructed 45 to 60 cm from the esophagojejunostomy. If a radical subtotal gastrectomy has been carried out, a Billroth I anastomosis (gastroduodenostomy), which is often performed for reconstruction after gastric resection for benign disease, is avoided because there is concern that recurrence at the line of duodenal transection will lead to obstruction of the anastomosis. A number of reconstructive techniques attempt to provide some reservoir capacity after gastrectomy.

At exploration, Mr. Lee undergoes a radical gastrectomy and Roux-en-Y esophagojejunostomy. The pathology results show poorly differentiated adenocarcinoma that extends through all the layers of the stomach to the serosa, with 3 of 20 lymph nodes positive for cancer. The margins of the resection are free of tumor.

Which early complication unique to radical gastrectomy must be avoided?

Other than bleeding and infection, perhaps the most feared complication of radical gastrectomy is a leak at the esophagojejunostomy site. Clinically, this may manifest as fever, abdominal tenderness, and leukocytosis. An anastomotic leak in the chest can be catastrophic and requires prompt recognition, immediate drainage, and institution of parenteral hyperalimentation. In spite of aggressive therapy, the mortality from an anastomotic leak remains high.

How soon after surgery can feedings by mouth be reinstituted?

Opinions vary on the postoperative management of patients who have undergone a radical gastrectomy. Some surgeons obtain an oral contrast radiograph, usually on postoperative day 5 or 6, and if no leak is demonstrated, the nasoenteral feeding tube is removed and oral intake begun. Other surgeons defer the radiographic studies and use clinical criteria alone (i.e., no signs of leak and return of bowel function) to determine when oral feeding can be resumed.

What postgastrectomy dietary measures prevent dumping syndrome?

Any operation that bypasses, ablates, or alters the pyloroantral pump mechanism of the stomach can lead to the so-called dumping syndrome. (See Selected Topics at the end of this chapter.) Several dietary measures can obviate this problem. The postgastrectomy diet generally consists of six small daily meals that are high in protein and low in carbohydrate. In addition, fluid intake with meals should be restricted. Generally, dumping is not common after a Roux-en-Y reconstruction, and, in fact, delayed emptying of the Roux-en-Y limb, also known as Roux-en-Y stasis syndrome, may occur if the limb is made too long (21).

What is the most common staging system for gastric cancer in the United States, and what stage is Mr. Lee's tumor?

A precise staging system is required for any malignancy for accurate comparison of various treatments. The most common staging system used in the United States is the American Joint Committee for Cancer (AJCC) tumor, node, and metastases (TNM) system (Tables 8.1 and 8.2). Mr. Lee's stage is T3N1M0 or

TABLE 8.1.

AJCC TUMOR, NODE, METASTASIS SYSTEM FOR GASTRIC CANCER

Primary Tumor (T)

Tis	Carcinoma in situ
T1	Invasion of lamina propria or submucosa
T2	Invasion of muscularis propria
T3	Invasion of serosa
T4	Invasion of adjacent structures

Lymph Node (N)

N0	No regional lymph node involvement
N1	Metastases to 1–6 regional lymph nodes
N2	Metastases to 7–15 regional lymph nodes
N3	Metastases to >15 regional lymph nodes

Metastatic Disease

M0	No distant metastasis
M1	Distant metastasis present

TABLE 8.2.

STAGING FOR GASTRIC CANCER

Stage			
0	Tis	N0	M0
IA	T1	N0	M0
IB	T1	N1	M0
	T2	N0	M0
II	T1	N2	M0
	T2	N1	M0
	T3	N0	M0
IIIA	T2	N2	M0
	T3	N1	M0
	T4	N0	M0
IIIB	T3	N2	M0
IV	T4	N1-3	M0
	T1-3	N3	M0
	T1-4	N0-2	M1

stage IIIA. A different staging system is used in Japan but has not been adopted in the United States (22).

What is the long-term prognosis for patients with gastric carcinoma?

The overall 5-year survival for adenocarcinoma of the stomach in the United States is only 5% to 15%. In the absence of lymph node involvement with tumor, the 5-year survival is 30% to 40%; with lymph node involvement, survival is reduced to 15% to 20%. The survival rates for gastric cancer are superior in Japan. That may be the result of numerous factors, including the following:

1. Inherent biologic differences of gastric cancer in Japan and the United States
2. Mass screening for earlier detection of gastric cancer in Japan
3. Better staging of gastric cancer in Japan owing to aggressive nodal dissection and intensive histopathologic examination
4. Technical superiority of Japanese surgeons with gastric cancer because of their enormous experience
5. The Japanese body habitus (i.e., less body fat), which facilitates a more radical dissection

What is the role of postoperative adjuvant therapy in the treatment of this patient?

Most studies in the United States do not show that there is any clear advantage to adjuvant chemotherapy. In a prospective randomized trial, the Gastrointestinal Tumor Study Group reported an improvement in survival in patients receiving 5-fluorouracil and semustine after curative resection. However, these results were not substantiated by two other prospective randomized multicenter trials conducted by the Eastern Cooperative Oncology Group and the Veterans Administration Surgical Oncology Group.

Japanese surgeons have been much more aggressive with chemotherapy, often initiating therapy in the operating room or immediately afterward. In addition, they have reported some success with hyperthermic intraperitoneal chemotherapy (17). The rationale for the use of intraperitoneal chemotherapy is the high incidence of peritoneal recurrences, particularly with transmural tumors, as in Mr. Lee's case. Also, higher drug levels can be reached in the peritoneal cavity with less systemic toxicity. Hyperthermia enhances the effectiveness of intraperitoneal chemotherapy. These results are preliminary and should be evaluated within the context of a controlled study; therefore, the routine use of adjuvant chemotherapy for gastric cancer has not been proved beneficial.

Is there any role for adjuvant radiation therapy in the treatment of this patient?

Gastric cancer has historically been considered a relatively radioresistant tumor. The dose of radiation that is required is often limited by the toxicity to the surrounding tissues. Radiation therapy delivered after curative resection has no proven benefit. In an attempt to lessen toxicity, some centers have tried delivering radiation therapy in the operating room. This technique requires specialized equipment and therefore is limited to a few major centers. External beam radiation therapy is given as a palliative measure, predominantly for locally unresectable tumors or for recurrent cancer.

What follow-up care should be provided to patients who have undergone a curative resection for gastric cancer?

There are no rigid guidelines for follow-up, but patients are monitored closely for the first 3 years because most recurrences fall within this period. Initially, patients are seen monthly and questioned about dysphagia, abdominal pain, weight loss, and blood in the stools. In addition, physical examination focuses on the appearance of any abdominal tenderness, masses, or ascites, and a digital rectal examination is performed to check for occult blood loss. Laboratory studies may include hemoglobin determinations and liver function tests. Although it has a low yield, a chest radiograph may be obtained yearly.

Some physicians perform a barium swallow study or endoscopy postoperatively to obtain baseline results and at arbitrary intervals thereafter. The opposing view is that postoperative tests that screen for recurrent disease neither are cost-effective nor improve survival and that it is, therefore, more prudent simply to investigate symptomatic patients with barium swallow studies of endoscopy. A consequence of gastrectomy is that the patients lack intrinsic factor and therefore require vitamin B_{12} injections to prevent megaloblastic anemia.

A year after surgery, Mr. Lee develops dysphagia associated with a 20-pound weight loss. A barium swallow study and endoscopy confirm a recurrence of tumor (proved by biopsy) at the anastomosis. CT scan reveals a 4- to 5-cm mass in the area of the esophagojejunostomy and suggests considerable adenopathy around the celiac axis, but the liver appears to be free of tumor. A chest radiograph is also clear. Mr. Lee is still very active, but he can swallow only liquids.

What is the pattern of recurrence of gastric cancer after a presumably curative resection?

Although many patients eventually develop distant disease, local regional disease recurs alone or as a component of treatment failure in as much as 80% of patients after apparently curative resection. Local regional recurrence is a tumor at the site of anastomosis, in the bed of resection, or in adjacent lymph nodes. The reported magnitude of local regional recurrence depends on how it is detected: by nonoperative means, during reoperation, or at autopsy. The stage of the initial tumor influences the incidence of local regional recurrences; lesions that extended through the wall and lesions with lymph node involvement have the highest incidence. Local regional recurrences are associated with a poor prognosis and are rarely resectable.

What are some options for treatment after recurrence of tumor?

Although resection of recurrent gastric cancer is rarely curative, selected patients may benefit from surgical palliation. The goal in the case of patients such as Mr. Lee is to offer palliation to control the dysphagia with the least harm to quality of life. These are the options for palliation of Mr. Lee's symptoms:

1. Surgical exploration with re-resection or surgical bypass (i.e., palliative esophagojejunostomy)
2. Endoscopic pneumatic dilation or laser ablation and placement of an expandable metallic endoprosthesis
3. Palliative chemotherapy or radiation therapy
4. Some combination of these therapies (e.g., endoscopic dilation and stent placement combined with intraluminal brachytherapy and systemic chemotherapy)

Mr. Lee is treated with endoscopic pneumatic dilation and stent placement, which is well tolerated and palliates his dysphagia. Eventually, however, he develops metastases and dies 3 months after the detection of his recurrent cancer.

SELECTED TOPICS

Postgastrectomy Syndromes

The postgastrectomy syndromes are a collection of disorders that are the sequelae of ablation or bypass of the pylorus and of truncal vagotomy. Fortunately, these disorders are relatively uncommon and, when they do occur, can be managed successfully without surgery. However, remedial operations may be required in patients who remain refractory to nonoperative measures.

Dumping Syndrome

Dumping syndrome consists of vasomotor and GI symptoms that follow a meal; it is often divided into an early and a late component. The vasomotor component consists of diaphoresis, weakness, dizziness, and palpitations. The GI symptoms consist of nausea, abdominal fullness, pain, cramping, and diarrhea. Early dumping manifests within the first 30 minutes after ingestion of a meal and is thought to result from rapid passage of hyperosmolar chyme into the small bowel. The resulting fluid shifts cause a rapid decrease in circulating plasma volume and are partially responsible of the vasomotor symptoms. In addition, hormones such as serotonin, bradykinin, and enteroglucagon play a role. Most patients can be managed with dietary measures (i.e., small, frequent low-carbohydrate, high-protein meals, with restriction of fluid intake with meals). Pectin (a gel-forming starch), serotonin antagonists, and somatostatin analogs have also been used to treat dumping syndrome. Operative intervention is rarely required; the best results are obtained with a Roux-en-Y diversion or, alternatively, a reversed jejunal segment.

Late dumping, which is less common, characteristically occurs 2 to 4 hours after meals, with vasomotor symptoms predominating. Late dumping is thought to result from insulin hyperresponsiveness to a carbohydrate load, and profound hypoglycemia ensues. Pectin can also ameliorate some of the symptoms associated with late dumping. Pectin can normalize the glucose tolerance curve.

Alkaline Reflux Gastritis

Alkaline reflux gastritis is associated with epigastric pain and sometimes with bilious vomiting. It is attributed to reflux of bile into the gastric pouch or esophagus. Endoscopy reveals erythematous, bile-stained mucosa. However, the severity of the gastritis seen endoscopically does not correlate well with the extent of symptoms. Some physicians favor the measurement of the degree of enterogastric reflux by using technetium-labeled sulfur colloid. Medical therapy involves administration of bile salt-binding agents such as cholestyramine and metoclopramide to facilitate gastric emptying. Nonoperative measurements of genuine alkaline reflux gastritis frequently fail. The procedure of choice for operative repair is the creation of a 45- to 60-cm Roux-en-Y limb.

Afferent Loop Syndrome

Afferent loop syndrome is manifested by postprandial epigastric fullness and pain that is relieved by bilious vomiting. It is caused by intermittent obstruction of the afferent limb of the gastrojejunostomy after eating. Pancreaticobiliary secretion distends the afferent loop causing pain. With time, the pressure in the limb builds up and is finally released in the form of projectile bilious vomiting. Endoscopy and radionuclide scans can aid in diagnosis. Afferent loop syndrome is often the consequence of an excessively long afferent loop. The treatment is operative, including a variety of procedures such as conversion of the gastrojejunostomy to a Billroth I anastomosis (gastroduodenostomy) or creation of a Roux-en-Y limb of a distal enteroenterostomy.

Postvagotomy Diarrhea

Postvagotomy diarrhea is an increase in stool frequency that occurs after truncal vagotomy. This diarrhea subsides in most patients, but in a few patients it persists and can be disabling. Although the cause of diarrhea is not fully understood, cholestyramine has therapeutic value. Remedial surgery is necessary in a few cases; it consists of interposition of a 10-cm reversed jejunal loop to slow intestinal transit.

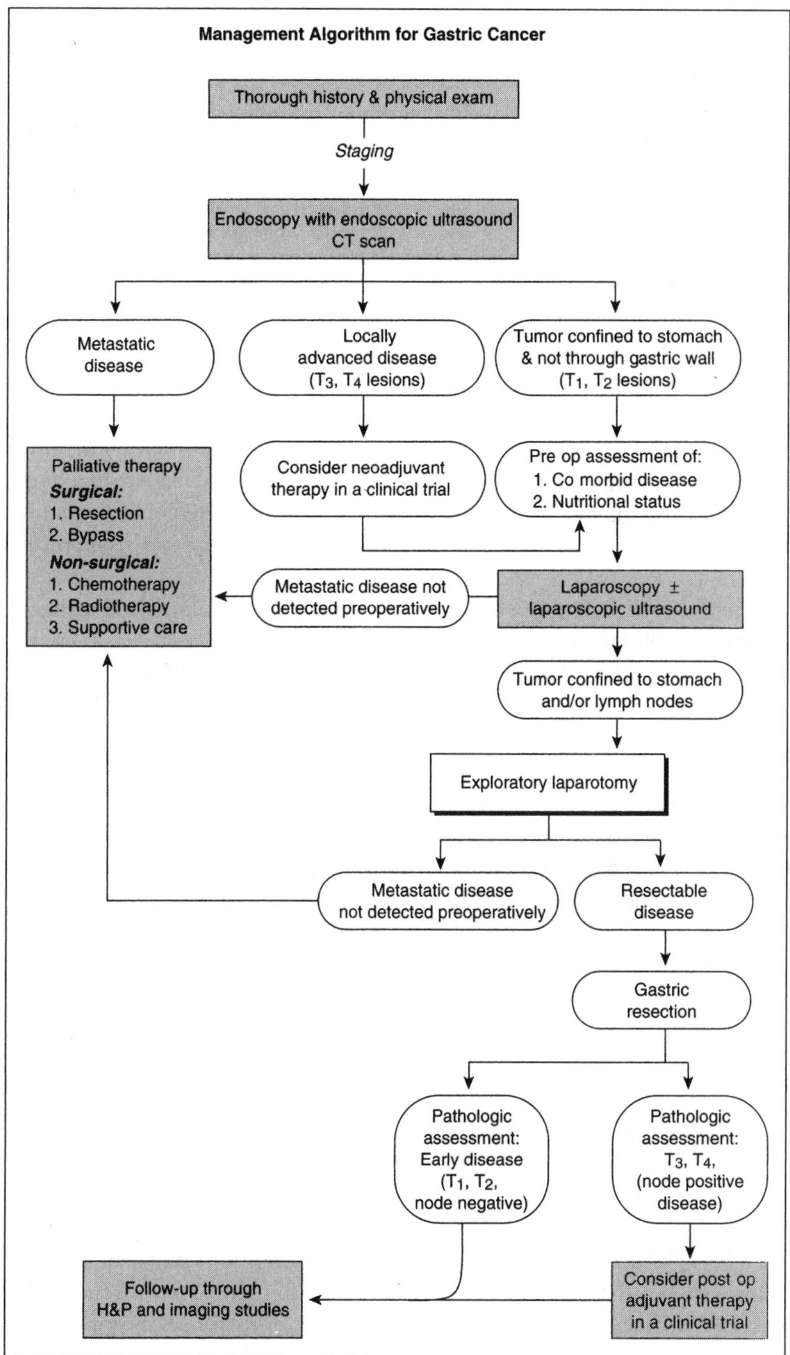
Management Algorithm for Gastric Cancer
Thorough history & physical exam
Staging
Endoscopy with endoscopic ultrasound CT scan
Metastatic disease
Locally advanced disease (T_3, T_4 lesions)
Tumor confined to stomach & not through gastric wall (T_1, T_2 lesions)
Palliative therapy
Surgical:
1. Resection
2. Bypass
Non-surgical:
1. Chemotherapy
2. Radiotherapy
3. Supportive care
Consider neoadjuvant therapy in a clinical trial
Pre op assessment of:
1. Co morbid disease
2. Nutritional status
Metastatic disease not detected preoperatively
Laparoscopy ± laparoscopic ultrasound
Tumor confined to stomach and/or lymph nodes
Exploratory laparotomy
Metastatic disease not detected preoperatively
Resectable disease
Gastric resection
Pathologic assessment: Early disease (T_1, T_2, node negative)
Pathologic assessment: T_3, T_4, (node positive disease)
Follow-up through H&P and imaging studies
Consider post op adjuvant therapy in a clinical trial

Algorithm 8.1.

REFERENCES

1. Jemal A, Murray T, Samuels A, et al. Cancer statistics, 2003. CA Cancer J Clin. 2003;53:5–26.
2. Hohenberger P, Gretschel S. Gastric cancer. Lancet. 2003;362:305–315.
3. Laufer I, Mullens J, Hamilton J. The diagnostic accuracy of barium studies of the stomach and duodenum: correlation with endoscopy. Radiology. 1975;115: 569–573.
4. Insko E, Levine M, Birnbaum B, et al. Benign and malignant lesions of the stomach: evaluation of CT criteria for differentiation. Radiology. 2003;228:166–171.
5. Sawyers JL. Gastric carcinoma. Curr Prob Surg. 1995;32:101–178.
6. Parker SL, Tongs T, Bolden S, et al. Cancer statistics. CA Cancer J Clin. 1996;46:5–27.
7. Hughes RW Jr. Diagnosis and treatment of gastric polyps. Gastroenterol Endocrinol Clin North Am. 1992;2:457–467.
8. Thompson GB, Van Heerden JA, Sarr MG. Adenocarcinoma of the stomach: are we making progress? Lancet. 1993;342:713–718.
9. Pointner R, Wetscher G, Gadenstatter M, et al. Gastric remnant cancer has a better prognosis than primary gastric cancer. Arch Surg. 1994;129:615–619.
10. Lunet H, Barros H. *Helicobactor pylori* infection and gastric cancer: facing the enigmas. Int J Cancer. 2003;106:953–960.
11. Wotherspoon AC, Doglioni C, Diss TC, et al. Regression of primary low-grade B-cell lymphoma of mucosal-associated lymphoid tissue type after eradication of *Helicobactor pylori*. Lancet. 1993;342:575–577.
12. Rocco A, Staibano S, Ottini L, et al. Is there a link between environmental factors and a genetic predisposition to cancer? A lesson from a familial cluster of gastric cancers. Eur J Cancer. 2003;39:1619–1624.
13. Theuer CP. Asian gastric cancer patients at a southern California comprehensive cancer center are diagnosed with less advanced disease and have superior stage-stratified survival. Am Surg. 2000;66:821–826.
14. Yano M, Tsujinaka T, Shiozaki H, et al. Appraisal of treatment strategy by staging laparoscopy for locally advanced gastric cancer. World J Surg. 2000;24: 1130–1136.
15. Kelsen DP. Adjuvant and neoadjuvant therapy for gastric cancer. Semin Oncol. 1996;23:379–386.
16. Pierie J, Ott M. Gastric cancer. In: Cameron JL, ed. Current Surgical Therapy. 7th ed. St. Louis, Mo: Mosby; 2001:105–112.
17. Sugarbaker P, Yu W, Yonemura Y. Gastrectomy, peritonectomy, and perioperative intraperitoneal chemotherapy: the evolution of treatment strategies for advanced gastric cancer. Semin Surg Oncol. 2003;21:233–248.
18. Peeters K, van de Velde C. Improving treatment outcome for gastric cancer: the role of surgery and adjuvant therapy. J Clin Oncol. 2003;21:272s–273s.
19. van de Velde C. The gastric cancer treatment controversy. J Clin Oncol. 2003;21:2234–2236.

20. Cuchieri A. Surgical treatment of patients with invasive gastric cancer: dogma, debate, and data. Eur J Surg Oncol. 1999;25:205–208.
21. Fromm D. Complications of gastric surgery. New York, NY: John Wiley and Sons; 1977:35–49.
22. Stomach. In: American Joint Committee on Cancer. AJCC Cancer Staging Manual. 6th ed. New York, NY: Springer-Verlag New York; 2002:99–106.

CHAPTER 9

OBESITY SURGERY

Mohammad K. Jamal and Eric J. DeMaria

Mrs. Greene is a 43-year-old white woman referred by her primary care physician for evaluation for a bariatric procedure. She has tried several weight loss programs and diet pills without much success.

She has significant comorbidities, including non-insulin-dependant diabetes mellitus, hypertension, degenerative joint disease, and chronic venous insufficiency. She also has sleep apnea for which she uses continuous positive airway pressure at night. She takes several medications including glipizide (Glucotrol), hydrochlorothiazide, and nonsteroidal anti-inflammatory drugs (NSAIDs). Her psychiatrist recently diagnosed her with clinical depression and started her on paroxetine HCl (Paxil).

Mrs. Greene's surgical history is significant for a total abdominal hysterectomy and appendectomy. She has had several right knee arthroscopies for evaluation of a torn meniscus as well as back surgery for a herniated disc.

Mrs. Greene is an obese female in no apparent distress with normal vital signs on examination. She weighs 326 pounds and is 5 feet 4 inches tall, giving her a body mass index (BMI) of 56 kg/m^2. Examination of her respiratory and cardiovascular system is unremarkable. Her abdominal examination reveals well-healed scars from prior surgeries as well as a small, easily reducible umbilical hernia. Her rectal examination is normal, and the stool is guaiac negative. Her lower extremities show changes of chronic venous disease. A preliminary diagnosis of morbid obesity–related comorbidities is made on the basis of history and physical examination findings.

What is the genetic basis of obesity?

Obesity is a complex disease influenced by the interaction of several genetic, endocrine, metabolic, and environmental factors. One of the major breakthroughs in obesity research was the identification of the mutated *ob* gene in mice. The protein encoded by this gene is leptin, which is a glycoprotein secreted primarily from adipose tissue that is thought to be a primary regulator of metabolism. Leptin functions in several ways. It acts as a satiety signaler by suppressing neuropeptide Y expression from the hypothalamus, impairs insulin-mediated glucose uptake in skeletal muscle, stimulates lipogenic enzymes in adipocytes, and alters hypothalamic-pituitary-adrenal balance, all of which contribute to obesity.

Although leptin trials in humans have been disappointing, the findings described have generated tremendous interest in the link between genetic factors and obesity. Elevated leptin blood levels in humans are associated with an increased percentage of body fat, a higher BMI, insulin resistance characterized by high blood pressure, low levels of high-density lipoprotein cholesterol, and elevated fasting insulin levels. Elevated leptin levels may be directly related to increased risk of heart disease.

The human obesity gene and the leptin receptor genes have been cloned, and several members of families with a mutation in the coding sequence of the leptin receptor gene have been identified. Other genetic mutations that may play some role in the development of obesity in humans include those of the glucocorticoid receptor gene responsible for glucocorticoid promotion of visceral fat accumulation, the beta-adrenergic receptor responsible for catecholamine effect on energy metabolism, and the sulfonylurea receptor gene responsible for glucose-stimulated insulin secretion.

How is obesity defined according to the National Institutes of Health (NIH) Consensus Panel on Gastric Surgery for Severe Obesity?

The most accurate way to define the relationship between body weight and frame size is to use the BMI, which is calculated by dividing the patient's weight in kilograms by the patient's height in meters squared. *Obesity* is defined as a BMI of greater than 30 kg per m^2. The 1991 NIH Consensus Panel on Gastric Surgery for Severe Obesity defined *morbid obesity* as a BMI of 35 kg per m^2 or greater with severe obesity–related comorbidities or as a BMI of 40 kg per m^2 or greater without comorbidities. *Super-obese* patients are defined as having a BMI of 50 kg per m^2 or greater. Other definitions of morbid obesity include patients who weigh at least 200% of their ideal body weight (IBW).

What is the prevalence of morbid obesity in the United States?

Obesity is a serious health problem in the United States; nearly 20% of the adult population is obese. An estimated 32.6 million Americans are overweight and 11.5 million are morbidly obese.

What are some of the obesity-related comorbidities and their impact on health care?

Significant obesity-related illnesses include adult-onset diabetes mellitus, hypertension, hypercholesterolemia, obesity hypoventilation and sleep apnea syndrome, cholelithiasis, cardiovascular disease, renal disease, and osteoarthritis. Others include necrotizing panniculitis, hypercoagulable states, and psychosocial problems as well as an increased risk of uterine, colon, and breast cancer. Several obesity-related illnesses may cause significant physical and emotional disability, including overflow incontinence, pseudotumor cerebri, sex-hormone imbalance, and gastroesophageal reflux. Overall, obesity-related illnesses consume nearly 5% of the total health care costs in the United States, a staggering $100 billion.

Does dietary treatment have a long-term success rate in the treatment of obesity?

No dietary approach has achieved long-term success in the treatment of morbid obesity. Two diet pills (phentermine and phenformin) were associated with an unacceptably high incidence of cardiac valvular disease and pulmonary hypertension and were removed from the market by the Food and Drug Administration (FDA). Currently available sibutramine (Meridia) and orlistat (Xenical) are associated with only a 10% weight loss in most studies. Surgery has been the only method proven to maintain long-term weight loss, and current options include restrictive procedures, malabsorptive procedures, or a combination of both.

What are the current surgical options, their associated complications, and the outcome data for the treatment of morbid obesity?

Surgical options for the treatment of morbid obesity can be divided into a combination of both restrictive and malabsorptive procedures or purely restrictive procedures. An example of the former is the Roux-en-Y gastric bypass, whereas vertical band gastroplasty, horizontal gastroplasty, and gastric banding are purely restrictive gastric procedures.

Roux-en-Y Gastric Bypass

This is currently the gold standard procedure. It developed based on the observation that patients who underwent partial gastrectomy for peptic ulcer disease tended to remain underweight. The proximal gastric bypass procedure uses a 30-mL pouch, a gastroenterostomy stoma of 1 cm, and a 45-cm long Roux-en-Y limb. The long-limb gastric bypass procedure for super-obese patients (BMI $\geq$50) involves a 150-cm long Roux limb (Fig. 9.1).

The gastric bypass works both by restricting the amount of food eaten and by intentionally inducing a dumping syndrome that pertains to high-fat, high-carbohydrate liquids. This procedure has been highly successful with several

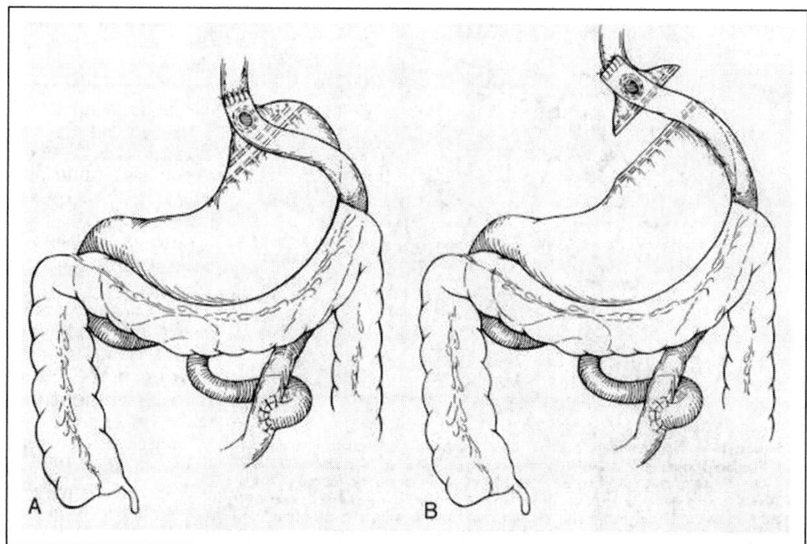

Figure 9.1. Roux-en-Y gastric bypass. A Roux limb, created by dividing the proximal jejunum 60-cm distal to the ligament of Trietz, is anastomosed end-to-side to a 30-mL gastric pouch. The proximal jejunal (biliopancreatic) limb is anastomosed end-to-end to the Roux limb 60-cm distal to the gastroenterostomy. The proximal gastric pouch and distal stomach can be stapled in continuity (**A**) or stapled and divided (**B**). (From Brunicardi F Charles, Reardon Patrick R, Mathew Brent D. The surgical treatment of morbid obesity. In: Townsend C, ed. Sabiston Textbook of Surgery. 16th ed. Philadelphia, Pa: WB Saunders; 2001, with permission.)

large series of patients over a long period who have demonstrated superior excess weight loss (EWL) when compared with patients who underwent gastric restrictive procedures. Long-lasting weight loss is typically 66% EWL at 2 years, 60% EWL at 5 years, and 50% EWL at 10 years.

Several noteworthy complications of gastric bypass include hernias (16%), marginal ulcers (13%), stomal stenosis (15%), wound infections (4.4%), and anastomotic leaks (1.2%). The mortality in most clinical series is low at 0.5%. Other complications include acute gastric dilatation, Roux-en-Y obstruction, vitamin and calcium deficiency, deep venous thrombosis (DVT), and pulmonary embolism. Minimally invasive techniques have similar complication rates except they have lower incidences of wound infections and hernias.

Biliopancreatic Diversion

This is both a gastric restrictive and intestinal malabsorptive procedure that involves a subtotal gastrectomy and ileo-ileal anastomosis (Fig. 9.2). It has excellent

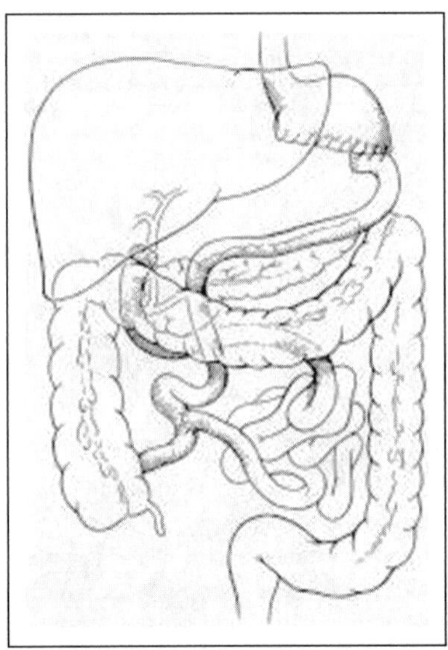

Figure 9.2. Biliopancreatic diversion. After a subtotal gastrectomy, the distal alimentary (Roux) limb, created by dividing the ileum 250 cm proximal to the ileocecal valve, is anastomosed to the 200-mL proximal gastric remnant. The biliopancreatic (jejunum to proximal ileum) limb is anastomosed end-to-side to the distal ileum 50-cm proximal to the ileocecal valve, leaving a 50-cm common channel between the biliopancreatic and the distal alimentary limbs. (From Brunicardi F Charles, Reardon Patrick R, Mathew Brent D. The surgical treatment of morbid obesity. In: Townsend C, ed. Sabiston Textbook of Surgery. 16th ed. Philadelphia, Pa: WB Saunders; 2001, with permission.)

weight loss results with 72% EWL maintained for 18 years. The mortality is low at 0.8%. However, serious complications occur in a vast majority of patients, including severe protein calorie malnutrition (15%), steatorrhea, and fat-soluble vitamin and iron deficiencies (3% to 14%). About 4.1% of patients eventually require reversal to a less malabsorptive procedure. The biliopancreatic diversion may be combined with the duodenal-switch procedure, which includes resecting a portion of the greater curvature of the stomach and dividing the proximal duodenum with a Roux limb reconstruction to the distal ileum. The long-term results of this modification are still under active investigation.

Distal Gastric Bypass

This is a variant of biliopancreatic diversion and involves construction of a 50-mL gastric pouch and a 150-cm common channel. It may also result in severe protein calorie malnutrition and fat-soluble vitamin deficiency. It is currently recommended in super-obese patients with failed Roux-en-Y gastric bypass (loss of <50% EWL at 3 or more years after surgery).

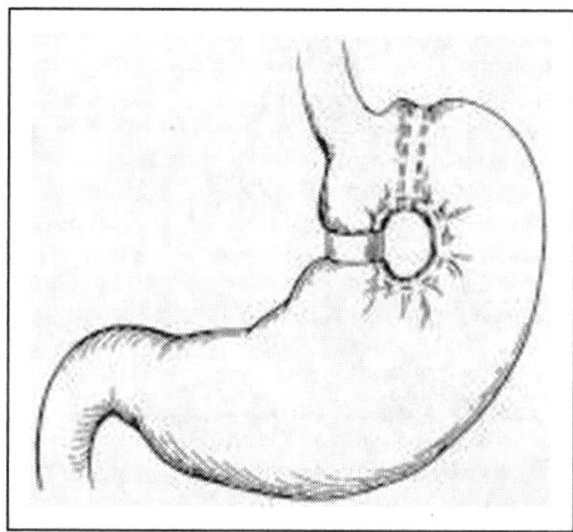

Figure 9.3. Vertical banded gastroplasty. A stapled vertical gastric pouch is constructed by firing a stapler at a point 3 cm from the lesser curve and 6 cm below the angle of His and by firing a linear noncutting stapler between the angle of His and the gastric window created by the EEA end-to-end anastamosis stapler. The gastric pouch outlet (stoma) is reinforced with a 1.5-cm-wide and 5.0-cm-circumference mesh collar. (From Brunicardi F Charles, Reardon Patrick R, Mathew Brent D. The surgical treatment of morbid obesity. In: Townsend C, ed. Sabiston Textbook of Surgery. 16th ed. Philadelphia, Pa: WB Saunders; 2001, with permission.)

Vertical Band Gastroplasty

This purely restrictive procedure with no malabsorptive component involves creating a 14-mL vertical gastric pouch and placing a polypropylene band (Marlex Mesh) around the lower end of the pouch (Fig. 9.3). The surgical variant of the vertical band gastroplasty is the Silastic ring vertical gastroplasty (SRVG). Weight loss is only 40% for the first 2 years, as compared to Roux-en-Y gastric bypass, in which weight loss is 66% for the first 2 years.

Gastric Banding

This procedure involves placing a polypropylene or Silastic band below the gastroesophageal junction using either open or minimally invasive techniques (Fig. 9.4). There are several varieties of gastric banding (e.g., Lap-Band and SAGB) with markedly variable results between European and U.S. investigators. The reported reduction in BMI is anywhere from 27 to 46 kg per m^2. Common complications of gastric banding include slippage or gastric herniation, obstruction, esophageal dilatation and esophagitis, and vomiting. There is a high frequency of re-operations and conversion to other bariatric procedures in patients undergoing gastric banding. Currently, only a few centers in the United States are performing this procedure.

The gastric bypass and biliopancreatic diversion with duodenal switch are currently the most common bariatric procedures performed in the United States using both open and minimally invasive techniques.

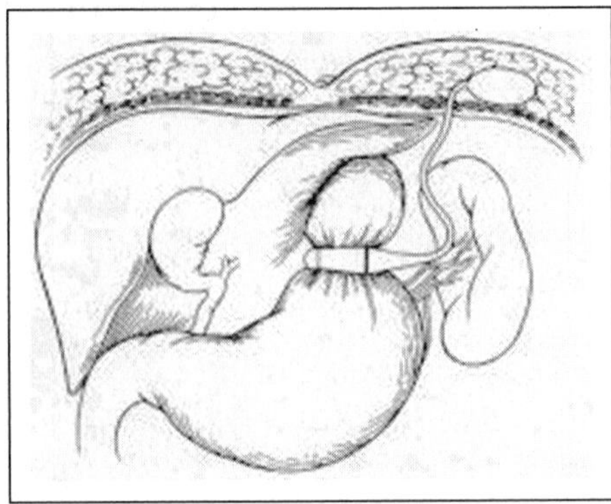

Figure 9.4. Gastric banding. A saline-injectable locking gastric band placed around the proximal stomach. The reservoir is buried subcutaneously and sutured to the anterior rectus sheath. (From Brunicardi F Charles, Reardon Patrick R, Mathew Brent D. The surgical treatment of morbid obesity. In: Townsend C, ed. Sabiston Textbook of Surgery. 16th ed. Philadelphia, Pa: WB Saunders; 2001, with permission.)

What are the essential preoperative investigations before a bariatric procedure?

Bariatric surgery is typically performed in large centers specially designed for evaluation and treatment of morbidly obese patients. The preoperative evaluation of patients undergoing bariatric surgery is tailored according to their symptomatology but should include a thorough consultation with a nutritionist, a psychiatrist, and a medical internist when deemed necessary. Furthermore, upper gastrointestinal (GI) contrast examination, upper endoscopy, and screening for *Helicobacter pylori* should be obtained whenever indicated. If not done already, consider pulmonary function testing, sleep apnea study, and cardiac workup on an individual basis. Screening for sweets-eating behavior is crucial for patients undergoing the gastric bypass procedure because sweets-eaters have a significantly higher failure rate from this procedure. A pre- or intraoperative gall bladder ultrasound is also essential to identify cholelithiasis that would necessitate a concomitant cholecystectomy.

Typical preoperative workup of these patients includes a thorough history and physical examination, hematologic studies (e.g., complete blood count, coagulation profile, basic metabolic liver function tests, and lipid profile), urinalysis, arterial blood gas analysis, thyroid function tests, chest radiograph, and electrocardiogram. Specialized studies for pulmonary, cardiac, and sleep apnea evaluation are performed when indicated. These include cardiac stress testing and echocardiography for cardiac disorders, pulmonary function testing for the obesity hypoventilation syndrome, polysomnography for the sleep apnea syndrome, lower extremity Doppler ultrasound for DVT, and glucose tolerance testing for diabetes.

When are pulmonary function testing and sleep apnea studies indicated?

A thorough history and physical examination will, in most cases, identify the need for these tests. A history of smoking, emphysema, asthma, or bronchitis should prompt further evaluation with pulmonary function tests. A history of snoring at night or excessive daytime somnolence is indicative of sleep apnea syndrome and requires investigation with a sleep apnea study.

Most studies show the incidence of obstructive sleep apnea to be 12- to 30-fold higher in the morbidly obese than in the general population. In obese patients, fat deposition in soft tissues of the neck as well as the oropharynx is the predominant mechanism causing narrowing of the upper airway. Apneic episodes occur as a result of upper airway obstruction, although other mechanisms may be involved. Obese patients are also at risk for the obesity hypoventilation syndrome, characterized by a PaO_2 less than 55 mm Hg, $PaCO_2$ greater than 47 mm Hg on an arterial blood gas, and restrictive lung disease on pulmonary function testing. Hypoxic episodes occurring from sleep apnea and chronic hypoventilation, combined with a decreased total lung capacity and pulmonary compliance resulting from the abdominal adiposity and increased intraabdominal pressure, all result in significant cardiovascular complications. These complications include systemic hypertension, left or right ventricular hypertrophy, pulmonary hypertension, cor pulmonale, polycythemia, and sudden cardiac death.

Mrs. Greene undergoes extensive preoperative counseling and evaluation for a laparoscopic long limb gastric bypass and is subsequently scheduled for surgery.

What are some of the important pre- and perioperative preparations for a bariatric procedure?

The choice of a specific procedure is dependant on the presenting symptoms of the patient and surgeon's familiarity with the procedure. This procedure should be thoroughly discussed with the patient during the preoperative visits and all possible risks and expected benefits of the operation explained in detail.

Standard preoperative management includes antibiotics and prophylaxis for DVT. Other perioperative preparations include adjustment in the doses of medications and anesthetic agents and intraoperative monitoring of peak airway pressures, end-tidal carbon dioxide, and arterial blood gases. Proper positioning of the patient on a footboard with adequate padding at all pressure points is essential to prevent iatrogenic nerve injuries, especially during placement in steep reverse Trendelenburg position.

Mrs. Greene undergoes an uneventful gastric bypass procedure and is monitored in the intensive care unit postoperatively. She is extubated the next morning and undergoes an upper GI series with water-soluble contrast that is negative for anastomotic leak or obstruction.

What is the typical postoperative course after a gastric bypass?

Patients are continued on prophylaxis for DVT and encouraged in the proper use of the incentive spirometer in the postoperative period. An upper GI series is obtained on the first postoperative day to evaluate for anastomotic leak. Following a negative study, patients are started on a clear liquid diet that is typically advanced to a purée on the second postoperative day. Soft-suction drains are removed before discharge. All patients are prescribed H_2 blockers and multivitamins and given six monthly intramuscular vitamin B_{12} injections. Patients with intact gall bladders are prescribed ursodiol to prevent cholelithiasis. Patients are typically seen 2 weeks after surgery and then regularly at 1- to 3-month intervals for the first year and every 6 months thereafter. Regular visits with the nutritionist, the psychiatrist, and the internist are also scheduled for frequent monitoring of dietary patterns and resolution of comorbid conditions.

How do some of the complications of gastric bypass present and how are they managed?

Anastomotic Leak

Although it has an incidence of 1% to 2% in most clinical series, anastomotic leak after gastric bypass is the most feared complication because it has a high mortality. Leaks can occur at both the gastroenterostomy and the entero-enterostomy sites. It is usually difficult to identify anastomotic leaks in morbidly obese patients because signs of peritonitis are delayed until it has developed into an abdominal catastrophe. Patients with anastomotic leaks may complain of mild abdominal pain without actual tenderness, guarding, rebound, or rigidity. Signs including tachycardia with a sustained heart rate of 125 or greater and hypotension are typically associated with an anastomotic leak in several clinical series.

Other symptoms characteristic of a leak include shoulder pain, back pain, scrotal pain, tenesmus, marked anxiety, and an impending "feeling of doom." It is imperative to identify and appropriately manage this condition before hemodynamic collapse, shock, and death. It is also imperative to differentiate this condition from pulmonary embolism because both have a similar presentation in this patient population.

If the patient's hemodynamic status permits, a water-soluble upper GI series is emergently performed to identify the anastomotic leak. Sometimes, despite a negative upper GI series, patients with a high index of suspicion and classic signs of a leak as well as impending hemodynamic instability should be immediately explored and the problem corrected.

Acute Gastric Distention

This problem is usually secondary to development of edema at the jejuno-jejunostomy with consequent build-up of massive gaseous distention, which, if untreated, can lead to gastric necrosis, perforation, staple line dehiscence, and disruption of the gastrojejunal anastomosis. Patients usually present with hiccups, severe left shoulder pain, and even shock. Diagnosis is confirmed with an upright abdominal radiograph following which urgent decompression of the distal stomach is carried out. This can be accomplished either by ultrasound-guided needle decompression or a surgically placed pigtail catheter in the excluded stomach.

Internal Hernia

This generally presents with chronic abdominal pain and symptoms of bowel obstruction. There are three potential sites for the development of internal hernias after a gastric bypass:

1. Through the mesenteric defect at the jejuno-jejunostomy
2. Through the opening in the transverse mesocolon where the Roux limb is brought ante- or retro-colic
3. The Peterson defect, located behind the Roux limb before it passes through the mesocolon.

Patients usually present with repeated attacks of periumbilical pain. An upper GI series may be diagnostic, necessitating an exploration and closure of the mesenteric defect.

Staple-Line Disruption and Marginal Ulceration

The incidence of this complication is quoted to be anywhere from 11% to 19%. Staple-line disruptions typically present with weight gain and marginal ulceration. They are more common in patients who have undergone gastric bypass in continuity as compared to isolated gastric bypass.

Marginal ulcer after gastric bypass is the result of acid production in the bypassed stomach in the presence of a gastrogastric fistula following staple-line disruption. Separation of the gastric pouch from the excluded stomach decreases the incidence of fistula formation and marginal ulcer. Interposition of a well-vascularized organ, such as the jejunum, between the pouch and main stomach is an attractive solution for patients who require remedial operations on the stomach and possibly for primary operations as well.

The ulceration typically occurs at the gastrojejunostomy site and presents with abdominal pain, nausea, and heartburn. An upper GI series followed by an endoscopy are usually diagnostic. An isolated marginal ulcer (incidence of 3%) usually responds to high-dose proton pump inhibitor therapy. However, in the presence of a staple-line disruption, treatment usually consists of re-exploration and takedown of the Roux limb with resection of the gastrogastrostomy and the ulcer.

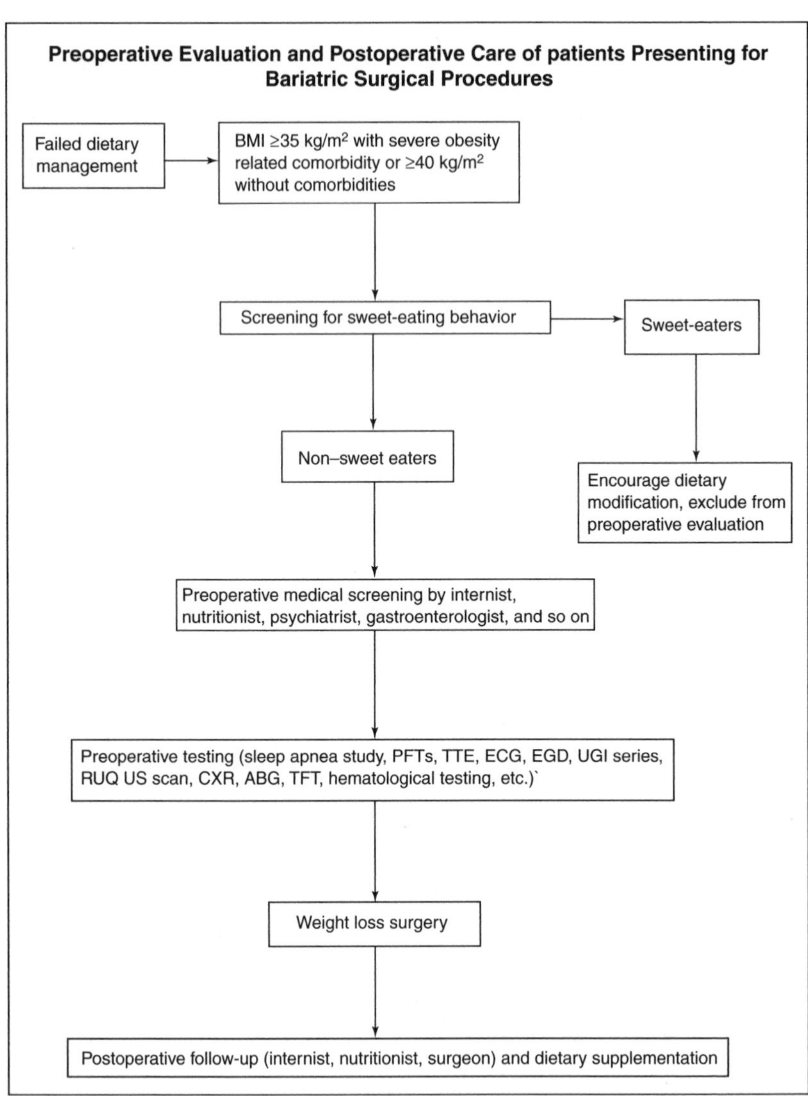

Algorithm 9.1. (ABG, arterial blood gas; CXR, chest radiograph; ECG, electrocardiogram; EGD, esophagogastroduodenoscopy; PFT, pulmonary function test; RUQ US, right upper quadrent ultrasound; TFT, thyroid function test; TTE, trans thoracic echo; UGI, upper gastrointestinal series.

Anastomotic Stricture

The incidence of this complication is about 15%. Stomal stenosis of the gastrojejunal anastomosis usually presents with nausea and dysphagia. An upper endoscopy with balloon dilation of the stricture is both diagnostic and therapeutic in most cases.

REFERENCES

Buchwald H, Buchwald JN. Evolution of operative procedures for the management of morbid obesity 1950–2000. Obes Surg. 2002;12:705–717.

Sugerman HJ, De Maria EJ. Gastric Surgery for Morbid Obesity, Mastery of Surgery. 4th ed. Philadelphia, Pa: Lippincott Williams & Wilkins; 2001.

Shahi B, Praglowski B, Deitel M. Sleep-related disorders in the obese. Obes Surg. 1992;2:157–168.

Brunicardi, F Charles, Reardon, Patrick R, Mathews Brent D. The surgical treatment of morbid obesity. In: Townsend C, ed. Sabiston Textbook of Surgery. 16th ed. Philadelphia, Pa: WB Saunders; 2001.

Vallis MT, Ross MA. The role of psychological factors in bariatric surgery for morbid obesity: identification of psychological predictors of success. Obes Surg. 1993;3:346–359.

Liu YJ, Araujo S, Recker RR, et al. Molecular and genetic mechanisms of obesity: implications for future management. Curr Mol Med. 2003;3:325–340.

Aitman JA. Genetic medicine and obesity. N Engl J Med. 2003;348:2138–2139.

CHAPTER

SMALL-BOWEL OBSTRUCTION

K. Francis Lee

George Chapman is a 42-year-old man who presents to the emergency department complaining of 3 days of crampy abdominal pain, nausea, and vomiting. Prior to the onset, he has had occasional abdominal colic that was relieved by intermittent bowel movement. However, for the past 3 days he has not had a bowel movement, and his abdominal pain has become diffuse and crampy, relieved only by emesis. He states that his vomitus is somewhat foul-smelling and dark green. His last meal was 3 days ago, and he has been having difficulty tolerating even liquids for the past 12 hours. His medical history is significant for appendectomy for ruptured appendicitis followed by intraabdominal abscess treated by percutaneous drainage tube approximately 5 years ago.

What is the differential diagnosis?

The patient's history of crampy abdominal pain relieved by emesis and a previous abdominal surgery suggests that this patient has small-bowel obstruction (SBO) until proven otherwise. Other possibilities include adynamic ileus, large-bowel obstruction (LBO), volvulus, gastroenteritis, pancreatitis, and mesenteric vascular occlusion.

What are the most common causes of SBO?

In adults, postoperative adhesions are the most common cause of SBO, producing up to two thirds of cases (26% to 64%); next are incarcerated hernia (6% to 21%) and neoplasms. Inflammatory bowel disease, diverticulitis, gallstone ileus, and bezoars are other less common causes of SBO (1).

What are the three most salient features of SBO on history, and why is it important to recognize them?

A history of abdominal pain, obstipation, and emesis typify SBO. More frequently than not the diagnosis must be made by history alone because the physical examination and laboratory tests are not diagnostic. A delay in diagnosing SBO can lead to catastrophe.

On physical examination, Mr. Chapman's vital signs are as follows: blood pressure, 140/92 mm Hg; heart rate, 100 beats per minute; respirations, 18 per minute; temperature, 98.2°F. Cardiopulmonary findings are within normal limits. His abdomen is noteworthy for a well-healed 10-cm scar in the right lower quadrant, moderate distention, and somewhat hyperactive bowel sounds. Except for some discomfort upon palpation, there is no significant tenderness or abnormal mass. The rectal examination is normal and heme negative.

Why is testing for blood important?

Heme-positive stool may be an early indication of ischemic bowel. The mucosal layer of the bowel wall is most susceptible to ischemia and may bleed before full-thickness bowel injury occurs. Also, in elderly patients, one should keep in mind cancer as a possible cause of bowel obstruction.

What is the significance of the quality of the bowel sounds?

In the early period of obstruction, peristalsis is increased, and hyperactive bowel sounds can be heard as the intestines attempt to overcome the obstruction. As the bowel distends, reflex inhibition of bowel motility results in a quiet abdomen (2). The quality of the bowel sounds does not help in differentiating between a partial and a complete obstruction.

What are the most common physical findings associated with SBO?

The most common physical abnormalities found in a patient with SBO are those associated with dehydration (e.g., low-grade fever, dry skin turgor or mucosa, tachycardia). Other than distention, the abdominal examination is most commonly *equivocal* (i.e., moderate subjective discomfort upon palpation without a bona fide tenderness or rebound).

Why does SBO not usually produce significant abdominal tenderness? How is this related to the pathophysiology of SBO?

Regardless of the cause, SBO results in either (a) simple distal intestinal obstruction with proximal distention and no vascular compromise or (b) strangulation of bowel or closed-loop intestinal obstruction. The consequences of intestinal obstruction and distention are decreased luminal fluid resorption and increased intraluminal fluid secretion (e.g., intestinal distention, nausea, emesis), overall fluid and electrolyte abnormality from fluid shifting into the interstitial third space, and dehydration, and luminal fluid stasis and overgrowth of bacteria (i.e., foul-smelling vomitus). Intestinal obstruction and proximal distention alone cause crampy abdominal pain. Mesenteric vascular occlusion due to strangulation or closed-loop bowel ischemia causes significant pain but not the same degree of tenderness. It is critically important that severe and increasing abdominal pain, even without significant tenderness, is treated surgically. Waiting for signs of peritonitis such as abdominal tenderness, rebound tenderness, or systemic signs of inflammation (e.g., fever or increased leukocyte count) leads to catastrophic delay, as these signs portend that the ischemic bowel may have already progressed to necrosis or perforation.

The emergency department physician reports that the patient's laboratory test and abdominal radiograph results are pending.

Which laboratory abnormalities are anticipated?

Signs of dehydration from emesis and shifting of fluid into the third space are common, such as mildly elevated hematocrit and normal or upper normal white blood cell count. Blood chemistries may show prerenal azotemia (blood urea nitrogen–creatinine ratio [BUN-Cr] above 20) and hypochloremic, hypokalemic metabolic alkalosis from ongoing emesis of acidic gastric juice.

What are the salient features of SBO on the kidney, ureter, and bladder and upright abdominal radiographs?

Radiographic examination of a patient with SBO indicates (a) multiple loops of distended small bowel in a stepladder pattern, which (b) layer out on the upright film showing air-fluid levels, and (c) absence of colonic air or stool. Other findings, such as free air under the right diaphragm from bowel perforation, are looked for as part of the routine radiographic evaluation.

Is it possible for the abdominal radiographs of SBO not to show any air-fluid levels?

Yes. Sometimes early in the course of SBO, effective emesis and relief of intraluminal fluid can give a normal-appearing bowel gas pattern. Also, completely fluid-filled loops of bowel can give a ground glass appearance on radiograph without the air-fluid levels.

What is the significance of loops of distended small bowel and air in the colon and rectum if they are visible on abdominal radiographs?

Air in the colon and rectum raise the possibility of adynamic ileus or partial SBO.

If the abdominal radiographs show loops of distended small bowel, distended cecum, and colon up to the descending colon, yet no rectal air or stool, what is the significance?

The possibility of LBO increases in the differential diagnosis. However, colonic air does not rule out SBO because colonic air is sometimes seen in the early phase of SBO.

What causes LBO, how does one work it up, and what are the treatments?

Causes of Large-Bowel Obstruction

Causes of LBO include sigmoid or cecal volvulus, obstructive colon cancer, obstruction from inflammatory reactions to diverticulitis or ulcerative colitis, fecal impaction or foreign body obstruction, sliding hernia, intraperitoneal adhesions (e.g., postsurgical adhesions, endometriosis). Children face a host of congenital problems, such as Hirschsprung's disease, imperforate anus, and meconium ileus.

Workup for Large-Bowel Obstruction

In addition to review of history, workup includes rectal examination and proctosigmoidoscopy to look for distal rectosigmoid disease. If the distal segment is normal in the presence of LBO, barium enema or colonoscopy is helpful to determine the more proximal colonic lesions.

Treatments for Large-Bowel Obstruction

The treatments must achieve two therapeutic goals: relieving the obstruction and addressing the underlying problem. For example, in the case of a septic and metabolically deranged patient with obstructive colon cancer, the obstruction can be dealt with by placing a diverting colostomy proximal to the point of obstruction, and the definitive resection may be performed as a second procedure. Or, if the bowel preparation status and the patient's physiologic state are optimal, the cancerous segment may be resected and a primary anastomosis performed. A complete knowledge of the entire colon is necessary before beginning any definitive treatment for obstructive colon cancer. In cecal volvulus, on the other hand, the bowel may simply be untwisted and cecopexy performed. The management of LBO is very different from that of SBO, thus it is important to distinguish the two.

The abdominal radiographs show distended loops of small bowel with air-fluid levels. There is some air, although scant, in the colon. There is no free air under the diaphragm, and the chest radiograph is unremarkable. The laboratory test results are still pending. The working diagnosis is now SBO.

What is the next step?

1. The patient's bowel must be decompressed with a nasogastric tube (NGT).
2. The patient is most likely dehydrated and needs aggressive intravenous (IV) fluid resuscitation. A urinary catheter is inserted to monitor urine output. Boluses of IV fluid are administered until the urine output becomes adequate (0.5 to 1 mL per kg per hour). If the patient is frail and elderly with a complicating cardiac disease, fluid resuscitation is done with central venous pressure monitoring.
3. Most importantly, a decision must be made as to whether this patient requires surgery.

How does a physician decide whether the patient is a candidate for surgery?

The decision to operate depends on the index of suspicion for bowel strangulation, closed-loop obstruction, and ischemic bowel. It is difficult to make the diagnosis of strangulation and ischemic bowel with just history and physical examination.

Clearly, abdominal pain associated with fever, leukocytosis, acidosis, peritoneal sign, and shock are all indications of bowel necrosis and necessitate surgical exploration. Generally speaking, even in the absence of these physical signs, unrelenting and increasing abdominal pain with obstipation and radiographic signs of SBO indicate surgery. Unless there are extenuating circumstances to the contrary, complete bowel obstruction should not be dismissed without exploratory surgery.

What is the difference between complete and partial SBO?

Partial SBO is distinguished from complete SBO by passage of flatus through the rectum and radiographic presence of air or stool in the colon despite the loops of distended small bowel. These indicate partial blockage of the intestines, allowing distal passage of some air and fluid.

Complete SBO is associated with a significant risk of strangulation and bowel ischemia. The incidence of necrotic bowel in patients with complete SBO has been reported to be as high as 30% (3). Patients with partial obstruction have a much lower incidence of ischemic complications. Accordingly, partial SBO may be treated conservatively, whereas a complete SBO requires timely operative intervention.

Does complete SBO always require operation?

Complete SBO does not always require operation. For patients who have had multiple episodes of SBO and who have been successfully managed without operation, it may be worthwhile to try an initial period of conservative management with nasogastric decompression. In such patients, proceed to surgery if pain becomes worse or if obstipation continues for 3 or 4 days without clinical progress. Generally speaking, however, the maxim "do not let the sun set or rise on bowel obstruction" holds true for complete SBO.

The patient undergoes insertion of the NGT and Foley catheter. He receives approximately 1 L of IV lactated Ringer's solution, and he produces 80 mL of urine in the subsequent hour. When the patient is interviewed again, he reveals that he has just passed a large amount of flatus following the NGT insertion. In addition, the radiologist confirms that the patient has some air and stool in the colon. The radiologist asks whether he should perform a contrast study of the upper gastrointestinal

tract with small bowel follow through to confirm the presumptive diagnosis.

What is the role of contrast studies in the diagnosis of SBO?

Contrast studies, which take up to 6 hours of bowel transit time, should never substitute for clinical judgment and should not delay timely operation. However, contrast studies do play a role in patients who have been on NGT decompression for a trial period without significant pain yet have not resolved their obstructive symptoms. These studies also play a role in patients who have been admitted repeatedly for the same obstructive symptoms, even if the patient's symptoms resolve. Overall, however, the role of contrast-enhanced radiographic studies in acute presentation of SBO is limited.

When told that a contrast radiologic study would not be necessary, the radiologist suggests that an abdominal computed tomography (CT) scan be considered because it is accurate for diagnosing SBO as well as many other intraabdominal abnormalities in cases in which the diagnosis is not absolutely clear.

What is the role of abdominal CT scan in the evaluation of SBO?

It is reasonable to obtain a CT scan if there is sufficient reason to suspect specific diagnoses other than SBO.

How accurate are the various radiographic studies in diagnosing SBO?

The overall sensitivity of plain abdominal radiograph is only 66%. Low-grade SBO can be interpreted as normal 21% of the time. Only 13% of complete SBO is interpreted as "definite SBO."

Barium enteroclysis is very accurate. Enteroclysis has a sensitivity of 100% and specificity of 88%. It can also predict the distance and etiology of obstruction in 86% to 88% of patients.

Abdominal CT scan appears to be more inconsistent in terms of accuracy. There have been reports touting that its accuracy is as high as 90%. For high-grade or complete SBO, the sensitivity may be as high as 88%. But for a low-grade SBO, the sensitivity is as low as 48%. Overall, the accuracy has been found to be as low as 66%, with sensitivity of 68% and specificity of 78%.

Considering such inconsistent accuracy with abdominal CT alone, some have advocated the use of CT enteroclysis with the oral contrast infused directly into the intestines through a long NGT. CT enteroclysis is suggested to have an accuracy as high as the barium enteroclysis with the added benefits of visualizing closed loop obstructions and localizing the lesions in a three-dimensional map, a piece of information helpful to a laparoscopic surgeon (4).

The presumptive diagnosis of partial SBO is made and Mr. Chapman is admitted for nasogastric decompression and observation. The nurse asks what IV fluids you would like to use.

How does one determine the IV fluid requirement for a 70-kg patient?
Fluid volume, sodium, and potassium requirements are determined separately. The following are rough estimations (5):

Daily Fluid Volume Requirement

Adults: 35 mL per kg per day × 70 kg = 2450 mL per day
Children: 100 mL per kg per day for first 10 kg body weight (0 to 10 kg)
+50 mL per kg per day for second 10 kg body weight (10 to 20 kg)
+20 mL per kg per day for each kg greater than 20 kg body weight (>20 kg)

Daily Sodium Requirement

Adults: 1.5 to 2 mEq per kg per day × 70 kg = 100 to 140 mEq per day
Children: 3.5 mEq per kg per day

Daily Potassium Requirement

Adults: 0.5 mEq per kg per day × 70 kg = 35 mEq per day
Children: 2 to 3 mEq per kg per day

Caloric Replacement Through Peripheral IV

Adults: 100 g glucose per day produces protein-sparing effects; that is, it minimizes endogenous muscle breakdown so that the body can generate glucose (gluconeogenesis) for the brain during the first few days of starvation (6).

The usual IV solution is 5% dextrose in water with 0.45% normal saline (NS) and 20 mEq potassium chloride at 100 mL per hour (D_5 ½ NS + 20 KCl at 100 mL per hour). This order will provide the following:

- 120 g dextrose per day, which is presumably adequate for protein sparing and minimizing the nitrogen loss and muscle breakdown
- 2400 mL fluid per day, which is adequate volume replacement
- 184 mEq sodium per day, which is more than adequate for sodium replacement (some physicians prefer to give 25% NS instead, which would provide 92 mEq of sodium per day)

TABLE 10.1.

NORMAL CONTENT OF GASTROINTESTINAL SECRETIONS

	Volume (mEq)	Na (mEq)	K (mEq)	Cl pH	HCO_3 (ml/day)	(mEq)
Gastric						
pH >4	2000	100	10	100	0	>4
pH 4	1500	60	10	130	0	<4
Duodenum	100–2000	140	5	80	0	<4–8
Bile	50–800	145	5	100	35	7.8
Pancreas	100–800	140	5	75	115	8–8.3
Small bowel	3000	140	5	104	30	7.8–8
Colon	200	80	30	40	40	
Feces	100	60	30	4	15	
Sweat		40	8	50		

- 48 mEq potassium per day, which is more than adequate for potassium replacement

Thus, D_5 ½ NS + 20 KCl at 100 mL per hour has become the usual IV order for a healthy 70-kg adult patient. However, each component of the IV therapy must change according to the following additional clinical factors:

- Third-space losses (increase fluid and electrolyte requirements)
- Operative blood and fluid losses (increase fluid and electrolyte requirements)
- Specific body secretory losses (increase fluid and electrolyte requirements)

Table 10.1 lists the specific secretory losses that must be replaced with supplemental IV therapy (7).

It is likely that this patient has had a period of gastric emesis resulting in severe salt and water deficit. Depending on the electrolyte profile, the IV order must be modified accordingly from the standard solution. Table 10.2 lists commonly used IV fluid preparations. The nurse also informs the physician that the laboratory has called her to report the following serum test results:

Sodium, 130 mEq
Chloride, 96 mEq
Potassium, 3.1 mEq
Bicarbonate, 33 mEq
BUN, 38 mg per dL
Creatinine, 1 mg per dL

TABLE 10.2.

COMPOSITION OF PARENTERAL FLUID (ELECTOLYTE CONTENT, mEq/L)

	Cations				Anions		
Solutions	Na	K	Ca	Mg	Cl	HCO_3	Osmolality (mO)
Extracellular fluid	142	4	5	3	103	27	280–310
Lactated Ringer's	130	4	3	—	109	28[a]	273
0.9% Sodium chloride	154	—	—	—	154	—	308
D_5 45% Sodium chloride	77	—	—	—	77	—	407
D_5W	—	—	—	—	—	—	253
M/6 Sodium lactate	167	—	—	—	—	167[a]	334
3% Sodium chloride	513	—	—	—	513	—	1026

[a] Present in solution as lactate that is converted to bicarbonate.

D_5W, 5% dextrose in water.

Reprinted with permission from Schwartz SI, Shires GT, Spencer FC, eds. Principles of Surgery. New York, NY: McGraw-Hill; 1994:75.

Hematocrit, 48%
White blood cell count, 9,200 per mL
Platelet count, 354,000 per mL

The patient receives D_5 NS + 40 KCl at 150 mL per hour.

How are this patient's blood chemistry abnormalities summarized?
Mr. Chapman's blood chemistry abnormalities are consistent with hypochloremic hypokalemic metabolic alkalosis due to hypovolemia from gastric fluid emesis and third-spacing (Table 10.3).

What is the significance of the elevated blood urea nitrogen (BUN) and creatinine levels?
A BUN–creatinine ratio greater than 20:1 is typical of hypovolemia and prerenal azotemia.

How does prerenal azotemia differ from renal failure on laboratory tests?
Table 10.4 compares renal failure and prerenal azotemia.

TABLE 10.3.

ELECTROLYTE ABNORMALITIES, SYMPTOMS AND SIGNS, CAUSES, AND TREATMENT

Electrolyte Abnormality	Symptoms, Signs, and Complications	Differential Diagnosis	Treatment
Hyponatremia	Usually asymptomatic if mild ($Na_s > 125$ mEq) or slow in onset. Neuromuscular effects: muscle spasms, hyperactive DTRs, seizures	Increased extracellular fluid: heart failure, renal failure, liver failure, malnutrition	(1) Treat underlying cause. (2) Asymptomatic: water restriction; symptomatic: hypertonic 3% saline (caution: overrapid correction of serum Na^+ level may cause central pontine myelinolysis).
		Normal extracellular fluid: SIADH, myxedema, adrenal insufficiency, hypothyroidism, stress, sickle cell disease	(1) Treat underlying cause. (2) Water restriction with or without diuretics.
		Decreased extracellular fluid: diuresis, adrenal insufficiency, renal tubular acidosis	(1) Treat underlying cause. (2) Saline infusion (total mEq Na^+ needed) = $(140 - Na_s) \times$ (total body weight in kg) $\times (0.6)$
		Pseudohyponatremia: hyperglycemia, hyperproteinemia, hyperlipidemia	Treat underlying cause
Hypernatremia	Thirst, fever, dry mucosal membranes, agitation, seizure, coma	DI (central neurogenic versus nephrogenic)	(1) Central DI responds to DDAVP; Nephrogenic DI does not respond to DDAVP. (2) Oral intake or IV infusion of free water.

continued

TABLE 10.3.

ELECTROLYTE ABNORMALITIES, SYMPTOMS AND SIGNS, CAUSES, AND TREATMENT—*Continued*

Electrolyte Abnormality	Symptoms, Signs, and Complications	Differential Diagnosis	Treatment
		Hypovolemia from inadequate water intake, excessive excretory or secretory free water loss	If hypovolemic, free water repletion. (Correct less than 50% deficit in first 8 hours, then remaining 50% in 16–24 hours. If too rapid, cerebral edema occurs.) If hypervolemic, diuretics and hypotonic fluid.
		Excessive Na intake or infusion (e.g., iatrogenic sodium bicarbonate, IV drug vehicle)	Same as above.
		Hyperadrenalism, hyperaldosteronism	Same as above. Note: Calculation of free water deficit = (Normal body water) − (Current body water) = (TBW × 0.6) − [(140 × TBW × 0.6)/Na_s].
Hypokalemia	ECG changes (low-voltage QRS, T, ST waves; increased P or U waves); weakness; fatigue; decreased DTR; ileus; increased tendency for arrhythmias or digitalis toxicity; nephrogenic DI if severe	Intracellular shift: alkalosis, rapid glucose metabolism associated with insulin administration in diabetic ketoacidosis, β-adrenergic agonists	(1) Treat underlying cause (e.g., alkalosis). (2) Oral or IV potassium repletion (caution if renal failure present).

		Potassium depletion through GI tract (diarrhea, emesis), diuretics, renal tubular disease, hyperaldosteronism	
Hyperkalemia	ECG changes (widened QRS, peaked T waves, first-degree heart block); bradycardia or asystole if severe; nausea; vomiting; diarrhea; weakness	Intracellular shift: acidosis β-adrenergic antogonists, reperfusion tissue necrosis, traumatic tissue necrosis	(1) Treat underlying cause. (2) Exchange resin (e.g., Kayexalate). (3) IV insulin + dextrose 50% water. (4) Sodium bicarbonate. (5) IV calcium. (6) Diuretics if appropriate. (7) Dialysis if acute and severe.
		Pseudohyperkalemia: hemolysis, leukocytosis (>70 K), thrombocytosis (>1000 K)	Same as above
		Renal failure, adrenal insufficiency, spironolactone overuse, impaired renal tubular function, GI bleeding	Same as above
Hypocalcemia	Neuromuscular irritability [hyperreflexia, muscle cramps, periorbital twitching (Chvostek's sign), carpopedal spasm to relative ischemia (Trousseau's sign), tetany, seizure], decreased myocardial relaxation and contractility, ECG: prolonged QT interval	Hypoalbuminenia (normal ionized calcium), acute alkalosis, hypoparathyroidism, pancreatitis, hypomagnesemia, hyperphosphatemia, pancreatitis, sepsis, fat embolism, shock, renal failure, rhabdomyolysis, renal tubular acidosis	Acute: IV calcium chloride or IV calcium gluconate Chronic: calcium carbonate; lactate; glubinate; vitamin D; phosphate-binding antacids (improve calcium absorption)

continued

TABLE 10.3.

ELECTROLYTE ABNORMALITIES, SYMPTOMS AND SIGNS, CAUSES, AND TREATMENT—*Continued*

Electrolyte Abnormality	Symptoms, Signs, and Complications	Differential Diagnosis	Treatment
		Pseudohypoparathyroidism, anticonvulsants (phenytoin, phenobarbital), aminoglycosides	
Hypercalcemia	Stones, bones, moans, and groans: renal stones, osteolytic lesions, bone pains, psychiatric disorders, lethargy, confusion, abdominal pain with or without organ dysfunction (e.g., peptic ulcers or pancreatitis)	HAP SCHMIT, MD: Hyperparathyroidism, Addison's disease, Paget's disease, sarcoidosis, cancer (osteolytic bone metastasis, humoral hypercalcemia or malignancy, paraneoplastic syndrome), hyperthyroidism, milk-alkali syndrome, immobilization, thiazides, myeloma, vitamin D intoxication	(1) Saline rehydration. (2) Furosemide. (3) Correct hypokalemia. (4) Mithramycin. (5) Calcitonin. (6) Glucocorticoids for malignancy. (7) Dialysis. (8) Also, treat underlying cause (e.g., parathyroidectomy for parathyroid hyperplasia).
Hypomagnesemia	Similar to hypocalcemia	Malnutrition (alcoholism, starvation, malabsorption, GI fistulas), GI losses from chronic emesis or diarrhea, burns, pancreatitis, SIADH, diuresis, primary hyperaldosteronism, insulin treatment of DKA, hypoparathyroidism	Treat underlying cause. Replacement therapy: IV $MgSO_4$ or oral magnesium oxide. Monitor replacement progress with monitoring of DTRs and serum levels.

Hypermagnesemia	Nausea, vomiting, weakness, ECG changes (AV block and prolonged QT)	Renal failure, overdose of magnesium = containing antacids, severe acidosis, adrenal insufficiency, hypothyroidism, DKA, severe burns or crush injury, iatrogenic (treatment of eclampsia)	Treat underlying cause (generally, the same as the treatment of hypercalcemia).
	Note on symptoms: (1) Serum levels >4 mEq, decrease of DTR. (2) Level >6 mEq hypotension and vasodilation. (3) Level >8 mEq, respiratory failure.		
Hypophosphatemia	Anorexia; weakness; tremors; decreased DTR; paresthesias; mental obtundation; rhabdomyolysis or hemolysis; impaired WBC, platelet, RBC functions, including decreased oxygen saturation due to decreased 2,3-DPG levels; decreased liver function	Reduced oral intake, nutritional recovery following starvation, alcoholism, acute renal tubular necrosis, anabolic state (treatment of DKA or nutritional recovery following starvation), alkalosis, decreased GI resorption due to vitamin D inadequacy	Treat underlying cause. Administer phosphate as needed [e.g., during nutritional phase following starvation (8 mM PO_4 for each 1000 calories)], IV phosphate if oral is unfeasible; fleets phosphate enema if oral or IV not available.
Hyperphosphatemia	Consequences of renal failure; acidosis, and consequent hypocalcemia; hypomagnesemia	Renal failure, hypoparathyroidism, acidosis, vitamin D intake, increased phosphate intake	Treat underlying cause. phosphate-binding antacid (e.g., Amphogel). Increase renal excretion with saline or acetazolamide. Renal dialsysis as needed.

DKA, diabetic ketoacidosis; DDAVP, 1-deamino-8-D-arginine vasopressin; DI, diabetes insipidus; DTR, deep tendon reflex; GI, gastrointestinal; IV, intravenous; Na_s, serum sodium; ECG, electrocardiogram; SIADH, syndrome of inappropriate secretion of antiduretic hormone; 2,3-DPG, 2,3-diphosphoglycerate; WBC, white blood cell; RBC, red blood cell; $MgSO_4$, magnesium sulfate; PO_4, phosphate.

TABLE 10.4.

PRERENAL AZOTEMIA VERSUS RENAL FAILURE

	Prerenal	Renal
Urine osmolality (mO/kg H_2O)	>500	<350
Urine sodium (mEq/L)	<20	>40
BUN/serum creatinine	>15	<10
Urine/plasma urea	>8	<3
Urine/plasma creatinine	>40	<20

Adapted with permission from Miller TR, Anderson RJ, Linas SL, et al. Urinary diagnosis indices in acute renal failure: a prospective study. Ann Intern Med. 1978;89:47.

What is paradoxic aciduria?

In surgical patients, metabolic alkalosis commonly occurs because of nasogastric suction of gastric acid and other compounding factors. It may appear logical that in the face of systemic alkalosis, the kidney would compensate by actively secreting the bicarbonate ion and resorbing the hydrogen ion, producing relatively alkaline urine. However, the opposite is observed. In the face of hypochloremic, hypokalemic alkalosis compounded by physiologic stress, the kidney attempts to retain water and sodium. In exchange for avid sodium retention, the kidney excretes other cations, such as hydrogen ion, into the tubules. Thus, the urine becomes paradoxically acidotic.

What are the differential diagnoses for hyponatremia and hypokalemia? What are the respective treatments?

Table 10.3 covers electrolyte abnormalities; symptoms, signs, and complications; differential diagnoses; causes; and treatments.

Over the following several hours, the crampy abdominal pain returns and acutely worsens. The patient has stopped passing flatus. Repeat abdominal radiographs show increased loops of small bowel with air–fluid levels and virtually no air in the colon. The patient is now writhing in pain and asks for pain medication.

What should be done for this patient now?

Although patients with partial SBO should have a period of observation on nasogastric decompression, continued evidence of obstruction or worsening abdominal pain necessitates emergent surgery.

The patient is advised to undergo surgery. When discussing the surgical options, the patient asks whether it is possible to perform a laparoscopic

surgery, thereby minimizing additional surgical incisions on his abdomen.

What is the role of the laparoscopic exploration of the abdomen and adhesiolysis for acute SBO?

Most studies of open versus laparoscopic surgery for SBO are retrospective, single center studies with relatively few patients. For emergent, acute cases of SBO, the success rate (without conversion to open surgery) is roughly between 45% and 55%. For elective cases of adhesiolysis without acute SBO, the success rate is much higher, reportedly up to 80%. The success rate appears to be higher when the prior surgical procedure is limited and when the patient has less time of delay before surgery.

However, there is some suggestion of a greater chance for intraoperative complications with the laparoscopic approach. When laparoscopy is performed successfully, however, patients' hospital length of stay is nearly half that of patients with open surgery (8–10).

Open exploratory celiotomy is offered and Mr. Chapman consents.

What is the optimal incision in this case?

When the cause of SBO is unclear and intraperitoneal adhesions are expected, a midline incision facilitates the best exposure and access to all quadrants of the abdomen.

What should the surgeon seek during exploration?

First, the cause of obstruction should be determined. Most commonly, it is due to surgical adhesions. If that is not the case, the physician should search for other causes, such as hernias or neoplasms.

Second, the point of obstruction should be determined. This is the point at which the proximal dilated bowel collapses distally. Sometimes the transition zone is abrupt, as in the case of kinking or twisting, but it can spread over a segment, at which point the cause may be less certain. The possibility of multiple points and closed-loop obstruction must be entertained and ruled out. The entire bowel must be visualized.

Third, evidence of bowel necrosis must be evaluated.

How can viable bowel be distinguished from the nonviable segment?

Although the pink peristaltic bowel is obviously viable and the bluish-black necrotic bowel is easily recognized to be nonviable, it can be difficult to distinguish ischemia from necrosis. The presence of peristalsis, the color of the bowel, and vigorous bleeding from cut edges are all clinical clues of viability. Intraoperative Doppler examination, fluorescein staining, and monitoring of the myoelectric activity of the bowel are all tests aimed at making the recognition of viable bowel easier. When bowel viability is questionable, the bowel may be left in place and the patient taken back to the operating room 12 to 24 hours later for a second look (7).

There are dense adhesions all over the peritoneum that require long tedious dissections to take down. Finally, in the right lower quadrant, clustered scar tissues tightly adhering around the midjejunum are discovered. The adhesions have kinked off the bowel lumen. The transition zone is acute at this point, with the proximal distended bowel and the distal collapsed segment apparent. After release of the scar, the bowel content passes freely into the distal segment. There is no evidence of bowel ischemia, and the rest of the bowel appears normal. While closing the abdomen, the medical student asks whether anything can be done at the time of surgery to minimize the future occurrence of adhesions and SBO.

Do biosynthetic products reduce the chance of adhesion formation?

The use of hyaluronic acid–carboxymethylcellulose membrane (Seprafilm) reduces the severity of dense adhesions following abdominal and pelvic surgeries. Theoretically, this would minimize the future occurrence of SBO. Wide adoption of these "anti-adhesion" products has not been the case, however. The product is expensive, and usually between 4 to 10 units of application are required.

There has been some question as to whether an anti-adhesion product increases the infectious complications. In a large prospective randomized trial, the product was found to be safe with respect to abscess formation; however, fistula and peritonitis occurred more frequently in the group using the product.

Finally, there is no long-term data on the reduction of the incidence of future bowel obstruction. This remains an area of controversy with divergent opinions among experts (11–13).

What are possible complications following surgery for SBO?

Recurrence, postischemic bowel stenosis, and other postsurgical complications such as wound infection, atelectasis, pneumonia, and urinary tract infection may follow surgery for SBO.

What is the incidence of recurrent SBO after the first episode from postsurgical adhesions is treated by celiotomy and lysis of adhesions?

The recurrence rate is probably 10% to 15%, which is higher than the incidence of the first episode.

What is the incidence of developing the first episode of SBO after an initial abdominal surgery?

Over a lifetime, the incidence of developing SBO following abdominal surgery is approximately 5%.

What is the risk of mortality from surgery for SBO?

The risk of mortality depends on the patient's comorbid factors (e.g., age, cardiopulmonary status); the preoperative hemodynamic and electrolyte derangement; and the extent of bowel ischemia, necrosis, and sepsis. Surgical mortality from uncomplicated SBO in a relatively healthy patient is less than 1%. Mortality from complicated septic SBO in compromised patients, on the other hand, can be much, much higher, such that the overall mortality from surgical decompression of SBO averages 9% to 13% (2).

In the recovery room, the patient's vital signs are as follows: blood pressure, 90/50 mm Hg; heart rate, 140 beats per minute; temperature, 100.2°F. He is still on the ventilator and has not fully awakened from long operative anesthesia. The patient is receiving 50% FIO_2 and 700 mL breaths (tidal volume) 10 times per minute as intermittent mandatory ventilation. His urine is dark brown and scant. The recovery room nurse informs the physician of the arterial blood gas (ABG) results: partial pressure of oxygen (PO_2), 160 mm Hg; partial pressure of carbon dioxide (PCO_2), 28 mm Hg; pH, 7.28; bicarbonate, 13 mEq.

What is the acid-base status of this patient, what are possible causes of his condition, and what is the treatment?

This patient has acute metabolic acidosis. (Table 10.5 provides a differential diagnosis.) Most likely, this is due to lactic acidosis from acute hypovolemic shock and hypoperfusion of distal organs. The treatment is volume resuscitation.

After 2 L of IV lactated Ringer's solution, the patient's hemodynamic profile is improved, and the urine output increases to 100 mL per hour. The new ABG is normal: PO_2, 150 mm Hg; PCO_2, 38 mm Hg; pH, 7.38; bicarbonate, 23 mEq. However, as the patient awakens, he begins to breathe on his own in addition to the ventilator. The ABG results are then PO_2, 150 mm Hg; PCO_2, 25 mm Hg; pH, 7.50; bicarbonate, 22 mEq.

What is the patient's acid-base status, what are possible causes of his condition, and what is the treatment?

The patient has acute respiratory alkalosis. (Table 10.5 provides a differential diagnosis.) In this case, the patient hyperventilated as he awoke, and the ventilator maintained its support. The treatment is to decrease the minute ventilation or, in this case, to wean the patient from the mechanical ventilator.

TABLE 10.5.

ACID-BASE ABNORMALITIES

Acid-Base	Primary Change**	Secondary Change**	Effect**	Cause	Treatment
Metabolic acidosis	$\downarrow HCO_3$	$\downarrow P_{CO_2}$	Last two digits pH = P_{CO_2} HCO_3 + 15 = Last two digits pH	High anion gap: KUSSMAL: ketoacidosis (diabetic, alcoholic, nutritional), uremia, salicylates, spirits (ethanol, ethylene glycol), methanol, (par)aldehyde, lactate (ischemia from shock or hypoxia, hepatic insufficiency)	Treat underlying cause. If mild acidosis (pH >7.25), no treatment needed. If moderate-to-severe acidosis (pH <7.20), consider IV bicarbonate injections if absolutely needed.
				Normal anion gap with normal or high serum potassium: exogenous chloride infusion as in TPN, posthypocapnia, rapid hydration and dilutional acidosis, adrenal insufficiency, early uremia, carbonic anhydrase inhibitors (e.g. acetazolamide)	Give 1/2 of acute base deficit and recheck laboratory test. Acute base deficit = 50% × body weight (in kg) × (25 − serum HCO_3).
				Normal anion gap with low serum potassium: diarrhea, fistulas (small bowel, pancreas, biliary), ureteral diversions, renal tubular acidosis	

Metabolic alkalosis	↑HCO_3	↑P_{CO_2}	$HCO_3 + 15 =$ Last two digits pH	Chloride responsive: excessive diuresis (acid loss through kidney tubules) or excessive vomiting (acid loss through emesis of gastric juice), contraction alkalosis, exogenous bicarbonate loading, villous adenoma	(1) Treat underlying cause. (2) Correct hypovolemia with chloride solution (e.g., normal saline). Sufficient for most chloride-responsive causes. (3) Correct hypokalemia with IV or oral potassium as appropriate to renal function, especially if chloride unresponsive. (4) Carbonic anhydrase inhibitor (Diamox) to increase renal excretion of bicarbonate. (5) Slow infusion of acid for chloride unresponsive refractory alkalosis. (6) H_2 antagonist to minimize acid loss through gastric tube.
				Chloride unresponsive: severe potassium depletion, hyperaldosteronism, Cushing's disease, exogenous glucocorticoid injection.	

continued

TABLE 10.5.

ACID-BASE ABNORMALITIES—*Continued*

Acid-Base	Primary Change**	Secondary Change**	Effect**	Cause	Treatment
Respiratory acidosis					
Acute	$\uparrow P_{CO_2}$	$\uparrow HCO_3$	Δ pH, 0.08 per 10 Δ in P_{CO_2}	Hypoventilation and subsequent hypercapnia	(1) Treat underlying cause. (2) Increase ventilation; intubate if needed; increase ventilatory rate, tidal volume, pressure support.
Chronic	$\uparrow P_{CO_2}$	$\uparrow\uparrow HCO_3$	$\leftarrow \Delta$ pH, 0.03 per 10 Δ in P_{CO_2}		
Respiratory alkalosis					
Acute	$\downarrow P_{CO_2}$	$\downarrow HCO_3$	$\Delta HCO_3 = 0.2 \times \Delta$ in P_{CO_2}	Hyperventilation and subsequent hypocapnia	(1) Treat underlying cause. (2) Decrease ventilation; increase dead space (bag partially over mouth in anxious patient); decrease ventilatory rate, tidal volume, pressure support.
Chronic	$\downarrow P_{CO_2}$	$\downarrow\downarrow HCO_3$	$\leftarrow \Delta HCO_3 = 0.3 \times \Delta$ in P_{CO_2}		

P_{CO_2}, partial pressure of carbon dioxide; P_{O_2}, partial pressure of oxygen; HCO_3, bicarbonate; Δ, change; IV, intravenous; TPN, total parenteral nutrition.

**O'Brien Wj. Fluids and electrolytes. In: Berry SM et al., eds. Mont Reid Surgical Handbook. St. Louis: Mosby, 1997:20–31.

The patient is weaned from the ventilator, and as he awakens and follows commands, he is extubated. He receives large volumes of IV fluid for the first 48 hours to maintain adequate urine output. On the fourth postoperative day, he complains of dyspnea. Chest radiograph shows a small left pleural effusion and mild pulmonary edema. The central venous pressure is 15 mm Hg. He appears to be in fluid overload. With IV furosemide around the clock, vigorous diuresis is achieved. While he is undergoing diuresis, the following laboratory results are obtained: Po_2, 75 mm Hg; Pco_2, 46 mm Hg; pH, 7.48; bicarbonate, 33 mEq.

What is the patient's acid-base status, what are possible causes of his condition, and what is the treatment?

Mr. Chapman now has contraction metabolic alkalosis. (Table 10.5 provides a differential diagnosis.) This is a common sequela in a postsurgical patient who undergoes vigorous diuresis, losing both salt and water. Sodium is lost in the

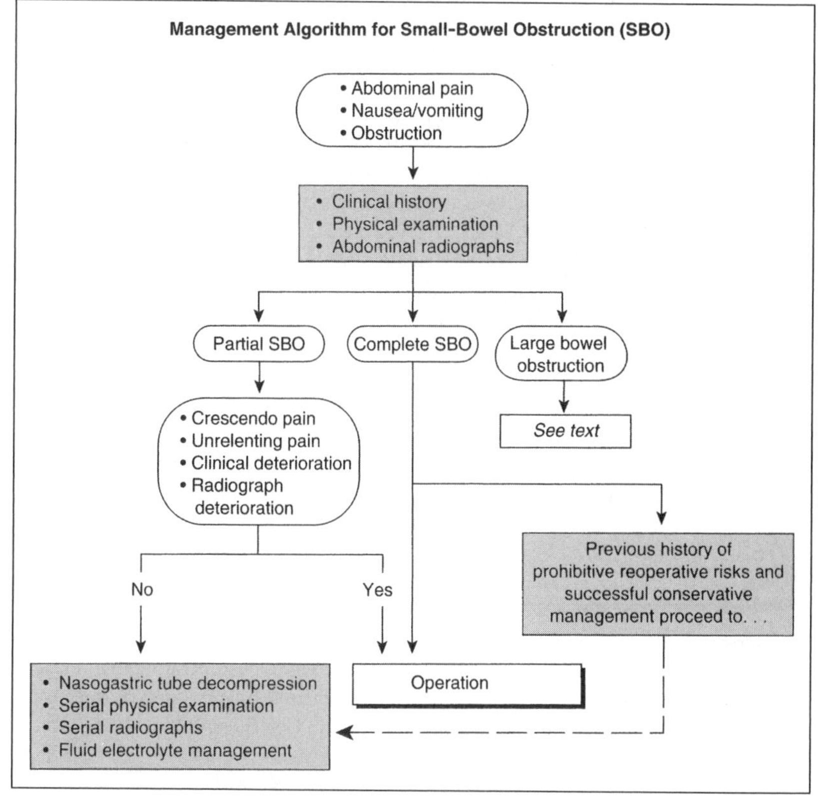

Algorithm 10.1.

proximal tubule, much of which is resorbed in the distal tubule. Resorption of sodium in the distal tubule is counterbalanced by active excretion of hydrogen, which leads to acidic urine and metabolic alkalosis. The treatment is to decrease the diuretic dose, infuse saline as appropriate for the overall goal of volume status, and supplement potassium.

Mr. Chapman's IV furosemide dose is reduced, he receives IV potassium supplementation, and his fluid status returns to normal. He reports flatus on the fourth postoperative day; the NGT is discontinued. He is advanced on diet, and on the sixth postoperative day, he is discharged home.

REFERENCES

1. Ellis H. Acute intestinal obstruction. In: Schwartz SI, Ellis H, eds. Maingot's Abdominal Operations. 9th ed. Norwalk, Conn: Appleton & Lange; 1989: 885–904.
2. Schwartz SI, Storer EH. Manifestations of gastrointestinal disease. In: Schwartz SI, Shires GT, Spence FC, et al., eds. Principles of Surgery. 4th ed. New York, NY: McGraw Hill; 1984:1021–1062.
3. Bulkley GB. Small bowel obstruction. Curr Surg. 1986;43:57.
4. Maglinte DDT, Kelvin FM, Rowe MG, et al. Small bowel obstruction: optimizing radiologic investigation and nonsurgical management. Radiology. 2001;218:39–46.
5. O'Brien WJ. Fluids and electrolytes. In: Berry SM, ed. Mont Reid Surgical Handbook. St. Louis, MO: Mosby; 1997:17–19.
6. Shires GT, Shires GT III, Lowry SF. Fluids, electrolyte, and nutritional management of the surgical patient. In: Schwartz SI, Shires GT, Spencer FC, eds. Principles of Surgery. New York, NY: McGraw Hill; 1994:61–93.
7. Mast B, Dyke CM. Small bowel obstruction. In: Lee KF, Dyke CM, eds. Surgical Attending Rounds. Malvern, PA: Lea & Febiger; 1992:85–94.
8. Levard H, Boudet MJ, Msika S, et al. Laparoscopic treatment of acute small bowel obstruction: a multicenter retrospective study. Aust N Z J Surg. 2001;71:641–646.
9. Wullstein C, Gross E. Laparoscopic compared with conventional treatment of acute adhesive small bowel obstruction. Br J Surg. 2003;90:1147–1151.
10. Navez B, Arimont JM, Guiot P. Laparoscopic approach in acute small bowel obstruction. A review of 68 patients. Hepatogastroenterology. 1998;45:2146–2150.
11. Vrijland WW, Tseng LN, Eijkman HJ, et al. Fewer intraperitoneal adhesions with use of hyaluronic acid-carboxymethylcellulose membrane: a randomized clinical trial. Ann Surg. 2002;235:193–199.
12. Beck DE, Cohen Z, Fleshman JW, et al. A prospective, randomized, multicenter, controlled study of the safety of Seprafilm barrier adhesion in abdominopelvic surgery of the intestine. Dis Colon Rectum. 2003;46:1310–1319.
13. Becker JM, Dayton MT, Fazio VW, et al. Prevention of postoperative abdominal adhesions by a sodium hyaluronate-based bioresorbable membrane: a prospective, randomized, double-blind multicenter study. J Am Coll Surg. 1996;183:297–306.

CHAPTER

APPENDICITIS

K. Francis Lee

Tammy Jenkins is a 24-year-old woman who goes to the emergency department on Sunday evening with lower abdominal pain. The pain started on Saturday afternoon as a general discomfort in her abdomen. She attributed the discomfort to beer and chips she consumed at a football game, but she became concerned when she woke up Sunday morning with a sharp pain in her right lower abdomen. She had no appetite for breakfast and had increasing pain throughout the day.

In the emergency department, her temperature is 37.9°C. Abdominal examination shows a nondistended abdomen with hypoactive bowel sounds. There is involuntary guarding, and the right lower quadrant (RLQ) is exquisitely tender to palpation. The leukocyte count is 11,500 with 78% segmentation. Serum electrolytes, blood urea nitrogen–creatinine ratio (BUN–Cr), bilirubin, and amylase are within normal limits. Kidney, ureter, and bladder (KUB) radiograph shows normal gas pattern without any free intraperitoneal air. Urinalysis is unremarkable. The patient asks for "some pain medication," stating that she "can't stand it anymore," and the nurse nods her head approvingly in sympathy.

Is it safe to administer intravenous (IV) analgesia in Ms. Jenkins' situation?

The concern has always been that IV analgesia will mask an ongoing intraabdominal catastrophe, leading the surgeon to miss the diagnosis and potentially endanger the patient. This dogma has been challenged recently, however. In fact, it has been demonstrated that IV analgesia results in a significant pain reduction without concurrent normalizing effects on the abdominal examination. There is strong evidence suggesting that contrary to traditional teaching, it is, in fact, safe to administer opioid analgesics in the setting of surgical evaluation of acute abdomen without increasing the chance of misdiagnosis (1–4).

Is this presentation typical or atypical of appendicitis?

Typical. Appendicitis typically occurs in people in their second or third decade, is slightly more common in men than women (3:2), and usually affects previously healthy patients (5). The classic pain begins as a dull periumbilical discomfort, then settles in the RLQ of the abdomen as a sharp pain occurring over a short time, as in the present case. Typical appendicitis is often diagnosed by the patient; roughly half of the cases are atypical, however, and can elude even the most experienced surgeon.

What are other possible diagnoses in this young woman?

In addition to appendicitis, there are a number of gynecologic conditions that can cause RLQ pain. These include pelvic inflammatory disease (PID), ectopic pregnancy, ovarian cyst rupture, Mittelschmerz, endometriosis, ovarian torsion, and ovarian vein thrombosis. Other possible diagnoses include Crohn's disease, right colon diverticulitis, cholecystitis, perforated ulcer, and renal or ureteral calculi.

Ms. Jenkins reveals that she has had an active sexual life for the past several months and has had more than one partner. Her last period was 1 week ago. She has had midcycle pain before, but this pain seems to be different. Upon closer inquiry, she also reveals that she has had infections in her abdomen for which she has taken antibiotics. She denies any other gynecologic history, previous pregnancy, and personal or family history of inflammatory bowel disease. She asks if this can be another infection.

What are the salient clinical features useful for differentiation between PID and appendicitis?

In a prospective study of 118 women, several factors were found to be associated with PID: longer duration of symptoms; nausea, vomiting, or both; history of venereal disease; cervical motion tenderness; adnexal tenderness; isolated peritoneal signs in RLQ abdomen.

What is the chandelier sign?

The chandelier sign describes exquisite tenderness of the cervix during pelvic examination.

What data must one always obtain on history and laboratory examination when evaluating a young woman with abdominal pain?

It is necessary to obtain the following information from a woman in her childbearing years who has abdominal pain:

- *Menstruation history:* A suspiciously prolonged menstrual cycle may indicate an ectopic pregnancy. Midcycle pain and mucous discharge may signify mittelschmerz, a syndrome of pain associated with ovulation.

- *Pregnancy history:* A human chorionic gonadotropin (βhCG) level should be obtained to determine whether the woman is pregnant. Women who are in their third trimester of pregnancy may have atypical appendicitis and therefore warrant a high index of suspicion.
- *Sudden RLQ or left lower quadrant (LLQ) pain without significant prodrome:* This presentation suggests ovarian cyst rupture or torsion of the ovary.

What are the anatomic reasons that acute appendicitis may mimic a variety of abdominal diseases?

The appendix is a 10-cm hollow tube attached to the cecum. Its intraabdominal location depends on the way it is attached by the mesoappendix. The symptoms vary according to the location of the inflamed portion and the affected contiguous structures, in the order of frequency: the low cecal position, the pelvic position, and the retrocecal position (5).

What is the clinical significance of McBurney's point, and where is it?

Charles McBurney (1845–1914) was an American surgeon who, in 1889, described the classic location of sharp pain on the spot "very exactly between an inch and a half and two inches from the anterior spinous process of the ilium on a straight line drawn from the bony prominence to the umbilicus" (5).

Pelvic examination does not reveal cervical motion tenderness or purulent discharge. There is some discomfort in the right adnexal area. The physician states that the main differential diagnosis is appendicitis versus PID.

Is it a reasonable option to obtain a radiologic study to increase the probability of a correct diagnosis?

Maybe. Some surgeons maintain that the clinical diagnosis of appendicitis by a surgeon is sufficient without any radiologic study before surgery. The occasional discovery of normal appendix at the time of surgery may be considered an acceptable false positive clinical diagnosis in order to minimize the occasional error of false negative diagnosis that would result in delayed operation, ruptured appendicitis, and associated complications.

On the other hand, ultrasonography (US) and computed tomography (CT) scans have demonstrated efficacy. US has a sensitivity of 75% to 90%, a specificity of 86% to 100%, a positive predictive value of 89% to 93%, and an overall accuracy of 90% to 94%. CT scanning is even more accurate, with a sensitivity of 90% to 100%, a specificity of 91% to 99%, and a positive predictive value of 95% to 97%. For the vast majority of patients who present with typical appendicitis, however, obtaining a CT scan may only delay the time of operation and may prove to be unnecessary in the end. It also adds to the cost of care (6).

What, then, is a reasonable way to incorporate radiologic studies in the diagnosis and management of patients with possible acute appendicitis?

A reasonable approach is to reserve the use of radiologic studies for patients with an atypical presentation or in patient populations in whom the possibility of a misdiagnosis is greater: young sexually active females with high likelihood of PID, pregnant women (US), and elderly patients with confounding factors. For patients with a classic presentation of appendicitis, radiologic studies are unnecessary (7,8).

As the possibility of surgery is being explained to her, Ms. Jenkins wants to know about the option of "video camera surgery through a scope" that she has seen on television.

How does the laparoscopic approach to appendectomy compare with that of the open approach?

Laparoscopic appendectomy is superior to the open approach in terms of decreased postoperative wound infections and recovery time. In a large review, patients who underwent laparoscopic appendectomy were found to be as follows when compared with patients who underwent open appendectomy:

- Are about half as likely to develop postoperative wound infections (odds ratio 0.47, 95% confidence interval between 0.36 and 0.62)
- Have decreased pain on postoperative day 1 by the visual analog score of 8 mm on a scale of 100 mm (95% confidence interval between 3 and 13 mm)
- Have reduced length of hospital stay by 0.7 days (95% confidence interval between 0.4 and 1.0)
- Have reduced time of recovery in terms of earlier return to normal activity, work, and sport by 6 days (95% confidence interval between 4 and 8 days), 3 days (95% confidence interval between 1 day and 5 days), and 7 days (95% confidence interval between 3 days and 12 days), respectively
- Have increased cost of the operation, but decreased cost outside the hospital
- Have reduced rates of negative appendectomies or unestablished final diagnosis

But the laparoscopic appendectomy was inferior to the open appendectomy in the following ways:

- Nearly three times as likely to develop postoperative intraabdominal abscesses (odds ratio 2.77, 95% confidence interval between 1.61 and 4.77)
- Increased duration of surgery by 14 minutes (95% confidence interval between 10 minutes and 19 minutes)

The reviewers concluded that the laparoscopic appendectomy would be advantageous over the open appendectomy in most cases of suspected appendicitis, except in patients in whom laparoscopy is contraindicated or unfeasible, in patients with gangrene, and patients with perforated appendicitis. In these patients, the laparoscopic approach carries a higher risk of intraabdominal infections (9).

In patients with perforated appendicitis, is there an alternative to immediate appendectomy?

Percutaneous drainage and interval appendectomy may be an alternative. If the appendiceal abscess is known to be well loculated and walled off on CT and the patient is not septic, one may percutaneously drain the abscess cavity in lieu of immediate appendectomy, laparoscopic or open, and treat with antibiotics for a few weeks. The patient returns later to have the appendix resected when the inflammation has decreased. Reports indicate a success rate of 70% to 90%.

The benefits of percutaneous drainage under radiologic guidance include precise anatomic identification of complex, multiloculated abscess; avoidance of operation for drainage without appendectomy; temporization of high-risk patients; and temporization of emergency appendectomy for an elective appendectomy (10). Interval appendectomy reportedly has been performed with the laparoscopic approach safely and effectively (11). Not all surgeons support this approach, however, and they continue to prefer open appendectomy and drainage.

The patient agrees to a laparoscopic evaluation in the operating room and possible appendectomy. She was warned of a conversion from laparoscopic to open appendectomy. Before the operation, she asks what will happen if it is discovered that the appendix is normal. Should her appendix be taken out anyway (incidental appendectomy)?

What are the arguments for and against performing an incidental appendectomy during this patient's laparoscopic examination? What evidence supports incidental appendectomy in this patient?

Removing the appendix during a negative exploration is controversial. The argument for incidental appendectomy is that the absence of the organ obviates any future question of appendicitis should the patient develop recurrent abdominal pain. The argument against incidental appendectomy is largely the risk of peritoneal or wound infection, especially during clean procedures in which resection through the appendiceal stump may spill the contents of the cecum.

In a prospective randomized study of 139 trauma patients, there was no significant difference in intraperitoneal or wound infections between the patients who received incidental appendectomy and the control group who did not (12). The factors that would sway the surgeons to perform incidental appendectomy include easy access to the appendix and technical feasibility, contaminated peritoneum (i.e., concomitant bowel content spillage), young age, and the likelihood of future abdominal pains (e.g., history of PID, family history of Crohn's disease).

In this young patient with a strong history of recurrent RLQ abdominal pain, an incidental appendectomy is justified.

The patient undergoes general anesthesia and endotracheal intubation for laparoscopy. With visualization through the infraumbilical laparoscope, dissection of the RLQ is performed through two 5-mm ports in the LLQ and the suprapubis. Densely inflamed tissue and desmoplastic reaction in the right pericolic gutter comes into view. A perforated appendix appears to be densely adherent to the cecum and the lateral abdominal wall. After several futile attempts to dissect the base of the appendix, it is decided to convert to the open procedure. A 5-cm skin incision is made in the RLQ directly over the cecum and appendix.

What layers of the abdomen does an RLQ incision go through?
The incision is made through the following layers in this order: skin, subcutaneous fat, external oblique muscle, internal oblique muscle, transversalis abdominis, and peritoneum.

When the peritoneum is opened, cloudy intraperitoneal fluid is noted. A culture and sensitivity sample of the fluid is sent to the microbiology laboratory. Further dissection reveals a gangrenous appendix with distal perforation in the pelvic brim.

How valuable is the practice of sending a sample of the intraperitoneal fluid for bacterial culture and sensitivity?
Not valuable. In a retrospective study of 308 pediatric patients, the results of routine culture and sensitivity did not lead to improvement in patient management. Only 16% of the patients had their antibody management changed as a result of the culture and sensitivity. However, specific antibiotic treatment based on culture result was associated with increased infectious complications. The use of empiric antibiotics without modification to culture results was associated with a lower incidence of infectious complications, fever duration, and length of hospitalization. The practice of routine culture is not helpful in most cases of acute appendicitis, and empiric broad-spectrum antibiotic coverage should be adequate (13).

What are the differences between uncomplicated appendicitis and perforated appendicitis in terms of morbidity and mortality? What are Ms. Jenkins's chances of developing complications?
The risk of mortality is 0.1% in patients with uncomplicated appendicitis, 0.6% in patients with gangrenous appendicitis, and 5% in patients with perforated appendicitis. With perforation, morbidity increases fourfold to fivefold, and wound infection increases 15% to 20%.

Does perforation of the appendix occur commonly among elderly patients with appendicitis?

Yes. The rate of perforation in the elderly is higher (30%) than in the general population for three main reasons. First, impaired structure and poor blood supply tend to cause early gangrene and early perforation. Second, there appears to be greater hesitancy to proceed with surgery in the elderly, who have high perioperative risks (5). Third, appendicitis in the elderly presents atypically more often than in the general population.

Are there any other patient populations in whom diagnosis of appendicitis is particularly difficult and is associated with increased incidence of delayed diagnosis and perforation?

Yes, there are three other groups: infants and young children, young sexually active women of childbearing age, and pregnant women.

Why is it difficult to diagnose appendicitis in infants and young children? What is the incidence of perforation among children?

The rate of perforation in patients younger than 1 year of age is 100%; below 2 years of age, 70% to 80%; and up to 5 years of age, 50% (5). This correlation to age is because the younger the infant, the less well he or she can communicate abdominal discomfort. Another reason is that many nonsurgical pediatric diseases cause abdominal pain, leading to a greater tendency to delay surgical diagnosis and initially attempt medical therapy.

In children, what are the two most common medical conditions that mimic appendicitis?

The leading differential diagnoses are gastroenteritis and mesenteric lymphadenitis.

How does one manage a pregnant woman suspected of having appendicitis?

Pregnant women suspected of having appendicitis are managed the same as nonpregnant women. Diagnosis and surgery must not be delayed because of fear of the anesthetic's effects on the fetus. A retrospective study of 12 pregnant women with appendicitis showed that delay in treatment is common because of uncertainty in making the diagnosis and hesitancy to proceed with surgery. Patients without perforation had no complications. However, there was a 50% perforation rate, with death of one mother and three fetuses (14).

Does the presentation of appendicitis change during pregnancy?

Yes. The farther along in the pregnancy, the larger the uterus and the more atypical the pain. In the first two trimesters, the pain tends to be typically in the RLQ. During the third trimester, the appendix is displaced upward, and the pain tends to be in the right flank or even in the right upper quadrant (RUQ). Generally speaking, one may assume that in the first two trimesters, diagnosis of appendicitis should proceed in the same manner as in a nonpregnant woman.

With some effort, the patient's appendix is bluntly dissected free from its dense adherence and brought out of the abdomen into the surgical field. The mesoappendix is ligated and divided. The appendix is then resected following double ligature around the stump. The pericolic gutter and the pelvis are copiously irrigated with warm normal saline.

Should a drain be placed in this patient's abdomen during the operation and left? What are the indications for drains after appendectomy?

Leaving a drainage tube is not indicated if there is no perforation, even if the appendix was found to be gangrenous. If an abscess is present, drainage is indicated. In the face of diffuse peritonitis, multiple prophylactic drainage tubes are not indicated; one should drain only loculated areas. The most important measure is copious irrigation of the contaminated area with normal saline with or without antibiotics before closure.

What type of drainage tube should be used?

Most people use simple drainage such as a Jackson-Pratt drain.

What are the various types of surgical drains?

See Selected Topics at the end of the chapter for descriptions of various surgical drains.

There is no loculation or abscess cavity; therefore, a drain is not considered necessary. The peritoneum and the muscular and fascial layers are closed. The subcutaneous tissue above the external oblique fascia is packed with Betadine-soaked gauze.

For Ms. Jenkins's case of perforated appendicitis, what is the best technique for wound closure?

Delayed primary closure is the best technique for closing this wound.

What is delayed primary closure? What are the types of wound closure?

- *Primary closure:* Healing by first intention, that is, to approximate the skin edges of the wound primarily in the operating room.
- *Secondary closure:* Healing by second intention, that is, to leave the wound open for chronic wound dressing changes. Secondary closure usually depends on granulation tissue for eventual skin closure.

- *Delayed primary closure:* Healing by third intention, that is, to delay approximating the edges of the wound by packing the wound with moist gauze until the third to fifth postoperative day, when there is a decrease in the bacterial count within the wound. Delayed primary closure is used for moderately to severely contaminated wounds.

Dressing is applied to the wound, general anesthesia is reversed, and the patient is extubated. As the patient awakens from the operation, she receives IV analgesia and is sent to the recovery room in stable condition.

What step would have been taken if laparoscopic or open exploration had revealed the appendix and the cecum to be normal?

If the appendix appears normal, the abdomen must be explored systematically. The small intestine is examined retrograde for regional enteritis or Meckel's diverticulum. The cecum and the ascending colon are examined for any tumor, especially in older patients. Exploration is much easier with laparoscopy; however, it is possible to explore the majority of the abdomen through the RLQ skin incision. If difficulty arises because of inadequate exposure, the incision must be extended. The pelvic organs and genitourinary system are examined for the appropriate differential diagnoses. The peritoneal fluid is cultured and sent to the microbiology laboratory. In the RUQ, the duodenum and gallbladder are examined. The stomach is examined for ulcer. Mesentery and omentum are examined, as are any enlarged lymph nodes.

What is Meckel's diverticulum?

Meckel's diverticulum is an omphalomesenteric remnant that did not fully retract during embryonic development. It is present in approximately 2% of the population. Within 2 feet proximally of the ileocecal valve, Meckel's diverticulum causes clinical complications in approximately 2% of the patients who have it. It contains ectopic tissue in the mucosa, most commonly gastric cells. The most common complications are ulceration, perforation, bleeding, and obstruction. A narrow-necked diverticulum may be treated with wedge resection, but a broad-necked Meckel's diverticulum may require a full diverticulectomy and ileal anastomosis.

What would have been done if Crohn's disease of the terminal ileum had been discovered in this patient? What would have been done with the appendix?

There is controversy as to whether the appendix should be left alone in the patient with Crohn's disease. Theoretically, appendectomy amidst severe granulomatous inflammation may increase the risk of complication (e.g., fistula formation). However, the literature has not yet clearly substantiated this. If the base of the appendix and the cecum are not involved in the inflammatory process, appendectomy is probably safe.

What would have been done if a tumor had been discovered in Ms. Jenkins's appendix? How often are tumors found in the appendix? What is the most common tumor of the appendix? What is the usual presentation of appendiceal tumor?

The most common type of appendiceal tumor is carcinoid, usually on the tip of the appendix. Carcinoid, comprising 77% of appendiceal tumors (15), was discovered in only 1.4% of 1,000 consecutive appendectomies (16). If the carcinoid tumor is small, a simple appendectomy is adequate; if the tumor is large, a more extensive resection is indicated. A retrospective literature review noted that tumors larger than 2 cm had a much higher incidence of regional metastasis than smaller ones. For this reason, simple appendectomy for tumors smaller than 2 cm and right hemicolectomy for tumors larger than 2 cm is recommended (17). Primary adenocarcinoma of the appendix is exceedingly rare (0.1%) (16). The usual presentation of an appendiceal tumor is similar to that of appendicitis.

Postoperatively, Ms. Jenkins is ordered NPO (nothing by mouth) with IV hydration and antibiotics. The course is entirely unremarkable except that on the first postoperative day, she has a fever of 39.1°C.

What is the differential diagnosis of postoperative fever?

The five W's—*w*ind, *w*ater, *w*ound, *w*alk, *w*onder drugs—is a popular mnemonic for common causes of postoperative fever. In the first 48 postoperative hours following abdominal procedures, atelectasis (wind) is the most common cause because pain prevents deep breathing. Urinary tract infection (water) occurs usually 3 to 5 days after surgery and is associated with indwelling Foley catheters and urinary symptoms. Wound infection occurs later, on postoperative days 5 to 7, and it is usually evident from local signs. Deep vein thrombosis (walk) can occur at any time; it is associated with calf tenderness and swelling. One must also consider superficial phlebitis from IV lines and line sepsis from central venous lines or hyperalimentation lines. Last, hypersensitivity to wonder drugs, such as antibiotics, can cause fever, rash, or pruritus at any time and is easily controlled by antihistamines and discontinuation of the culpable agents. In Ms. Jenkins's case, bacteremia from the RLQ abdomen is another possible source, although her clinical condition should improve after adequate irrigation and surgical drainage.

With vigorous respiratory therapy, including early walking and coughing, Ms. Jenkins's fever subsides. She receives a 3-day course of IV antibiotic therapy. The wound is closed after 4 days without any difficulty. Diet is advanced to clear liquids on postoperative day 2, then to regular diet on postoperative day 3. She is discharged on postoperative day 5 with a clinic appointment in 1 week.

SELECTED TOPICS

Surgical Drains

Each surgical drainage system is distinctive and may be described by a set of three features: location, type, and material.

Location

The location of the drain usually determines its name, as evidenced by the following examples:

Nasogastric tube
Esophagostomy tube
Gastrostomy tube
Duodenostomy tube
Jejunostomy tube
Long intestinal tube
Cecostomy tube
Biliary tube
Nephrostomy tube
Ureterostomy tube
Chest tube

Types

There are two general types of surgical drainage systems, *open* and *closed,* depending on whether the distal end of the drain communicates with the outside environment.

Open Drainage Systems

Most superficial abscess cavities are drained openly; the benefits include simplicity and age-old familiarity. In fact, open drainage of an abscess cavity with simple tubes is one of the oldest and most effective surgical techniques known. A major disadvantage is the possibility of retrograde infection into the body cavity because of free communication with the external environment. For areas where retrograde infection portends a serious complication (e.g., the splenic bed following splenectomy), it is best to use a closed drainage system with the hope of maintaining sterility.

Closed Drainage Systems

Closed systems may evacuate the fluid collection by either gravity or suction. Straight drainage by gravity suffices for some drains (e.g., urinary catheters). However, negative pressure applied on a drainage tube provides the additional benefit of facilitating closure of dead space. For example, the subcutaneous space

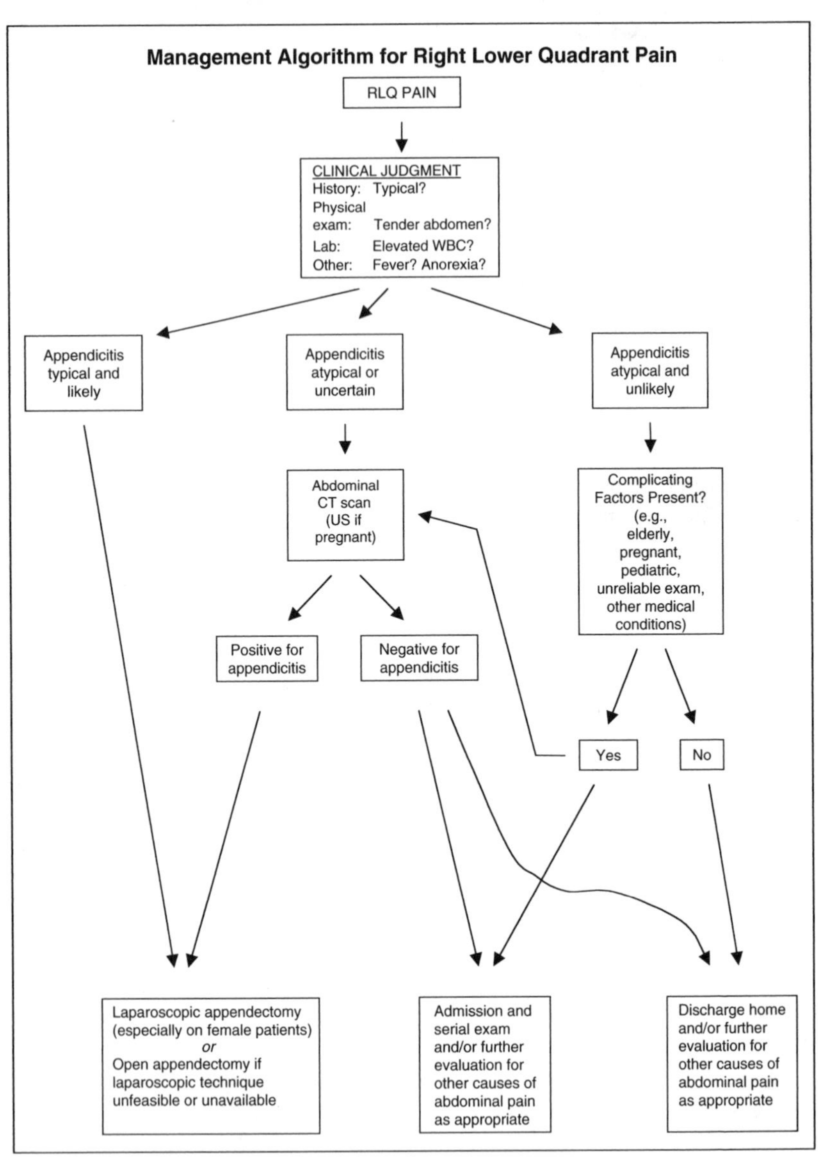

Algorithm 11.1.

in the axillae following axillary lymph node dissection may close and heal better with continuous suction applied to the drainage tubes. A special type of closed system may provide an additional port, enabling one to irrigate the body cavity while suctioning the irrigant. Another special type of closed drainage system may use a water seal at the distal end of the tube to protect against inadvertent influx of air or bacteria into the body cavity. A typical ubiquitous example is a chest tube.

Material

A drainage system is characterized by the material, often named after the company or the inventor. These include Foley catheter, Red Rubber Robinson catheter, Salem-Sump catheter, Penrose drain, Jackson-Pratt drain, and Hemo-Vac drain. If percutaneous drainage of a periappendiceal abscess is necessary, a closed drain system may be considered. In a patient with bladder atony, one may use a closed Foley urinary catheter, which is drained by gravity. A patient with gastric dilation usually receives a closed Salem-Sump nasogastric tube drained by wall suction. A patient with malignant gastric outlet obstruction may receive decompression through a closed Foley-gastrostomy drainage system.

REFERENCES

1. Mahadevan M, Graff L. Prospective randomized study of analgesic use for ED patients with right lower quadrant abdominal pain. Am J Emerg Med. 2000;18:753–756.
2. McHale PM, Lo Vecchio F. Narcotic analgesia in the acute abdomen—a review of prospective trials. Eur J Emerg Med. 2001;8:131–136.
3. Wolfe JM, Lein DY, Lenkoski K, et al. Analgesic administration to patients with an acute abdomen: a survey of emergency medicine physicians. Am J Emerg Med. 2000;18:250–253.
4. Graber MA, Ely JW, Clarke S, et al. Informed consent and general surgeons' attitudes toward the use of pain medication in the acute abdomen. Am J Emerg Med. 1999;17:113–116.
5. Condon RE. Acute appendicitis. In: Sabiston DC. Davis Christopher Textbook of Surgery. Vol 13. Philadelphia, PA: WB Saunders; 1986:967–982.
6. Paulson EK, Kalady MF, Pappas TN. Suspected appendicitis. N Engl J Med. 2003;348:236–242.
7. Patrick DA, Janik JE, Janik JS, et al. Increased CT scan utilization does not improve the diagnostic accuracy of appendicitis in children. J Pediatr Surg. 2003;38:659–662.
8. Naoum JJ, Mileski WJ, Daller JA, et al. The use of abdominal computed tomography scan decreases the frequency of misdiagnosis in cases of suspected appendicitis. Am J Surg. 2002;184:587–589.
9. Sauerland S, Lefering R, Neugebauer EAM. Laparoscopic versus open surgery for suspected appendicitis (Cochrane Review). In: The Cochrane Library. Chichester, UK: John Wiley and Sons; 2004:2.

10. van Sonnenberg E, Wittich GR, Casola G, et al. Periappendiceal abscesses: percutaneous drainage. Radiology. 1987;163:23–26.
11. Vargas HI, Averbook A, Stamos MJ. Appendiceal mass: conservative therapy followed by interval laparoscopic appendectomy. Am Surg. 1994;60:753–758.
12. Strom PR, Turkleson ML, Stone HH. Safety of incidental appendectomy. Am J Surg. 1983;145:819–822.
13. Kokoska ER, Silen ML, Tracy TF, et al. The impact of intraoperative culture on treatment and outcome in children with perforated appendicitis. J Pediatr Surg. 1999;34:749–753.
14. Horowitz MD, Gomez GA, Santiesteban R, et al. Acute appendicitis during pregnancy: diagnosis and management. Arch Surg. 1985;120:1362–1367.
15. Dunn JP. Carcinoid tumors of the appendix: 21 cases with a review of the literature. N Z Med J. 1982;95:73–76.
16. Dymock RB. Pathological changes in the appendix: a review of 1000 cases. Pathology. 1977;9:331–339.
17. Thirlby RC, Kasper CS, Jones RC. Metastatic carcinoid tumor of the appendix: report of a case and review of the literature. Dis Colon Rectum. 1984;27:42–46.

CHAPTER

12

INFLAMMATORY BOWEL DISEASE

Jan Wojcik

CROHN'S DISEASE

Debra Goldberg is a 34-year-old unemployed woman with a history of psychiatric illnesses. She arrives in the emergency department complaining of several months of intermittent abdominal pain, which has become more severe during the past several weeks. It occurs postprandially throughout the lower abdomen but appears to be mainly right sided. The pain is crampy and is usually associated with nausea. She reports the presence of loose bowel movements during the past 6 months. A review of systems reveals a moderate weight loss, increased malaise, and fatigue during the same period.

Physical examination reveals a thin, somewhat gaunt young woman who is normotensive and afebrile. The abdomen is mildly distended, and a sense of fullness is appreciated in the right lower quadrant. The bowel sounds appear to be hyperactive. Rectal digital examination reveals guaiac-positive stool and no masses. The laboratory values are remarkable for an elevated white blood cell (WBC) count of 15,300 mL^{-1}, hematocrit of 31.1 mg per dL, an albumin level of 2.6 g per dL, and an erythrocyte sedimentation rate of 59 mm per hour.

Plain radiographs of the abdomen reveal several moderately dilated loops of small intestine with rare air–fluid levels and air in the colon. A subsequent barium enema reveals a normal colon but a significant stricture in the distal ileum, which is proximally dilated.

What is the most likely diagnosis? How was this disease initially described?
At the 1932 meeting of the American Medical Association, Burrill B. Crohn described 14 cases of what he termed *terminal ileitis.* Later that year, 52 cases were

reported in a classic paper by Crohn et al. (1). Its traditional name in American literature is *regional enteritis;* in Britain it is called *Crohn's disease* (CD). CD of the colon was first recognized as a separate entity by Lochart-Mummery and Morson in 1960 (2).

What causes CD?

Although many investigators have sought an infectious agent in CD, there has never been any conclusive evidence that such an agent will ever be isolated. For many years, there has been speculation that the immune system may be involved in the pathogenesis of the disease.

D.C. is told that she may have inflammatory bowel disease. She reports that one of her nursing school friends has ulcerative colitis.

In terms of causation, how is ulcerative colitis (UC) different from CD?

UC may be caused by a transmissible agent that results in a theoretic immunologic response in the colon, although nobody has been able to elucidate a possible agent. Patients with UC also have a defect in the protective mucous glycoprotein secretion that is not present in patients with CD (3).

Is there a genetic component in either CD or UC?

In reported series of CD patients, the percentage of people with a family history is 10% to 20% (4). The proband concordance rate among monozygous twins is 54% for CD. Heredity may be quite strong in those who develop CD before early adulthood. The hereditary link is much stronger in UC. More recently, much attention has been focused on splitting CD back into subgroups defined by clinical features such as anatomic location of disease, extent of disease, and disease behavior (i.e., inflammatory, fistulizing, or fibrostenotic). High concordance rates for anatomic location of CD and disease behavior have been reported in CD-affected relatives, suggesting that these clinical features may be genetically determined (5).

Does CD occur more frequently in some parts of the world than in others?

CD is common in northwestern Europe and North America. Low prevalence rates are reported in Hispanics and Asians. Areas of low incidence include Japan and southern Europe. CD is infrequent in South America, Asia, and tropical Africa.

Is the geographic distribution of UC similar?

Yes, UC is most common in Scandinavia, the United States, Great Britain, Australia, New Zealand, and South Africa. In addition, UC appears five times as often in Jews as in non-Jews living in Western countries. As with CD, there is a predilection for women, and there is a bimodal age distribution, with the greatest peak in the second and third decades and a minor peak in the elderly (6,7). The term *ulcerative colitis* was in common use by the end of the Civil War. In 1885, Pitt and Durham described pseudopolyps as a complication of UC.

D.C. becomes a bit anxious and asks for specific details about CD.

What are the anatomic features of CD?

The hallmark of CD is its segmental distribution in the terminal ileum, often with rectal sparing but frequently with perianal disease. The transmural nature of the inflammatory process is characterized by deep fissures that penetrate adjacent structures, causing abscesses and fistulas. Fat wrapping of involved bowel segments and mesenteric lymphadenopathy are common stigmata. The principal microscopic features are noncaseating granulomas with multinucleate giant cells, microabscesses, fissures, a chronic inflammatory cell infiltrate, lymphoid hyperplasia, edema, and fibrosis. Identification of noncaseating granulomas is possible in 70% of patients; in the remaining 30%, the diagnosis is made by a combination of overall gross and microscopic features.

How is this different from UC?

Unlike CD, UC is a continuous disease, maximally involving the rectum and spreading proximally. There are no true skip lesions; the involved segment in UC is contagious; and areas that may appear normal on endoscopic examination are always abnormal when examined microscopically. In 10% to 20% of patients with pancolitis, the ileum is also involved in a process that is indistinguishable from the colonic disease for 5 to 15 cm. UC is predominantly a mucosal disease characterized by epithelial ulceration and regeneration. In active disease, polymorphonuclear infiltration with crypt abscesses is the hallmark of the disease. Depletion of the goblet cell mucin is characteristic, and its extent is related to the severity of the disease.

Clinically, how does one differentiate CD from UC?

The features characteristic of CD in the large intestine are rectal sparing; distal ileal involvement; focal aphthous ulcers; deep ulceration with a cobblestone pattern; and fistula, abscess, or stricture. In contrast, UC produces intermittent attacks of rectal bleeding in combination with granular mucosal disease.

What is the natural history of CD?

CD, unlike UC, rarely goes into complete remission. Once the disease becomes symptomatic, it tends to progress to its hallmark complications of obstruction, local sepsis, and fistulas. Patients with inactive disease may develop the mechanical complications but not usually sepsis, and the course of the disease is relatively benign. Active disease is associated with florid and diffuse small-bowel disease or active colitis that has associated metabolic sequelae and sepsis.

The survival rate in patients with CD does not differ from that of the general population. Chronic active small-bowel disease tends to progress toward obstruction. The most common presentation of colonic disease is diarrhea and weight loss. Anorectal strictures tend to be progressive and may eventually require proctectomy. Anorectal fistulas have a variable course. Recurrence of CD is almost inevitable, and recurrent disease tends to have the same presentation as the original episode. Recurrence is more common in perforating disease than in nonperforating (i.e., obstruction, bleeding) disease.

D.C. asks whether there was evidence of obstruction on the barium enema study and what the radiograph showed. She is told that a mild to moderate degree of obstruction was seen in the terminal ileum, along with several other radiographic features.

What are the radiographic features of CD?

CD is usually demonstrated by the use of contrast radiographs. The diagnosis of small-bowel disease is best demonstrated either by upper gastrointestinal contrast study with modified follow-through examinations or by use of enteroclysis studies. The classic string sign is usually from edema and spasm rather than fibrosis. Colonic disease can be demonstrated by double contrast studies. The general radiologic features can be best summarized as edema, ulceration, fibrosis, and fistulas. Fistulas are more common in small-bowel than in large-bowel disease. Traditionally, colonic CD affects the proximal colon, usually with ileal involvement. Approximately 50% of patients with CD have rectal disease. The coalescence of ulcerated areas leads to the formation of the cobblestone pattern. The terminal ileum is involved in 50% to 70% of patients with Crohn's colitis. Strictures in CD tend to have tapered margins in contrast with carcinomas, which have abrupt narrowing.

What are the radiographic features of UC?

Plain radiographs can be useful in patients with acute fulminant colitis, in whom the affected segments of the colon are widened and distended with air. Toxic megacolon usually affects the transverse colon, but it also may involve the sigmoid colon. Contrast radiology should never be used in patients with acute colitis because of concerns about septicemia, perforation, and megacolon. The earliest radiographic changes are an irregular mucosal line that is thick and indistinct.

As the disease progresses, more severe superficial ulcerations or erosions appear. The presence and extent of ulceration correlates well with the disease activity. Eventually, the denuded mucosa is replaced by granulation tissue, leaving only islands of intact mucosa. These pseudopolyps are the result of severe colitis; they indicate an inflammatory process and virtually never become malignant. Although the rectum is usually the most involved structure, there is some relative rectal sparing in 20% of patients. Any stricture must be differentiated as benign or malignant.

What are the typical endoscopic features of CD?

Endoscopy shows the mucosal surface in CD as granular or nodular with friability, erosions, and aphthous ulcers. Discontinuous disease, especially with aphthous ulceration or serpiginous linear ulceration, is pathognomonic of Crohn's colitis. Aphthous ulceration is believed to be the first macroscopically recognizable sign of CD. Deep linear ulcers give rise to a cobblestone pattern. True cobblestoning occurs only in patients with CD. As a general rule, cobblestoning, discontinuous disease, and anal lesions suggest CD.

How does this contrast with the findings in UC?

Endoscopy is essential for obtaining biopsies and making the diagnosis of UC. The findings at endoscopy are usually more pronounced than can be seen radiographically.

Is it always possible to classify a patient as having either CD or UC?

No. Despite the differences outlined, in approximately 10% to 15% of cases there is doubt about diagnosis. Eventually, the patient's history dictates the final diagnosis. Recurrence in the small bowel, perianal disease, fistulas, and abscesses are hallmarks of CD, regardless of what the original biopsies may have indicated.

The patient is encouraged to start medications right away.

What is the appropriate initial therapy for CD?

Medical therapy is the first-line treatment in patients with uncomplicated CD. Corticosteroids have been beneficial for acute CD. Azathioprine and 6-mercaptopurine have a steroid-sparing effect that may require months before the effect can be noted. Cyclosporine also has been shown to be somewhat useful in maintaining remission. Metronidazole has been used extensively in patients with perianal disease and to a certain extent in those with left-sided colonic disease (8). Sulfasalazine has a limited role in Crohn's colitis and no therapeutic benefit for ileal CD. It does not appear to have a corticosteroid-sparing effect. Adverse reactions to the sulfapyridine moiety of sulfasalazine occur in 15% of patients.

How does medical therapy differ for patients with UC?

As with Crohn's colonic disease, steroid therapy is initiated to control the disease, and as the steroids are reduced, sulfasalazine is added to prevent relapse. The active ingredient of sulfasalazine, 5-aminosalicylic acid, can be delivered orally or in enemas or suppositories. In contrast to CD, the immunosuppressive agents have not been shown to have singular benefit.

How is sulfasalazine used?

Sulfasalazine consists of sulfapyridine bound to 5-aminosalicylic acid. It was first used in 1942, and clinical benefit was demonstrated by 1948. Unfortunately, sulfasalazine may be associated with dose-related side effects such as nausea, vomiting, headache, and malaise. Side effects rarely occur when the dose is less than 4 g per day. Sulfasalazine crosses the placental barrier and can impede the absorption of albumin-bound drugs. Most of the side effects of sulfasalazine are due to the sulfapyridine fraction of the molecule; therefore, pharmacologic research has concentrated on removing that moiety. Maintenance therapy with sulfasalazine usually consists of 2 g per day.

Are there any other therapies?

Carry out metabolic surveillance in anyone with inflammatory bowel disease. Electrolyte and nutritional abnormalities are common and should be aggressively sought. Complete bowel rest by total parenteral nutrition has not been shown to reduce the colectomy rate or offer clinical benefit to patients with UC or CD. Nutritional support should be carried out, however, to allow for repair of the diseased bowel.

Studies on the clinical utility of monitoring thiopurine metabolites and preliminary investigations into the potential therapeutic role of 6-thioguanine have helped improve our understanding and use of azathioprine and 6-mercaptopurine. It appears that repetitive infliximab infusions may be used to maintain remission in CD, and every 8-week infliximab infusions do not result in increased side effects. Trials using other antibodies directed at tumor necrosis factor (TNF)-α have not shown the same clinical benefit as infliximab.

D.C. is prescribed a combination medical regimen with corticosteroids as the core agent. (For comparative dose-equivalency of corticosteroids, see Table 12.1.) In the ensuing several weeks in an outpatient setting, her symptoms improve steadily. One day, however, she complains of severe right lower quadrant pain, and she presents to the emergency department with a tight obstruction of the terminal ileum and evidence of complete small-bowel obstruction. Surgical consultation is obtained.

How should one proceed with surgical management of a patient with CD?

Adhere to certain principles. First, reserve surgical treatment for symptoms and not for radiologic findings. The presence of internal fistulas is not necessarily an indication for surgical intervention because not all internal fistulas cause symptoms. Fistulas most commonly develop in the distal ileum. Second, surgical treatment should avoid extensive small-bowel resection. Third, surgical management should avoid rendering patients incontinent. It often has been stated that

TABLE 12.1.

BIOLOGIC ACTIVITY PROFILES OF SYNTHETIC ANALOGS OF CORTISOL

	Equivalent Dose (mg)	Sodium Retention	Biologic Half-Life (Hours)	Steroid Potency
Cortisol	1	20.0	1.0	8–12
Fluorocortisol	10	—	125	—
Short-acting analogs				
Prednisolone	4	5.0	0.8	12–36
Methylprednisolone	5	4.0	0.5	12–36
Triamcinolone	5	4.0	0.0	12–36
Long-acting analogs				
Betamethasone	25	0.6	0.0	36–54
Dexamethasone	25	0.6	0.0	36–54

Adapted from Tepperman J. Metabolic and Endocrine Physiology. Chicago, Ill: Year Book; 1980:193, with permission.

incontinent Crohn's patients are the result of overaggressive surgeons, not of the disease itself. Last, surgical management is preferred for patients developing complications from medical therapy or sepsis from delayed surgery.

With nasogastric decompression and medical treatment, the patient's symptoms improve. Over the ensuing 2 weeks, she resumes a solid diet and has satisfactory bowel movements. However, 3 weeks after discharge she returns to the emergency department with obstructive symptoms. Radiologic workup indicates obstruction at the same area in the terminal ileum.

What are the indications for surgical intervention in CD?

The principal indications for operating on a patient with CD are complications, namely recurrent obstruction, abscess formation, severe colitis, anal destruction, or malignancy. Complications requiring urgent surgical intervention include profuse blood loss, free perforation, acute progressive ileitis, intestinal obstruction, and toxic dilation. An attempt should be made to avoid using suture material that might cause tissue reaction and promote the formation of strictures or recurrent disease at the site of anastomosis. Current techniques favor extramucosal polypropylene sutures or staples.

At this point, the surgeon recommends abdominal exploration to identify and treat the intestinal obstruction.

What type of incision should be used for a patient with CD?

In open abdominal procedures, a midline incision is preferred for all operations in patients with CD. It does not transgress possible stoma sites on the lateral abdomen, and it can be reopened relatively easily. Most patients with CD have fewer adhesions than normal, but they can have significant intrabowel adhesions. It is usually advisable to have the patient in Allen stirrups because access to the vagina, anus, or rectum may be necessary.

Laparoscopic surgery can be considered in certain cases. The proposed advantages of laparoscopic surgery make it particularly attractive for patients with CD. These theoretical advantages include minimal physiologic insult, which may be especially important for the Crohn's patient already under significant physiologic stress; less adhesion formation and superior cosmesis, which may benefit a Crohn's patient likely to undergo multiple operations over time; short postoperative ileus; and rapid return to normal activity, which can be a significant advantage for someone with a chronic, sometimes disabling disease such as Crohn's (9).

Resort to open laparotomy in a timely manner if the anatomy is unclear because of adhesions or obesity or other miscellaneous reasons. Complete dissection and visualization of the mesenteric vessels, early identification of the ureter, intraoperative colonoscopy to mark the site of obscure pathology, and secure closure of the fascial opening at the site of the ports of insertion are important technical considerations. Although the laparoscopic approach requires longer surgical time and utilizes more expensive instruments, these additional costs to the institution may be recovered through earlier discharge.

In the operating room, exploration of the abdomen reveals a 6-inch area of terminal ileum that is densely inflamed, with fatty mesentery encroaching around the bowel. The area is tightly narrowed and is the obvious cause of bowel obstruction. An attempt is made to resect the least amount of small bowel, and a primary side-to-side anastomosis is made.

Why is small-bowel preservation so important?

More than 80% of patients with ileal CD require surgical treatment. The likelihood of resection increases with the duration of follow-up. The risk of reoperation for recrudescence of CD is approximately 50% at 10 years. Most patients need three or four operations in their lifetime, which makes small-bowel conservation essential in order to avoid the development of short-bowel syndrome.

Are there special techniques to promote small-bowel conservation?

Because small-bowel recurrence rates are independent of the extent of resection or lymphatic clearance, one need only resect to soft, pliable bowel. Although resection is the correct first surgical approach, stricturoplasty may be useful in the setting of recurrent disease accompanied by stricture formation (10). Strictures can be assumed to be symptomatic if the luminal diameter is less than 15 to 20 mm. One must make a longitudinal incision across the full thickness of the stricture and suture the opening at an orthogonal angle transversely. Extramucosal suturing in a single layer is preferred. Recurrence rates are approximately 2% in a 5-year period. Certain principles allow for the safe operation on a CD patient:

- Surgical treatment is used only for symptoms.
- Resection is not advisable for diffuse or acute disease.
- Surgical treatment should avoid rendering the patient incontinent.
- Surgical management must keep the safety of the patient foremost.

Are there any areas in the management of patients with CD that require special consideration?

Yes, surgery has a limited role in the management of perianal CD. Coexisting rectal disease is an unfavorable sign because most of those patients eventually require diversion. The use of metronidazole is advised, and any abscess must be drained. Establishing drainage is an essential means of preserving long-term function. Setons made from vessel loops and mushroom catheters are useful for establishing drainage. Anorectal fistulas should be opened only in the absence of rectal disease, only if the tract is superficial, and only if they are symptomatic. All other fistulas should be treated conservatively (11). Colonic disease portends a worse outcome than small-bowel disease. In addition, the more complex the fistula, the less likely it is to heal after a surgical fistulotomy. Anorectal strictures rarely lend themselves to dilation, and most eventually require proctocolectomy because of the progressive disease.

What does one do in the setting of presumed appendicitis if acute ileitis is discovered instead at the time of laparotomy?

Acute appendicitis is exceedingly rare in patients with CD; in fact, it is so rare that it is hard to justify a prophylactic appendectomy. If during laparotomy, the appearance is more consistent with acute ileitis, terminate the procedure and institute medical therapy postoperatively (12). If, however, the appearance is typical of chronic CD, ileal resection with ileocolonic anastomosis is appropriate.

D.C. recovers without any major complications except for postoperative atelectasis and fever. She receives pulmonary toilet and walks vigorously. On the third day after surgery, she passes flatus and begins to tolerate diet well. She is discharged on the sixth postoperative day, after which she is followed-up by her internist. On medications, she enjoys a quiescent period without many abdominal symptoms.

About 3 months later, she is referred to the gastroenterologist for pain in the lower abdomen and bloody stool. Colonoscopic evaluation shows evidence of a severe inflammatory process in the right colon and in the

midsigmoid colon. The patient requests to be seen by a surgeon, who discusses with her the merits of medical versus surgical treatment of Crohn's colitis.

Does the medical management of CD differ with location?

Yes. There is no specific therapy for CD in the true sense of the word. All therapy is directed at controlling symptoms rather than the disease. Although sulfasalazine has an effect on Crohn's colitis, it has no effect on small-bowel disease. Delayed-release medications have been used in ileocolonic disease and are effective at high doses. Corticosteroids are effective in the treatment of acute CD, regardless of the location of the disease. In addition, 6-mercaptopurine and azathioprine have been used as corticosteroid-sparing agents and to treat recurrent CD after multiple resections. There is a lengthy period before the agents exert their optimal effect. Cyclosporine may be useful in an acute setting. All these medications do have adverse side effects that should be discussed with the patient before treatment begins.

Are there any special considerations in the surgical treatment of colorectal CD?

The proportion of patients requiring surgical intervention in CD of the colon is slightly less than that in ileal disease, but nearly two thirds of them require an operation. If the colon is involved, several overriding factors must be addressed:

- The likelihood of a permanent stoma if the disease is diffuse or involves the rectum
- The hazards of a total colectomy in a malnourished patient
- The high morbidity and mortality from intraabdominal sepsis

Those with right-sided disease have the highest operative rate; those with rectal disease have the lowest operative rate. Approximately 5% to 10% require an emergency operation for fulminant colitis. Between 40% and 50% of patients with colonic CD eventually have an ileostomy. Of all patients with fulminant colitis, 20% to 30% will be found to have Crohn's colitis rather than UC. Surgical intervention is warranted whenever medical therapy fails to effect demonstrable improvement in signs and symptoms. Progressive dilation of the transverse colon to more than 5.5 cm is reason for concern. Any deterioration or lack of improvement within 72 hours while under maximal medical therapy mandates an urgent laparotomy.

The surgical options are limited in such situations, consisting mostly of subtotal colectomy and ileostomy. In the absence of rectal disease, an ileosigmoid anastomosis maximizes the rectal reservoir function and offers the best functional outcome. If there is rectal involvement, active perianal disease, or skip lesions in the small bowel, restoration of intestinal continuity is unlikely. Recurrence rates after ileorectal anastomosis are significantly higher than after proctocolectomy;

hence proctocolectomy with ileostomy appears to be warranted. Steroids seem to have little influence on the eventual functional outcome. In the setting of a proctocolectomy, CD may lead to delayed healing of the perineal wound, sometimes for up to a year.

Are there special complications associated with ileostomies?

Yes. The incidence of ileostomy dysfunction is high and may be associated with disease recurrence. Complications may include but are not limited to retraction, prolapse, and obstruction. Most ileostomy complications may be managed by local revision, but if recurrent CD is the issue, a formal resection is mandated.

On the surgeon's recommendation, D.C. undergoes aggressive medical treatment consisting of sulfasalazine enema and corticosteroids. Her symptoms wane, and once again she is relatively symptom-free. She is quite satisfied with her medical and surgical care.

ULCERATIVE COLITIS

Rebecca Tetrault is a 30-year-old woman who has had UC for 9 years. She is recovering from a 10-day hospital stay during which she was treated for a severe bout of acute UC. The patient requests a second opinion on the treatment she received for her acute colitis.

How is acute colitis treated in patients with UC?

Acute fulminating colitis often occurs without any history of disease. Optimal medical management is instituted with intravenous steroids, bowel rest, and repetitive examinations. Toxic colitis, with or without megacolon, is an emergent life-threatening complication of inflammatory bowel disease. In up to 30% of cases it may occur as the initial presentation of the disease, although it may occur at any time during its course. The overall incidence in patients with UC is about 10%. Although in the past toxic colitis was thought to be a rare complication of CD compared with UC, recent studies have shown that Crohn's colitis is the etiology in approximately 50% of the cases. The overall incidence of complicated CD is about 6%, with an increasing number occurring in Crohn's colitis. The counterpoint is that failure to heed the signs and symptoms of impending perforation is associated with a mortality of 35% to 75%.

Once the diagnosis of toxic colitis is suspected, aggressive medical therapy is initiated. A team approach is required involving both gastroenterologists and surgeons. Optimal medical management and preparation for surgery are the hallmarks of therapy. Narcotics, if required, must be used with caution so as to not mask the signs of peritonitis. Antidiarrheal agents are contraindicated. Fluid and electrolyte losses should be corrected promptly and blood transfusions given if needed. Broad-spectrum antibiotics are given because the bowel wall is both thin and ulcerated, which may predispose to enteric organisms translocating through the bowel wall and invading the portal or systemic circulation. The key to management is compulsive monitoring of vital signs, hydration, abdominal girth, and twice daily plain films of the abdomen. This is supplemented with both serial laboratory testing and serial abdominal examinations.

There is compelling evidence that early colectomy is the single most important factor in maintaining low mortality in patients with acute fulminant colitis. The timing of the operation is crucial, and failure to respond clearly to maximal medical therapy over 72 hours is an indication for an emergency colectomy. Prompt surgery is indicated for patients with toxic colitis or megacolon if there is evidence of free perforation, peritonitis, or massive hemorrhage. Surgery may also be indicated to avoid perforation if no clinical improvement occurs with aggressive medical management within 48 to 72 hours. A persistently dilated colon on plain films is also often an indication for operative intervention. If perforation occurs, mortality may be greater than 40%, whereas if surgery is completed before perforation, the mortality is between 2% and 8%. Because the diagnosis of UC versus Crohn's colitis may not be firmly established, subtotal colectomy with ileostomy is the procedure of choice. The rectum is divided above the pelvic brim so as not to open the pelvic planes of dissection with the associated risk of sepsis.

R.T. is satisfied with the fact that she has recovered from her acute bout of colitis, but she wants to know what issues she should be concerned about now.

What are the concerns in chronic UC?

There is an increased risk of colorectal cancer in patients with UC. It is linked to the duration of the disease, the age of onset, and the severity of the first attack of the disease. The risk of cancer is significantly greater in those with pancolitis as opposed to those with predominantly left-sided disease. Whether there is a genetic predisposition to cancer in patients with extensive colitis is not known. The distribution of cancers probably does not differ from that of the sporadic carcinoma seen in the general population. The incidence of synchronous cancers in patients with UC is higher than that seen in sporadic disease. Detection of dysplastic areas is the key to early detection and treatment of chronic UC. An effective screening policy is essential, and the retained rectum after a colectomy without a proctectomy is often neglected.

How significant is the risk of malignancy in patients with chronic UC?

The increased risk of colorectal cancer in the setting of chronic UC is, as mentioned earlier, related to the extent of the disease, the age of onset, the severity of the first attack, and the duration of follow-up. The usual method of screening is surveillance colonoscopic examinations with appropriate biopsies, which are searched for dysplastic changes in the regenerative mucosa. Dysplasia is thought to be a marker for cancer. Because of the slow evolution of dysplasia and its patchy nature, biopsies should be multiple and repeated regularly. The optimal frequency of surveillance is not known. Most studies confirm that the risk of cancer is greater in those whose colitis extends at least into the right transverse colon as opposed to those with isolated rectosigmoid involvement.

The incidence of cancer arising in a patient who has had colitis for fewer than 10 years is negligible. The incidence after 15 years of extensive colitis rises to 3%, to 5% after 20 years of disease, and to nearly 10% after 25 years of disease. The risk of developing carcinoma is highest in patients who were diagnosed with UC before age 30 years. The best cohort study reveals that those diagnosed before age 30 had a risk of carcinoma eight times that of the general population, and pancolitis raises that risk to a factor of 19. The incidence of synchronous lesions is greater among patients with chronic UC than in the general population. Contemporary reports indicate that the survival rate of patients with colorectal cancers and UC is comparable with that seen in persons with sporadic lesions.

What are the features of dysplasia?

Dysplasia is a histopathologic marker for patients who are likely to develop carcinoma. It is patchy and an imperfect marker, but it may help in the decision as to when to recommend a prophylactic colectomy. The following features are the cardinal signs of dysplasia:

- Variation in the size and shape of epithelial cell nuclei, which have prominent nucleoli and are hyperchromatic and distorted
- Possibly hyperchromatic cell cytoplasm
- Mucin at the base of the cell rather than at the apex, as is normal
- Abnormal mitosis in the upper third of the crypts
- Budding of the crypts (adenomatous changes)
- Elongation of the crypts (villous change)
- Loss of nuclear polarity (pseudostratification)

There are three gross features of dysplasia: polypoidal lesions, low elevated plaques, and stricture or ulcer (13). The low elevated plaques are the most difficult to detect during colonoscopy. Rectal biopsies for the detection of dysplasia or cancer are often negative, even in the presence of a malignancy, which limits its usefulness.

R.T. is concerned that her disease was diagnosed when she was 23 years of age and that, in some episodes, her internist said that her entire colon was inflamed. In addition, she soon will be in her 10th year of UC. She asks whether she should undergo surgery to "get rid" of her disease.

What are the surgical options of patients with chronic UC?

Restorative proctocolectomy with ileal pouch anal anastomosis has become the standard surgical option for the definitive treatment of mucosal UC. The performance of a total proctocolectomy and ileostomy has remained an option on those individuals deemed not candidates due to fecal incontinence or associated medical issues. There is no routine upper age limit for restorative proctocolectomy.

As the cumulative clinical data have shown over the years, the restorative proctocolectomy with ileal pouch anal anastomosis has become the standard of care for patients seeking a cure without a permanent stoma. Parks and Nicholls first reported the procedure in 1978 (14). There is a reoperative rate of 15% to 25% and an overall failure rate of 5% to 15% after a median of 8 years. Also, there usually remains a small amount of mucosa at the top of the anal canal that is still at risk for carcinoma. Advanced techniques have led to the use of stapling to anastomose the pouch to the anal segment, obviating mucosectomy and its technical issues. Whether this will continue to be optimal in the long run remains to be assessed, but for now this has revolutionized the manner and time required to perform these procedures. The type of pouch created does not actually correlate with outcome. The majority of cancers arising in the anal transitional zone after restorative proctocolectomy have been after mucosectomy. What is sought is a pliable, moderate-capacity pouch that is capable of distending and allowing the patient to defer the urge to defecate (Fig. 12.1). The common complications include pelvic abscess, intestinal obstruction, anal anastomotic stricture, and pouchitis.

The role of laparoscopic surgery in UC is still somewhat unclear. Subtotal and total colectomy for CD and UC and restorative proctocolectomy for UC can be performed. However, clear advantages have not yet been demonstrated with the exception of cosmesis. Although the results are more encouraging now than they were 10 years ago, these procedures are still associated with lengthy operative times and long hospitalizations. None of the benefits repeatedly demonstrated after laparoscopic surgery for segmental CD have been proven after total abdominal colectomy or restorative proctocolectomy (15).

Is total proctocolectomy with an everted stoma (Brooke's ileostomy) also a surgical option for chronic UC?

This procedure has fallen out of favor for a variety of reasons. First and foremost is the issue of the permanent ileostomy. Second is the issue of a prolonged healing of the perineal wound, with wound failure rates ranging from 17% to 85%, even after a year. The third drawback relates to the sexual complications of proctocolectomy. Many women complain of dyspareunia at the perineal scar, and men note poor ejaculatory function. Finally, there is the permanency of the procedure, which is a difficult mental hurdle for young patients. Although this is almost never indicated as an emergency procedure, rectal bleeding may dictate

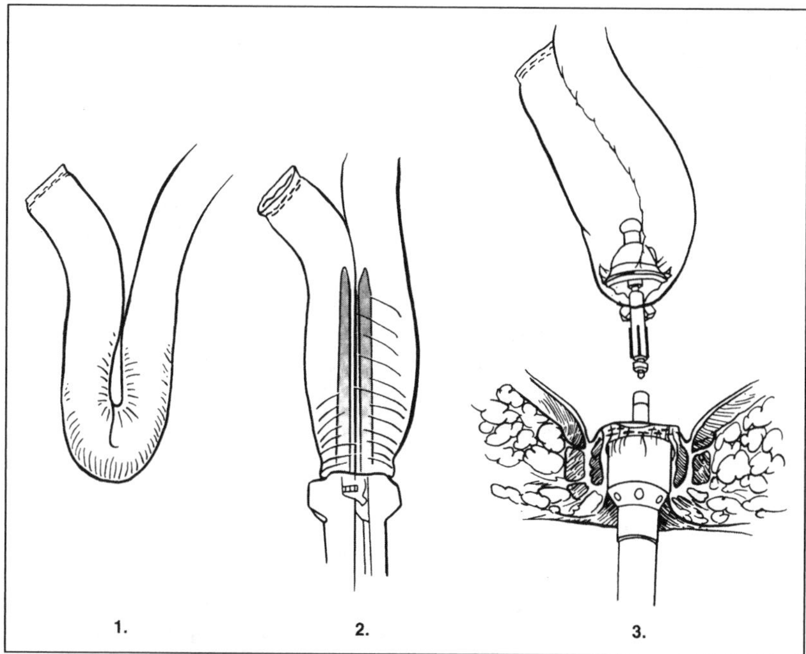

Figure 12.1. J-pouch ileoanal anastomosis following proctocolectomy. **1.** Terminal ileum configured in J shape. **2.** Stapled ileum into a J pouch. **3.** Ileoanal anastomosis using an end-to-end anastomosis stapler. (Adapted from Fazio VW, Tjandra JJ, Lavery IC. Techniques of pouch construction. In: Nicholls J, Bartolo D, Mortensen N, eds. Restorative Proctocolectomy. Oxford, UK: Blackwell; 1993, with permission.)

an emergency proctocolectomy. The rate of revision of Brooke's ileostomy over 5 years ranges from 10% to 20%. It has a role in patients who have poor sphincter function or a low-lying rectal cancer, as well as those who are unwilling to commit themselves to the restorative proctocolectomy.

Is a total proctocolectomy with a continent ileostomy (e.g., Kock pouch) a surgical option for patients with chronic UC?

This procedure offers only historical interest because of its high reoperative rate (upward of 25% to 50% within 5 years) and poorer performance characteristics than the restorative proctocolectomy.

R.T. decides to undergo restorative total proctocolectomy with a J-pouch ileoanal anastomosis. The operation is performed without difficulty. She has a relatively benign postoperative course and is discharged on the ninth postoperative day. Initially, she has more than 20 bowel movements

per day, but over time this decreases to a manageable frequency of about four times per day. However, 6 weeks after the operation she presents with fever, blood-tinged diarrhea, and severe pain upon defecation. The surgeon diagnoses pouchitis.

What is pouchitis?

Inflammation of the ileal reservoir is a recognized complication of restorative proctocolectomy. Interestingly, this almost always occurs in the setting of UC, with familial adenomatous polyposis being exceedingly rare. Within 5 years of creation of the pouch, approximately 35% of patients develop at least one episode of local inflammation leading to increased bowel movements, tenesmus, and bleeding. Two thirds of these persons have only a single episode. Pouchitis can be classified as acute, acutely relapsing, subacute, or chronic. The cause is unknown. The endoscopic findings are hemorrhagic and edematous mucosa with very minute ulcerations. The inflammation may extend into the proximal ileum. A neutrophil infiltrate is revealed on biopsy. Treatment with metronidazole appears to be most effective, with a response rate of 80% to 90%. Pouchitis alone rarely necessitates pouch excision (16) (Algorithm 12.1).

With metronidazole and other symptomatic management, the patient's pouchitis resolves. Her bowel movements are once again manageable, and she is quite satisfied with her care. She is satisfied that she no longer has to deal with the inflammatory colon. However, she wonders whether there are other effects of UC that are cause for concern.

Are any other disorders associated with UC?

Hepatobiliary complications of UC or its treatment include fatty liver, gallstones, primary sclerosing cholangitis, primary biliary cirrhosis, biliary strictures, bile duct carcinoma, chronic active hepatitis, and intermittent cholestasis. These are its characteristics:

- There is a marked incidence of chronic active hepatitis in patients with UC.
- Gallstones occur more frequently if there has been an ileal resection.
- The incidence of cirrhosis varies from 1% to 5% and is usually associated with extensive colitis. Varices may develop, and, in the presence of an ileostomy, stomal varices can become a significant morbidity. If a colectomy is required, avoidance of a stoma should be a prime consideration, and a restorative proctocolectomy should be considered.
- Primary sclerosing cholangitis is a rare disorder (affecting 1% to 4% of patients with inflammatory bowel disease) that affects all parts of the biliary tree in a chronic inflammatory process. It appears to be related to cross-reactivity of anticolon and antineutrophil antibodies; 70% of cases are associated with UC (17). Men are more commonly affected than women, and most

patients are 25 to 45 years of age. Diagnosis is usually by endoscopic retrograde cholangiopancreatography. There is no specific effective treatment, and patients may require liver transplant when liver failure supervenes. The diffuse and extensive nature of the disease usually prohibits the performance of any bypass procedures. Although primary sclerosing cholangitis is a progressive disease, the rate of progression is quite variable. There is no evidence that colectomy affects the natural history of the disease.

Approximately 5% to 10% of patients with UC develop *cutaneous manifestations* at some point. The most common manifestations are erythema nodosum, pyoderma gangrenosum, exfoliative dermatitis, and vasculitis. These are its characteristics:

- Pyoderma gangrenosum is probably the most bothersome of the cutaneous manifestations, with an incidence of 1% to 5%. Approximately 50% of the patients who initially complain of pyoderma gangrenosum eventually are diagnosed with UC (18). Although it is not related to the severity of the colitis, pyoderma gangrenosum often rapidly improves upon colectomy. Rapidly enlarging deep areas of ulceration develop, usually over a lower limb, after initially appearing as a papule; it can also occur on the trunk. There is a predilection for areas previously traumatized, and the lesions tend to be extremely tender. Treatment of the underlying colitis is essential, and hyperbaric oxygen therapy offers some benefit. Retention of the rectal stump may prevent resolution of the lesions.
- Erythema nodosum occurs in 2% to 4% of patients with colitis and is more common in women than in men. Lesions, which generally present over the anterior surface of the tibia, consist of raised red tender nodules. Erythema nodosum usually improves after colectomy without any significant scarring. Its clinical course essentially parallels that of the colitis.
- Exfoliative dermatitis may occur as a complication of sulfasalazine therapy, but it also can result from severe colitis. It appears to resolve after proctocolectomy.

The incidence of *ocular lesions* in patients with UC varies from 1% to 12%, with episcleritis (predominantly in CD) and uveitis being the most common.

Colitic arthritis is usually associated with asymmetric migratory arthropathy. The most commonly affected joints, in order, are the knees, wrists, and elbows. Treatment usually is conservative and related to symptoms.

Ankylosing spondylitis also is associated with UC and is 20 to 30 times as common as in the general population. There is a genetic pathogenesis and association with the HLA-B27 antigen. One or more vertebrae and a sacroiliac joint are inflamed. The development of a rigid spine often leads to pulmonary complications. Various nonsteroidal pain medications are used for the management of the associated pain, and physical therapy is indicated to minimize the disability. Surgical treatment of the inflammatory bowel disease has no influence on the course of the axial arthropathy.

Should ulcerative proctitis be considered as a part of the spectrum of UC, or should it be viewed in a different light?

Ulcerative proctitis, initially described by Thaysen in 1934, is quite different from UC. The risk of proximal extension into the sigmoid colon is less than 30% at 20 years of disease. The likelihood that surgery will be required is approximately 6% at 20 years of disease. Most patients respond to topical steroids or sulfasalazine. There appears to be a male preponderance, and it appears to occur in an older population.

The inflamed mucosa begins at the dentate line and proceeds proximally for 5 to 15 cm. The histologic appearance is identical to that of UC. The presenting

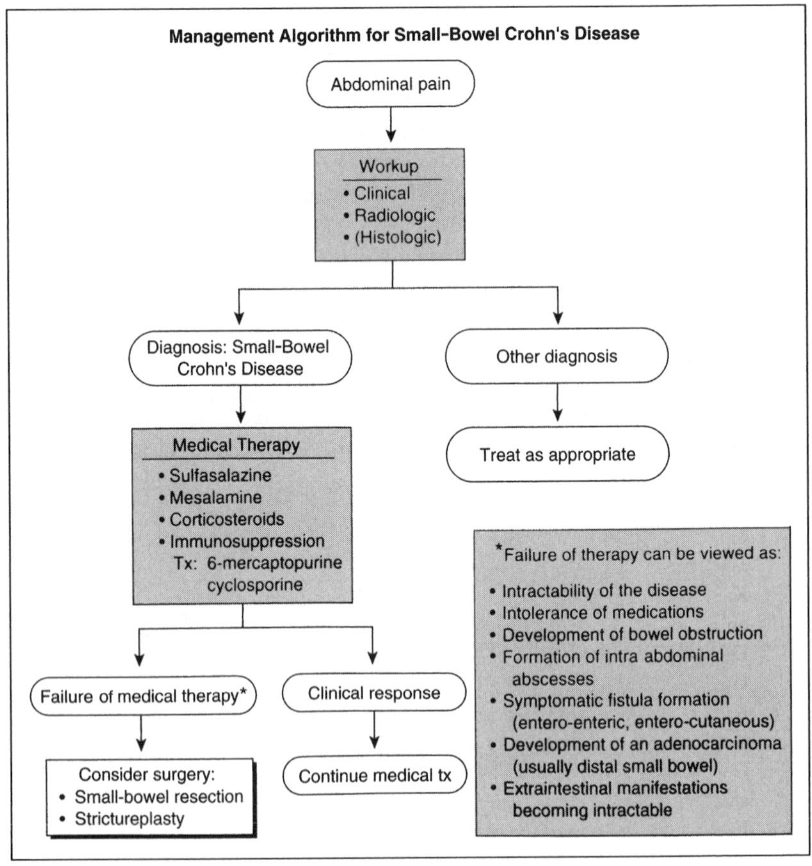

Algorithm 12.1.

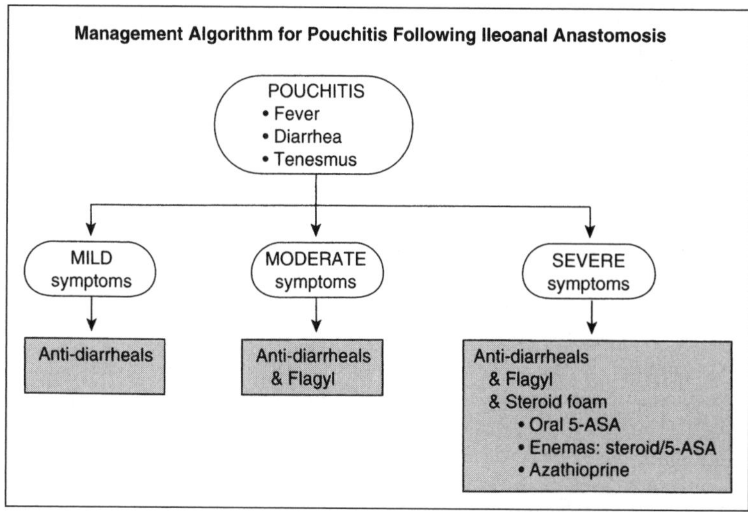

Algorithm 12.2.

symptoms are bleeding, urgency, mucous discharge, and tenesmus. There are no general symptoms, as there are in colitis. Treatment is usually in the form of topical steroids, whether by enemas or foams. There is a spontaneous remission rate of 40%, making no treatment possibly a viable option. If no spontaneous remission has been noted within 6 weeks, a course of steroid enemas or suppositories is indicated.

REFERENCES

1. Crohn BB, Ginzburg L, Oppenheimer GD. Regional ileitis: a pathologic and clinical entity. JAMA. 1932;99:1323–1329.
2. Morson BC, Lockhart-Mummery HE. Crohn's disease of the colon. Gastroenterologia. 1959;92:168–173.
3. Gold DV, Miller F. Comparison of human colonic mucoprotein antigen from normal and neoplastic mucosa. Cancer. 1978;38:3204–3208.
4. Keighley MRB, Williams NS. Crohn's disease: aetiology, incidence and epidemiology. 1993;49:1592–1630.
5. Duerr RH. Update on the genetics of inflammatory bowel disease. J Clin Gastroenterol. 2003;37:358–367.
6. Kirsner JB, Spencer JA. Family occurrences of ulcerative colitis, regional enteritis, and ileocolitis. Ann Intern Med. 1963;59:133–144.
7. Corman ML. Nonspecific inflammatory bowel disease. In: Corman ML. Colon and Rectal Surgery. Philadelphia, PA: JB Lippincott Co; 1989:741–887.
8. Farmer RG, Whelan G, Fazio VW. Long-term follow-up of patients with Crohn's disease: relationship between the clinical pattern and prognosis. Gastroenterology. 1985;88:1818–1825.

9. Ludwig KA, Milson JW, Church JM, et al. Preliminary experience with laparoscopic intestinal surgery for Crohn's disease. Am J Surg. 1996;171:52–56.
10. Alexander-Williams J. The technique of intestinal strictureplasty. Int J Colorectal Dis. 1986;1:54–57.
11. Allan A, Keighley MRB. Management of perianal Crohn's disease. World J Surg. 1989;12:198–202.
12. Strong SA, Fazio VW. Crohn's disease of the colon, rectum and anus. Surg Clin North Am. 1993;73:933–963.
13. Nugent FW, Haggitt RC, Colcher H, et al. Malignant potential of chronic ulcerative colitis. Gastroenterology. 1979;76:1–5.
14. Parks AG, Nichols RJ. Proctocolectomy without ileostomy for ulcerative colitis. BMJ. 1978;2:85–88.
15. Gurland BH, Wexner SD. Laparoscopic surgery for inflammatory bowel disease: results of the past decade. Inflamm Bowel Dis. 2002;8:46–54.
16. Pemberton JH, Kelly KA, Beart RW Jr. Ileal-pouch anastomosis for chronic ulcerative colitis: long-term results. Ann Surg. 1987;206:504–513.
17. LaRusso NF, Wiesner RH, Ludwig J, et al. Primary sclerosing cholangitis. N Engl J Med. 1984;310:899–903.
18. Mir-Madjlessi SH, Taylor JS, Farmer RG. Clinical course and evolution of erythema nodosum in chronic ulcerative colitis: a study of 42 patients. Am J Gastroenterol. 1985;80:615–620.

CHAPTER

13

DIVERTICULAR DISEASE OF THE COLON

Ciaran J. Walsh

DIVERTICULAR DISEASE

Helen Witt is a 65-year-old moderately obese woman who presents to the emergency department complaining of left lower quadrant abdominal pain associated with anorexia and nausea for the past 2 days. She says she had this type of pain once last year and was told she probably had diverticular disease. At that time, her symptoms settled down very quickly, no investigations were performed, and nothing more was done about her condition.

On this occasion, her pain started gradually with intermittent gripping that became constant and more severe. She felt as though she had a fever and noted that going over the speed bumps on the way into the hospital caused her pain in the lower abdomen. Her history is significant for an appendectomy and open cholecystectomy many years ago, and recently her primary care physician prescribed ranitidine for a hiatal hernia diagnosed on upper gastrointestinal (GI) endoscopy. She is not diabetic. She denies any recent change in her bowel habit, blood from the rectum, or weight loss. She has no urinary frequency or dysuria and has no history of urinary tract infections.

On examination, she looks a little flushed. Her temperature is 37.9°C, her pulse is 92 beats per minute, and her blood pressure is 156/88 mm Hg. Her abdomen is obese but not distended. Abdominal examination reveals local left lower quadrant tenderness and guarding but no palpable mass. The rest of her abdomen is soft and not tender. Her bowel sounds are normal. Digital rectal examination is normal. Her laboratory values are normal, as is her acute abdominal radiograph series. The emergency

department staff members think she has acute diverticulitis, and they want to know what investigations should be performed and whether Mrs. Witt should be admitted.

What is diverticular disease?

It is a benign disease of the colon characterized by the development of pulsion-type outpouchings. These are really false diverticula because they consist of mucosa lined only by serosa. They most often occur between the mesenteric and antimesenteric taenia coli, where the colonic blood vessels pierce the muscle. They indicate herniation of the mucosa through weak points in the colon wall. They are most common in the sigmoid and left colon but may occur anywhere in the colon.

What is the difference between diverticulosis and diverticulitis?

Diverticulosis is diverticula in the colon. *Diverticulitis* is an infective complication of these diverticula.

What causes diverticulosis?

Diverticulosis most likely develops as a result of a low-fiber diet. As food becomes more refined and processed, the amount of dietary fiber decreases. This is particularly prevalent in Western societies, which consume only one-tenth the amount of fiber consumed 100 years ago, before refined diets were so prevalent. In rural Africa and other societies not exposed to a Western diet, diverticular disease is almost nonexistent (1). Rural Africans reportedly consume 60 to 100 g of fiber a day, whereas Americans consume only 10 to 15 g per day.

How does a high-fiber diet prevent diverticulosis?

Fiber increases stool weight, decreases whole gut transit time, and lowers colonic intraluminal pressure. A high-fiber diet requires less contraction by the bowel to propel the stool onward. There is less segmentation, and muscle hypertrophy does not occur.

What is the prevalence of diverticular disease?

Approximately 30 million Americans have diverticulosis. Only 1% to 2% of people younger than 30 years of age are affected; one third of Americans older than 45 years are affected. The incidence rises with age; two thirds of the population older than 85 years is affected (2). Most people are asymptomatic, but 15% to 30% eventually develop diverticulitis.

What is Saint's triad?

Saint's triad is the constellation of cholelithiasis, hiatal hernia, and diverticulosis.

What is the most likely diagnosis for Mrs. Witt? What is the differential diagnosis?

Acute diverticulitis with local peritonitis is the most likely diagnosis for this patient. She has had an appendectomy, which means that the most likely differential diagnoses are colon carcinoma, inflammatory bowel disease, and ischemic colitis.

What are the most common complications of diverticular disease?

Perforation (micro or macro) causing pericolic infection with formation of a phlegmon, pericolic abscess, fistula formation, and frank peritonitis are the most common complications of diverticular disease. Acute inflammation can also lead to ulceration or erosion into a colonic wall blood vessel (remember where on the bowel diverticula most commonly occur) and cause bleeding. Chronic inflammation may lead to stricture formation and colon obstruction. Small-bowel obstruction is a common but not frequently mentioned complication of acute diverticulitis. Up to 20% of patients with acute diverticulitis may have small-bowel obstruction as a result of a loop of small bowel getting snared in the inflammatory nest. This is to be distinguished from an ileus, which may develop as a result of acute diverticulitis.

What is the Hinchey classification of acute diverticulitis?

This is a classification of severity of acute diverticulitis (3). There are four stages:

- *Stage I:* Includes a pericolic abscess
- *Stage II:* Includes a distant or remote abscess
- *Stage III:* Includes purulent peritonitis
- *Stage IV:* Includes fecal peritonitis

These classifications permit a realistic comparison of treatment outcomes and formulation of management guidelines for each stage of the disease. The basic pathophysiology of acute diverticulitis is perforation. Whereas microperforations seal and may lead to an abscess or phlegmon, a large perforation may cause fecal peritonitis.

What fistulas are associated with diverticulitis?

A fistula may develop between the inflamed colon and any surrounding structure. Colovesical fistulas are the most common, accounting for nearly 60% of fistulas associated with diverticular disease (4). Approximately 2% of patients with acute diverticulitis develop a colovesical fistula. They are more common in men than in women, probably because in women the uterus lies between the colon and the bladder. Colocutaneous fistulas are the next most common type associated with diverticulitis. A women who has had a hysterectomy may develop a colovaginal fistula.

What are the symptoms and signs of a colovesical fistula?

Dysuria (90%), pneumaturia (70%), and fecaluria (70%) are the most common symptoms. Chronic urinary tract infections may occur. There are no physical signs related to the fistula per se, although one third of patients have evidence of a systemic infection.

How is a diagnosis of colovesical fistula confirmed?

Barium enema, cystoscopy, or both may demonstrate the communication between the colon and bladder. Radiography of the urine after a barium enema is described. Often the fistula cannot be demonstrated and the diagnosis is made based on history. The patient may be asked to urinate while in the bathtub to see if bubbles appear in the water.

How should Mrs. Witt's diagnosis be confirmed? What investigation should be ordered?

The investigation of choice at this point is computed tomography (CT) of the abdomen and pelvis with intravenous (IV) and water-soluble oral contrast. This not only helps to confirm the diagnosis but also demonstrates the extent of the disease, including any abscess collections or free intraperitoneal air or fluid. In general, the diagnosis can be made clinically with sufficient confidence to permit treatment without more definitive investigation.

What are the criteria used to diagnose acute diverticulitis by CT?

Colonic wall thickening, stranding of pericolic fat, pericolic or distant abscesses, and extraluminal air are characteristics of diverticulitis seen on CT (5). Colonic diverticula seen on CT are not diagnostic of acute diverticulitis.

Should Mrs. Witt have a barium enema or colonoscopy?

Mrs. Witt definitely should not have a barium enema or colonoscopy. Both procedures could worsen the situation. Colonoscopy could blow open a sealed perforation. Barium enema could provoke free perforation and lead to extravasation of barium into the peritoneal cavity, causing barium peritonitis.

Mrs. Witt's CT shows significant thickening of the sigmoid colon, stranding of the pericolic fat with colonic diverticulosis, and a very small fluid collection in the pouch of Douglas.

Should the fluid be drained percutaneously? What should be done at this point?

The films should be reviewed with the radiologist. CT-guided percutaneous drainage is an excellent option for identifiable pericolic abscesses in patients with acute diverticulitis. The potential for CT-guided percutaneous drainage is one of the reasons CT is so attractive in patients with acute diverticulitis. Approximately

75% of peridiverticular abscesses can be drained in this way. The advantages are that it facilitates resolution of the sepsis without surgical drainage, and it permits a one-stage elective operation later. There is no evidence that Mrs. Witt has an abscess, thus there is no merit in percutaneous drainage in her case.

While the physician is reviewing the CT, a staff member of the emergency department calls and says the cubicle is needed. They want to send Mrs. Witt home with antibiotics.

Is sending Mrs. Witt home with an antibiotic prescription appropriate?
No. Mrs. Witt should be admitted for bowel rest, IV fluids, IV antibiotics, pain relief, and observation. In general, outpatient management is appropriate for patients who can tolerate diet, who do not have systemic symptoms, and who do not have peritoneal signs. Mrs. Witt fails to meet all of these criteria.

What percentage of people with diverticular disease need surgery? Is Mrs. Witt likely to need surgery on this admission?
Approximately 1% of patients with diverticular disease eventually require surgery. Approximately 15% to 30% of patients admitted to the hospital with acute diverticulitis need surgery. Mrs. Witt is not likely to need surgery on this admission.

Mrs. Witt's condition settles quickly with conservative management, and she is sent home after 3 days with a prescription for a course of oral antibiotics.

How should Mrs. Witt's follow-up be handled?
Mrs. Witt should be seen in the clinic in a few weeks to make sure that the acute episode has settled. At that time, full assessment of her colon, either by flexible sigmoidoscopy and barium enema or by colonoscopy, should be arranged.

Mrs. Witt says she fears colonoscopy because her sister underwent colonoscopy and then needed an operation for a perforated colon. She agrees to a barium enema, which is performed 6 weeks after her acute attack. It confirms sigmoid and left-colon diverticulosis but is otherwise normal. There is no stricture or fistula noted, only minimal muscle hypertrophy and mild spasm.

What further treatment is advised for Mrs. Witt? Is she going to have another attack, and should she undergo surgery?
Mrs. Witt should be advised to continue with conservative treatment. After the acute inflammation has settled, she should start a high-fiber diet. Up to 45% of patients have recurrent symptoms after an attack of acute diverticulitis. Long-term dietary supplementation with fiber after a first attack of diverticulitis may

prevent recurrent attacks in up to 70% of patients. With each recurrent attack, the patient is less likely to respond to medical treatment. In general, elective surgery is advised after two well-documented attacks of acute diverticulitis. However, if the first attack is complicated by abscess, stricture, obstruction, or fistula, surgery should be considered after the first attack. Mrs. Witt has not had two well-documented attacks nor was this attack complicated by abscess, stricture, obstruction, or fistula.

What constitutes a high-fiber diet?

A high-fiber diet contains 20 to 35 g of fiber per day. This may be unpalatable to patients, and the fiber should be increased gradually (e.g., increase by 5 g per week). These patients also should be advised to drink at least six glasses of noncaffeinated beverages a day.

Does age have any bearing on the treatment of patients with acute diverticulitis?

Yes. Diverticular disease tends to be most virulent in patients under 50 years of age. Acute attacks tend to be more severe than in older patients, and a higher percentage of these younger patients need surgery on the first admission. Moreover, many surgeons advocate elective surgery after one attack of acute diverticulitis in a young patient, even if the attack was uncomplicated.

Mrs. Witt says she does not like bran and cannot drink very much because she gets bloated. She really wants to consider an operation.

What elective operation is a surgeon likely to choose for her case? Would she need a stoma?

The elective operation of choice is a one-stage left colectomy with colorectal anastomosis. She had an uncomplicated attack and therefore is not likely to need a protecting stoma upstream of the anastomosis.

PERITONITIS

Charles Moran is a 54-year-old man who goes to the emergency department complaining of severe lower abdominal pain. His history is unremarkable except for taking nonsteroidal antiinflammatory drugs for "rheumatism." He admits to having had three previous attacks of lower abdominal pain, similar to this although not as severe. On the first occasion, 7 years ago, he remembers having gripping left lower quadrant pain that settled spontaneously after 3 days. The next occasion was 5 years ago, at which time he went to his primary care physician. The physician wanted to send him to the emergency department, but Mr. Moran refused. He says the pain went away when he took the antibiotics his doctor gave him and stuck to fluids only by mouth.

His most recent attack was 2 years ago. He was on vacation overseas and developed severe left lower quadrant abdominal pain and fever. He said he had chills and felt so poorly that he had to go to the local hospital. He said they did CT and told him he had diverticulitis with an abscess on the bowel. He says they put "a tube in it under the scanner," administered IV fluids and antibiotics, and discharged him 5 days later. He has no records of his hospital admission.

On direct questioning, he admitted to a change in his bowel habit during the past few months, saying his stools had become "like a pencil," more difficult to pass. He said that he had been feeling fine until this morning, when he was sitting on the toilet straining to pass a stool. He suddenly developed excruciating left lower quadrant abdominal pain, which has now spread to the right side. He says that he has to lie very still or the pain gets worse. On examination, his face is pale, his pulse rate is 110 beats per minute, his blood pressure is 160/90 mm Hg, and his temperature is 38.7°C. A head and neck examination is normal. He is not jaundiced. Chest examination reveals reduced air entry in both bases. His abdomen is slightly distended, and he is very tender, with guarding in both the left and right lower quadrant. He has markedly reduced bowel sounds on auscultation. Digital rectal examination is normal. Laboratory values, including serum amylase level, are normal except for a white blood cell (WBC) count of 17,000 with evidence of left shift. Urinalysis is normal. A chest radiograph is normal, without evidence of free air under the diaphragm. Abdominal films show a few dilated loops of small bowel in the lower abdomen.

What is this patient's diagnosis?

Mr. Moran has peritonitis. His history strongly suggests perforated diverticular disease.

If Mr. Moran has a perforated viscus, why is there no free air on the plain radiographs?

The emergency department physician did not order an erect chest radiograph. Either an erect chest radiograph or a lateral decubitus abdominal film is required to demonstrate free air under the diaphragm. Furthermore, only 70% to 80% of patients with a perforated viscus have free air on preoperative radiographs.

What test should Mr. Moran undergo next?

Mr. Moran should have an exploratory laparotomy as soon as possible after adequate resuscitation and stoma marking.

Laparotomy confirms the preoperative diagnosis of perforated diverticular disease. There is diverticular disease throughout the left colon

and a free perforation of the distal sigmoid with associated purulent peritonitis (Hinchey stage III).

What other disease must be considered at this time?

Perforated sigmoid colon cancer is a possibility in this patient. Both diverticular disease and colon cancer are common, and they may coexist. It can be very difficult to distinguish whether a phlegmon is caused by diverticulitis or sigmoid colon cancer, particularly in the presence of peritonitis.

What operation should Mr. Moran undergo?

The surgeon should perform Hartman's operation, a resection of the diseased sigmoid colon with an end left-sided colostomy and closure of the distal rectal stump (2).

Are there any other surgical options?

A one-stage resection and colorectal anastomosis, as would be performed during elective surgery for diverticular disease, is performed by some surgeons for patients with Hinchey stages I and II. It is not appropriate in Mr. Moran's case because the risks of anastomotic breakdown are too high. The Hartman operation is the safer and more traditional approach. When the patient is fully recovered, intestinal continuity may be restored, usually 4 to 6 months after the initial procedure.

What are the complications of the Hartman operation?

Complications specific to this procedure include damage to the left ureter, stomal necrosis or retraction, disruption of the rectal stump suture line, and, in the long term, failure to restore bowel continuity.

Sylvia Noro, a 69-year-old retired librarian, is brought to the emergency department by her daughter, who reports that Mrs. Noro passed a large amount of blood into the toilet bowl that morning and complained of being dizzy afterward. The patient denies any nausea, vomiting, or abdominal pain. She is uncertain whether she ever passed blood from the rectum in the past because she has very poor eyesight. She denies anal pain or prolapse of tissue in the rectum. She says that 10 years ago, she had surgery and radiation treatment for cancer of the cervix. Her only medicine is a "water tablet," which she takes each morning. She is not taking warfarin, aspirin, or other nonsteroidal antiinflammatory drugs. She does not smoke or drink alcohol.

On examination, she looks pale, her pulse is regular at 98 beats per minute, and her blood pressure is 150/70 mm Hg when reclining; when standing, her pulse is 110 beats per minute and her blood pressure is 130/50 mm Hg. Her head, neck, and chest examinations are normal.

There are no bruises, petechiae, or areas of abnormal skin pigmentation. She is not jaundiced. The abdomen is not distended and is completely nontender, with normal bowel sounds. There are no pulsatile masses, and peripheral pulses are all normal. Perianal examination is normal. She is able to tolerate digital rectal examination without any pain. There are no rectal masses, and anal sphincter tone is normal, but there is frank red blood on the glove. Urinalysis findings are negative; however, her urine is very concentrated.

Did Mrs. Noro have a significant bleed?

A little blood can look particularly impressive when mixed with the amount of water in a toilet bowl. However, Mrs. Noro most likely had a significant bleed. She gives a history of being dizzy, and she demonstrated orthostatic hypotension on examination in the emergency department. Orthostatic hypotension is common among the elderly, particularly those taking diuretic agents.

Why not measure her hemoglobin level and, if it is normal, send her home from the emergency department?

Mrs. Noro is tachycardic with a wide pulse pressure when lying down. In the context of her presentation, it would be dangerous to attribute her pulse and blood pressure to anything other than an acute bleed. Time and subsequent investigation may prove otherwise, but this is the safe approach. An acute bleed may not affect the hemoglobin level if there has not been time for equilibration of the intravascular volume. Also, it would be dangerous to say that the bleed was not significant because the hemoglobin level was normal. Mrs. Noro should be admitted and a workup performed.

Is the color of the blood significant?

Although there are exceptions, knowing the color of the blood can help to narrow the possible sources of the blood loss. Blood from any site, no matter how old, can turn red when it is dropped into a bowl of water. Blood that is red on the glove is truly red. The descriptive terms of others may be misused. An example is the term melena, which should be reserved for the classic black, sticky, tarry, and foul-smelling stool caused by bleeding in the upper GI tract. However, if the bleeding is particularly brisk or if the colon has been shortened by a colectomy, there may not be time for the bowel to produce typical melena. Maroon stools suggest distal ileal or right colonic blood, whereas true red blood usually comes from the left colon or anorectal area. The most common causes of massive bleeding from the upper GI tract that present with red blood from the rectum are peptic ulcer disease, esophagogastric varices, GI erosions, and an aortoduodenal fistula.

What is the initial working diagnosis?

Mrs. Noro most likely has bleeding in the lower GI tract.

What is the differential diagnosis in this case?

The most likely alternatives are angiodysplasia (6) and diverticular disease. Considering her history, radiation proctitis is also a possibility. Other possibilities include hemorrhoids, inflammatory bowel disease, ischemic colitis, and a benign or malignant colonic neoplasm. Less likely causes are anal fissure, Meckel's diverticulum, and bleeding in the upper GI tract. Mrs. Noro does not drink alcohol, has never smoked, does not take aspirin or other nonsteroidal antiinflammatory drugs, and has no history of aortic surgery.

Does the fact that the patient denies any pain associated with this episode help narrow the differential diagnosis?

The absence of abdominal pain is against ischemic colitis. Moreover, this patient has never smoked and has no stigmata of atherosclerotic vascular disease. The absence of anal pain makes bleeding from an anal fissure unlikely. Both diverticular bleeding and bleeding due to angiodysplasia are usually painless, as is the bleeding caused by radiation proctitis.

Why isn't colorectal cancer high on the list of differential diagnoses?

This sort of brisk bleeding is uncommon in patients with colorectal malignancies. Patients with colorectal cancer usually present with more gradual or even occult blood loss. Colonic polyps can bleed briskly on occasion, particularly if the patient is taking warfarin.

Why is radiation proctitis part of the differential diagnosis?

Radiation therapy for carcinoma of the cervix in women and carcinoma of the prostate in men is the most common cause of radiation proctitis, which can cause very significant lower GI tract bleeding. The fact that this is a first presentation and that Mrs. Noro's radiation treatment was 10 years ago does not preclude the diagnosis.

What is the first step in Mrs. Noro's management?

Mrs. Noro should have a large-bore peripheral IV line placed, have some crystalloid fluid to resuscitate her, and have blood drawn for the following tests: full blood cell count, platelet count, serum electrolyte levels, coagulation screen, blood type, and cross-match.

Is a nasogastric tube appropriate for this patient?

Yes. Although an upper GI tract bleed is unlikely, a nasogastric tube helps to detect one. Blood in the nasogastric aspirate raises the possibility of upper GI bleeding. Absence of blood in a bile-tinged nasogastric aspirate makes upper GI bleeding very unlikely. Another indication of bleeding in the upper GI tract is an elevation of the serum blood urea nitrogen (BUN) level out of proportion to the serum creatinine level.

Mrs. Noro's laboratory tests are all normal except the hemoglobin of 11.1 g per dL and a WBC count of 14.4.

How do Mrs. Noro's laboratory results help with the differential diagnosis?

The absence of coagulopathy suggests a primary lesion within the GI tract rather than bleeding from the GI tract as a manifestation of a systemic illness. The hemoglobin of 11.1 g per dL helps very little. The elevated WBC count is consistent with an acute bleed but does not narrow the differential diagnosis.

The patient remained stable in the emergency department with no further bleeding. Her pulse returns to 82 beats per minute with 500 mL of normal saline given over the hour that it took the laboratory work to come back.

What is the next step in Mrs. Noro's care? What tests should be done first?

The next step is to start the search for the source of bleeding. Mrs. Noro should undergo anoscopy and proctoscopy. Anoscopy reveals any hemorrhoids or anal fissure. Digital examination does not diagnose hemorrhoids. Proctoscopy permits assessment of the mucosal lining of the rectum. Proctitis, whether caused by radiation or by inflammatory bowel disease, can be identified, as can rectal cancer. It is important to have suction and irrigation on hand so that blood or clots can be removed to allow proper vision of the mucosa.

Mrs. Noro's anoscopy and proctoscopy revealed red blood in the rectum, which was easily evacuated. There was no evidence of proctitis, and no bleeding source was identified.

What is in the management plan now?

Lower GI tract hemorrhage stops spontaneously with supportive management alone in up to 90% of cases. Mrs. Noro should be admitted for continued resuscitation and observation. When the bleeding stops, a colonoscopy is performed after bowel preparation.

Does the absence of signs and symptoms of diverticulitis mean that her bleeding is more likely to be caused by angiodysplasia than by diverticular disease?

No. Bleeding diverticulosis is rarely associated with inflammatory changes. It is a different clinical scenario from that of acute diverticulitis.

What investigations may be useful in a patient with a lower GI tract hemorrhage?

Aside from the investigations already mentioned, nuclear scintigraphy, angiography, and colonoscopy have all been beneficial. These patients should not have a barium enema because barium precludes scintigraphy, confuses angiography, and impedes colonoscopy.

On the way to the nursing floor, Mrs. Noro passes a large amount of red blood and clots from the rectum, and her blood pressure is now 90/40 mm Hg.

How does this affect the treatment plan?
Mrs. Noro is now unstable, with evidence of a large lower GI tract bleed. She needs aggressive resuscitation and more urgent investigation. The physician must make sure there is enough cross-matched blood for Mrs. Noro, and at least 4 units should be kept in reserve.

What is the most likely diagnosis now?
Mrs. Noro most likely has diverticular disease or angiodysplasia.

How should Mrs. Noro be investigated now? Should she go straight to the operating room for a colectomy?
Every effort should be made to find the source of bleeding. Blind colectomies (i.e., without knowing the bleeding site) yield poor results. A segmental colonic excision may miss the source of bleeding, whereas subtotal colectomies and ileorectal anastomoses tend to have a poor functional outcome in this elderly population. Furthermore, these patients typically have comorbid medical conditions that put them at high risk for surgery.

What investigation should be performed at this time?
Nuclear scintigraphy, angiography, or both should be performed (7).

What are the two common forms of nuclear scintigraphy performed in the investigation of lower GI tract hemorrhage?
Technetium-labeled sulfur colloid and technetium-labeled red blood cell are the two most common forms of nuclear scintigraphy used to detect bleeding in the lower GI tract. Technetium-labeled sulfur colloid is cleared rapidly from the bloodstream and has limited value in the patient with intermittent bleeding. However, in the actively bleeding patient, such as Mrs. Noro, it is quicker to perform, is likely to be positive, and can direct selective angiography. Technetium-labeled red blood cell scans require a number of hours for completion and are less suitable in the unstable patient. However, these scans have the advantage of being able to detect intermittent bleeding because the labeled red blood cells remain in the vascular compartment for longer periods. Therefore, this scan is the technique of choice in the stable intermittently bleeding patient. It can detect bleeding rates as low as 0.1 to 0.5 mL per minute.

Mrs. Noro's sulfur colloid scan shows a lesion in the ascending colon.

What should be done next?

Mrs. Noro should now proceed to selective arteriography, which not only can accurately identify the source but also may be therapeutic.

Why not proceed directly to angiography and forgo the nuclear scan?

This is a reasonable strategy in the patient with a large bleed. Angiography requires a bleeding rate of 0.5 to 2 mL per minute to be positive. First doing a nuclear scan allows the physician to be more selective with the mesenteric vascular catheterization, and this has a number of advantages. First, if appropriate, gel embolization can be performed. Second, a catheter can be introduced into the bleeding mesenteric vessel for selective vasopressin infusion.

Mrs. Noro is confirmed to have a bleeding diverticulum in the proximal ascending colon.

Should the radiologist remove the vascular catheter and send Mrs. Noro to surgery?

No. This type of lesion may respond to treatment with intraarterial vasopressin. This technique is successful in up to 70% of patients and avoids surgery in this high-risk group.

Despite vasopressin treatment, Mrs. Noro continues to bleed. She has now had 6 units of blood since admission.

What should be done next?

Mrs. Noro should proceed to surgery for a right hemicolectomy.

Does Mrs. Noro need an ileostomy or can she undergo a primary anastomosis?

Although she has not had a formal bowel preparation, resection and primary anastomosis of the right colon can be done safely. Many surgeons would also perform a primary anastomosis on left-sided bleeding lesions, although this is somewhat less conservative.

Is the course of bleeding diverticulosis in this patient typical of this condition?

No. As mentioned previously, most patients stop bleeding spontaneously (8). Most of those who do not stop spontaneously respond to angiographic intervention.

What is the role of colonoscopy in patients with major lower GI tract hemorrhage?

Colonoscopy is technically difficult in these circumstances and is not the investigation of choice. Colonoscopy is better used for patients with intermittent

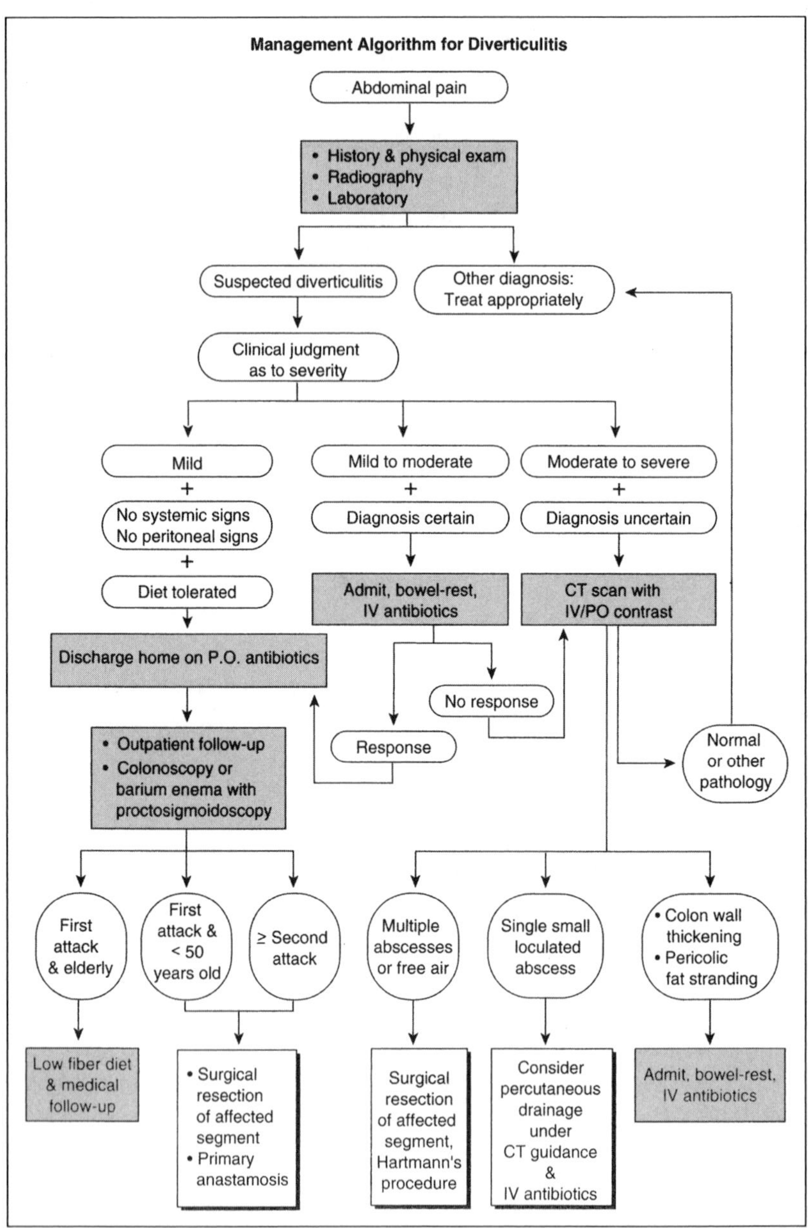

Algorithm 13.1.

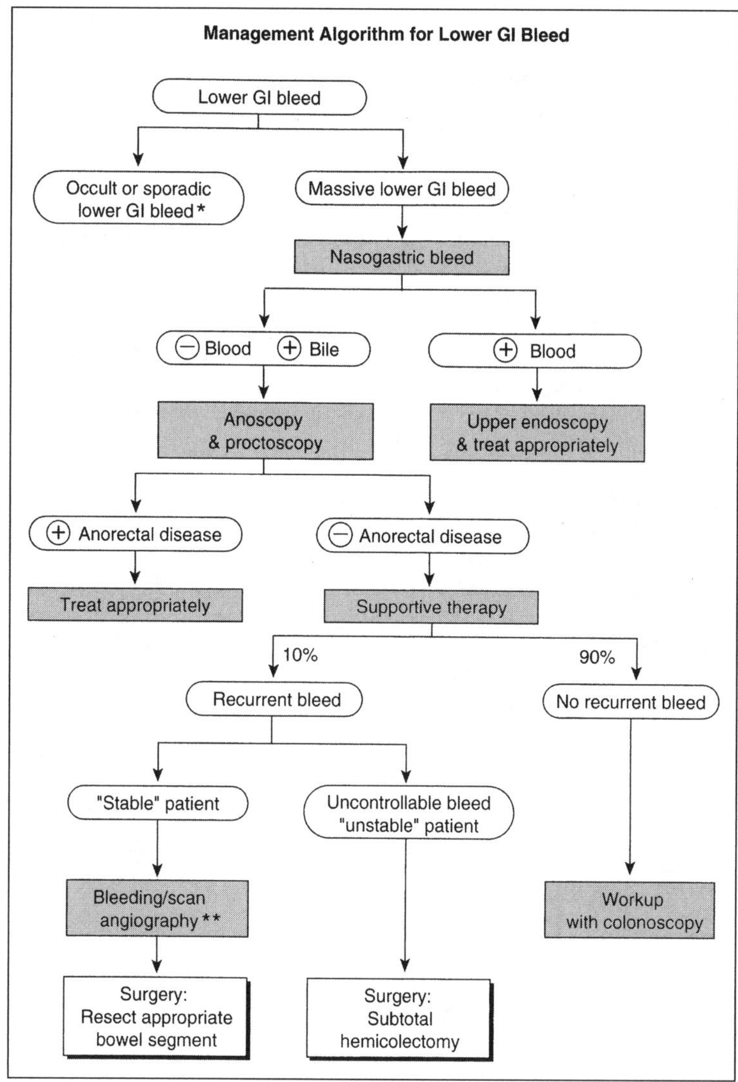

Algorithm 13.2.

bleeding who are stable enough to permit bowel preparation. Colonoscopy may be helpful intraoperatively in patients who proceed to surgery without localization of the bleeding site.

Mrs. Noro recovered uneventfully and was discharged home on the sixth postoperative day. She is tolerating a general diet.

What is the natural history of bleeding diverticulosis in patients not undergoing surgery?

Recurrent episodes of hemorrhage requiring a second admission to the hospital occur in 25% of patients. After a second episode, the chance of a third episode rises to 50%.

REFERENCES

1. Painter NS, Burkitt DP. Diverticular disease of the colon: a deficiency disease of Western civilization. BMJ. 1971;2:450–454.
2. Roberts PL, Veidenheimer MC. Current management of diverticulitis. Adv Surg. 1994;27:189–208.
3. Hinchey EF, Schaal PG, Richards GK. Treatment of perforated diverticular disease of the colon. Adv Surg. 1978;12:85–109.
4. Colcock BP, Stahmann FD. Fistulas complicating diverticular disease of the sigmoid colon. Ann Surg. 1972;175:838–846.
5. Hulnick DH, Megibow AJ, Balthazar EJ, et al. Computed tomography in the evaluation of diverticulitis. Radiology. 1984;152:491–495.
6. Boley SJ, Brandt LJ. Vascular ectasias of the colon. Dig Dis Sci. 1986;31(9 Suppl): 265–425.
7. Treat MR, Forde KA. Colonoscopy, technetium scanning and angiography in active rectal bleeding: an algorithm for their combined use. Surg Gastroenterol. 1983;2:135–138.
8. Cheskin LJ, Bohlman M, Schuster MM. Diverticular disease in the elderly. Gastroenterol Clin North Am. 1990;12:391–403.

CHAPTER

14

CANCER OF THE COLON AND RECTUM

D. Lee Gorden and Todd M. Tuttle

Isaac Jones is a previously healthy 66-year-old man who arrives at the emergency department with a complaint of light-headedness when standing. He describes passing black tarry stools three to four times in the past week. He has lost nearly 20 pounds in the past 6 months. He does not smoke, and he drinks alcohol only occasionally. His only medication is ibuprofen for mild arthritis.

What are the distinctions among melena, hematochezia, bright red blood per rectum, and heme-positive when describing a patient's stools?

All of these terms describe bleeding from the gastrointestinal (GI) tract.

- *Melena:* The passage of tarry, reddish-black stools
- *Hematochezia:* Bloody stools
- *Bright red blood per rectum:* Implies bleeding from a distal source or a massive hemorrhage from a proximal source
- *Heme-positive bleeding:* Bleeding that is not grossly visible; however, stools test positive on hemoccult cards

The correct description of a patient's stools may give important clues as to the source and rate of bleeding.

At the initial physical examination, Mr. Jones' vital signs are as follows: blood pressure, 140/80 mm Hg; heart rate, 104 beats per minute; temperature, 37°C; respiratory rate, 12 breaths per minute. His chest is clear to auscultation bilaterally, and a mild, regular, tachycardia is revealed. The abdomen is soft, not tender, and not distended, with normal bowel sounds. The rectal examination is significant, with hemoccult-positive melanotic stool in the vault. His neurologic examination produces normal findings.

Laboratory studies show a normal electrolyte profile. The white blood cell count is 7.4×10^3 cells per mm^3 (normal count, 4.5 to 11 cells per mm^3), hemoglobin level is 8.1 g per dL (normal level, 14 to 18 g per dL), with a mean corpuscular volume (MCV) of 72 fL (normal range, 86 to 98 fL), and the platelet count is 240,000 per mL (normal count, 150,000 to 450,000 per mL). Liver function test findings are within normal limits.

Which conditions should be considered in the differential diagnosis of lower GI tract bleeding?

The most common causes of lower GI bleeding are, in order of decreasing frequency, diverticular disease, carcinoma of the colon, inflammatory bowel disease, colonic polyps, vascular ectasias, ischemic colitis, rectal ulcers, and hemorrhoids, together with several very rare disorders (1). Algorithm 14.1 outlines a management algorithm for the workup for heme-positive stools.

Mr. Jones is anemic, and the low MCV suggests that his blood loss results from a chronic, not an acute, process. He undergoes colonoscopy, which reveals a fungating mass proximal to the hepatic flexure. The lesion is not amenable to endoscopic removal, and surgery is recommended.

What types of tumors occur in the colon and rectum?

Adenocarcinomas are the most common malignant colorectal tumors. Other malignant tumors are carcinoids, GI stromal tumors, primary lymphomas, and metastatic tumors originating from other organs (2). The most frequently encountered neoplasms are adenomas and adenomatous polyps (discussed later in this chapter).

How common is colorectal cancer?

Cancer of the colon and rectum is the third most commonly diagnosed malignancy and the second leading cause of cancer deaths in men and women in the United States. In 2002, an estimated 107,300 new cases of colon cancer and 41,000 new rectal cancers occurred. An estimated 56,600 patients died in 2002 from colorectal cancer. Importantly, nearly 50% of patients diagnosed develop metastases within 5 years. However, mortality from colorectal cancer has decreased over the past several decades (3).

What are some important anatomic considerations of the blood supply to the colon and rectum?

The arteries that supply the colon are paralleled by veins of the same names. The superior and inferior mesenteric veins join the splenic vein, which drains into the portal vein to the liver. Thorough review and knowledge of this anatomy is essential to a successful surgical resection.

The lymphatic drainage of the colon parallels the venous channels. Lymph nodes may be found in the colonic mesentery, the mesorectum, and the para-aortic area.

Low-lying cancers of the anal canal may spread to the deep inguinal nodes, and tumors of the anus may spread to the superficial inguinal nodes.

How should individuals be screened for colorectal cancer?

Average-risk, asymptomatic patients should undergo colorectal cancer screening at age 50. The most commonly used method is annual fecal occult blood test plus flexible sigmoidoscopy every 5 years. Colonoscopy can be performed every 5 to 10 years or double-contrast barium enema every 5 years. Virtual colonoscopy using computed tomography (CT) or other imaging modalities is not yet recommended (4–6).

What are the surgical options for the treatment of colon cancers?

The surgical treatment of colon tumors depends on their location. For single lesions, a segmental resection is usually performed, whereas for synchronous lesions, a more extensive resection may be required. Standard surgical procedures according to the location of the tumor include right hemicolectomy, transverse colectomy, left hemicolectomy, and sigmoid colectomy, with the corresponding mesentery and mesenteric lymph nodes included in the resection. A surgical margin of at least 2 cm is desirable, both proximal and distal to the tumor (7).

Should laparoscopic resection be performed for colon cancer?

Laparoscopic treatment for many nonmalignant diseases now is preferred over a traditional open operation. For laparoscopic-assisted colectomy, several small ports are introduced into the peritoneal cavity and pneumoperitoneum is established. Laparoscopic staging is performed, the colon is mobilized, and the vascular pedicle ligated and divided. The tumor-containing colon is then exteriorized through a small incision. Standard extracorporeal techniques are used to divide the colon and perform the anastomosis. Weeks et al. described the results of a multicenter prospective randomized trial comparing laparoscopic-assisted versus open colectomy for colon cancer. Only minimal short-term quality of life benefits were found in patients undergoing laparoscopic-assisted colectomy. Survival data from this study are not available (8,9).

The role of laparoscopic colectomy for colon cancer remains controversial and is continuing to be evaluated in trials. In the 2003 guideline, the National Comprehensive Cancer Network did not recommend laparoscopic colectomy.

Mr. Jones is scheduled to undergo a right hemicolectomy.

Is any additional diagnostic or staging information required before surgery?

An appropriate preoperative staging evaluation for colon cancer patients includes chest radiograph, colonoscopy, complete blood count, platelet count, carcinoembryonic antigen (CEA) level, and pathology review. The routine use of abdominal–pelvic CT is controversial. For rectal cancer, abdominal–pelvic CT is useful because the finding of metastatic disease may alter treatment decisions. In addition, endorectal ultrasound (ERUS) should be performed on patients with rectal cancer.

The CEA level, an important tumor marker, should be established preoperatively so that subsequent levels can be monitored. Abnormal preoperative liver function tests in patients with colonic malignancy are of concern and may suggest metastatic disease in the liver.

In patients with rectal cancer, the most important step is preoperative determination of the stage of the patient's disease. Again, history and physical examination, including a digital rectal examination and, for women, a pelvic examination, are very important. Patients with rectal tumors should undergo CT of the abdomen and pelvis.

ERUS is the most accurate method for staging local tumors. When performed by an experienced surgeon or radiologist, this procedure can disclose the depth of invasion with an accuracy of 85% to 90% and predict any nodal metastases with an accuracy of 85%. ERUS can help identify candidates for local therapy, patients who need radical surgery, and patients who would benefit from preoperative radiation therapy.

How should the bowel be prepared before colorectal surgery?

Three principles direct preparation of the colon for surgery:

1. Mechanical preparation of the colon to cleanse it of stool
2. Intraluminal antibacterial treatment
3. Systemic antibiotic therapy. The addition of oral antibiotics to the standard mechanical bowel preparation reduces complications after colonic surgery by as much as 40%.

An accepted preoperative bowel preparation procedure is as follows:

1. The patient is maintained on a clear liquid diet for 24 hours before surgery.
2. A balanced electrolyte solution, such as GoLYTELY or magnesium citrate, is used for mechanical cleansing and lavage of the bowel until the output is clear. A tap water or phosphate enema is a possible addition.
3. Oral antibiotics are administered 19, 18, and 9 hours before scheduled surgery. A widely used preparation is neomycin 1 g plus metronidazole with the possible addition of erythromycin. The use of parenteral antibiotics is somewhat controversial, but most surgeons recommend at least one dose of parenteral antibiotic, such as a second- or third-generation cephalosporin, within 30 minutes before incision to help reduce postoperative wound infection rates.

Mr. Jones undergoes a right hemicolectomy with no intraoperative complications. His postoperative course is uneventful.

What are the common staging systems for colon and rectal cancers?
Many staging systems have been devised and modified in an attempt to standardize and improve predictive outcomes. The most currently accepted staging method is the TNM system (Table 14.1).

The pathology findings confirm that Mr. Jones has stage T2N0M0 adenocarcinoma of the colon.

TABLE 14.1.

TUMOR, NODE, METASTASIS STAGING SYSTEM FOR COLORECTAL CANCER

Primary Tumor (T)

TX	Primary tumor cannot be assessed
T0	No evidence of primary tumor
Tis	Carcinoma in situ: Intraepithelial or invasion of lamina propria
T1	Tumor invades submucosa
T2	Tumor invades muscularis propria
T3	Tumor invades through muscularis propria into the subserosa, or into non-peritonealized, pericolic, or perirectal tissues
T4	Tumor directly invades other organs or structures, and/or perforates visceral peritoneum

Regional Lymph Nodes (N)

NX	Regional lymph nodes cannot be assessed
N0	No regional lymph node metastases
N1	Metastases in 1–3 regional lymph nodes
N2	Metastases in 4 or more regional lymph nodes

Distant Metastases (M)

MX	Distant metastasis cannot be assessed
M0	No distant metastasis
M1	Distant metastasis

Stage Grouping

Stage	T	N	M
0	Tis	N0	M0
I	T1	N0	M0
	T2	N0	M0
IIA	T3	N0	M0
IIB	T4	N0	M0
IIIA	T1–T2	N1	M0
IIIB	T3–T4	N1	M0
IIIC	Any T	N2	M0
IV	Any T	Any N	M1

Which clinical or pathologic factors predict survival of patients with colorectal cancers?

In addition to the staging system, several other factors are important determinants of survival after treatment for colorectal cancer:

- Vascular or lymphatic microinvasion
- Perineural invasion
- Presence of signet ring cells
- Mucin content
- Neuroendocrine differentiation of the tumor
- Tumor ploidy

Is sentinel lymph node (SLN) biopsy useful for colorectal cancer?

Not yet. SLN biopsy has replaced routine lymph node dissection in most patients with breast cancer and melanoma. For those diseases, the two main advantages of SLN biopsy are that it (a) reduces the side effects of lymph node dissection, and (b) provides more accurate nodal staging information. Because mesenteric lymph node dissection is not associated with any long-term side effects, the main benefit of SLN biopsy for colorectal cancer would be improved staging information.

In the standard method of evaluating lymph node dissections, the pathologist examines one or two levels of each lymph node. This method underestimates the incidence of lymph node metastases. If each lymph node is examined with serial sectioning (five to six levels for each lymph node) and special stains (immunohistochemistry), then occult metastases can be identified in about 10% to 20% of node-negative patients. However, the average mesenteric lymph node dissection yields about 15 lymph nodes. An intense pathologic analysis of all lymph nodes is not feasible. Instead, SLN biopsy provides the pathologist with one or two SLNs that can be examined with serial sectioning and immunohistochemistry.

The SLN for colon cancer is identified by injecting 2 to 3 mL of a vital blue into the subserosa surrounding the tumor. The blue SLNs are then tagged with a suture. Standard colectomy and mesenteric lymph node dissection are performed. The tagged SLNs are removed and undergo serial sectioning and immunohistochemistry. The rest of the specimen is analyzed in the usual fashion. Even though SLN biopsy can identify occult metastases in 10% to 20% of patients, the prognostic significance of occult metastases is not known. Presently, SLN biopsy for colorectal cancer is investigational (10).

Would Mr. Jones benefit from either adjuvant chemotherapy or radiation?

Adjuvant therapy is treatment of clinically inapparent microscopic disease. Randomized clinical trials have demonstrated that adjuvant chemotherapy improves the survival of patients with stage III colon cancer. Most oncologists recommend 6 months of 5-fluorouracil (5-FU) plus leucovorin. Adjuvant chemotherapy is not indicated for stage I colon cancer. Selected patients with stage II (grade 3 or 4 tumors, bowel obstruction, lymphatic or vascular invasion, T4 tumors) may benefit from chemotherapy. Either preoperative or postoperative chemoradiation is recommended for patients with stage II or III rectal cancer (11). Second-line chemotherapeutic agents, such as oxaliplatin and irinotecan, are currently being used to treat recurrent colorectal cancers.

What are the surgical options for the treatment of rectal cancers?

Rectal cancers may be treated with transanal excision, low anterior resection, or abdominoperineal resection, depending on tumor size and location, depth of bowel wall penetration, and lymph node involvement. Importantly, excision of the mesorectum provides the best chance for cure. Patients with rectal tumors may be candidates for local resection if there is no evidence of fixation to adjacent structures, transmural invasion of the tumor, or nodal spread, and if the histology of a biopsy specimen is favorable.

Primary anastomosis of the bowel is routine unless there is obstruction with significant distention of the colon or perforation from a tumor. The exception is abdominoperineal resection, in which an end-colostomy must be performed. For very low anastomoses, many surgeons recommend a temporary proximal diverting stoma to protect the distal anastomosis from the fecal stream. The technical considerations of the various procedures are not discussed in this chapter.

Many patients with rectal cancer can be treated with sphincter preservation. Abdominoperineal resection with end-colostomy is required to treat low rectal cancers invading the sphincter muscles. An anterior resection with either colorectal or coloanal anastomosis is appropriate treatment for selected patients with mid-rectal cancers. Carefully selected patients with rectal cancer may be candidates for transanal excision. Acceptable criteria for transanal excision include the following:

- Tumor less than 30% circumference of bowel
- Size less than 3 cm
- Clear margins
- Location near the anal verge
- Well to moderately differentiated tumors

Do patients with rectal cancers benefit from adjuvant therapy?

Adjuvant chemotherapy improves the survival of patients with node-positive rectal cancer. Moreover, adjuvant radiation therapy improves local recurrence rates in patients with stage II or III rectal cancer. However, whether preoperative or postoperative radiation is more beneficial is a subject of controversy. Recent evidence suggests that the outcome after radiation therapy may be improved by the addition of low-dose 5-FU to the treatment regimen; 5-FU acts as a radiosensitizer and potentiates the effects of the radiation therapy.

After discharge from the hospital, Mr. Jones requires follow-up and long-term surveillance for recurrence of colon cancer.

Surveillance procedures that can aid in early detection of recurrences include the following:

1. *History and physical examination.* Weight loss and GI bleeding are important indicators of possible recurrence.
2. *Routine flexible sigmoidoscopy and colonoscopy.* Its use is debatable, but it is useful for detecting metachronous lesions.
3. *Monitoring the levels of CEA.* An elevated CEA level may be the first clue to tumor recurrence. Serum CEA levels, measured at scheduled intervals, should be compared to a baseline CEA level measured several weeks after the initial surgical resection. CEA is not a good screening marker for colorectal cancer in the general population, but it is useful in surveillance for recurrent disease.
4. *Positron emission tomography (PET) imaging.* PET is useful for staging patients with known recurrent disease in the liver. It has a sensitivity of 90% to 100% and a specificity of 67% to 98%.

A suggested follow-up schedule from the National Comprehensive Cancer Network for patients with colorectal cancers is shown in Table 14.2 (12).

TABLE 14.2.

SUGGESTED FOLLOW-UP AFTER CURATIVE RESECTION FOR COLORECTAL CANCER: GUIDELINES OF THE NATIONAL COMPREHENSIVE CANCER NETWORK

History and physical	Every 3 mo × 2 yr then every 6 mo for a total of 5 yr
CBC	Not recommended
Liver function test	Not recommended
CEA	Every 3 mo × 2 yr then every 6 mo for a total of 5 yr (for T2 or greater lesions)*
Abdominal ultrasound	Not recommended
Abdominal CT scan	If indicated for certain clinical situations
Chest radiograph	If indicated for certain clinical situations
Colonoscopy	1 yr postop (or for obstructing lesion and unprepped bowel, after 3–6 mo), repeat in 1 yr if abnormal or every 3–5 yr if negative for polyps
Flexible proctosigmoidoscopy	Not recommended

* If the patient is a potential candidate for surgical resection of isolated metastasis.

CBC, complete blood count; CEA, carcinoembryonic antigen; CT, computed tomography.

At his 1-year follow-up visit, Mr. Jones is feeling well, but his alkaline phosphatase level is elevated and his CEA level is twice that of the measured baseline level. Colonoscopy shows no recurrence of tumor, but CT of the abdomen reveals a single low-density lesion 3 cm in diameter in the left lobe of the liver.

What is the survival rate for patients with isolated liver metastases from a primary colorectal tumor?

Patients with untreated liver metastases have an expected median survival of less than 1 year. Systemic chemotherapy has not significantly improved the survival in this group of patients. Hepatic resection in patients with isolated lesions in the liver leads to a 30% to 40% 5-year survival. Many advances have been made to enhance the safety and efficacy of liver resection for metastatic disease.

What are the criteria for successful resection of liver metastases?

To be considered for resection of liver metastases from colorectal cancer, a patient must be medically fit to undergo a major operation. In addition, there must be no evidence of extrahepatic metastases, and the lesions must be completely resectable, with tumor-free margins. Thus, re-staging of the patient's tumor is important to ensure that metastases are confined to the liver. This can be done with CT imaging of the chest, abdomen, and pelvis. Patients with recognized metastases in the liver should undergo PET staging to determine if there are any extrahepatic metastases in centers where this modality is available. Biopsy of lesions identified on CT is not necessary in the setting of planned curative liver resection. Surgery combined with modalities such as radiofrequency ablation, portal vein embolization, and adjuvant chemotherapy have increased the numbers of patients benefiting from surgical treatment of metastases. After liver resection, follow-up should include a physical examination, complete blood count, chemistry profile including CEA level, chest, radiography, and abdominal CT every 6 to 12 months, in addition to the routine colonoscopy follow-up for metachronous colon cancer.

Although there is some disagreement on this subject, the features of hepatic metastases that are associated with a poor prognosis include (a) more than four metastases, (b) positive margins at the time of resection of the tumor, (c) markedly elevated CEA levels, (d) lymph node–positive primary tumor, and (e) a short disease-free interval (less than 12 months) from the time of initial resection.

What are some of the etiologic factors of colorectal cancer?

Environmental risk factors include a high-fat, low-fiber diet, and probably cigarette smoking. Diseases that predispose to cancer of the colon and rectum include ulcerative colitis and Crohn's disease. Patients who have had colorectal, breast, ovarian, or uterine cancer are also at increased risk.

Molecular regulatory mechanisms play an important role in the pathogenesis of colorectal cancer. Oncogenes associated with colorectal cancer include K-*ras*, H-*ras* (most prevalent), N-*ras*, C-*myc*, and C-*src*. These mutated genes regulate the proliferation of tumor cells. In addition, the loss of tumor suppressor genes, including *APC*, *MCC*, and *DCC*, leads to decreased regulation of tumor cell growth. In the future, identification of mutated genes may be an important tool for screening, staging, and surveillance for colorectal malignancies (13,14).

What are the familial polyposis syndromes?

Familial adenomatous polyposis (FAP) is an autosomal dominant condition in which the patients are diagnosed by the presence of at least 100 adenomatous polyps in the colon and rectum. The incidence of malignant degeneration of polyps in these patients approaches 100% by the third or fourth decade of life. FAP is a general growth disorder associated with extracolonic manifestations, and this broad category is subdivided into groups with characteristic clinical manifestations. For example, *Gardner's syndrome* is associated with osteomas of the skull and desmoid tumors, whereas *Turcot's syndrome* is characterized by brain tumors. Other extracolonic manifestations of FAP are gastric or duodenal polyps and periampullary cancers. Hereditary polyposis syndromes account for approximately 1% of colorectal cancers. Total proctocolectomy is recommended for FAP patients who have a high lifetime risk of developing colorectal cancer.

Hereditary nonpolyposis colorectal cancers (HNPCC), also known as *Lynch syndromes*, are characterized by colon cancer arising at an early age in the absence of polyposis. HNPCC accounts for 2% to 5% of all colorectal cancers. The lifetime risk of colorectal cancer is nearly 80% in individuals carrying a mutation in an HNPCC gene. Patients with HNPCC are at increased risk for other malignancies such as endometrial, stomach, and ovarian cancer.

What is the importance of polyps in colorectal cancer?

Polyps of the colon and rectum may be divided into those that have potential for malignant degeneration and those that are benign. The most common type of benign colonic polyps is hyperplastic. Other benign polyps include hamartomas, inflammatory polyps, and lipomas. Peutz-Jeghers polyps and juvenile polyps have very low malignant potential. Polyps with malignant potential may be associated with familial syndromes or sporadic. The most common are adenomatous polyps that are categorized according to type—tubular, villous, or tubulovillous—and the degree of dysplasia. The cancer risk for these polyps is related to size: less than 1 cm, 1% to 10%; 1 to 2 cm, 7% to 10%; and more than 2 cm, 35% to 53%.

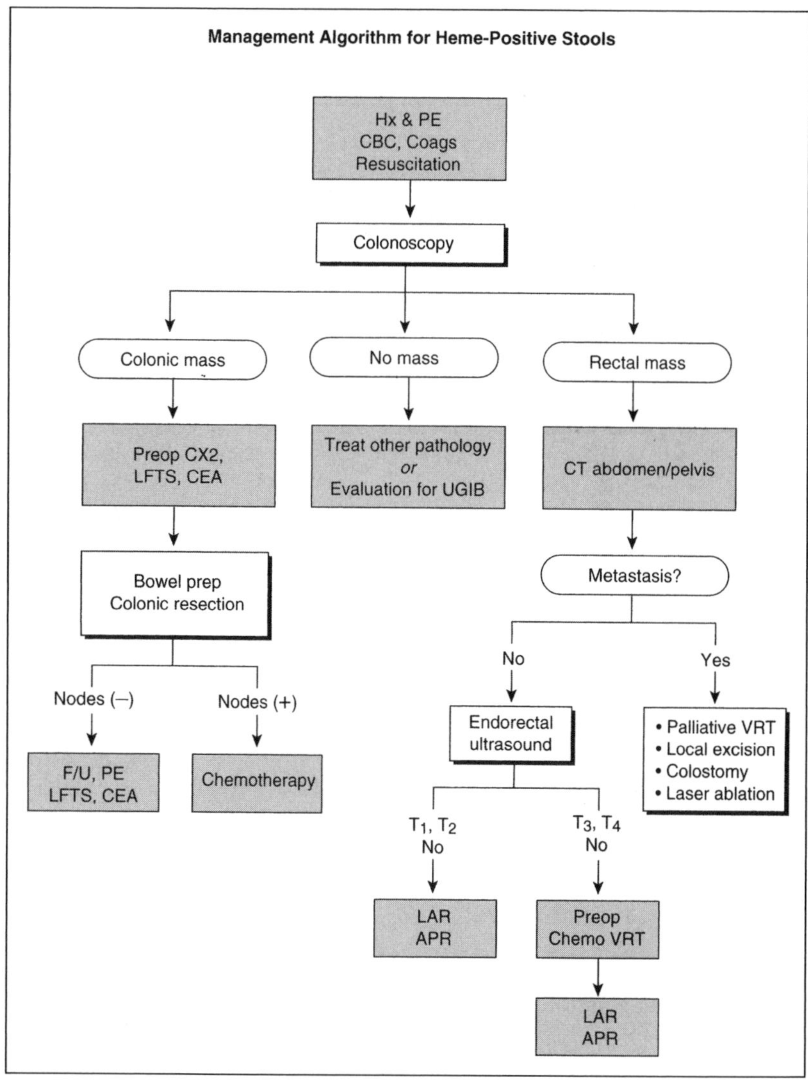

Algorithm 14.1.

REFERENCES

1. Farrands PA, Taylor I. Management of acute lower gastrointestinal haemorrhage in a surgical unit over a 4 year period. J Royal Soc Med. 1987;80:79–82.
2. Sabiston DC. Textbook of Surgery. 14th ed. Philadelphia, PA: WB Saunders; 1991.
3. Jemal A, Thomas A, Murray T, et al. Cancer Statistics, 2002. CA Cancer J Clin. 2002;52:23–47.

4. Mandel JS, Bond JH, Church TR, et al. Reducing mortality from colorectal cancer by screening for fecal occult blood. Minnesota Colon Cancer Control Study. N Engl J Med. 1993;328:1365.
5. Hardcastle JD, Chamberlain JO, Robinson MH, et al. Randomised controlled trial of faecal-occult-blood screening for colorectal cancer. Lancet. 1996;348:1472–1477.
6. Selby JV, Friedman GD, Quesenberry CP Jr, et al. A case-control study of screening sigmoidoscopy and mortality for colorectal cancer. N Engl J Med. 1992;326:653–657.
7. Cohen MC, Winawer SJ. Cancer of the Colon, Rectum, and Anus. New York, NY: McGraw–Hill; 1995.
8. Weeks JC, Nelson H, Gelber S, et al. Clinical Outcomes of Surgical Therapy (COST) Study Group. Short-term quality-of-life outcomes following laparoscopic-assisted colectomy vs. open colectomy for colon cancer: a randomized trial. JAMA. 2002;287:321–328.
9. Lacy AM, Garcia-Valdecasas JC, Delgado S, et al. Laparoscopy-assisted colectomy versus open colectomy for treatment of non-metastatic colon cancer: a randomised trial. Lancet. 2002;359:2224–2229.
10. Saha S, Wiese D, Badin J, et al. Technical details of sentinel lymph node mapping in colorectal cancer and its impact on staging. Ann Surg Oncol. 2000;7:120–124.
11. Moore HCF, Haller DG. Adjuvant therapy of colon cancer. Semin Oncol. 1999;26:545–555.
12. Meyerhardt JA, Mayer RJ. Follow-up strategies after curative resection of colorectal cancer. Semin Oncol. 2003;30:349–360.
13. Maddoff RD. Colorectal cancer genetics. Bull Am Coll Surg. 1996;81:26–32.
14. Kinzler KW, Vogelstein B. Lessons learned from hereditary colorectal cancer. Cell. 1996;87:159–170.

CHAPTER

15

ANORECTAL DISEASE

Kelli M. Bullard, Daniel A. Saltzman, and Todd M. Tuttle

Lucas Boyd is a 47-year-old man who seeks medical attention for a 10-day complaint of progressive rectal pain, perianal swelling, and foul-smelling drainage. He complains of a constant ache that is exacerbated by sitting and walking. He denies having fever, chills, constipation, diarrhea, or abdominal pain. His medical history is unremarkable, he takes no medications, and he has no allergies. Mr. Boyd's vital signs are normal, and his temperature is 37°C. Examination of the perianal region reveals a fluctuant tender mass measuring 3 × 2 cm in the left perianal region. The overlying skin is indurated and erythematous. He is too tender to tolerate a digital rectal examination (DRE). Significant laboratory data include a hemoglobin level of 13.2 g per dL, a white blood cell count of 7,000, and a normal platelet count.

What is the most likely diagnosis for Mr. Boyd's complaint on the basis of the history and physical examination?

Mr. Boyd has a perirectal abscess.

Where do perirectal abscesses originate?

The majority of perirectal abscesses result from infections of the anal glands and crypts (cryptoglandular infection). The glands are found in the intersphincteric plane, traverse the internal sphincter, and empty into the anal crypts at the level of the dentate line. Infection of an anal gland results in the formation of an abscess that enlarges and spreads along one of several planes in the perianal and perirectal spaces. More unusual causes of perirectal abscess (especially recurrent abscess and fistula) include Crohn's disease, malignancy, radiation, and opportunistic infection.

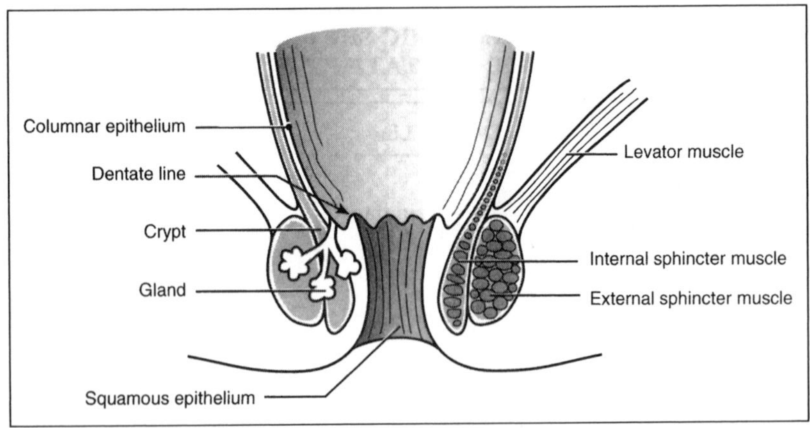

Figure 15.1. Anatomy of the anal canal.

What is the anatomy of the anal canal?

A basic knowledge of anorectal anatomy is fundamental to understanding perirectal disease (Fig. 15.1). The anal canal, the terminal end of the alimentary tract, measures approximately 2 to 4 cm (2 to 3 cm in most women, 3 to 4 cm in most men). In the anal canal, the *internal sphincter* is the continuation of the inner circular smooth muscular layer of the rectum and the *external sphincter* is the continuation of the outer longitudinal skeletal muscular layer of the rectum. The superior border of the external sphincter fuses with the puborectalis muscle and forms a sling originating at the pubis and joining behind the rectum. The intersphincteric plane, the space between the internal and external sphincters, is a fibrous continuation of the longitudinal smooth muscle of the rectum. Normally, 6 to 10 anal glands lie in this intersphincteric space.

What is the dentate line, and what is its anatomic significance?

The dentate line is an important surgical landmark at the union of the embryonic ectoderm with the gut endoderm. The line is recognizable as the line demarcating the transitional and squamous epithelium below and the rectal mucosa above. The columns of Morgagni begin at this line and extend cephalad. The dentate line divides the nervous system, vascular supply, and lymphatic drainage of the anal canal into two routes (Table 15.1).

What is the typical presentation of a perirectal abscess?

Severe anal pain is the most common presenting complaint. Walking, coughing, or straining can aggravate the pain. A palpable mass is often detected by inspection of the perianal area or by DRE. In the absence of systemic sepsis, fever and

TABLE 15.1.

ANATOMIC SIGNIFICANCE OF THE DENTATE LINE

	Above Dentate Line	Below Dentate Line
Innervation	Autonomic (anorectal mucosa is insensate)	Somatic (anoderm is sensate)
Venous drainage	Superior rectal vein → Inferior mesenteric vein → Portal circulation	Middle and inferior rectal veins → Internal iliac and internal pudendal veins → Systemic circulation
Lymphatic drainage	Inferior mesenteric, internal iliac lymph nodes	Inguinal lymph nodes

leukocytosis are rare. The diagnosis of a perianal or perirectal abscess usually can be made with physical examination alone (either in the office or in the operating room); however, complex or atypical presentations may require imaging studies such as computed tomography or magnetic resonance imaging to fully delineate the anatomy of the abscess. Rarely, patients will present with fever, urinary retention, and signs of sepsis. These findings should raise the suspicion of a severe, necrotizing soft tissue infection (often called *Fournier's gangrene*), which can be life threatening.

How does the original infection of the anal glands spread?

As infection in an anal gland enlarges, the resulting abscess spreads in one of several directions:

- *Perianal abscess:* most common; appears as a painful swelling at the anal verge, resulting from the spread of pus downward between the two sphincters.
- *Intersphincteric abscesses:* occur in the intersphincteric space and can be notoriously difficult to diagnose, often requiring an examination under anesthesia.
- *Ischiorectal abscess:* forms if the growing intersphincteric abscess penetrates the external sphincter below the puborectalis. Infection can spread into the fat of the ischiorectal fossa, and the abscess can become quite large. An ischiorectal abscess may involve both sides of the ischiorectal fossa, forming a *horseshoe abscess*. DRE will reveal a painful swelling laterally in one or both ischiorectal fossae.
- *Supralevator abscess:* uncommon; may result from extension of an intersphincteric or ischiorectal abscess upward or extension of an intraperitoneal abscess downward.

What is the differential diagnosis of a perirectal inflammatory process?

The differential diagnosis includes pilonidal abscess, hidradenitis suppurativa, infected sebaceous cyst, folliculitis, periprostatic abscess, Bartholin abscess, inflammatory bowel disease (Crohn's disease), or unusual infection (e.g., actinomycosis, tuberculosis).

Mr. Boyd is admitted to the hospital and taken to the operating room for incision and drainage of the abscess. Creating a small incision parallel to the anus drains the abscess. Anoscopy is performed and no internal opening (i.e., infected gland) is found. Mr. Boyd's postoperative care includes sitz baths and analgesia. He is discharged the day after surgery.

What is appropriate treatment for a perirectal abscess?

Perianal and perirectal abscesses should be treated by surgical drainage as soon as the diagnosis is established. If the diagnosis is in question, an examination under anesthesia is often the most expeditious way to both confirm the diagnosis and treat the problem. Delayed or inadequate treatment may occasionally cause progression to serious, life-threatening infection.

The site of the surgical incision depends on the location of the abscess:

- A perianal abscess is best drained through a small incision parallel to the anal verge to avoid injury to the sphincter, which could occur with a radial incision.
- An ischiorectal abscess is drained in a similar fashion, but may require a larger incision.
- An intersphincteric abscess is drained into the anal canal by creating a limited sphincterotomy.

A supralevator abscess can be extremely complex and drainage depends on the origin of the abscess:

- If the abscess is secondary to an upward extension of an intersphincteric abscess, it should be drained through the rectum.
- If a supralevator abscess arises from the upward extension of an ischiorectal abscess, it should be drained through the ischiorectal fossa.
- If the abscess is secondary to intraabdominal disease, the primary process requires treatment and the abscess is drained via the most direct route (i.e., transabdominally, rectally, or through the ischiorectal fossa).

Postoperatively, sitz baths and analgesia are the mainstay of treatment. Packing is rarely required and can increase pain. Stool softeners and bulk agents (fiber) can be helpful. Treatment of a perianal or perirectal abscess by drainage alone cures about 50% of patients. The remaining 50% develop persistent fistulas in ano (1).

Although often administered for the treatment of perirectal abscesses, antibiotics are only indicated if there is extensive overlying cellulitis or if the patient is immunocompromised, has diabetes mellitus, or has valvular heart disease. Antibiotics alone are ineffective in treating perianal or perirectal infection.

Mr. Boyd's recovery is uneventful, but 6 months later he returns with a complaint of persistent perirectal drainage. Physical examination reveals left perianal induration and an external opening at the site of the prior incision that is draining pus.

What is a fistula in ano?

A fistula is an abnormal communication between two epithelium-lined surfaces. A fistula in ano has its external opening in the perirectal skin and its internal opening in the anal canal at the dentate line. The fistula usually originates in the infected crypt (*internal opening*) and tracks to the *external opening*, usually the site of prior drainage.

What are the most common symptoms of fistula in ano?

The most common symptom of fistula in ano is persistent drainage. Recurrent abscesses may occur, especially if the external opening heals. Pain is rare with fistula in ano and suggests the presence of an undrained abscess. Patients may also complain of perirectal itching, irritation, and discharge (2).

What is the pathogenesis of fistula in ano?

A fistula in ano forms during the chronic phase of an acute inflammatory process that begins in the intersphincteric anal glands. The course of the fistula can often be predicted by the anatomy of the previous abscess. Fistulas are categorized based on their relationship to the anal sphincter complex (3):

- *Intersphincteric fistula:* tracks through the distal internal sphincter and intersphincteric space to an external opening near the anal verge
- *Transsphincteric fistula:* often results from an ischiorectal abscess and extends through both the internal and external sphincters
- *Suprasphincteric fistula:* originates in the intersphincteric plane and tracks up and around the entire external sphincter
- *Extrasphincteric fistula:* originates in the rectal wall and tracks around both sphincters to exit laterally, usually in the ischiorectal fossa

How is the internal opening of a fistula in ano located? What is Goodsall's rule?

Goodsall's rule relates the location of the internal opening to the external opening of a fistula in ano. Although the external opening is often easily identifiable, identification of the internal opening may be more challenging. Goodsall's rule can be used as a guide in determining the location of the internal opening.

In general, fistulas with an external opening *anteriorly* connect to the internal opening by a *short, radial tract.* Fistulas with an external opening *posteriorly* track in a *curvilinear fashion to the posterior midline.* However, an exception to this rule occurs if an anterior external opening is greater than 3 cm from the anal margin; these fistulas usually track to the posterior midline (4).

What other diseases are included in the differential diagnosis of fistula in ano?

The majority of fistulas are cryptoglandular in origin, but trauma, Crohn's disease, malignancy, radiation, or unusual infections (e.g., tuberculosis, actinomycosis, or chlamydia) may also produce fistulas. A complex, recurrent, or nonhealing fistula should raise the suspicion of one of these diagnoses.

What is the appropriate treatment for a patient, such as Mr. Boyd, who has an intersphincteric fistula?

Treatment of a fistula in ano is based on *eradication of infection* and *preservation of continence.* Simple intersphincteric fistulas can often be treated by *fistulotomy* (opening the fistulous tract), curettage, and healing by secondary intention. Treatment of a transsphincteric fistula depends on its location in the sphincter complex. Fistulas that include less than 30% of the sphincter muscles can usually be treated by sphincterotomy without risk of incontinence. High transsphincteric and suprasphincteric fistulas that encircle a greater amount of muscle are more safely treated by initial placement of a *seton,* which is a drain placed through a fistula to maintain drainage and induce fibrosis. A fistulotomy can often be performed 6 to 8 weeks later without compromising continence. Extrasphincteric fistulas are rare, and treatment depends on both the anatomy and etiology of the fistula.

High fistulas may be treated by *endorectal advancement flap. Fibrin glue* has also been used to treat persistent fistulas with variable results. Complex fistulas with multiple tracts may require numerous procedures to control sepsis and facilitate healing. Proctoscopy should be performed in all cases of complex or nonhealing fistulas to assess the health of the rectal mucosa. Biopsies of the fistula tract should be taken to rule out malignancy.

Sandra Smith is an otherwise healthy 42-year-old woman who comes to the office with a complaint of "hemorrhoids." Her symptoms consist of severe perianal pain and bleeding after having a bowel movement. She describes the pain as sharp and says it lasts for several hours after she moves her bowels. She also notices spots of bright red blood on the toilet paper. She has had no drainage from the perinanal area. She has been using several over-the-counter hemorrhoid treatments without relief. She has a long history of constipation. Perianal examination reveals a posterior midline crack in the anoderm and a small skin tag. There are

no masses, fluctuance, erythema, or drainage present. She is too tender to tolerate a DRE.

What is an anal fissure?

An anal fissure is a tear in the anoderm, thought to result from the passage of hard stool or prolonged diarrhea. The fissure occurs most often in the posterior midline and may be associated with a skin tag or sentinel pile. Characteristic symptoms include tearing pain with defecation and hematochezia (usually described as blood on the toilet paper). Patients may also complain of a sensation of spasm for several hours after a bowel movement. On physical examination, the fissure can often be seen in the distal anal canal by gently separating the buttocks. Patients are often too tender to tolerate DRE, anoscopy, or proctoscopy.

What are the therapeutic options for treating an anal fissure?

First-line therapy includes bulk agents, stool softeners, and warm sitz baths. Lidocaine jelly can provide additional relief. Nitroglycerin ointment (5) and topical diltiazem (6) have also been used. Medical therapy is effective in most acute fissures but will heal only approximately 50% to 60% of chronic fissures (7).

Lateral internal sphincterotomy is often recommended for chronic fissures that have failed medical treatment. The aim of this procedure is to decrease spasm of the internal sphincter by dividing a portion of the muscle. Healing is achieved in over 95% of patients using this technique, and most patients experience immediate pain relief. Recurrence occurs in less than 10% of patients, but the risk of incontinence (usually to flatus) ranges from 5% to 15% (7). Injection of botulinum toxin has recently been proposed as an alternative to surgical sphincterotomy for chronic fissure (7–9).

What are hemorrhoids?

The upper anal canal is lined by anal cushions consisting of three thick, vascular, submucosal bundles that lie in the left lateral, right posterior lateral, and right anterior lateral positions. The function of these cushions is not entirely clear, but they aid in continence and engorge during defecation to protect the anal canal from abrasions. Excessive straining, increased abdominal pressure, and hard stools increase venous engorgement of the hemorrhoidal plexus and produce abnormal hemorrhoidal tissue, which may become symptomatic. Because hemorrhoids are a normal part of anorectal anatomy, treatment is only indicated if they become symptomatic.

What are the most common presenting symptoms of a patient with internal hemorrhoids?

The most common manifestation of internal hemorrhoids is painless rectal bleeding. *Internal hemorrhoids* are located above the dentate line and covered by

TABLE 15.2.

CLASSIFICATION OF HEMORRHOIDAL DISEASE

Class of Hemorrhoid	Attributes
First degree	Does not protrude through anus
Second degree	Protrudes; reduces spontaneously
Third degree	Protrudes; reduces with manual pressure
Fourth degree	Protrudes; does not reduce; prone to strangulation and may require urgent or emergent surgery

insensate anorectal mucosa. Internal hemorrhoids may prolapse or bleed, but they rarely become painful unless they develop thrombosis and necrosis (usually related to severe prolapse, incarceration, and/or strangulation). The severity of internal hemorrhoids is graded according to the severity of prolapse. The standard classification of hemorrhoidal disease, as outlined by Buls and Goldberg, is presented in Table 15.2 (10).

If a patient presents with rectal bleeding and internal hemorrhoids are found, can the workup be considered complete?

Internal hemorrhoids are the most common cause of rectal bleeding; however, other causes of rectal bleeding should be excluded. Anoscopy is the procedure of choice for diagnosing internal hemorrhoids. Proctoscopy or flexible sigmoidoscopy can diagnose lesions in the rectum and descending colon. Colorectal carcinoma occasionally presents with hematochezia and, for this reason, patients with persistent unexplained bleeding should undergo colonoscopy.

Does portal hypertension cause internal hemorrhoids?

No. The incidence of hemorrhoids in the adult population with portal hypertension is no higher than in the normal population (11). *Rectal varices,* however, can result from portal hypertension and can occasionally present with massive hemorrhage. Treatment of rectal varices focuses on decreasing portal venous pressure (e.g., transjugular intrahepatic portosystemic shunt [TIPS] or surgical shunt procedure). Local measures almost never control bleeding from rectal varices.

What are the most common presenting symptoms of a patient with external hemorrhoids?

External hemorrhoids are located below the dentate line and are covered with anoderm. Because the anoderm is richly innervated, thrombosis of an external hemorrhoid may cause significant pain. A *skin tag* is redundant fibrotic skin at the anal verge, which may result from a thrombosed external hemorrhoid and may be confused with symptomatic hemorrhoids. External hemorrhoids and skin tags may cause itching and difficulty with hygiene if they are large. Treatment of external hemorrhoids and skin tags is only indicated for symptomatic relief.

What is the preferred treatment for hemorrhoids?

Bleeding from first- and second-degree internal hemorrhoids often improves with the addition of dietary fiber, stool softeners, increased fluid intake, and avoidance of straining. Pruritus may often resolve with improved hygiene. Over-the-counter topical medications are desiccants and are relatively ineffective for treating hemorrhoidal symptoms. Persistent bleeding from first- and second-degree internal hemorrhoids may be treated using rubber band ligation. Infrared photocoagulation and sclerotherapy are also effective procedures for controlling bleeding (1). Third- and fourth-degree hemorrhoids and mixed internal-external hemorrhoids require surgical hemorrhoidectomy (excisional hemorrhoidectomy). Because of the significant postoperative pain associated with excisional hemorrhoidectomy, *stapled hemorrhoidectomy* has been proposed as an alternative surgical approach (12,13).

Thrombosed external hemorrhoids can be effectively treated with excision during the first 24 to 48 hours after acute thrombosis. This procedure can usually be performed in the office under local anesthesia. Because the clot is usually loculated, simple incision and drainage is rarely effective. After 48 hours, the clot begins to resorb, and sitz baths and analgesics are usually adequate.

Maurice Sellers is a 32-year-old homosexual man who has been complaining of perirectal pain, bleeding, and occasional discharge. He has also noticed numerous perianal growths. A proctoscopic examination reveals numerous anal warts in the perianal region and in the anal canal.

What is the etiology of Mr. Seller's problem?

Mr. Sellers has condylomata acuminata (anogenital warts) of the anorectum. Condyloma acuminata are caused by the human papillomavirus (HPV), and sexual transmission is the most common source of infection. Condyloma usually occur in the perianal area or in the squamous epithelium of the anal canal. HPV infection is associated with anal intraepithelial neoplasia and squamous cell carcinoma. There are approximately 30 serotypes of HPV. HPV types 16 and 18 appear to predispose to malignancy.

Treatment of anal condyloma depends on the location and extent of disease. Small warts on the perianal skin and distal anal canal may be treated in the office with topical application of bichloracetic acid or podophyllin. Although 60% to 80% of patients will respond to these agents, recurrence and reinfection are common. Imiquimod (Aldara) is an immunomodulator that has recently been introduced for topical treatment of several viral infections including anogenital condyloma (14).

Larger and/or more numerous warts require excision and/or fulguration in the operating room. Excised warts should be sent for pathologic examination to rule out dysplasia or malignancy. It is important to note that prior use of podophyllin may induce histologic changes that mimic dysplasia. Condyloma acuminata is often associated with other sexually transmitted diseases; therefore, examination and testing for herpes or chlamydial infection, gonococcal proctitis, anorectal syphilis, and HIV is prudent.

Which neoplasms occur in the anorectal region?

Cancers of the anal canal are uncommon and account for only about 2% of all colorectal malignancies. Neoplasms of the anal canal can be divided into those affecting the *anal margin* (below the dentate line) and those affecting the *anal canal* (above the dentate line). In many cases, therapy depends on whether the tumor is located in the anal canal or at the anal margin.

Epidermoid carcinoma is the most common malignancy of the anorectum and includes squamous cell carcinoma, cloacogenic carcinoma, transitional carcinoma, and basaloid carcinoma. The clinical behavior and natural history of these tumors are similar. Squamous cell carcinoma in situ is often called *Bowen's disease.* Epidermoid carcinoma is a slow growing tumor and usually presents as an anal or perianal mass. Pain and bleeding may be present. Epidermoid carcinoma of the anal margin may be treated in a similar fashion as squamous cell carcinoma of the skin in other locations, and wide local excision is usually adequate treatment for these lesions. Epidermoid carcinoma occurring in the anal canal or invading the sphincter cannot be excised locally, and first-line therapy relies on chemotherapy and radiation (the *Nigro protocol:* 5-fluorouracil, mitomycin C, and 3000 cGy external beam radiation) (15). Over 80% of these tumors can be cured using this regimen.

More uncommon tumors of this region include basal cell carcinoma, adenocarcinoma, extramammary Paget's disease (adenocarcinoma in situ), melanoma, and metastatic lesions.

What are the complications of anorectal surgery?

Urinary retention is the most common complication following anorectal surgery. The risk of urinary retention can be minimized by limiting intraoperative and perioperative intravenous fluids and by providing adequate analgesia.

Pain can lead to fecal impaction. Risk of impaction may be decreased by preoperative enemas or a limited mechanical bowel preparation, liberal use of laxatives postoperatively, and adequate pain control.

Bleeding may also occur postoperatively. A small amount of bleeding, especially with bowel movements, is to be expected, but massive hemorrhage can

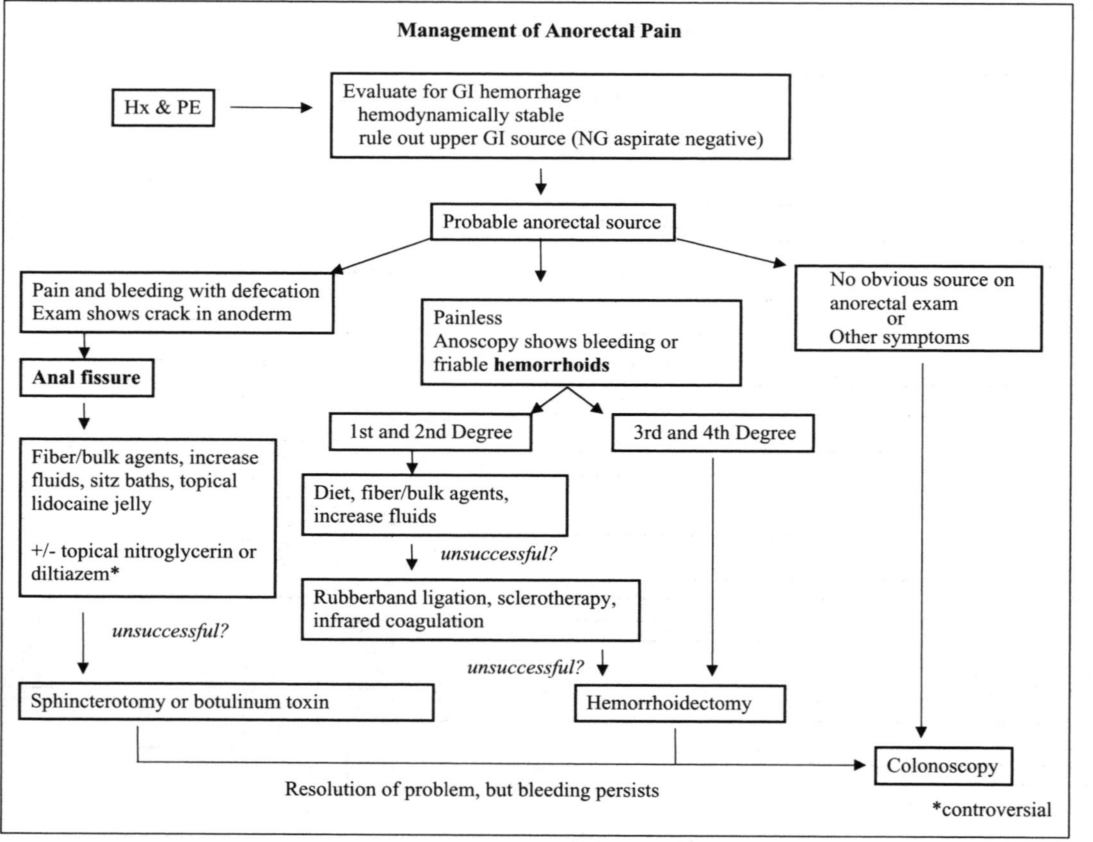

Algorithm 15.1.

Management of Anorectal Bleeding

Hx & PE → Anoscopy or Exam under anesthesia (if very tender)

- Pain, swelling, +/- drainage? → Perirectal Abscess → Incision and drainage → Wound care
- Fistula? → Fistula in ano
  - Low/superficial? → Fistulotomy
  - High/deep? → Seton drainage → Second stage fistulotomy, advancement flap, fibrin glue*
- Fissure? → Anal Fissure → Fiber/bulk agents, increase fluids, sitz baths, topical agents → *unsuccessful?* → Sphincterotomy or botulinum toxin injection*
- Hemorrhoids? → Hemorrhoids
  - Thrombosed external hemorrhoid?
    - <48 hours → Excise
    - >48 hours → Sitz baths, analgesia → *unsuccessful?* → Hemorrhoidectomy
  - Incarcerated, strangulated, gangrenous? → Hemorrhoidectomy

*controversial

Algorithm 15.2.

occur, particularly after hemorrhoidectomy. Bleeding may occur in the immediate postoperative period (often in the recovery room) due to inadequate ligation of the vascular pedicle. Bleeding may also occur 7 to 10 days after hemorrhoidectomy, when the necrotic mucosa overlying the vascular pedicle sloughs. Although some patients who are bleeding may be safely observed, most require an examination under anesthesia to ligate the bleeding vessel.

Infection is uncommon after anorectal surgery; however, necrotizing soft tissue infection can have devastating consequences. Severe pain, fever, and urinary retention may be early signs of infection. If infection is suspected, an emergent examination under anesthesia, drainage of abscess, or débridement of all necrotic tissue is required. Long-term sequela of anorectal surgery include incontinence, anal stenosis, and anal mucosal ectropion (1,16).

REFERENCES

1. Bullard K, Rothenberger D. Colon, rectum, and anus. In: Brunicardi C, ed. Schwartz's Principles of Surgery. 8th ed. New York, NY: McGraw-Hill; 2004.
2. Garcia-Aguilar J, Belmonte C, Wong W, et al. Anal fistula surgery: factors associated with recurrence and incontinence. Dis Colon Rectum. 1996;39: 723–729.
3. Parks AG, Gordon PH, Hardcastle JD. A classification of fistula-in-ano. Br J Surg. 1976;63:1–12.
4. Goodsall D. Diseases of the Anus and Rectum. London, UK: Lonmans; 1900.
5. Bailey H, Beck D, Billingham R, et al. A study to determine the nitroglycerin ointment dose and dosing interval that best promote the healing of chronic anal fissures. Dis Colon Rectum. 2002;45:1192–1199.
6. Jonas M, Speake W, Scholefield J. Diltiazem heals glyceryl trinitrate-resistant chronic anal fissures: a prospective study. Dis Colon Rectum. 2002;45: 1091–1095.
7. Madoff RD, Fleshman JW. AGA technical review on the diagnosis and care of patients with anal fissure. Gastroenterology. 2003;124:235–245.
8. Minguez M, Herreros B, Benagees A. Chronic anal fissure. Curr Treat Options Gastrenterol. 2003;6:257–262.
9. Mentes B, Irkorucu O, Akin M, et al. Comparison of botulinum toxin injection and lateral internal sphincterotomy for the treatment of chronic anal fissure. Dis Colon Rectum. 2003;46:232–237.
10. Buls J, Goldberg S. Modern management of hemorrhoids. Surg Clin North Am. 1978;58:469–478.
11. Jacobs D, Bubrick M, Onstad G, et al. The relationship of hemorrhoids to portal hypertension. Dis Colon Rectum. 1980;23:567–569.
12. Pescatori M, Favetta U, Dedola S, et al. Transanal stapled excision of rectal mucosal prolapse. Tech Coloproct. 1997;1:96–98.
13. Sutherland LM, Burchard AK, Matsuda K, et al. A systematic review of stapled hemorrhoidectomy. Arch Surg. 2002;137:1395–1406.

14. Staley M. Imiquimod and the imidazoquinolones: mechanism of action and therapeutic potential. Clin Exp Dermatol. 2002;27:571–577.
15. Nigro N, Vaukevicius V, Considine B. Combined therapy for cancer of the anal canal: a preliminary report. Dis Colon Rectum. 1974;17:354–356.
16. Schoetz D. Complications of anorectal operations. Surg Clin North Am. 1983;63:1249–1257.

CHAPTER

16

CHOLELITHIASIS AND ACUTE CHOLECYSTITIS

Viriato M. Fiallo

Consuelo Rodriguez is a 40-year-old woman with right upper quadrant pain that started 2 months ago. The pain is precipitated by fatty meals; it begins approximately 60 minutes after eating and lasts for several hours. On occasion, she feels the pain in the inferior aspect of the scapula, the shoulder, and the epigastrium. She frequently feels nauseous with the pain, and she has occasional emesis. Her primary care physician orders an ultrasound of the right upper quadrant that shows multiple stones in the gallbladder. The patient is referred to be evaluated for surgery.

Can cholelithiasis cause any other symptoms?

A significant number of patients with cholelithiasis do not have postprandial pain but instead have dyspepsia, vague upper gastric discomfort, or even mildly increased flatulence as primary symptoms (1).

How many types of gallstones are known?

There are three types of gallstones: cholesterol, pigmented, and mixed. Approximately 10% of stones are pure cholesterol, 15% are pigmented, and the remaining 75% are mixed (1).

What are the factors in the formation of gallbladder stones?

Factors in the formation of cholesterol stones include supersaturation of bile acid micelles, formation of abnormally high-cholesterol–containing biliary vesicles, and ileal disorders or ileal resections. The gallbladder also plays a role in the pathogenesis of cholesterol stones by favoring *nucleation* (the process by which cholesterol monohydrate crystals form and agglomerate) and crystal growth by abnormal absorption or secretion, by a defective surface pH, or by providing essential nucleating factors including mucin, desquamated cells, bacteria, and reflux intestinal contents (1–3).

Are stones the only cause of symptoms related to gallbladder disease?
No. Functional disorders of the gallbladder and the sphincter of Oddi can give rise to clinical manifestations similar to those of cholelithiasis. These motility disorders have been called *chronic acalculous cholecystitis,* or *gallbladder dyskinesia.*

The most specific test for these disorders is cholecystokinin-enhanced cholescintigraphy with assessment of gallbladder ejection fraction. An ejection fraction of less than 35% is considered abnormal (4). Other than biliary dyskinesia, undetectable small stones or cholesterolosis also can be symptomatic. For these patients, duodenal drainage studies demonstrating abnormal bile-containing cholesterol or calcium bilirubinate crystals have been useful. Approximately 80% of patients with abnormal cholecystokinin-cholescintigraphy or abnormal duodenal drainage studies have significant improvement of their symptoms after cholecystectomy (1).

What is the significance of biliary sludge?
A study in the 1990s looked at the clinical significance of gallbladder sludge. Diagnosis of gallbladder sludge was made by ultrasound in 286 patients followed up for a mean of 20 months. Although sludge disappeared spontaneously within a relatively short time in 71% of the patients, gallbladder sludge was significant because cholelithiasis or other complications occurred in 19% of the patients. Acute calculus cholecystitis developed in 7.1% of the patients (5).

Are any people more likely to form gallstones than others?
An increased incidence of gallstone disease has been observed in elderly patients, certain ethnic groups, women, immediate family members of a patient with cholelithiasis, obese patients, diabetic patients, cirrhotic patients, patients with truncal vagotomy, and patients receiving long-term total parenteral nutrition (1).

What is the natural history of gallstones?
Asymptomatic patients with gallstones generally have a benign course. Approximately 2% of asymptomatic patients with gallstones develop symptoms every year. One study of 123 patients with asymptomatic cholelithiasis and an actuarial follow-up period of up to 20 years showed that only 5.7% of these patients developed severe complications, including obstructive jaundice, acute cholecystitis, gallstone ileus, and pancreatitis. Only 13% eventually developed mild symptoms that required elective cholecystectomy (2,6,7).

Should asymptomatic gallstones be treated?
It is a general practice not to treat cholelithiasis until symptoms develop. The morbidity and mortality rates of asymptomatic patients treated with observation versus cholecystectomy are similar (8).

Indications for prophylactic cholecystectomy follow (8,9):

- *Children with gallstones:* they almost always develop symptoms
- *Sickle cell disease:* this condition poses diagnostic difficulties, and approximately 25% of these patients develop symptoms
- *Calcified gallbladder:* Approximately 50% of these patients have an associated gallbladder cancer
- *Stones larger than 2.5 cm:* they are frequently associated with acute cholecystitis, and a prophylactic cholecystectomy may be warranted
- *Nonfunctioning gallbladder:* this indicates advanced disease, and 25% of patients develop symptoms

Is diabetes mellitus an indication for prophylactic cholecystectomy?

A prospective study of non–insulin-dependent diabetic patients who were followed for 5 years showed that a cumulative percentage of 10.8% of patients developed symptoms and 4.2% developed complications (9). Another prospective review comparing diabetic and nondiabetic patients who underwent cholecystectomy did not show a difference in the incidence of perforation, wound infection, overall morbidity, or mortality (1). Therefore, in general, prophylactic cholecystectomy in an asymptomatic diabetic patient may not be recommended (2,10). However, it is important to consider individual factors such as age and comorbidities, and surgery may be appropriate in selected asymptomatic diabetic patients.

What are the possible complications of untreated symptomatic cholelithiasis?

Possible complications include acute cholecystitis, obstructive jaundice, acute cholangitis, gallstone ileus, and gallstone pancreatitis. Less than 1% of patients with initial complication of cholelithiasis have a fatal outcome during that hospitalization (1).

Now that Mrs. Rodriguez has a good understanding of the pathogenesis of gallstones and the possible complications of cholelithiasis, she wants to know her treatment options.

What are the treatment options for symptomatic cholelithiasis?

The treatment options include operative management consisting of open or laparoscopic cholecystectomy, percutaneous cholecystostomy, extracorporeal shock wave lithotripsy (ESWL), oral gallstone dissolution agents (ursodeoxycholic acid), and contact dissolution agents through a percutaneous approach with methyl *tert*-butyl ether (MTBE).

How effective are the nonoperative options in the management of symptomatic cholelithiasis?

ESWL is usually combined with oral bile acid dissolution. Complete stone clearance rates vary from 60% to 90%. The factors that determine the complete clearance of the stones are the isodensity with bile and the computed tomography (CT) score (Hounsfield units below 75). The main causes of failure are acquired stone calcification and impaired gallbladder motility (11). When calculated by actuarial analysis, the probability of stone recurrence has been 5.5% to 7% after 1 year, 11% to 12% after 2 years, 13% after 3 years, 20% after 4 years, and 31% after 5 years (11,12).

Gallbladder emptying is an important factor in the recurrence of gallstones. One study showed that the recurrence rate was 53% at 3 years when the gallbladder ejection fraction was less than 60% but only 13% in patients with an ejection fraction above 60% (13). The cumulative risk of gallstone recurrence by actuarial analysis has been shown, after complete direct contact dissolution with MTBE, to be as follows (14):

1 year, 23%
2 years, 34%
3 years, 55%
4 years, 70%

When are nonsurgical options indicated?
These modalities are indicated for symptomatic patients who are poor risks for laparoscopic cholecystectomy. Most protocols for ESWL are limited to symptomatic patients with one to three radiolucent stones with a diameter of 30 mm or less and a functioning gallbladder according to CCK hepatobiliary iminodiacetic acid (CCK HIDA) scan. ESWL is safe and effective for patients with a single stone not more than 20 mm in diameter, but the efficacy for larger single stones and multiple stones is poor (12,14,15). Long-term use of ursodeoxycholic acid is associated with reduced risk of biliary pain and acute cholecystitis (16).

For cholelithiasis, how should symptomatic gallstones be treated?
The preferred method of treating symptomatic gallstones is laparoscopic cholecystectomy. It has the advantages of little postoperative discomfort, short hospital stay, and short postoperative disability. This procedure can be performed safely with an overall morbidity that ranges from 3% to 10%, and mortality rates are 0 to 0.1%. Injury to the bile ducts occurs in 0.2% to 0.6% of patients undergoing this procedure. The incidence of complication decreases with increased surgeon experience and with careful attention to laparoscopic surgical technique. The incidence of major bile duct injury can decrease to rates comparable with those of open cholecystectomy.

What are the chances of having calculi in the common bile duct (CBD) in routine cholecystectomy?
CBD stones are found in 8% to 15% of patients undergoing cholecystectomy for symptomatic cholelithiasis (1). The incidence seems to be greater in patients older than 60 years of age (25%).

Should intraoperative cholangiography be performed routinely during laparoscopic cholecystectomy?

This topic is controversial. Advocates of routine intraoperative cholangiography during laparoscopic cholecystectomy argue that this practice gives a better definition of the anatomy by providing a road map for the surgeon and by identifying anomalous insertion of the cystic duct or other anatomic aberrations of the bile ducts. Only those performing it routinely become proficient in cannulating the cystic duct and in interpreting the fluoroscopic images. Also, a routine intraoperative cholangiogram enables the surgeon to detect an injury to the bile tract early during operation, allowing a prompt repair and reducing the morbidity associated with delayed diagnosis and repair of injuries made to major bile ducts (2,16).

Other surgeons argue against the routine use of cholangiography because they say it is too technical, it wastes time and expense, there are false-positive studies (4%), and it has not been proven that routine intraoperative cholangiography prevents bile duct injury (1,16,17). A retrospective nationwide cohort analysis of Medicare patients undergoing cholecystectomy and a retrospective population-based cohort study looking at the Washington State Hospital discharge database showed that the rate of CBD injury was significantly lower when intraoperative cholangiography was used. Use of intraoperative cholangiography does not, however, completely prevent injuries (18,19).

In what circumstances should an intraoperative cholangiogram be performed?

An intraoperative cholangiogram should be performed if there is cholangitis or pancreatitis or a history thereof; if preoperative evaluation shows a dilated or thick CBD; if there are multiple small stones in the gallbladder and the cystic duct; or if the liver function tests are abnormal. An intraoperative cholangiogram is also performed if the surgeon is unable to identify all the structures of the triangle of Calot.

Mrs. Rodriguez agrees to have her gallbladder removed via laparoscopy. While awaiting surgery, she develops severe, constant right upper quadrant pain accompanied by nausea and vomiting. The pain increases rapidly in intensity and is referred to the epigastrium, the right shoulder, and the tip of the scapula.

What is wrong with Mrs. Rodriguez?

The patient may have acute cholecystitis or biliary colic. Biliary colic causes pain that reaches a plateau lasting minutes to hours. In patients with acute cholecystitis, the pain persists after several hours and may last days. With time, the pain tends to localize more in the right upper quadrant because of the inflammation irritating the peritoneum (1).

What causes inflammation of the gallbladder in acute cholecystitis?
It is believed that the initial inflammatory process is a biochemical phenomenon as opposed to an infectious event. The mediators that have been shown to cause cellular injury and inflammation are the bile acids, lithogenic bile, pancreatic juice, lysolecithin, phospholipase A, and prostaglandins. The bacterial invasion is a secondary process (1).

During physical examination, Mrs. Rodriguez is found to have a tender right upper quadrant with mild guarding and a positive Murphy's sign. Her temperature is 37.8°C orally. Laboratory examination reveals a leukocyte count of 10,000 per mL, normal electrolyte levels, and a total bilirubin of 1.8 mg per dL. Plain radiograph of the abdomen shows a normal bowel pattern but no stones.

What is Murphy's sign?
A classic physical sign of cholecystitis, Murphy's sign is elicited by pressing the right upper quadrant with one's hand and asking the patient to inhale. The sign is present when the patient suddenly stops the inspiratory effort because of the exquisitely painful contact of the inflamed gallbladder with the examiner's hand.

What is the significance of a palpable mass in the right upper quadrant when acute cholecystitis is suspected?
The palpable mass may represent hydrops (mucocele) or a pericholecystic abscess. Hydrops occurs when a gallbladder obstructed by an impacted stone fills with a clear or white mucoid material. The wall usually is not inflamed. The mucoid fluid results from altered secretion of the gallbladder epithelium. Symptoms suggesting cholecystitis may or may not be present (1,2).

In the case of pericholecystic abscess, the patient usually is toxic. Empyema, pus in the lumen of the gallbladder, frequently accompanies this condition. The abscess is secondary to a subacute perforation of the inflamed gallbladder. Intervention in the form of cholecystectomy or cholecystostomy is mandated.

Does the lack of an elevated white blood cell count and high fever rule out acute cholecystitis?
No. A recent retrospective study of 100 consecutive patients suspected of having acute cholecystitis who were seen in the emergency department revealed that only Murphy's sign had a high sensitivity (97.2%) and a high positive predictive value (93.3%) in diagnosing acute cholecystitis compared with biliary scintigraphy (21). These results are similar to those of another retrospective study of 198 patients, which showed that patients with acute cholecystitis (confirmed at surgery) frequently lacked fever and leukocytosis (22).

Does a negative abdominal radiograph rule out gallstones?

No. Because gallstones consist largely of the radiolucent cholesterol pigments, only 15% of them are radiopaque. In contrast, kidney stones are 85% radiopaque, a consequence of the higher composition of calcium in kidney stones.

What is the significance of air in the gallbladder revealed by plain radiograph?

Emphysema of the gallbladder is a result of infection by gas-producing organisms (e.g., clostridia) and is a surgical emergency. It also may arise from a fistula between the intestine and the gallbladder, allowing air into the latter.

How does ultrasound compare with radionuclide imaging, such as HIDA scan? In which situations is one preferred over the other?

Ultrasound is simple, fast, and 95% accurate for demonstrating gallstones (i.e., cholelithiasis) (20). It cannot, however, demonstrate the acute infection of the gallbladder as well as HIDA (accuracy of ultrasound, 79% to 86%) (21). Ultrasound diagnosis of acute cholecystitis is inferred from the ultrasonic images of thickened wall, pericystic fluid, and the presence of intracavitary sludge or stones, intramural gas, and sloughed mucosal membrane.

However, a radionuclide scan has almost 100% sensitivity for diagnosing acute cholecystitis (23). Intravenously (IV) injected isotopes (e.g., HIDA) are secreted into the bile, revealing the biliary tract. The test is reliable with the serum bilirubin level of up to 8 to 10 mg per dL; above those levels, the reliability decreases. The gallbladder is usually visible within 20 to 30 minutes. Failure to reveal the gallbladder implies obstruction of the cystic duct and infection of the organ. Acute cholecystitis is highly likely if the gallbladder is not visible at 1 hour and is certain if the gallbladder is not visible at 4 hours. Acute cholecystitis is mostly a clinical diagnosis; therefore, ultrasound is an adequate test to demonstrate it in a patient with a high clinical suspicion. In patients whose clinical presentation for acute cholecystitis is equivocal or in whom preoperative diagnosis is mandatory because of a significant surgical risk, HIDA scan is more appropriate because of its higher accuracy.

What is the problem with the HIDA scan?

It can have false-positive results, especially in critically ill patients on total parenteral nutrition with prolonged fasting and in patients with acute pancreatitis.

Can the specificity of HIDA scan be improved in these circumstances?

Yes. Pretreatment with cholecystokinin is helpful in the presence of functional resistance to tracer flow into the gallbladder (24). Administration of IV morphine causes spasm of the sphincter of Oddi, thereby causing reflux of bile with radionuclide in the gallbladder. This technique is recommended when the gallbladder is not visible after 1 hour (24). Morphine also increases the visibility of gallbladder in patients pretreated with cholecystokinin (25).

Mrs. Rodriguez has a mildly elevated total bilirubin.

What does this test result mean in her case?

Because the patient does not have a history of liver disease, the two possible explanations are the presence of a stone or stones in the CBD and Mirizzi's syndrome.

What is Mirizzi's syndrome?

Mirizzi's syndrome is characterized by obstruction of the common hepatic duct (CHD) or CBD due to contiguous inflammation in the gallbladder or the cystic duct or to compression of the CHD by an impacted large stone in the adjacent cystic duct. The chronic inflammation can result in a stricture. Mild jaundice is present in up to 20% of patients with acute cholecystitis (1). It is usually the result of contiguous inflammation.

Can acute cholecystitis occur in the absence of cholelithiasis?

Yes. The condition known as *acalculous cholecystitis* comprises 4% to 8% of cases of acute cholecystitis (26). Classically, this condition is found in critically ill patients. Recent evidence suggests that the incidence is increasing and that it can be found outside the critical care setting. Most of these patients suffer from atheromatous vascular disease or diabetes mellitus (2). Risk factors include blood volume depletion, prolonged ileus, opioid administration, total parenteral nutrition, severe trauma, sepsis, severe burns, and starvation. The inflammation may arise from prolonged distention of the gallbladder or stasis and inspissation of bile, with subsequent mucosal injury and thrombosis of the vessels of the seromuscular layer of the gallbladder (2). A microangiographic study of 15 patients with acutely inflamed gallbladders showed poor and irregular capillary filling in acalculous cholecystitis versus dilation of arterioles and regular filling of capillaries in calculous cholecystitis (27).

Where do biliary fistulas most commonly form? What are some of the complications?

Fistulas are formed frequently between the gallbladder or the CBD and the skin (e.g., biliary cutaneous), duodenum (e.g., cholecystoduodenal), and pleura. Problems with fistulas are infection (e.g., cholangitis from the retrograde infection from the bowel, peritonitis from bile leakage, and infection of the affected organ), electrolyte abnormalities (from the continual loss of electrolytes in the bile, most commonly resulting in hyponatremia), malabsorption syndrome (from the lack of bile, which is critical in the intestinal absorption of fat and fat-soluble vitamins), and gallstone ileus.

What is the radiographic interpretation of air in the gallbladder, dilated proximal loops of bowel, and a calcified mass in the right lower quadrant of the abdomen?

The interpretation includes the diagnosis of gallstone ileus, which occurs when a large stone formed in either the gallbladder or the CBD passes through a biliary–enteric fistula. In the intestine, it may cause obstruction at a narrow lumen, most commonly at the ileocecal valve, which causes dilation of the proximal bowel.

What is the proper treatment of gallstone ileus?

Gallstone ileus is treated surgically. The gallstone is removed through a small enterotomy. Concomitant cholecystectomy and repair of the fistula are indicated because the patent biliary–enteric fistula may cause recurrent episodes. However, if the patient is too ill, the definitive therapy may be performed later. Enterolithotomy alone has a mortality rate of 5%, in contrast to a mortality rate of 15% for enterolithotomy and cholecystectomy (1).

If inflammation of the gallbladder and the surrounding tissue is anticipated in the setting of acute cholecystitis, is laparoscopic cholecystectomy technically feasible? Is it a good choice?

Yes. With increasing experience, laparoscopic cholecystectomy can be performed safely with complication rates and mortality rates comparable with those of open surgery for acute cholecystitis (30–32). Acute cholecystitis has a higher conversion rate and incidence of accidental opening of the gallbladder than does laparoscopic cholecystectomy for chronic disease (32,33).

What are the factors that determine the conversion to an open cholecystectomy?

The two main factors determining conversion from laparoscopic to open operation for acute cholecystitis are any gangrenous cholecystitis and the timing of the operation (28–30,32). Conversion rates are lower if the operation is performed within 96 hours of the start of the attack (28,29). The operation is performed as soon as possible after admission to prevent the development of significant inflammation, which increases the technical difficulty of the procedure (30,31).

Mrs. Rodriguez, a well-informed patient, raises the point that perhaps she should see a gastroenterologist first, especially if there is any doubt that there is a stone in her CBD.

Should Mrs. Rodriguez undergo a preoperative endoscopic evaluation of her biliary anatomy? What is the role of endoscopic retrograde cholangiopancreatography (ERCP) in the era of laparoscopic cholecystectomy?

A study of one series of selected patients shows that the positive yield for CBD stones during ERCP ranged from 14% to 55%, with an average of 35%. The clearance of CBD stones varies between 74% and 100%. This indicates that 65% of patients have a negative study with its attendant costs, additional hospitalization, and inherent risk of unnecessary complications. Evidence in the literature suggests that the highest yield for preoperative ERCP detection and treatment of CBD stones is in patients who are jaundiced, whose ultrasound shows CBD stones, who have acute cholangitis, and who have worsening gallstone pancreatitis.

Patients with a moderate risk of having CBD stones are those with a CBD diameter of 8 mm; those with worsening liver function tests, particularly bilirubin, alkaline phosphatase, serum glutamic-oxaloacetic transaminase (SGOT), and serum glutamate-pyruvate transaminase (SGPT); and high-risk elderly patients because of the possibility of prolonged operation. Patients with a less than 2% risk of having CBD stones are those with no history of jaundice, normal bile duct diameter in ultrasound, and normal liver function studies (34).

Is there an alternative to ERCP?

Yes. Magnetic resonance cholangiopancreatography (MRCP) is a noninvasive imaging modality for detection of bile duct stones and other pathologies of the biliary tree and pancreas. It has a sensitivity of 84% to 93%, specificity of 96% to 98%, positive predictive value of 91% to 93%, negative predictive value of 93% to 98%, and diagnostic accuracy of 92% to 96% for detection of calculi (36,37).

Mrs. Rodriguez agrees to have her gallbladder taken out with laparoscopy without ERCP. A 10-mm trocar is placed inferior to the umbilicus with the open technique. The abdomen is insufflated with carbon dioxide, and the laparoscope is introduced into the abdominal cavity. Another 10-mm trocar is placed below the xiphoid process under direct visualization with the laparoscope. Then 5-mm trocars are placed below the costal margin at the midclavicular line and the anterior axillary line. An edematous and friable gallbladder wall is found, as are adhesions to the omentum.

What are the important technical steps of performing the laparoscopic cholecystectomy in this situation?

If the gallbladder is so distended that it is difficult to grab the fundus, it is drained of bile (or mucoid material in the case of hydrops) to allow good placement of the grasping forceps. The fundus is retracted over the liver and another grasping forceps used to grab the ampulla. The ampulla is retracted away from the liver, exposing the triangle of Calot. The most important step is to identify all of the structures in the triangle, including the cystic duct, the cystic artery, the junction of the cystic duct and the gallbladder, and the junction of the cystic duct with the CBD. The major contraindication to the laparoscopic approach is failure to expose all of the structures in the triangle (2).

Where is the cystic artery? What is the triangle of Calot?
It is important to attempt to ligate the cystic artery first so that the subsequent dissection upon the gallbladder is relatively bloodless. The cystic artery is usually found in the triangle of Calot. The boundaries of the triangle of Calot are the cystic duct, the right border of the CHD and right hepatic duct, and the inferior border of the liver.

What are the common variations of the arterial supply of the gallbladder?
The cystic artery arises from the common hepatic artery in 95% of cases. In the remaining cases, the variations include origination from the gastroduodenal artery, two cystic arteries, and coursing of the cystic artery anterior to the CHD instead of posterior (35).

What are the common anomalies of the biliary tree?
Usually, the cystic duct originates from the middle to the upper part of the CHD. However, common variations include origination from as high as the right hepatic duct to as low as just proximal to the ampulla of Vater; spiral anterior or posterior insertion to the CHD; and absent, short, or long cystic ducts (35).

What are accessory bile ducts? What are the sinuses of Luschka?
Accessory bile ducts are common; reported incidence ranges from 1% to 33%. They are bile ducts from the liver that course adjacent to the gallbladder and empty into a larger distal duct. Some of the smaller ducts (e.g., sinuses of Luschka) may empty directly into the gallbladder. Performing cholecystectomy without recognizing them may result in cutting across these ducts, which leads to persistent drainage of bile into the subhepatic bed and causes biloma or abscess.

What are the valves of Heister, and what is their significance?
The valves of Heister are mucosal folds (not true valves) in the cystic duct that may complicate attempts to pass a probe or a cholangiogram catheter into the gallbladder. During the laparoscopic exploration, all of the structures in the triangle of Calot are identified. An intraoperative cholangiogram is obtained because of the mild elevation of the total bilirubin. The cholangiogram reveals two small filling defects in the distal CBD.

Preoperative laboratories showed a mild elevation of the total bilirubin. An intraoperative cholangiogram is obtained. It reveals a 6-mm stone in the distal CBD.

At this point, what are the options for dealing with CBD stones?
Laparoscopic CBD exploration, laparoscopic antegrade sphincterotomy, open CBD exploration, and postoperative ERCP may be performed to remove the CBD stones (36). The precise indications for laparoscopic exploration, open

CBD exploration, and postoperative ERCP have not been clearly established. The laparoscopic transcystic exploration is performed after cannulation and dilation of the cystic duct with a balloon catheter or a ureteral dilator. The stones are dealt with under fluoroscopic or ureteroscopic guidance by flushing, pushing through the ampulla, basket retrieval, or electrohydraulic lithotripsy. The transcystic approach is preferred when stones are less than 6 mm in diameter, when the diameter of the cystic duct is greater than 4 mm, when the diameter of the CBD is less than 6 mm, and when the cystic duct entrance is lateral (37).

Laparoscopic choledochotomy with CBD exploration is preferred in the case of multiple stones, stones larger than 6 mm in diameter, stones in the CHD, a cystic duct smaller than 4 mm, a CBD smaller than 6 mm, and a posterior or distal cystic duct entrance. Laparoscopic choledochotomy should not be performed if there is marked inflammation or if the tissue is too weak to hold sutures (37). The exploration is conducted in a similar fashion to the open technique. AT-tube is left in place to drain the CBD.

The postoperative ERCP is a valuable option if the surgeon is reluctant to perform a laparoscopic exploration and if the institution has good endoscopists. A transcystic catheter can be passed into the duodenum through the cystic duct at the time of surgery to facilitate the retrograde approach to the ampulla (36).

How is an open CBD exploration conducted?

Through a small longitudinal incision on the anterior wall of the CBD, calculi are removed directly with forceps or scoops, extracted with tools such as Fogarty balloon-tipped catheters, or irrigated out. In this manner, the distal CBD, the proximal bile ducts, and right and left hepatic ducts are explored in that order. After all of the calculi are removed, a Bakes dilator is passed through the ampulla into the duodenum, confirming the patency of the sphincter. The tip of the T-tube is placed in the CBD through the incision to drain the bile postoperatively. The incision is closed with interrupted sutures, ensuring no leakage of bile around the T-tube. Postexploration cholangiography is performed to confirm the absence of retained stones in the CBD and passage of dye into the duodenum.

Following open CBD exploration as described here, how often do retained CBD stones occur?

Retained CBD stones occur in approximately 10% of patients (38).

What technique can reduce the incidence of retained stones following CBD exploration?

Use of choledochoscopy for direct visualization of the biliary ducts during stone extraction can reduce the likelihood of a missed or retained stone. Although the reported rates vary greatly, choledochoscopy can decrease the rate from approximately 10% to less than 2% (38).

What can be done to remove an impacted stone?

The Kocher maneuver can be used to remove an impacted stone. It is done by incising the lateral peritoneal reflection of the second portion of the duodenum for exposure. Afterward, a longitudinal incision on the anterior duodenum is made to expose the sphincter from within the lumen. The impacted stone may be removed directly, and if there is fibrosis at the orifice, a limited sphincterotomy may facilitate the extraction.

Before the abdomen is closed after open CBD exploration, should the gallbladder fossa be drained?

Routine drainage of the gallbladder fossae after any form of cholecystectomy is not warranted. In elective cholecystectomies, use of drains actually may increase the incidence of postoperative fever and wound infection. In cases of CBD exploration or excessive fluid accumulation, however, drainage may be employed. Drainage-related complications may be decreased by using a closed-suction drain, separating the drain exit wound from the incisional wound, and removing the drain within 48 hours of placement.

Mrs. Rodriguez undergoes a successful transcystic laparoscopic CBD exploration. After closure of the cystic duct and control of the cystic artery, the surgeon dissects the gallbladder off the liver bed. During this procedure, the gallbladder is punctured and bile and stones are spilled. The young scrub nurse and the medical students are aghast.

What is the significance of this incident?

A study of 52 patients who underwent laparoscopic cholecystectomy for acute cholecystitis did not show any increase in early complications after intraoperative spillage of bile and stones. Other studies have had similar results (32).Yet case reports of late complications after spillage of stones during laparoscopic cholecystectomy include intraabdominal abscesses, chronic suppuration of the umbilical incision secondary to entrapped infected stones, persistent abdominal wall sinuses, tracks from the port site abscesses, subhepatic inflammatory masses, cholelithoptysis, liver abscesses, and empyema. These complications present weeks or months after the original procedure. Most of them necessitate exploratory laparotomy. An experimental study suggested that infected bile in combination with multiple stones increases the chances of formation of intraabdominal abscesses as opposed to the spillage of stones in the absence of infected bile (39). It is recommended that if infected bile is spilled, attempts should be made to close the defect either by placing laparoscopic clips or by stitching the defect to avoid spillage of infected stones. The abdominal cavity is thoroughly irrigated, and, if the stones cannot be recovered, conversion to an open cholecystectomy is considered.

Are there any other options for the treatment of acute cholecystitis?

In critically ill patients and those with a very high risk of developing complications due to significant associated conditions, a simple drainage of the gallbladder without removal (i.e., cholecystostomy) can be performed. With the recent advances in interventional radiology, this procedure is done under local anesthesia, percutaneously, with ultrasound guidance. Both the transhepatic and the transperitoneal approaches are safe. The response rates vary from 59% to 93%, with morbidity rates of 0 to 18% and mortality rates of 0 to 12% (40,41). Complications include misplacement in the colon, exacerbation of sepsis, bile leakage, and bleeding (40–42).

The overall recurrence of cholecystitis is 15% (43). The procedure is thought to be definitive in patients with acalculous cholecystitis (41,42,44). Factors determining a good response include the presence of cholelithiasis, wall thickening, distention of the gallbladder, pericholecystic fluid, and absence of gangrene, indicating that the procedure is beneficial when the gallbladder is the source of sepsis (40,45,46). In patients who have a high operative risk and whose cardiorespiratory status prevents elective surgery, the procedure can be combined with contact dissolution with MTBE or with percutaneous extraction of the stones (41,47).

The defect in the wall of the gallbladder is repaired with laparoscopic clips, and the peritoneal cavity is copiously irrigated after the cholecystectomy is completed. No stones are left in the abdomen. Approximately 36 hours after completion of the laparoscopic cholecystectomy, Mrs. Rodriguez is still complaining of significant abdominal pain and nausea. The abdomen is moderately distended and somewhat tender. She has a low-grade fever, her white blood cell count is 12,000 per mm^3, and her bilirubin level is 1.9 mg per dL.

What is the differential diagnosis of these findings?

The differential diagnosis includes postoperative pancreatitis, retained CBD stone, cystic duct leak, accessory duct leak, and injury to the bile ducts. Bile leaks usually present 5.3 plus or minus 4.2 days after laparoscopic cholecystectomy. Manifestations, which are nonspecific, include unusual pain, nausea, vomiting, fever, and tenderness (48). Most bile leaks are from the cystic duct (77% of cases); 31% of patients with a cystic duct leak have a retained stone (48). Leaks from accessory bile ducts after cholecystectomy are also well known (discussed earlier).

The amylase and the lipase levels are normal. What is the next step in management of Mrs. Rodriguez?

The HIDA scan has a very good sensitivity and specificity for the diagnosis of bile leakage after laparoscopic cholecystectomy (49,50). Both ultrasound and CT are very good in assisting diagnosis of intraabdominal collections. The relative roles of these three tests have not been well defined in the literature. If any of these tests are positive, ERCP is performed to confirm the leak, identify the site and the cause, and plan the management. Minor leaks usually respond to sphincterotomy, bile duct stenting, or nasobiliary drainage. Percutaneous drainage of a biloma or of peritoneal bile is also indicated in these situations. In more severe injuries with intact ducts, endoscopic dilation and stenting may be useful in closing the leaks or preventing strictures.

For more severe injuries involving the CBD, a multidisciplinary approach that includes the interventional radiologist, the endoscopist, and the surgeon is always necessary (51–55). The best results are obtained when the injury is recognized early during surgery and is immediately repaired. For a surgical approach to CBD injury, hepaticojejunostomy seems to have a better outcome than primary end-to-end repair (55).

A HIDA scan raised suspicion of a bile leak. Mrs. Rodriguez underwent ERCP and sphincterotomy with stent placement combined with percutaneous drainage of a large biloma. She was found to have a leak from a patent cystic duct. The drainage decreased 5 days later, and a repeat HIDA scan showed no leakage. She was discharged.

What should be done if the pathology report reveals cancer of the gallbladder?

There are numerous reports of implantation of the cancer in the trocar sites and of peritoneal dissemination with manipulation of the gallbladder during laparoscopic cholecystectomy. It has been suggested that the risk is higher than with open cholecystectomy. If the cancer is confined to the mucosa of the organ (Tis, T1a) and the gallbladder was removed intact, laparoscopic cholecystectomy may be sufficient. If the malignancy invades the wall (T1b, T2, T3) or if the gallbladder was torn during the procedure, the patient should undergo laparotomy, radical cholecystectomy, and excision of the trocar sites (56–58). However, gallbladder cancer is found among the elderly, and the prognosis is extremely poor. An honest and open discussion of the value of additional surgery should be held with the patient.

Is laparoscopic cholecystectomy safe during pregnancy?

Recent reports of small numbers of patients suggest that laparoscopic cholecystectomy may be safe during pregnancy (59–61). Only one study of a small number of patients suggests otherwise (62). This study reported four fetal deaths among seven pregnant women who underwent laparoscopic procedures. Of the seven patients, three had acute appendicitis, three had gallstone pancreatitis, and one had acute cholecystitis. Postulated risks include trocar injury to the uterus, decreased uterine blood flow, premature labor from the increased intraabdominal pressure, and increased fetal acidosis (63).

The Society of American Gastrointestinal and Endoscopic Surgeons recommends the following maneuvers to enhance safety of the procedure (63):

- Defer the intervention until the second trimester of pregnancy
- Use pneumatic compression devices to prevent deep venous thrombosis
- Continuously monitor the fetal heart rate and maternal end-tidal carbon dioxide level
- Protect the fetus with a lead shield over the lower abdomen if intraoperative cholangiogram is planned
- Use the open technique for access to the abdomen
- Use the partial (15° to 30°) left decubitus position to shift the uterus off the vena cava
- Maintain the intraabdominal pressure at 8 to 12 mm Hg
- Always obtain an obstetric consultation before operating

Giles Sampson is a 73-year-old man who goes to the emergency department complaining of abdominal pain that started 3 days ago. It is now in the right upper quadrant. It is not associated with meals and does not respond to antacids. He states that he had a temperature of 38.3°C and that he has felt chills intermittently. He reports dark urine during the past 2 days. The patient had a laparoscopic cholecystectomy 2 years ago for acute cholecystitis.

What do the symptoms and history suggest?

These symptoms suggest acute cholangitis. With the history of a laparoscopic cholecystectomy, the patient may have a retained stone or an iatrogenic bile duct stricture.

What is Charcot's triad?

Charcot's triad is fever, right upper quadrant abdominal pain, and jaundice. Charcot's triad was described in 1987 by Jean M. Charcot, a French neurologist. Approximately 70% of patients describe three symptoms: 80% to 95% have fever; 80% to 86% have jaundice; and 67% to 80% have pain (64–66). Pain has become less common because of the increased incidence of cholangitis with obstruction of percutaneous draining biliary catheters and internal biliary stents. Pain is usually seen with cholangitis because of stones (67).

Physical examination reveals a well-developed and well-nourished man in no apparent distress. He is mildly tachycardic. His temperature is 38°C. The patient has jaundiced sclerae. Examination of the abdomen reveals a soft, nondistended abdomen that is mildly tender in the right upper quadrant. There are no peritoneal signs or palpable masses. Rectal examination shows guaiac-negative stools. Laboratory data show a total

bilirubin level of 13.8 mg per dL, alkaline phosphatase level of 381 mIU per mL, SGPT of 126 mIU per mL, SGOT of 101 mIU per mL, and a lactate dehydrogenase level of 122 mIU per mL. The white blood cell count is 20,800 per mm^3.

What is the pathophysiology of acute cholangitis?

Three key elements are necessary for the development of acute cholangitis: bacteriobilia, biliary stasis, and obstruction. The bile can be contaminated during percutaneous procedures, endoscopy, and biliary bypass procedures. Reflux through the ampulla of Vater has also been postulated. Bacteria also can reach the bile through lymphatics, arterial circulation, and portal venous circulation.

What causes the sepsis in acute cholangitis?

The biliary obstruction increases the intraluminal pressure in the bile ducts. With the increased pressure, bacteria regurgitate into the lymphatics and the portal system. From there, the infection enters the systemic circulation. With obstruction, the pressure is higher than 200 mm Hg. These pressures can be increased easily during percutaneous or endoscopic cholangiography (67).

How frequently is bacteriobilia present?

Bile has been found to be colonized in 20% to 40% of cases of cholelithiasis, 90% of cases of choledocholithiasis, and 12% to 20% of cases of malignant obstruction (67).

What is the most common cause of bile duct obstruction?

The most common cause is secondary stones from the gallbladder. Other causes of obstruction are primary bile duct stones; benign strictures caused by surgical procedures, congenital pathologies, or rare conditions such as sclerosing cholangitis; malignant strictures; pancreatitis, both acute and chronic; extrinsic compression such as in Mirizzi's syndrome; parasites; and obstructed biliary stents or percutaneous catheters.

What is the most common malignant obstruction?

Carcinoma of the head of the pancreas is the most common malignant obstruction. Other malignant causes are ampullary carcinoma, bile duct adenocarcinoma, duodenal carcinoma, and gallbladder carcinoma.

How are the CBD stones classified?

They are generally classified as primary or secondary. Primary stones are formed de novo in the bile duct. They are usually soft, smooth, yellowish tan, and not formed of cholesterol. They often conform to the shape of the bile duct. They are usually formed in the presence of biliary stasis and bacterial contamination.

Production of β-glucuronidase by the organisms catalyzes the hydrolysis of bilirubin diglucuronide to unconjugated bilirubin, which binds to calcium to form insoluble calcium bilirubinate. Secondary stones are formed in the gallbladder and pass to the CBD through the cystic duct or via a fistulous communication (68).

What organisms are most commonly found in the bile of patients with acute cholangitis?

Most patients are infected with gut organisms, the most common being *Escherichia coli* and *Klebsiella. Streptococcus faecalis* have been common in the past, but *Enterococcus* is now the most common gram-positive organism seen in biliary tract infections. Increasing numbers of cultures show *Enterobacter, Pseudomonas,* and *Serratia.* The most common anaerobes are the bacteroids. Approximately 50% of patients have more than one organism. Fungal infections are rare, but fungi are occasionally found in diabetics and in patients with enterobiliary stents. Since the 1990s, more patients have had recurrent cholangitis related to occluded stents and percutaneous drainage catheters. This has caused a shift toward resistant organisms (67).

What are the characteristic laboratory findings in patients with acute cholangitis?

There is elevation of the total bilirubin, direct bilirubin, alkaline phosphatase, SGOT, and SGPT. These enzymes begin to rise within 1 hour of the onset of obstruction and continue to rise for weeks. The increase in serum bilirubin results from blockage of excretion, and alkaline phosphatase rises because of increased synthesis of the enzyme by the canalicular epithelium. Consequently, serum alkaline phosphatase may be elevated, but bilirubin may be normal or slightly elevated in partial obstruction. The elevation of alkaline phosphatase is out of proportion to that of SGOT and SGPT. Blood cultures are positive in 25% of patients.

What is Courvoisier's law?

Courvoisier's law states that when the CBD is obstructed by a stone, dilation of the gallbladder is rare, but when it is obstructed in another way, dilation is common. For example, obstructive jaundice due to a CBD stone is not associated with a palpable mass in the right upper quadrant (i.e., a distended gallbladder) because the organ is either scarred from chronic inflammation or surgically removed. However, in patients with periampullary cancer, the jaundice is associated with a palpable mass because the gallbladder is dilated without scarring.

A diagnosis of acute cholangitis is made according to the history, physical examination, and laboratory tests.

What additional test may be useful at this point?

An ultrasound of the upper abdomen can differentiate obstructive from nonobstructive lesions with an accuracy of 99% for showing dilated bile ducts (67). Cholescintigraphy is not generally useful for cholangitis because the degree of anatomic precision needed to plan the treatment of this condition is not attainable with this technique (67).

What other tests are useful for this condition?

CT is complementary to ultrasound. It is excellent for the detection of dilated ducts, and it is very useful in cholangitis caused by malignancy because it may detect pancreatic masses, adenopathy, or liver metastases. Direct cholangiography via percutaneous technique or endoscopy provides essential diagnostic and anatomic information for determining the source of cholangitis and for treating the cause of obstruction (67).

An ultrasound of the right upper quadrant reveals a dilated CBD. This is followed by CT of the abdomen. There are no pancreatic masses, and there are no abscesses or metastases in the liver. Both the extrahepatic and intrahepatic bile ducts are dilated. The patient is admitted to a general surgical floor.

What is the initial approach to the management of a patient with cholangitis?

First and foremost is to support the patient hemodynamically and treat the infection. IV administration of fluids and ascertainment of adequate urine output are essential. Antibiotics that are effective on the biliary tract organisms are started immediately. The secondary aspect of management is to find the underlying cause of obstruction.

Upon admission to the ward, Mr. Sampson's fever rises to 39.1°C. IV fluids and antibiotics are started immediately.

What is the likelihood that the infection will be controlled by hydration and antibiotics?

Approximately 70% to 85% of patients with cholangitis respond to antibiotics and hydration. However, 15% progress to a more severe form of cholangitis with continued sepsis, shock, and central nervous system depression (69). Patients with malignancy respond to antibiotics alone in fewer than 50% of cases (67).

What is Reynolds' pentad?

Reynolds' pentad is mental status deterioration and severe shock in addition to the right upper quadrant pain, jaundice, and fever traditionally seen in patients with cholangitis.

What are the different types of cholangitis?

Ascending cholangitis has a wide spectrum of clinical manifestations depending on the location and the type of obstruction. Acute nonsuppurative cholangitis generally is the milder clinical presentation, which is commonly caused by partial obstruction of the biliary tract. Usually responsive to antibiotics, nonsuppurative cholangitis is most often seen with benign strictures, sclerosing cholangitis, extrinsic compression of the CBD, and CBD stones.

Acute toxic cholangitis (*suppurative cholangitis*) is a more aggressive process, usually caused by complete or nearly complete obstruction of the biliary tract, resulting in pus under pressure. Even when treated with systemic antibiotics, patients with suppurative cholangitis manifest a rapidly deteriorating condition, leading to high fever, hyperbilirubinemia greater than 4 mg/dL, septic shock, and eventual death if not treated (64). Reynolds' pentad of symptoms is associated with this form of the disease. Cholangiohepatitis, also known as recurrent pyogenic cholangitis, is endemic to Asia. It is a chronic, recurrent form of the disease characterized by intrahepatic stones, strictures, and infection. These patients also develop hepatic abscesses. The principles of management include delineation of ductal anatomy, extraction of stones, drainage of strictured segments, and resection of badly damaged liver parenchyma (68).

Sclerosing cholangitis is a progressive disease that causes inflammation and fibrosis of the bile ducts. It can involve the intrahepatic and extrahepatic segments of the biliary tract. It is thought to be immune related, and it is well documented in the setting of ulcerative colitis.

AIDS-related cholangiopathy is characterized by right upper quadrant and epigastric pain, cholestasis and dilated bile ducts, diffuse abnormalities on imaging of the biliary tree, papillary stenosis, and abnormal liver function tests. In 75% of cases, an opportunistic infection can be identified. In patients with biliary disease, pain is often relieved by endoscopic sphincterotomy, whereas cholecystectomy provides pain relief in patients with acalculous cholecystitis (69,70).

What is the appropriate treatment for progressively worsening ascending cholangitis?

Acute toxic cholangitis is treated with IV antibiotics and aggressive fluid therapy guided by monitoring of central pressures and cardiopulmonary indices to attain good tissue perfusion. Vasopressor medication may be necessary to achieve this goal. However, aggressive intensive care management should not delay the mainstay of treatment, which is the emergency decompression of the biliary obstruction.

On the morning after admission, Mr. Sampson's fever spiked to 39.4°C, and his blood pressure fell to 70/30 mm Hg. He was transferred to the

intensive care unit and was resuscitated aggressively. His blood pressure returned to 110/60 mm Hg, and preparations were made for emergency decompression of the biliary tract.

What are the modalities of emergency biliary duct decompression?

The three modalities are (a) percutaneous transhepatic cholangiography (PTC), (b) ERCP, and (c) surgical decompression. The choice of modality depends on the level of expertise of the operator, the degree of dilation of the bile ducts, the location and cause of the obstruction, and any previous surgical procedures (e.g., biliary enteric bypasses and gastric resections).

ERCP is the preferred method for emergency decompression for impacted CBD stones, for suspected proximal malignancies, and for nondilated bile ducts. A prospective randomized study comparing ERCP with surgical emergency decompression showed a lower mortality rate for ERCP (10 versus 32%; $p < 0.03$). Fewer patients in the ERCP group needed ventilatory support (12 versus 26 patients; $p < 0.005$), and residual stones were significantly less frequent (3 versus 12, $p = 0.03$) (71). A stent or a nasobiliary drainage tube can be left until definitive treatment is carried out.

Complications include bleeding (2%), pancreatitis (5%), and perforation. The rate of complications after sphincterotomy is related to the indications for the procedure (e.g., dysfunction of sphincter of Oddi and cirrhosis) and to the endoscopic technique (e.g., difficulty in cannulating the bile duct, achievement of access to the bile duct by precut sphincterotomy, and use of combined percutaneous-endoscopic procedure) (71,72).

PTC is preferred in patients with proximal obstruction with dilated ducts and in patients whose anatomy has been disrupted by previous biliary enteric bypass or gastric resections. Advantages include simplicity and safety, no need for general anesthesia, and a high rate of success. Possible complications include bacteremia, bile leak, formation of cholangiovenous communications, and blockage of the drainage catheter. The incidence of immediate complications is approximately 2% to 5% (67).

Surgical decompression in the presence of severe cholangitis with sepsis and coagulopathy carries reported mortality rates of 20% to 60% (71). It is now reserved for patients for whom ERCP and PTC are unavailable or were unsuccessful. A CBD exploration is carried out initially, and a T-tube is left in the CBD to allow drainage of the infected bile and to have a port of access for later study of the biliary tract. The role of laparoscopic CBD exploration in acute cholangitis has not been defined. Laparoscopic cholecystectomy after endoscopic clearance of CBD stones is recommended in the presence of cholelithiasis and if the patient has no significant operative risks. A prospective, randomized, multicenter trial in

120 patients who underwent endoscopic sphincterotomy and stone extraction, with proven gallbladder stones, showed an incidence of recurrent biliary pathology in 47% of the patients that did not undergo an interval cholecystectomy. Therefore, laparoscopic cholecystectomy is recommended after ERCP clearance of CBD stones if the patient is an acceptable surgical risk (78).

The surgical options for formal decompression of the biliary tract are transduodenal sphincteroplasty, choledochoduodenostomy, and choledochojejunostomy. A formal surgical decompression is absolutely indicated in patients with primary CBD stones because stasis plays a significant role in the pathogenesis of these stones (68,73). These procedures also have been recommended for recurrent stones after a second CBD exploration, multiple large stones, and stones in the hepatic ducts. A recent randomized study showed no difference in morbidity, mortality, or long-term results between choledochoduodenostomy and choledochojejunostomy. Choledochoduodenostomy may be preferable because it is technically easier and permits easy access for further endoscopic exploration or treatment if necessary (74).

What are the treatment options for benign strictures and for intrahepatic stones with recurrent cholangitis?

These conditions require a close interaction between surgeons, interventional radiologists, and endoscopists. ERCP can be used to define the anatomy and to stent distal lesions in the biliary tract. This modality has been particularly useful for the treatment of strictures after repairs of laparoscopic injuries of the bile ducts. PTC is used for definition of the anatomy and for definitive or adjunctive treatment. Radiologic treatment options include dilation of strictures, stent placement, and transhepatic cholangioscopy with lithotripsy or lithotomy (75,76). The interventional radiologist can place transhepatic catheters through strictures that surgeons can use as guides for locating the lesion and stenting biliary enteric bypasses.

The principles of successful repair of biliary strictures are exposure of healthy proximal bile ducts that provide drainage to the entire liver; preparation of a suitable segment of intestine that can be brought to the area of the stricture without tension, most frequently a Roux-en-Y jejunal limb; and creation of a direct biliary enteric mucosal-to-mucosal anastomosis. Excellent long-term results can be achieved in 70% to 90% of cases. Approximately two thirds of restrictures are evident within 2 years, and 90% are seen within 7 years (77).

Mr. Sampson had a successful ERCP and sphincteroplasty. He was found to have a retained stone from his previous laparoscopic cholecystectomy. No abnormalities of the bile ducts were identified. His overall condition improved with the antibiotics, and he was discharged a week after admission.

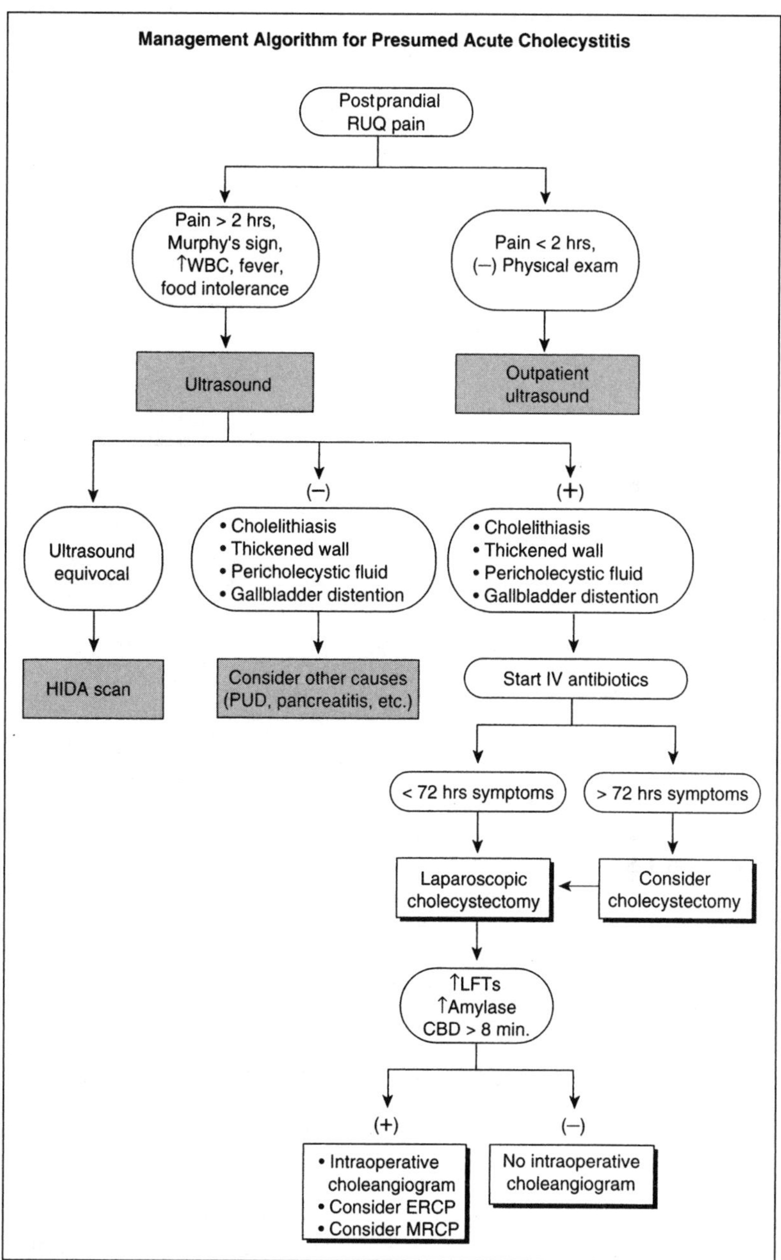

Algorithm 16.1.

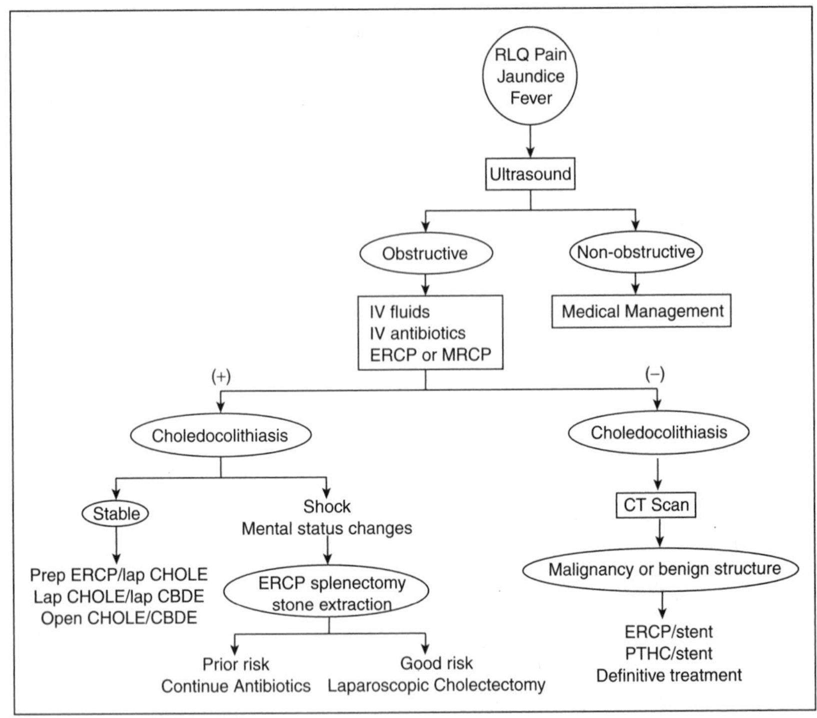

Algorithm 16.2.

REFERENCES

1. Gieugiu DIN, Roslyn JJ. Calculous biliary disease. In: Greenfield LJ, et al., ed. Surgery: Scientific Principles and Practice. 2nd ed. Philadelphia, PA: Lippincott–Raven Publishers; 1997.
2. Cuschieri A. Acute and chronic cholecystitis. In: Cameron JL. Current Surgical Therapy. 5th ed. St. Louis, Mo: Mosby; 1995.
3. Jazrawi RP, Pazzi P, Petroni ML, et al. Post prandial gallbladder motor function: refilling and turnover of bile in health and in cholelithiasis. Gastroenterology. 1995;109:582.
4. Soper NJ. Biliary anatomy and physiology. In: Greenfield LJ, et al., ed. Surgery: Scientific Principles and Practice. 2nd ed. Philadelphia, PA: Lippincott–Raven Publishers; 1997.
5. Janowitz P, Klatzer W, Zemnler T, et al. Gallbladder sludge: spontaneous course and incidence of complications in patients without stones. Hepatology. 1994;20: 291.
6. McSherry CK, Ferstenberg H, Calhoun WF, et al. The natural history of diagnosed gallstone disease in symptomatic and asymptomatic patients. Ann Surg. 1985;202:59.

7. Friedman GD, Raviola CA, Fireman B, et al. Prognosis of gallstones with mild or no symptoms: 25 years of follow up in a health maintenance organization. J Clin Epidemiol. 1989;42:127.
8. Gracie WA, Ransohoff DF. The natural history of silent gallstones. Gastroenterology. 1981;80:1161.
9. Del Favero G, Caroli A, Meggiato T, et al. Natural history of gallstones in non–insulin-dependent diabetes mellitus: a prospective 5-year follow up. Dig Dis Sci. 1994;39:1704.
10. Aucott JN, Cooper GS, Bloom AD, et al. Management of gallstones in diabetic patients. Arch Intern Med. 1993;153:1053.
11. Adamek HE, Jorg S, Bachor OA, et al. Symptoms of post-extracorporeal shock wave lithotripsy: long-term analysis of gallstone patients before and after successful shock wave lithotripsy. Am J Gastroenterol. 1995;90:1125.
12. Sackmann M, Niller H, Klueppelberg U, et al. Gallstone recurrence after shock-wave therapy. Gastroenterology. 1994;106:225.
13. Pauletzki J, Althaus R, Holl J, et al. Gallbladder emptying and gallstone formation: a prospective study on gallstone recurrence. Gastroenterology. 1996;111:765.
14. Pauletzki J. Gallstone recurrence after direct contact dissolution with methyl tert-butyl ether. Dig Dis Sci. 1995;40:1775.
15. Nahrwold DL. Gallstone lithotripsy. Am J Surg. 1993;165:431.
16. Tomida S, Abel M, et al. Long-term ursodeoxycholic acid therapy is associated with reduced risk of biliary pain and acute cholecystitis in patients with gallbladder stones: a cohort analysis. Hepatology. 1999;30:6.
17. Russell JC, Walsh SJ, Maltie AS, et al. Bile duct injuries 1989–93: a state-wide experience. Connecticut Laparoscopic Cholecystectomy Registry. Arch Surg. 1996;131:382.
18. Flum DR, Koepsell T, et al. Common bile duct injury during laparoscopic cholecystectomy and the use of intraoperative cholangiography: adverse outcome or preventable error? Arch Surg. 2001;136:1287.
19. Flum DR, Dellinger EP, et al. Intraoperative cholangiography and risk of common bile duct injury during cholecystectomy. JAMA. 2003;289:1639.
20. Kullman E, Borch K, Lindstrom E, et al. Value of routinely intraoperative cholangiography in detecting aberrant bile ducts and bile duct injuries during laparoscopic cholecystectomy. Br J Surg. 1996;83:171.
21. Singer AJ, McCracken G, Henry MC, et al. Correlation among clinical, laboratory, and hepatobiliary scanning findings in patients with suspected acute cholecystitis. Ann Emerg Med. 1996;28:267.
22. Gruber PJ, Silverman RA, Gottesfeld S, et al. Presence of fever and leukocytosis in acute cholecystitis. Ann Emerg Med. 1996;28:273.
23. Fink-Bennett D, Freitas JE, Ripley SD, et al. The sensitivity of hepatobiliary imaging and real-time ultrasonography in the detection of acute cholecystitis. Arch Surg. 1985;120:904.
24. Kim CK. Pharmacologic intervention for the diagnosis of acute cholecystitis: cholecystokinin pretreatment or morphine, or both? J Nucl Med. 1997;38:647.
25. Chen CC, Holder LE, Maunoury C, et al. Morphine augmentation increases gallbladder visualization in patients pre treated with cholecystokinin. J Nucl Med. 1997;38:644.

26. Nahrwold DL. The biliary system. In: Sabiston DC, ed. Textbook of Surgery. 13th ed. Philadelphia, PA: WB Saunders; 1986.
27. Hakala T. Microangiopathy in acute acalculous cholecystitis. Br J Surg. 1997;84:1249.
28. Eldar S. Laparoscopic cholecystectomy for acute cholecystitis: prospective trial. World J Surg. 1997;21:540.
29. Garber SM. Early laparoscopic cholecystectomy for acute cholecystitis. Surg Endosc. 1997;11:347.
30. Coo KP, Thirlby RC. Laparoscopic cholecystectomy in acute cholecystitis: what is the optimal timing for operation? Arch Surg. 1996;131:540.
31. Unger SW, Rosenbaum G, Unger HM, et al. A comparison of laparoscopic and open treatment of acute cholecystitis. Surg Endosc. 1993;7:408.
32. Rattner DW, Ferguson C, Warshaw AL. Factors associated with successful laparoscopic cholecystectomy for acute cholecystitis. Ann Surg. 1993;217:233.
33. Diez J, Arozamena CJ, Ferraina P, et al. Relation between postoperative infections and gallbladder bile leakage during laparoscopic cholecystectomy. Surg Endosc. 1996;10:529.
34. MacFadyen BV, Passi RB. The role of endoscopic retrograde cholangiopancreatography in the area of laparoscopic cholecystectomy. Semin Laparosc Surg. 1997;4:18.
35. Schwartz SI. Gallbladder and exerbiliary system. In: Schwartz SI, et al., ed. Principles of Surgery. 4th ed. New York, NY: McGraw-Hill; 1984.
36. Johnson AB, Hunter JG. Future treatment of common bile duct stones. Semin Laparosc Surg. 1997;4:45.
37. Petelin JB. Techniques and cost of common bile duct exploration. Semin Laparosc Surg. 1997;4:23.
38. King ML, String ST. Extent of choledoscopic utilization in common bile duct exploration. Am J Surg. 1983;146:322.
39. Zorluoglu A, Ozguc H, Yilmazlar T, et al. Is it necessary to retrieve dropped gallstones during laparoscopic cholecystectomy? Surg Endosc. 1997;11:64.
40. England RE, McDermott VG, Smith TP, et al. Percutaneous cholecystostomy: who responds? AJR Am J Roentgenol. 1997;168:1247.
41. Vauthey JN, Lerur J, Martini M, et al. Indications and limitations of percutaneous cholecystostomy for acute cholecystitis. Surg Obstet Gynecol. 1993;176:49.
42. Boland GW, Lee MJ, Leung J, et al. Percutaneous cholecystostomy in critically ill patients: early response and final outcome in 82 patients. AJR Am J Roentgenol. 1994;163:339.
43. Hamy A, Visset J, Likholatnikov D, et al. Percutaneous cholecystostomy for acute cholecystitis in critically ill patients. Surgery. 1997;121:398.
44. van Overhagen H, Meyers H, Tylanus HW, et al. Percutaneous cholecystostomy for patients with acute cholecystitis and an increased surgical risk. Cardiovasc Intervent Radiol. 1996;19:72.
45. Hultman CS, Hergst CA, McCall JM, et al. The efficacy of percutaneous cholecystostomy in critically ill patients. Am Surg. 1996;62:263.
46. Lo LD, Vogelzang RL, Braun MA, et al. Percutaneous cholecystostomy for the diagnosis and treatment of acute calculous and acalculous cholecystitis. J Vasc Intervent Radiol. 1995;6:629.

47. Hamy A, Visset J, Likholatnikov D, et al. Percutaneous cholecystostomy for acute cholecystitis in critically ill patients. Surgery. 1997;121:398.
48. Barkun AN, Rezieg M, Mehta SN, et al. Postcholecystectomy biliary leaks in the laparoscopic era: risk factors, presentation, and management. McGill Gallstones Treatment Group. Gastrointest Endosc. 1997;45:277.
49. Mirza DF, Narsimhan KL, Ferraznet BH, et al. Bile duct injury following laparoscopic cholecystectomy: referral pattern and management. Br J Surg. 1997;84:786.
50. Sandoval BA, Goettler CE, Robinson AV, et al. Cholescintigraphy in the diagnosis of bile leak after laparoscopic cholecystectomy. Am Surg. 1997;63:611.
51. Ponsky JL. Endoscopic approaches to common bile duct injuries. Surg Clin North Am. 1996;76:505.
52. Barton JR, Russell RC, Hatfield AR, et al. Management of bile leaks after laparoscopic cholecystectomy. Br J Surg. 1995;82:780.
53. Barthel J, Scheider D. Advantages of sphincterotomy and nasal biliary tube drainage in the treatment of cystic duct stump leak complicating laparoscopic cholecystectomy. Am J Gastroenterol. 1995;90:1322.
54. Raijman I, Catalano MF, Hirsch GS, et al. Endoscopic treatment of biliary leakage after laparoscopic cholecystectomy. Endoscopy. 1994;26:741.
55. Gough D, Donohue JH. Characteristics of biliary tract complications during laparoscopic cholecystectomy: a multi-institutional study. Am J Surg. 1994;167:27.
56. Jacobi CA, Keller H, Monig S, et al. Implantation of metastases of unsuspected gallbladder carcinoma after laparoscopy. Surg Endosc. 1995;9:351.
57. Copher JC, Rogers JJ, Dalton ML. Trocar-site metastasis following laparoscopic cholecystectomy for unsuspected carcinoma of the gallbladder: case report and review of the literature. Surg Endosc. 1995;9:348.
58. Wagholikar GD, Behari A, et al. Early gallbladder cancer. J Am Coll Surg. 2002;194:137.
59. Eichenberg BJ, Vanderlinden J, Miguel C, et al. Laparoscopic cholecystectomy in the third trimester of pregnancy. Am Surg. 1996;62:874.
60. Martin IJ, Dexter SP, McMahon MJ. Laparoscopic cholecystectomy in pregnancy: a safe option during the second trimester? Surg Endosc. 1996;10:508.
61. Wishner JD, Zolfaghari D, Wohlgemuth SD, et al. Laparoscopic cholecystectomy in pregnancy: a report of six cases and review of literature. Surg Endosc. 1996;10:314.
62. Amos JD, Schorr SJ, Norman PF, et al. Laparoscopic surgery during pregnancy. Am J Surg. 1996;171:435.
63. Guidelines for laparoscopic surgery during pregnancy. Society of American Gastrointestinal Endoscopic Surgeons. Surg Endosc. 1998;12:189–190.
64. Boey HA, Way LW. Acute cholangitis. Ann Surg. 1980;191:264.
65. O'Connor MJ, Schwartz ML, McQuarrie DG, et al. Acute bacterial cholangitis. Arch Surg. 1982;117:437.
66. Sievert W, Vakil N. Emergencies of the biliary tract. Gastroenterol Clin North Am. 1988;17:247.
67. Sharp KW. Acute cholangitis. In: Cameron JL. Current Surgical Therapy. 5th ed. St. Louis, MO: Mosby; 1995.

68. Roslyn JJ, Zinner MJ. Gallbladder and extrahepatic biliary system. In: Schwartz SI, et al. Principles of Surgery. 6th ed. New York, NY: McGraw-Hill; 1994.
69. Nash JA, Cohen SA. Gallbladder and biliary tract disease in AIDS. Gastroenterol Clin North Am. 1997;26:323.
70. Ducreux M, Buffet C, Lamy P, et al. Diagnosis and prognosis of AIDS-related cholangitis. AIDS. 1995;9:875.
71. Lai EC, Mok FP, Tan ES, et al. Endoscopic biliary drainage for severe acute cholangitis. N Engl J Med. 1992;326:1582.
72. Freeman ML, Nelson DB, Sherman S, et al. Complications of endoscopic biliary sphincterotomy. N Engl J Med. 1996;335:909.
73. Giurgiu DIN, Roslyn JJ. Calculous biliary disease. In: Greenfield LJ, et al., ed. Surgery: Scientific Principles and Practice. 2nd ed. Philadelphia, PA: Lippincott–Raven Publishers; 1997.
74. Panis Y, Faguiez PL, Brisser D, et al. Long term results of choledochoduodenostomy versus choledochojejunostomy for choledocholithiasis. French Association for Surgical Research. Surg Gynecol Obstet. 1993;177:33.
75. Yeh YH, Huang MH, Yang JC, et al. Percutaneous trans-hepatic cholangioscopy and lithotripsy in the treatment of intrahepatic stones: a study with 5 years follow-up. Gastrointest Endosc. 1995;42:13.
76. Jan YY, Chen MF. Percutaneous trans-hepatic cholangioscopic lithotomy for hepatolithiasis: long-term results. Gastrointest Endosc. 1995;42:1.
77. Lillemoe KD. Biliary strictures and sclerosing cholangitis. In: Greenfield LJ, et al., ed. Surgery: Scientific Principles and Practice. 2nd ed. Philadelphia, PA: Lippincott–Raven Publishers; 1997.
78. Boerma D, Rauws EA, et al. Wait-and-see policy or laparoscopic cholecystectomy after endoscopic sphincterotomy for bile-duct stones: a randomised trial. Lancet. 2002;360:761.

CHAPTER

17

LIVER DISEASE: PORTAL HYPERTENSION

Jeffrey L. Kaufman

Henry Norman is a 60-year-old man who goes to the emergency department because of intermittent vomiting of bright red blood over the previous 4 hours. For several days, he has not felt well, but he has not seen a doctor in over a year. His bowel movements have been normal in consistency, and both stool and urine have had normal color. He felt weak and slightly dizzy when moving around his house before the vomiting started. After vomiting, he felt so weakened that he could not get up to go to the bathroom to vomit again. He has no history of peptic ulcer disease. He has smoked 1 to 1.5 packs per day for years. For most of his working life, he has drunk a fifth of vodka every 2 days or consumed two six-packs of beer after work. He had jaundice once in his youth; a physician attributed it to hepatitis. He is a metal fabricator and has not missed work because of accidents or binge drinking; he has never had a drunk driving violation. His father was said to be alcoholic and died of liver failure at age 57. His siblings are alive and well, and none of them drinks alcohol.

Mr. Norman is a thin man who appears chronically ill. His vital signs are as follows: respiratory rate, 24 breaths per minute; supine pulse rate, 142 beats per minute; supine blood pressure, 80/45 mm Hg; and body temperature is normal. The muscles of his arms and temporal fossae appear wasted, his sclerae are mildly icteric, and there are prominent telangiectases over the nose and cheeks. The chest and cardiac examination are normal, but the abdominal examination reveals mild tympany. The liver edge is firm and is at the right costal margin. There is no visceral tenderness to palpation. The stool is dark, tarry, and guaiac positive. The genitalia are those of a normal man, but the testes are atrophic. His femoral pulses are 2+, but popliteal and pedal pulses are

absent. His fingers reveal yellow staining of the right index and middle fingernails, and he is right-handed. He has no asterixis. He is unable to produce a urine sample.

What are the key findings of the initial evaluation and treatment of Mr. Norman?

Mr. Norman's history indicates a recent and perhaps ongoing hemorrhage. Acute blood loss is indicated by the history and vital signs, which are best explained by significant hypovolemia. A priority is to resuscitate him by placing large-bore intravenous lines and rapidly infusing isotonic saline solution. Blood is drawn for typing and cross-matching. Additional tests include a complete blood count, platelet count, clotting studies (prothrombin time and partial thromboplastin time), and determination of electrolytes, blood urea nitrogen, and creatinine levels. Because of his history, liver function should be studied, including determination of albumin, total protein, bilirubin, alkaline phosphatase, aspartate transaminase, and alanine transaminase. The amylase level should also be checked.

What are the end points for volume infusion?

The pulse rate, blood pressure, and urine formation should be evaluated. If the ability to urinate is in doubt, a Foley catheter should be placed to guide resuscitation. With complete resuscitation, his blood pressure will rise to whatever is his normal, probably a systolic above 120 mm Hg; the heart rate will drop, probably to below 100 beats per minute; and his urine output will be more than 30 to 50 mL per hour. He would undoubtedly have orthostatic hypotension on admission to the emergency department, and this would disappear with full resuscitation. Note that he may manifest a tachycardia because of anemia.

What is the role of vasopressors in this patient?

Mr. Norman should not be treated with vasopressors because the hypovolemia is caused by hemorrhage; the shock is therefore treated with volume resuscitation, including blood transfusion when cross-matched blood is available.

Mr. Norman responds to infusion of 1.5 L saline: his pulse decreases to 115 beats per minute, and his blood pressure increases to 122/75 mm Hg. A nasogastric tube is passed, and lavage with warm saline partially clears clots and liquid blood with repeated rinses. Some of the rinses appear stained with bile.

What is the differential diagnosis for this patient?

The most likely diagnosis is gastric or duodenal ulceration with bleeding. Other possibilities include gastritis with bleeding, portal hypertension with esophageal varices that have hemorrhaged, gastric variceal bleeding from portal hypertension (portal hypertensive gastropathy), bleeding from gastric varices as a result of splenic vein thrombosis, gastric or duodenal neoplasm with extrahepatic portal obstruction, Mallory-Weiss tear with hemorrhage, esophagitis with bleeding, and a myeloproliferative disorder with sclerosis of the portal system (1). Underlying carcinomatosis, stomach, liver, esophageal, or even small bowel, can also occur. End-stage liver disease with varices can also occur in the context of hepatitis.

Despite the patient's history of alcohol consumption, peptic ulcer disease remains highest on the list because it accounts for one half to two thirds of cases of upper gastrointestinal (GI) bleeding. Gastritis accounts for another 15% of cases (2). *Helicobacter pylori* as a causative agent should be considered in the differential diagnosis.

Mr. Norman's initial laboratory tests show the following results: hematocrit, 21%; platelet count, 55,000 per mL; sodium, 147 mEq per L; potassium, 3.7 mEq per L; chloride, 101 mEq per L; CO_2, normal; blood urea nitrogen, 35 mg per dL; creatinine, 1.8 mg per dL; prothrombin time, 16 seconds (international normalized ratio [INR], 1.4); partial thromboplastin time, 44 seconds. The chest radiograph is normal. He continues to retch and vomit blood.

What diagnostic study is performed next?

Upper GI endoscopy should be performed as soon as possible.

Mr. Norman is given 3 U of blood. His blood pressure stabilizes at 120/75 mm Hg, his pulse is maintained at 75 to 85 beats per minute, and his urine volume increases. He undergoes upper GI endoscopy, which reveals active bleeding from large esophageal varices.

What therapeutic options does the endoscopist consider?

Endoscopic sclerotherapy should be performed if possible. The technique of sclerotherapy is to visualize the varices directly and to inject a sclerosant in and around them. As early as 1939, Crafoord considered using specially modified rigid esophagoscopes to inject esophageal varices with material that would cause them to scar and thrombose (3). The procedure did not become prominent because of its technical difficulty in comparison with shunting, but when fiberoptic endoscopes became clinically available in the 1970s, the procedure was revived. Because of its ease, most centers used sclerotherapy as the main procedure for early control of bleeding varices, especially in poor-risk patients (4).

The agents available for sclerotherapy in the United States is ethanolamine oleate. The procedure is successful in the initial control of bleeding varices in 80% to 90% of patients, in combination with other measures for medical management. In patients with acute bleeding, such as Mr. Norman, technical success depends on a clear view of the site of hemorrhage without interference from bleeding sites or persistent blood in the gastroesophageal lumen. Bleeding from gastric varices is more difficult to control with sclerotherapy because the upper stomach cannot be fixed in position for injection and because there are more veins that can bleed. Gastropathy from portal hypertension, including submucosal hyperemia, cannot be treated with sclerotherapy (5). The outcome is influenced by the Child classification of the patient at the time of sclerotherapy (6). An alternative surgical procedure, early portacaval shunting, has produced better results in the short- and long-term management of people with bleeding varices than has sclerotherapy (7). Additional studies favorably compare esophageal transection with sclerotherapy for control of acute bleeding (8).

What causes esophageal varices?

In normal conditions, blood flows through the portal veins under low pressure (less than 10 mm Hg), which is consistent with the low resistance in the portal circulation of the liver. Significant increases in portal venous blood flow can be accommodated (e.g., during digestion) without an increase in portal venous pressure. In a diseased liver, with alteration of the microscopic portal architecture, obstruction to portal venous flow leads to elevation of portal venous pressure. The physiologic response to this rise in pressure is the formation of alternative channels for blood flow from the intestine to the central venous system, which bypass the liver altogether. These varices occur in the retroperitoneum, along the esophagus and stomach, around the anal canal, and around the umbilicus. Patients with symptoms of portal hypertension have portal venous pressures typically higher than 20 mm Hg, sometimes higher than 40 mm Hg.

What causes portal hypertension?

The causation of portal hypertension is complex. Fibrosis of the liver, regeneration of liver nodules, and hepatocyte swelling all lead to distortion of portal architecture. The cause of rapid swings in portal pressure is uncertain. In North America and Europe, the most common cause of portal hypertension is alcoholic liver disease, or Laënnec's cirrhosis. Worldwide, extrahepatic obstruction and fibrosis from schistosomiasis (*Bilharzia*) are the leading causes. Other causes of portal hypertension include portal or splenic vein thrombosis, which can be spontaneous or iatrogenic (e.g., use of umbilical vein catheters in neonatal intensive care units was a significant cause in the past); hepatic vein or vena cava obstruction (Budd-Chiari syndrome); hypersplenism with secondary portal hypertension caused by massive increases in portal vein blood flow (the liver architecture is normal but overwhelmed).

Which findings on initial history and physical examination suggest that portal hypertension with cirrhosis is the cause of bleeding?

Alcohol abuse is common in the general population; practitioners should therefore check for warning signs by asking each patient about the quantity of alcohol used, binge drinking if any, and any societal adverse events such as being away from work or being arrested for drunk driving (9). Often, the most important history for the quantity of alcohol consumption comes from the patient's family. Almost always associated with alcohol abuse is smoking. The physical examination often shows a general loss of muscle mass, and wasting can be severe in the end-stage patient. The liver feels firm and is often enlarged below the costal margin. Ascites may be present, although it may be difficult to differentiate fluid in the abdomen from mesenteric adiposity combined with muscle laxity. Spider angiomata over the chest and upper back can occur, as can gynecomastia. Testicular atrophy is common. There are no direct signs of portal engorgement other than the rare appearance of caput medusa from periumbilical collateral venous channels.

How are patients with portal hypertension classified in terms of prognosis?
Child classified patients with alcoholic cirrhosis in terms of the expected morbidity and mortality from surgery for portal hypertension (2). The original intent was to stratify outcomes on the basis of a worst-case analysis. This classification was later modified by Pugh (2) to provide a general classification of the severity of disease. It describes the degree of liver damage in terms of protein synthetic function and ability to process digestive products (Table 17.1). A patient's classification is based on the worst criterion. For example, a patient who has fixed ascites but all other factors in the B group range is still placed in group C.

No single test assesses liver function overall in a manner analogous to the creatinine clearance for renal function or ejection fraction for cardiac function. Other tests that describe liver function include prothrombin time as a measure of synthetic function and the bromsulphalein clearance test as a measure of the ability to process products of digestion (10). A cofactor in the prognosis of these patients is alcoholic hepatitis as established by liver biopsy. Biopsy is not routinely

TABLE 17.1.

CHILD-PUGH CLASSIFICATION OF PATIENTS WITH CIRRHOSIS

Liver Function or Patient's Status	Group A	Group B	Group C
Bilirubin (mg/dL)	<2	2–3	>3
Albumin (g/dL)	>3.5	3–3.5	<3
Ascites	None	Some (easily controlled)	Fixed
Encephalopathy	None	Minimal	Significant
Nutritional status	Normal	Adequate	Poor (muscle wasting prominent)

performed for patients with portal hypertension, but when tissue is obtained, the architectural changes in the liver and the prominence of Mallory bodies correlate with the outcome of surgery (11).

Why do varices bleed?

The specific reason varices that have been stable for years suddenly hemorrhage is unknown. Portal pressure varies significantly over the day, especially with changes in the degree of inflammation of the liver. Other factors include esophageal or gastric erosion over varices. A prospective study of the predictors of bleeding from extant varices indicated that dominant risk factors are Child class, size of varices, and any abnormal markings over the varices (red wale markings) (12). Other factors that correlated with bleeding in other studies include the location of varices, other markings over the varices (cherry-red spots and hematocystic spots), color of varices, esophagitis, ascites, and prothrombin time.

Mr. Norman is admitted to the intensive care unit for stabilization. An hour later, his blood pressure falls to 90/60 mm Hg, and his heart rate increases to 120 beats per minute. He continues to pass melanotic stools that are more copious and more liquid. He receives a bolus of crystalloid, which normalizes the blood pressure, but he continues to have tachycardia.

How should a patient such as Mr. Norman be stabilized?

Recurrence of bleeding is very common, even after technically satisfactory sclerotherapy. The patient must be resuscitated with fluids and blood products. Any coagulopathy must be corrected. Fresh frozen plasma must be administered, as must vitamin K. If the platelet count is severely depressed, platelet transfusion may be needed. If there is the slightest suspicion that alcoholism is the cause of bleeding varices, precautions against acute alcohol withdrawal syndrome must be taken: the patient is treated with prophylactic doses of a sedative-hypnotic drug, commonly lorazepam, and is closely observed for signs of agitation or delirium (13). In addition, thiamine is given to prevent Wernicke's encephalopathy.

What is the role of drugs in the control of bleeding?

For many years, vasopressin was used to control acute bleeding from esophageal varices. Octreotide is now the favored drug because vasopressin at high doses causes coronary vasoconstriction, which may induce clinically significant myocardial ischemia, especially when there is underlying coronary artery disease. Both drugs cause vasoconstriction on the arterial side of splanchnic blood flow, which leads to reduction in portal pressure.

All vasoconstrictors should be considered stopgap measures that allow control of bleeding; no drug is effective long term. Studies with systemic vasopressin show that after the drug is withdrawn, hemorrhage recurs in more than 50% of patients

(14). In several controlled trials, administration of propranolol reduced long-term bleeding from esophageal varices (15–17). Some clinicians express concern about the potential for accentuation of shock by beta-blocking agents if significant rebleeding occurs in patients with esophageal varices; however, European studies have not confirmed this complication. The patient with both diabetes and bleeding esophageal varices may be difficult to manage with these medications, out of concern for an impaired autonomic response due to neuropathy involving the splanchnic nerves. Long-term use of propranolol may prevent rebleeding from stenosis in a transjugular intrahepatic portosystemic shunt (TIPS) (see What are the options for treatment?) by reducing portal pressure (18).

What are the mechanical techniques for stopping acute severe variceal bleeding?

A Sengstaken-Blakemore (SB) tube can be placed in the stomach and esophagus. This large-bore nasogastric tube has a 300-mL gastric balloon, a long esophageal balloon, and two aspiration ports. The tube is guided into place by fluoroscopy to ensure that the gastric balloon is safely in the stomach before it is inflated; blind placement carries risk of esophageal rupture. Initially, only the gastric balloon inflated to determine whether pressure on the varices at the gastroesophageal junction will lead to hemostasis. If this fails, the esophageal balloon can be inflated to put direct pressure on the varices. SB tubes are fixed to a helmet or over pulleys to provide gentle traction with weights. The airway must be controlled with intubation. Because the tube completely obstructs the esophagus functionally, aspiration of blood or saliva is a major risk. In addition, the tube is so uncomfortable that sedation may be needed. Also, encephalopathy may further compromise the patient's ability to protect the airway. For these reasons, the patient should be intubated when SB tubes are employed.

SB tubes can quickly lead to esophageal erosion and thus recurrent bleeding from varices. In general, the SB tube is used as a temporary measure after initial failure to control bleeding; endoscopic sclerotherapy should be repeated in 12 to 18 hours. If this is not possible, the esophageal balloon, if inflated initially, should be deflated as a trial within the first 24 hours, and the gastric balloon should be taken off traction thereafter. If hemostasis is maintained, the tube is left in place for 12 to 24 hours of observation and sedation; it can then be removed and further sclerotherapy can be performed. If bleeding recurs, the tube is available for reinflation in preparation for further intervention.

Mr. Norman is given octreotide and he has another sclerotherapy session. His condition stabilizes, and no further bleeding is noted for the next 48 hours. He is allowed small amounts of fluid by mouth, and his loose melanotic stools decrease in frequency. His hematocrit stabilizes, and the octreotide is successfully tapered off. He is sent to the general medical floor. His total protein level is 3.1 mg per dL and the prothrombin

time is 14 seconds (INR, 1.3); he has mild tenderness to deep palpation of the liver edge under the right costal margin. On the sixth day in hospital, he has another sclerotherapy session and is found to have some distal esophagitis, but the varices are still prominent halfway up the esophagus. Sclerotherapy is repeated. He is prescribed a histamine$_2$-antagonist and antacids by mouth and discharged home. A month later, he returns to the emergency department with nearly identical symptoms of bleeding, hematemesis, and melanotic stools. His family confirms that he consumed a pint of vodka on the day the bleeding recurred. He receives a blood transfusion, and endoscopy reveals bleeding esophageal varices. He is readmitted to the intensive care unit, where he is given octreotide again. The bleeding slows but it does not stop completely. He is now noted to have mild encephalopathy and jaundice, with a total bilirubin level of 4 mg per dL.

What are the options for treatment?

The options include more sclerotherapy, portasystemic decompression surgery, esophagogastric transection surgery (Sugiura procedure), TIPS, and liver transplantation (19). The condition of the patient guides the treatment decision (Algorithm 17.1). The Child class must be determined because it is an important prognosticator of surgical outcome, although it has been modified over the years to provide a more general estimate of liver function. In addition, the liver disease should be evaluated in the context of any other organ system that has failed because patients with multiple organ system failure have a poor prognosis. In most patients, the decision at this point is to intervene to decrease portal pressure or directly remove varices from the esophagus or stomach. In the case of patients with a particularly poor prognosis because of underlying liver disease, the clinician should discuss end-of-life issues with the family.

Are other tests and imaging studies important at this time?

At some point, the patient should be checked for the various types of hepatitis, especially if there is to be consideration of a liver transplant. A variety of computed tomographic and magnetic resonance techniques have been promoted as helpful in determining the status of the liver (20), but these should not be ordered unless there will be a therapeutic impact from them. Angiography is necessary to plan any portal decompressive surgery or to plan for a transplant.

What is a portasystemic shunt, and what are some common shunting techniques?

Portasystemic shunting consists of diverting high-pressure portal blood into the systemic circulation (Fig. 17.1). It is the oldest treatment for portal hypertension. The earliest model of this shunt was used by Eck in dogs in 1877. Pavlov

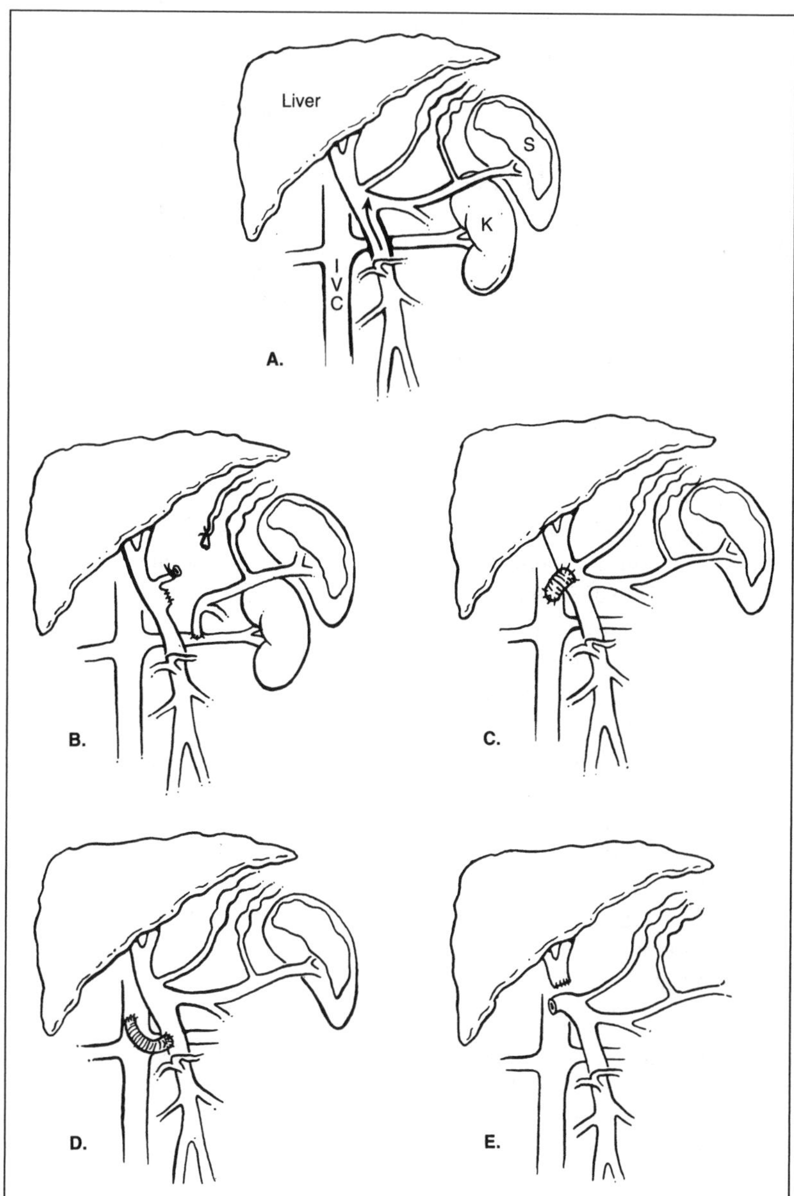

Figure 17.1. Portal anatomy and major shunt types. **A:** Baseline condition with varices. **B:** Distal splenorenal shunt. **C:** H-graft interposition portocaval shunt. D: Mesocaval shunt. **E:** End-to-side portocaval shunt. *IVC,* Inferior vena cava; *K,* kidney; *S,* spleen.

followed these experiments and determined that shunting was complicated by hepatic encephalopathy. The operation was unused until the 1930s, when Whipple and others revived the concept of portacaval shunting. The operation was modified after it was recognized that the development of encephalopathy depended on whether liver blood flow was completely or partially diverted and whether the patient used a low-protein diet after surgery. Because the liver normally receives 70% of its blood supply through the portal vein, total diversion of portal blood flow results in complete bypass of the liver's ability to metabolize various body metabolites. This leads to accumulation of harmful metabolites that cause encephalopathy. Ingestion of a protein-rich diet aggravates this condition.

These are the main shunt procedures:

End-to-side portacaval shunt was one of the two main operations used throughout the 1960s. The portal vein is totally diverted into the vena cava, leaving the liver to survive on hepatic artery flow.

Side-to-side shunt was the other commonly used procedure, in which the technique of Eck was applied to create a partial diversion of portal flow.

Mesocaval shunt, a modification of the partial diversion technique, was popularized by Drapanas. A graft is used to connect the side of the superior mesenteric vein to the vena cava (21).

Linton central splenorenal shunt is the procedure in which the splenic vein distally is turned into the left renal vein.

Distal splenorenal shunt was devised by Warren and Zeppa in the late 1960s in an attempt to reduce the rate of encephalopathy. The portal system is divided into two parts by dividing the splenic vein off the portal vein (at its junction with the superior mesenteric vein) and turning the splenic vein into an anastomosis with the left renal vein (22,23). This shunt diverts portal flow from the stomach, spleen, and esophageal varices but leaves portal flow from the small and large intestine intact.

H-graft bridge, used by Sarfeh to create a more facile central partial shunt that was, in effect, a side-to-side shunt, is a 10-mm H-graft to bridge the portal vein and vena cava (24).

All shunt procedures have complications in common; all are major abdominal or retroperitoneal operations and all carry significant risk for chronically ill patients. The main concerns in the immediate postoperative period are worsening of liver failure, worsening of ascites, exacerbation of hepatic encephalopathy, and shunt failure with recurrent hemorrhage.

What is the prognosis after shunt surgery?

Shunt surgery does not alter the long-term prognosis for survival, which is based on the Child class of the patient at the time of surgery. Shunt surgery is intended to stop variceal hemorrhage, which in the short term causes significant mortality—approximately 25% per major bleeding episode, even in recent studies (2). The operation chosen should stop the hemorrhage and have a low risk of short-term encephalopathy. Shunt surgery does not cure the liver disease, which remains a significant cause of death. Because the Child classification can be used easily with bedside criteria and tests that have been available for decades, it is possible to compare current survival with that in the 1940s and earlier. For patients with bleeding esophageal varices, 1-year survival has remained constant at 30% to 40%. This poor prognosis applies predominantly to alcoholic cirrhosis and to diseases in which hepatocellular functional reserve is destroyed. The prognosis is better for patients with a disease such as primary splenic vein thrombosis or schistosomiasis, in which hepatic reserve can be maintained.

What is the Sugiura procedure?

Dissatisfaction with the results of shunting, even in the 1960s and 1970s, led to a search for an alternative approach that preserved blood flow to the liver. Transesophageal open ligation of varices was attempted, but the mortality and morbidity from this procedure were high. Sugiura modified this approach by defining a multiple-stage devascularization of esophageal and gastric varices in a large cohort of Japanese patients. This procedure has been modified in the United States and Europe with use of a transabdominal approach and stapling. The Sugiura procedure is rarely used now in North America and Europe, except in patients in whom shunting or sclerotherapy is not possible, but it remains popular in Japan (25,26).

What is the role of TIPS?

In the late 1980s, interventional radiology gained importance in the treatment of portal hypertension. Images of the portal architecture are required before any shunt operation can be planned. Imaging was originally performed by direct puncture of the spleen and injection of radiopaque contrast medium. With improvements in digital angiography in the last 20 years, it has become easy to obtain selective angiograms of the celiac and superior mesenteric circulation by tracking the contrast through to the portal venous phase. Angiographers attempted transhepatic puncture into the portal system with direct injection of sclerosing material, thrombogenic agents, or even emboli into the largest varices, but these techniques generally failed to achieve a long-term benefit.

Finally, after the development of endovascular stents, it became possible to create an artificial channel between the hepatic veins and the portal vein, dilate the channel, and maintain it with a metal stent. This procedure, TIPS, has been moderately successful in recent years as an alternative to surgery in the highest risk patients (27–30). Nevertheless, TIPS has been associated with a problematic rate of recurrent portal hypertension because of stent thrombosis or fibrosis.

What is the role of hepatic transplantation?

The only curative procedure for primary liver disease is transplantation, which was introduced in the 1970s and has progressed to be an option today (31). Transplantation is the only procedure that treats portal hypertension and restores hepatic metabolic function, but it remains a problem for several reasons:

1. Livers remain in short supply; therefore, only a few thousand procedures can be performed each year in the United States.
2. The procedure is very expensive because of the cost of surgery and the ongoing cost of immunosuppression; many potential recipients do not have the needed insurance or personal finances.
3. Ethical concerns have been raised about the propriety of allowing transplantation for alcoholic cirrhosis, with opponents noting that the significant medical resources used for a transplant would be more properly distributed to people who have not abused alcohol.

Nevertheless, liver transplantation has generally been performed in centers that treat relatively large numbers of patients, and a high success rate has been achieved in the 1990s for this technically demanding operation (32).

When should surgery be considered in the management of liver failure and portal hypertension?

Surgery has a smaller role today than it did 20 years ago (33). Most medical consultants consider surgical portal decompression only after bleeding has not been controlled by other means. A shunt operation is uncommon, and, in general, the patients at the time of operation have significant risk factors and are in Child class B or C. In such situations, early surgical consultation is encouraged so that the surgeon is familiar with the patient in case a shunt is necessary, and the surgeon should encourage early portal system angiography for the patient in whom medical management seems to be failing.

Patients with severe hemorrhage are aggressively treated with medical therapy and sclerotherapy. Repeated endoscopic sclerotherapy is performed at short intervals to obliterate varices as quickly as possible (34). Failure to follow this procedure is likely to cause rebleeding. A problem for the surgeon is that the longer a patient with marginal liver function remains without proper nutrition and the greater the number of hemorrhagic episodes, the more likely that the patient's Child classification will deteriorate and the higher the mortality will be after surgery (35,36). Because some centers have obtained results with surgery that are equivalent to those with sclerotherapy, some authors strongly advocate early surgery, that is, surgery before the patient's status deteriorates (5,37).

Should patients with varices that have not yet hemorrhaged have surgery?

Approximately 30% of patients with asymptomatic esophageal varices go on to bleed (1). The outcome of a prospective study performed more than 20 years ago

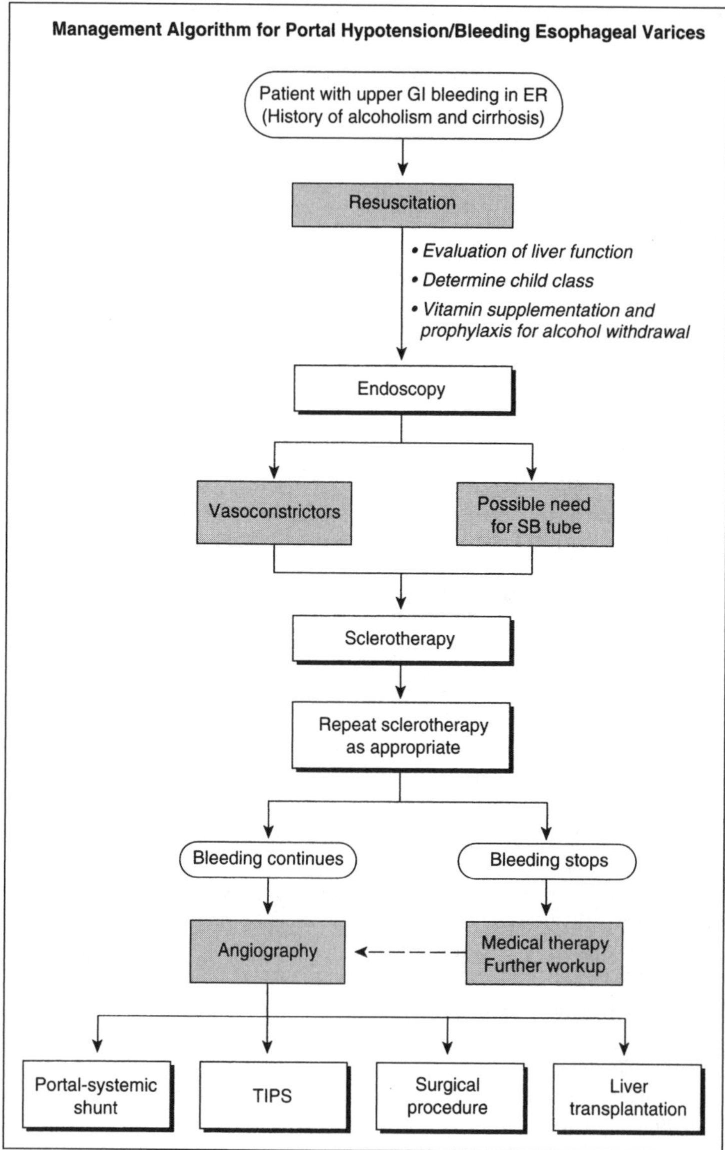

Algorithm 17.1.

did not favor preemptive surgery for nonhemorrhaging varices (38). Intervention with prophylactic medical therapy may be cost effective. Most patients who have incidental esophageal varices from portal hypertension should be evaluated to establish the cause of the liver dysfunction, if alcoholism is not the apparent cause. Measures to restore liver function include avoidance of the noxious stimulus, use of vitamins, and perhaps medication with a beta-blocker. A low-protein diet is used to avoid encephalopathy, and patients with ascites are treated with diuretics or repeated paracentesis (39). Consider those with refractory ascites for TIPS or for hepatic transplantation but rarely for a portacaval shunt. (Algorithm 17.1)

REFERENCES

1. Collini FJ, Brener B. Portal hypertension. Surg Gynecol Obstet. 1990;170:177–192.
2. Resnick RH. Portal hypertension. Med Clin North Am. 1975;59:945–953.
3. Terblanche J, Kahn D, Bornman P. Long-term injection sclerotherapy treatment for esophageal varices. Ann Surg. 1989;210:725–731.
4. Cello JP, Grendell JH, Crass RA, et al. Endoscopic sclerotherapy versus portacaval shunt in patients with severe cirrhosis and acute variceal hemorrhage. N Engl J Med. 1987;316:11–15.
5. Orloff MJ, Orloff MS, Orloff SL, Hanes KS. Treatment of bleeding from portal hypertensive gastropathy by portacaval shunt. Hepatology. 1995;21:1011–1017.
6. Garrett KO, Reilly JJ, Schade RR, van Thiel DH. Sclerotherapy of esophageal varices: long-term results and determinants of survival. Surgery. 1988;104:813–818.
7. Orloff MJ, Orloff MS, Rambotti M, et al. Is portal-systemic shunt worthwhile in Child's class C cirrhosis? Ann Surg. 1992;216:256–268.
8. Burroughs AK, Hamilton G, Phillips A, et al. A comparison of sclerotherapy with staple transection of the esophagus for the emergency control of bleeding from esophageal varices. N Engl J Med. 1989;321:857–862.
9. Adams WL, Barry KL, Fleming MF. Screening for problem drinking in older primary care patients. JAMA. 1996;276:1964–1967.
10. Galambos J. Evaluation of patients with portal hypertension. Am J Surg. 1990;160:14–18.
11. Andreoni B, Chiara O, Maggioni D, et al. Role of hepatic histologic findings in the prognosis and treatment of bleeding esophageal varices. Am J Surg. 1989;157:220–224.
12. North Italian Endoscopic Club for the study and treatment of esophageal varices. Prediction of the first variceal hemorrhage in patients with cirrhosis of the liver and esophageal varices. N Engl J Med. 1988;319:983–989.
13. Kosten TR, O'Connor PG. Management of drug and alcohol withdrawal. N Engl J Med 2003;48:1786–1795.
14. Burnett DA, Rikkers LF. Nonoperative emergency treatment of variceal hemorrhage. Surg Clin North Am. 1990;70:291.
15. Teran JC, Imperiale TF, Mullen KD, et al. Primary prophylaxis of variceal bleeding in cirrhosis: a cost-effectiveness analysis. Gastroenterology. 1997;112:473–482.

16. Bernard B, Lebrec D, Mathurin P, et al. Propranolol and sclerotherapy in the prevention of gastrointestinal rebleeding in patients with cirrhosis: a meta-analysis. J Hepatol. 1997;26:312–324.
17. Burroughs AK, Pangou E. Pharmacological therapy for portal hypertension: rationale and results. Semin Gastrointest Dis. 1995;6:148–164.
18. Bellis L, Moitinho E, Albraldes JG, et al. Acute propranolol administration effectively decreases portal pressure in patients with TIPS dysfunction. Gut. 2003;52:130–133.
19. Rosemurgy AS, Zervos EE. Management of variceal hemorrhage. Curr Probl Surg. 2003;40:263–343.
20. Reddy SI, Grace ND. Liver imaging. A hepatologist's perspective. Clinics in Liver Disease. 2002;6:297–310.
21. Lillemoe KD, Cameron JL. The interposition mesocaval shunt. Surg Clin North Am. 1990;70:379–394.
22. Warren WD, Zeppa R, Fomon JJ. Selective trans-splenic decompression of gastroesophageal varices by distal splenorenal shunt. Arch Surg. 1967; 168:437–455.
23. Millikan WJ Jr, Warren WD, Henderson JM, et al. The Emory prospective randomized trial: selective versus nonselective shunt to control variceal bleeding: ten-year follow-up. Ann Surg. 1985;201:712–722.
24. Sarfeh IJ, Rypins EB, Mason GR. A systematic appraisal of portacaval H-graft diameters. Ann Surg. 1986;204:356–394.
25. Abouna GM, Baissony H, Al-Nakib BM, et al. The place of Sugiura operation for portal hypertension and bleeding esophageal varices. Surgery. 1987;101:91–98.
26. Takenaka H, Nakao K, Miyata M, et al. Hemodynamic study after devascularization procedure in patients with esophageal varices. Surgery. 1990;107:55–62.
27. Zemel G, Katzen BT, Becker GJ, et al. Percutaneous transjugular portasystemic shunt. JAMA. 1991;266:390–393.
28. Pursnani KG, Sillin LF, Kaplan DS. Effect of transjugular intrahepatic portasystemic shunt on secondary hypersplenism. Am J Surg. 1997;173: 169–173.
29. LaBerge JM, Ring EJ, Gordon RL, et al. Creation of transjugular intrahepatic portasystemic shunts with the Wallstent endoprosthesis: results in 100 patients. Radiology. 1993;187:413–420.
30. Conn HO. Portal hypertension, varices, and transjugular intrahepatic portosystemic shunts. Clinics in Liver Disease. 2000;4:133–150.
31. Garrett KO, Reilly JJ, Schade RR, et al. Bleeding esophageal varices: treatment by sclerotherapy and liver transplantation. Surgery. 1988;104:819–823.
32. Henderson JM, Gilmore GT, Hooks MA, et al. Selective shunt in the management of variceal bleeding in the era of liver transplantation. Ann Surg. 1992;216: 248–254.
33. Conn HO, Lebrec D, Terblanche J. The treatment of oesophageal varices: a debate and a discussion. J Intern Med. 1997;241:103–108.
34. Chung RS, Dearlove J. The sources of recurrent hemorrhage during long-term sclerotherapy. Surgery. 1988;104:687–696.

35. Grossman MD, McGreevy JM. Effect of delayed operation for bleeding esophageal varices on Child's class and indices of liver function. Am J Surg. 1988;156: 502–505.
36. Pomerantz RA, Eckhauser FE, Knol JA, et al. Operative timing and patient survival following distal splenorenal shunt. Am Surg. 1989;55:333–337.
37. Rikkers LF, Jin G, Burnett DA, et al. Shunt surgery versus endoscopic sclerotherapy for variceal hemorrhage: late results of a randomized trial. Am J Surg. 1993;165:27–33.
38. Greig JD, Garden OJ, Carter DC. Prophylactic treatment of patients with esophageal varices: is it ever indicated? World J Surg. 1994;18:176–184.
39. Runyon BA. Care of patients with ascites. N Engl J Med. 1994;330:337–342.

CHAPTER

18

PANCREATITIS

Jeannie F. Savas

Anne Ryan is a 29-year-old woman who visits the emergency department with severe epigastric abdominal pain, nausea, and vomiting during the previous 2 to 3 days. She has a history of pancreatitis. She denies having fever, chills, or any other associated complaints. She denies the use of alcohol. Her medical history is significant for familial hypertriglyceridemia for which she is prescribed medication; she has a history of noncompliance. She has had no surgery. She is very thin and in moderate distress during physical examination. She has poor capillary refill; her blood pressure is 90/60 mm Hg; her heart rate, 120 beats per minute; her temperature, 38.3°C; her respiratory rate, 30 breaths per minute. The mid-epigastrium is quite tender, but there is no peritonitis or palpable mass.

What diagnosis is most likely?

Given Ms. Ryan's history of pancreatitis and her epigastric pain associated with nausea and vomiting, acute pancreatitis is the likely culprit. The differential diagnosis includes gastritis, peptic ulcer disease, biliary disease, pneumonia, and myocardial infarction.

What are the symptoms and signs of pancreatitis?

The classic history is epigastric pain radiating to the back. The pain is described as a constant boring or knifelike pain often associated with anorexia, nausea, vomiting, and occasionally fever. The patient may give a history of pancreatitis. The abdominal findings may range from mild epigastric tenderness to diffuse peritonitis. A mass or ascites may be found with complicated pancreatitis (e.g., pseudocyst, abscess, pancreatic duct leak, severe acute pancreatitis). Any ecchymosis in the flank (Grey-Turner's sign) or periumbilical area (Cullen's sign) should be noted. Although very rare, they are both signs of retroperitoneal hemorrhage, which may accompany severe acute pancreatitis (1).

What laboratory or radiologic tests support this diagnosis?

Elevated serum amylase, lipase, or urinary amylase is expected. However, many other conditions may result in hyperamylasemia. Abdominal film may show pancreatic calcification if the patient has chronic pancreatitis. The abdominal film often shows an ileus pattern of some dilated loops of small bowel with a few air–fluid levels. The ileus pattern may be diffuse or local, as with the sentinel loop, a single dilated jejunal loop in the upper abdomen, or colon cutoff sign. Here the colon is dilated to the mid-transverse colon, and little gas is seen distally. An upright chest film rules out pneumonia and free intraabdominal air. A left pleural effusion may be visible. Ultrasound may show an edematous pancreas and, more importantly, the presence or absence of gallstones or a dilated common bile duct (CBD). Abdominal computed tomography (CT) may show pancreatic edema, fluid collections, soft tissue stranding, necrosis, or associated complications of pancreatitis. However, CT generally is not recommended as a primary diagnostic tool in patients with simple acute pancreatitis.

What causes pancreatitis?

Pancreatitis is most frequently caused by gallstones or alcohol ingestion (Table 18.1). Other causes include congenital abnormalities of the pancreas and its ductal system, hypertriglyceridemia, trauma, drugs (e.g., thiazides, azathioprine) (Table 18.2), and iatrogenic causes (e.g., surgery, endoscopic retrograde cholangiopancreatography [ERCP]).

What is the treatment for acute pancreatitis?

Because oral intake stimulates the pancreas, the patient is given nothing by mouth (NPO). If the patient is vomiting or has gastric distention, nasogastric decompression alleviates these symptoms and prevents aspiration. Intravenous (IV) fluids are given, and parenteral nutrition is considered if enteral nutrition will not be an option for a prolonged period. Histamine$_2$ blockers may help suppress pancreatic secretion (2).

The patient receives a fluid bolus of 1 L normal saline (NS), after which her vital signs stabilize. A Foley catheter is placed and laboratory tests performed, yielding the following results: calcium, 5.9 mg per dL; carbon dioxide, 18 mEq per L; creatinine, 1.4 mg per dL; glucose, 250 mg per dL; amylase, 1200 U per L; lipase, 9200 IU per L; triglycerides, 31,000 mg per dL; liver function tests, normal; hemoglobin, 10 g per dL; white blood cell count, 12,000 per mm^3. She is given 2 g calcium IV and transferred to her room, where she is kept NPO and receives pain medication and

TABLE 18.1.

CAUSES OF ACUTE PANCREATITIS AND HYPERAMYLASEMIA

Acute Pancreatitis	Hyperamylasemia
Alcohol	Renal insufficiency
Biliary tract disease	Mumps
Hyperlipidemia	Macroamylasemia
Hypercalcemia	Mesentric thrombosis
Familial tendency	Perforated peptic ulcer
Trauma	Cardiopulmonary bypass
External disease	Tumors
Operative	Head trauma
Retrograde pancreatography	Peritonitis
Ischemia	Salivary hyperamylasemia
Hypotension	Drugs
Cardiopulmonary bypass	Small-bowel obstruction
Atheroembolism	
Vasculitis	
Pancreatic duct obstruction	
Tumor	
Pancreatic divisum	
Ampullary stenosis	
Ascaris infestation	
Duodenal obstruction	
Viral infection	
Scorpion venom	
Drugs	
Idiopathic	

maintenance IV fluids. She receives furosemide for oliguria. The next morning, she is in respiratory distress and has the following laboratory values: calcium, 4.2 mg per dL; creatinine, 4.9 g per dL; hemoglobin, 8 g per dL. She is transferred to the intensive care unit, intubated, and given more IV calcium and fluid boluses.

Why did Ms. Ryan deteriorate?

She was severely dehydrated and hypocalcemic. Although attempts were made to correct these deficiencies in the emergency department, she should have had more frequent monitoring of her vital signs and laboratory values to be sure that she was adequately resuscitated.

TABLE 18.2.

DRUGS IMPLICATED IN THE INITIATION OF ACUTE PANCREATITIS

Definite Association	Probable Association
Azathioprine	Thiazide diuretics
Estrogens	Furosemide
	Ethacrynic acid
	Sulfonamides
	Tetracycline
	L-Asparaginase
	Corticosteroids
	Phenformin
	Procainamide
	Valproic acid
	Clonidine
	Pentamidine
	Dideoxyinosine

Reprinted from Townsend C, ed. Sabiston's Textbook of Surgery. 15th ed. Philadelphia, Pa: WB Saunders; 1997, with permission.

What are Ranson's criteria?

Ranson (3) described a series of signs that help determine the severity of acute pancreatitis. They have recently been modified and are now known as the Glasgow criteria (4). One group of signs are assessed at the time of admission and the others are assessed within 48 hours (Table 18.3). At the time of Ranson's study, patients with fewer than two criteria had 1% mortality; those with three or four signs, 15%; those with five or six signs, 40%; and those with more than six signs, 100%. With the advances in monitoring and treatment, the mortality for each subgroup has probably decreased, but the study has not been repeated recently.

These criteria help identify severe pancreatitis and thus enable it to be treated aggressively. Because only five signs are assessed on admission, however, one should consider the possibility of severe pancreatitis if more than two or three signs are seen initially or if there are signs of hemodynamic instability or respiratory distress. Treatment should not wait until all criteria are met, which takes 48 hours.

Was this patient treated appropriately?

Ms. Ryan did not have all appropriate tests to determine how many Ranson's or Glasgow signs she had. With her hemodynamic compromise, severe hypocalcemia, tachypnea, and oliguria, Ms. Ryan required more aggressive monitoring and resuscitation, even without accurate assessment of her pancreatitis.

TABLE 18.3.

RANSON'S CRITERIA FOR PANCREATITIS

At Admission	During Initial 48 Hours
Age above 55 yr	Hematocrit falling >10%
WBC >16,000 cells/mm^3	BUN falling >5 mg/100 mL
Blood glucose >200 mg/100 mL	Serum calcium <8 mg/100 mL
Serum lactate dehydrogenase >350 IU/L	Arterial P_{O_2} <60 torr
AST >250 U/100 mL	Base deficit >4 mEq/L
	Estimated fluid sequestration >6 L

AST, aspartate transaminase; BUN, blood urea nitrogen; WBC, white blood cell.

From Townsend C, ed. Sabiston's Textbook of Surgery. 15th ed. Philadelphia, Pa: WB Saunders; 1997, with permission.

During the next 48 hours in the intensive care unit, Ms. Ryan requires 15 L crystalloid, 6 units blood, 8 g calcium, and emergency plasmapheresis to manage her severe hypertriglyceridemia. With this treatment, her hemoglobin and calcium levels return to normal, and her creatinine decreases to 2.9 mg/dL after reaching a high of 9. As her pancreatitis improves, she requires less respiratory support as well. Antibacterial prophylaxis with imipenem is started.

A week later, although hemodynamically improved, Ms. Ryan continues to require ventilatory support and begins to spike fevers to 39.4°C. Her white blood cell count rises to 22,000 per mm^3. She is now receiving total parenteral nutrition.

Is there a role for prophylactic antibiotics in patients with acute pancreatitis?

In a recent study, patients with severe acute pancreatitis who received prophylactic treatment with imipenem had fewer infectious complications (5). Imipenem is the only drug that has been studied for this indication, although other broad-spectrum antibiotics may be as effective.

What are the infectious complications of pancreatitis?

Pancreatic abscess, infected pancreatic necrosis, infected pancreatic pseudocyst, line sepsis, pneumonia, infected pleural effusion, catheter-related urinary tract infection, and pancreatic or enteric fistulas may result from severe acute pancreatitis.

How is the cause of infection diagnosed?

All indwelling catheters, urinary or vascular, should be changed, and a thorough physical examination should be performed in search of findings such as cellulitis, abdominal mass, and increased abdominal tenderness. A chest radiograph helps assess for pneumonia and large pleural effusion. Often, the abdominal examination is difficult in a patient with pancreatitis either because of preexisting tenderness or because the patient is sedated or receiving pain medication. Therefore, when infection is suspected, abdominal CT is often required. If available, dynamic or spiral CT with contrast is best because it will demonstrate abscess, pseudocyst, or pancreatic necrosis.

What is the treatment for pancreatic abscess or infected pseudocyst?

If possible, radiology-guided percutaneous drainage is best, especially in already compromised patients (6). If this cannot be done, surgical drainage is required.

What is the treatment for pancreatic necrosis?

Although it is controversial, most studies advocate nonoperative therapy for patients with only small areas of necrosis (less than 20% to 30%) or when no infection is suspected (7). However, when infection is suspected—because of marked fever and leukocytosis, bacteremia, failure to improve clinically, or positive Gram stain on aspirated necrosis—surgical management is indicated. Intraoperative findings are thick necrotic tissue surrounding the pancreas, sometimes extending into the transverse mesocolon, small-bowel mesentery, or retroperitoneum. Extensive débridement is performed. Most often, this requires multiple visits to the operating room with the abdomen packed between visits. When no further débridement is necessary, drains are placed and the abdomen is closed. A sample of the necrotic tissue is sent to the laboratory for Gram stain and culture to guide antimicrobial therapy. It is prudent to place a feeding jejunostomy so that an elemental diet may be given when tolerated.

What is the treatment for gallstone pancreatitis?

If a patient with pancreatitis has gallstones, even if there are other possible causes of pancreatitis, the gallbladder should be removed after the pancreatitis has clinically resolved. This is usually done before the patient is discharged from the hospital to prevent another attack of pancreatitis, which may be more severe than the initial attack. Some literature supports early ERCP to remove the stone or a sphincterotomy if there is suspicion of a persistent, obstructing distal CBD stone in a patient whose pancreatitis fails to improve (8,9). However, ERCP itself may worsen pancreatitis (10). Some centers use magnetic resonance cholangiopancreatography (MRCP) as a diagnostic maneuver before ERCP because MRCP is noninvasive (11). Although not a functional study, this technique has been shown to be very accurate in defining pancreatic and biliary structures and ductal anatomy, including the identification of choledocholithiasis, when performed by an experienced radiologist.

Ms. Ryan underwent six to eight surgical débridements for her infected pancreatic necrosis, which was diagnosed with dynamic abdominal CT. She also had a surgical jejunostomy feeding tube. Her enteral elemental diet was advanced over several weeks, and TPN was discontinued. She required a tracheostomy because of prolonged ventilator dependence. After long stays in the intensive care unit and hospital, she was able to tolerate a low-fat oral diet and was discharged home.

Gerald Stevens is a 45-year-old man who visits the hospital with acute onset of epigastric pain, hematemesis, and dizziness. He has a history of alcoholic pancreatitis. Mr. Stevens has mild epigastric tenderness. A nasogastric tube confirms fresh blood clots in his stomach. His vital signs are stable, although his hemoglobin is 8 g per dL. The IV access is obtained. Esophagoduodenoscopy reveals a large opening in the posterior gastric wall that is filled with clotted blood. No active bleeding is seen. Abdominal CT shows evidence of chronic pancreatitis and a large pseudocyst adherent to the posterior gastric wall.

What are the most common causes of gastrointestinal bleeding in a patient with pancreatitis?

The most common causes are not related to pancreatitis; they include alcoholic gastritis, peptic ulcer disease, varices, Mallory-Weiss tear, and tumor. Rarely, as in this patient, a large untreated pseudocyst may erode into an adjacent organ and cause bleeding.

What causes a pseudocyst?

A pancreatic pseudocyst forms as a result of a contained pancreatic duct leak, often the result of a proximal ductal obstruction. This usually occurs during a bout of acute pancreatitis, and the surrounding inflammatory reaction forms a wall and thus a pseudocyst.

What is the surgical treatment for a pseudocyst?

A pseudocyst may be treated with internal or external drainage. The pseudocyst is opened and sewn to an adjacent structure, usually the stomach (cystogastrostomy) or jejunum (cystojejunostomy). This is the preferred method of drainage if no infection is present. External drainage, which is the best option for an infected pseudocyst, may be performed percutaneously (with radiologic guidance) or surgically. The risk of external drainage is that the patient may develop a pancreatic-cutaneous fistula if there is still a connection between the pseudocyst and the pancreatic duct. It is customary to send a portion of the wall of a suspected pseudocyst to the pathologist to rule out cystic tumor of the pancreas, in which case there is a true epithelial-lined cyst wall. Another treatment option is resection of the pseudocyst. This is usually reserved for pseudocysts in the tail of the pancreas when no proximal strictures are present.

When is surgery indicated for a pseudocyst?

Surgery or percutaneous drainage is indicated for all infected pseudocysts. Uninfected pseudocysts should undergo surgical drainage if they are very large (more than 6 cm) or persist after the pancreatitis has resolved in order to avoid further complications, such as rupture or bleeding. Unless they are very large, most pseudocysts spontaneously resolve within 4 to 6 weeks after a bout of acute pancreatitis (12). Large pseudocysts may cause abdominal discomfort, bloating, and early satiety because they compress adjacent organs. They also may erode into an adjacent organ and present as an intestinal bleed, as in this patient, or rupture free into the peritoneal cavity, causing pancreatic ascites if the pseudocyst communicates with the pancreatic duct.

How is a pseudocyst diagnosed?

A pseudocyst should be suspected in a patient with a history of pancreatitis who has early satiety, abdominal distention, or an abdominal mass. Abdominal ultrasound or CT confirms the diagnosis and usually can rule out tumor. Infection is suspected if the patient has a high fever, marked abdominal tenderness, leukocytosis, or typical radiologic features. MRCP or ERCP may be useful to document ductal strictures or connection to the pseudocyst if therapy is contemplated. ERCP, if performed, should be done within 24 hours of surgery to avoid infecting the pseudocyst.

Mr. Stevens underwent operative exploration for his gastrointestinal bleeding. An anterior gastrotomy revealed that the pseudocyst had spontaneously ruptured into the posterior gastric wall. The edges of gastric mucosa, adjacent to the cystogastrostomy, were bleeding and therefore were oversewn. The clot was evacuated from the pseudocyst, and no further bleeding was noted. The anterior gastrotomy was closed. Mr. Stevens recovered uneventfully.

Dennis Keith is a 35-year-old man who visits the emergency department with abdominal pain and weakness of acute onset. During physical examination, he is notably pale, tachycardiac, and hypotensive, and he has a distended abdomen. After initial IV fluid boluses of 2 L lactated Ringer's solution, he remains unstable and is immediately taken to the operating room. A midline abdominal incision reveals 2 to 3 L of blood in his abdomen. The abdomen is packed in four quadrants while the anesthesiologist transfuses him and restores normal blood pressure. As the packs are removed, bleeding is noted to be coming from the left upper quadrant, and a splenectomy is performed. The bleeding continues and is found to originate from the splenic artery proximal to the site of its division. The bleeding artery is controlled, and the patient recovers uneventfully. The spleen appears grossly normal when inspected in the operating room after its removal. The physician later learns that Mr. Keith had a recent episode of gallstone pancreatitis.

What is the diagnosis?

This patient ruptured a splenic artery pseudoaneurysm that developed during pancreatitis. With no history of trauma, other possibilities include a perforated viscus; spontaneous splenic rupture; and rupture of an abdominal aortic, iliac, or visceral artery aneurysm.

What are the vascular complications of pancreatitis?

The most common complication is splenic artery pseudoaneurysm because of inflammation of the pancreas in proximity to the vessel. Other causes of bleeding include rupture of a pseudocyst, erosion of a pseudocyst into vascular structures or bowel, and varices arising from splenic vein thrombosis. Splenectomy is curative for management of bleeding varices in this situation, which is called *sinistral hypertension.*

Mr. Keith required no further intervention because the splenic artery pseudoaneurysm was repaired during surgery. He should have no future bouts of pancreatitis because his gallbladder was removed at the time of his initial attack.

While intoxicated, John Roberts, a 27-year-old man, sustains a stab wound to his midepigastrium and complains of severe abdominal pain. On exploration, he is found to have two gastrotomies, one anterior and one posterior, which are repaired. A thorough exploration reveals no other evidence of injury. He recovers well, except that on postoperative day 5 he still has a significant amount of abdominal pain, anorexia, and nausea. Mr. Roberts has no fever or leukocytosis, but his amylase level is elevated. The physician suspects that he has either alcoholic pancreatitis or some degree of injury to his pancreas not recognized at surgery. Two days later, Mr. Roberts has sudden onset of severe abdominal pain and massive distention that causes respiratory distress. After initial resuscitation, abdominal CT demonstrates ascites, a left pleural effusion, and a possible pancreatic laceration. Analysis of ascitic and pleural fluid demonstrates an amylase level above 50,000 U per L.

What is the diagnosis?

This patient had pancreatic ductal disruption leading to the development of pancreatic ascites and a pancreaticopleural fistula. He had likely suffered injury to the pancreas from the stab wound, which either was not recognized initially or resulted in a delayed rupture of the duct.

What is the treatment for pancreatic ascites?

Initial management is resuscitation of the patient: respiratory support if needed, IV fluids, nasogastric decompression, and pancreatic rest. Next, one must determine whether there is an ongoing pancreatic leak and, if so, its cause. When a leak is caused by a major disruption of the duct or gland, surgery is indicated to resect, repair, or drain the injury (13). When no major disruption is noted, ERCP with stenting or external drainage may be sufficient. MRCP or ERCP is usually necessary to diagnose the cause of the pancreatic ascites and determine whether there is an ongoing leak.

Is pancreatic juice corrosive to the peritoneal cavity and its organs?

Pancreatic enzymes are secreted in their inactive form into the duodenum, where they are activated. Therefore, when the ascites results from a pancreatic leak, no direct injury results. The major symptoms are pain from acute pancreatitis and discomfort or respiratory compromise due to massive abdominal distention.

How do pancreatic fistulas develop?

The pancreas is a retroperitoneal structure; if the leak does not rupture through the peritoneum, it can track along the retroperitoneum into the pleural cavities, mediastinum, or pericardium. When there is any open connection to the skin, such as a surgical incision or drain, a pancreatic-cutaneous fistula may develop.

How are pancreatic fistulas treated?

The treatment is similar to that of pancreatic ascites (Table 18.4). Any major ductal disruption requires surgery, whereas minor leaks may be treated with ERCP and stenting. Treatment also includes avoiding pancreatic stimulation; the patient should take NPO, instead receiving parenteral nutrition or, alternatively, an elemental diet administered via a jejunal feeding tube. The use of somatostatin analogs is expensive and controversial (14), but they have been shown to diminish the volume of pancreatic fluid secretion and, in many cases, result in quicker or higher rates of closure of pancreatic fistulas.

Mr. Robert underwent distal pancreatectomy (to remove the injured portion of the pancreatic duct) and resection of the fistulous tract with placement of drains. He soon recovered and tolerated a general diet.

Janet Morgan is a 13-year-old girl referred for a second opinion. She has a history of chronic relapsing pancreatitis, and a brother and two cousins have the same problem. She is not taking any medications and denies any drug or alcohol use. She gives no history of abdominal trauma.

How will the physician diagnose and treat Janet's pancreatitis?

With a young patient, one must consider familial pancreatitis and congenital anomalies such as pancreas divisum and cystic fibrosis. Abdominal CT, ERCP, or MRCP may help to define the anatomy and rule out complications of pancreatitis such as pseudocysts and stricture. MRCP is a relatively new technology not available in all centers, but it is quite accurate. Ultrasound is performed to rule out cholelithiasis. Treatment is conservative (i.e., NPO, pancreatic rest, analgesia) during the acute phase and in the long term may entail chronic dietary

TABLE 18.4.

MANAGEMENT OF PATIENTS WITH INTERNAL PANCREATIC FISTULA

- Nonoperative treatment
  - Prohibition of oral intake
  - Nasogastric tube suction
  - Paracentesis for pancreatic ascites
  - Thoracentesis or chest tube for pancreatic pleural effusion
  - Hyperalimentation
  - Somatostatin (octreotide)
- Operative treatment
  - Direct duct leak
    - Roux-en-Y drainage of duct leak
    - Pancreatic resection for distal duct leak with Roux-en-Y drainage of proximal pancreatic remnant for any proximal duct disease
  - Leaking pseudocyst
    - Roux-en-Y drainage of pseudocyst to jejunum
    - Small distal pseudocyst: possible resection with Roux-en-Y drainage of proximal pancreatic remnant for any proximal duct disease
    - External drainage

From Townsend C ed. Sabiston's Textbook of Surgery. 15th ed. Philadelphia, Pa: WB Saunders; 1997, with permission.

modifications, that is, low-fat diet with or without pancreatic enzyme supplementation.

Janet's ultrasound reveals no gallstones or dilated ducts. No masses or pseudocysts are seen on abdominal CT. MRCP demonstrates normal pancreatic ductal anatomy without dilation or stricture. It is determined that she has familial pancreatitis and is treated medically as described earlier.

Rhys Williams is a 45-year-old man who is a frequent visitor to the emergency department. He is a recalcitrant alcoholic who has repeated bouts of pancreatitis. His abdominal pain is exacerbated by a recent binge. He says this pain feels just the same as every time he has pancreatitis—a gradually worsening midepigastric pain that radiates to his back. He has been vomiting for 2 days, and he has no desire for any food or alcohol. He denies any other symptoms but demands pain medication. During physical examination, he appears thin, has mild tachycardia at 105 beats per minute, and has rebound tenderness in the upper abdomen. No masses are palpated, and he is heme-negative on rectal examination.

His laboratory tests are all within normal limits except for an elevated urinary amylase level and a white blood cell count of 12,000 per mm^3. The abdominal radiograph demonstrates pancreatic calcification. Last year, Mr. Williams had an ultrasound that showed no gallstones.

What is the diagnosis?

Mr. Williams has the classic presentation of chronic relapsing pancreatitis caused by alcohol use. The history and physical examination were performed to rule out other causes of pain, such as gastritis, gallstone pancreatitis, and peptic ulcer disease. The serum amylase level often is normal in patients with a history of chronic pancreatitis, but an elevated urinary amylase level confirms that there is an acute exacerbation. The serum lipase level is also a useful test for pancreatitis, as it is a more specific finding than an elevated serum amylase level.

What is the treatment for chronic relapsing pancreatitis?

In the acute setting, the treatment is pancreatic rest, nasogastric decompression if vomiting persists, analgesia, and fluid resuscitation. Serial abdominal examinations determine when the patient is improved. This usually requires 1 or 2 days, at which time the diet is advanced as tolerated and pain medicines are tapered.

After 2 days, Mr. Williams is tolerating a low-fat diet and requires only occasional acetaminophen with codeine (Tylenol with Codeine) for pain. He is discharged and given a follow-up appointment in 2 weeks. He misses this appointment but comes back in 2 months complaining of foul-smelling diarrhea, especially after eating greasy foods. He has no pain or nausea but is again drinking excessively.

What is the cause of his current symptoms?

Mr. Williams has steatorrhea, which is confirmed by finding fat in the stool. This is a result of pancreatic insufficiency.

What advice and treatment should this patient receive?

Mr. Williams needs counseling about his alcohol abuse. Pancreatic enzyme supplementation, to be taken with meals, will improve the steatorrhea, as will avoidance of fatty foods.

Does Mr. Williams need insulin or oral hypoglycemics because of his pancreatic insufficiency?

Endocrine insufficiency may result from severe or chronic pancreatitis, although exocrine deficiency is much more common. Diabetes mellitus may develop in up to 38% of patients with chronic pancreatitis (15).

The nutritionist speaks with Mr. Williams at length about a proper low-fat diet. He understands her recommendations and promises to try to

modify his diet. He is shocked when the physician tells him that his problem is a result of his alcohol use and says no one ever told him that. The physician explains that his pancreatitis will likely continue to get worse unless he abstains, and Mr. Williams agrees to quit. Six months later, Mr. Williams returns because he ran out of pills. He states they helped him with the diarrhea. He tried to quit drinking but says it was just too hard. He now has pain every day, although it has not been severe enough to get admitted to the hospital. He is angry at the physicians in the emergency department because they refuse to give him any more IV pain medication. He says he had some pain medication left over from a tooth extraction that took care of his pain, so he wants a prescription for more. The physician again counsels him about his need to abstain from alcohol and gives him information on several detoxification centers. His physical examination is significant only for a 10-pound weight loss, and there is no evidence of acute pancreatitis.

What is the cause of his chronic pain?

Mr. Williams suffers from chronic pancreatitis and will likely have progressive worsening of his pain if he continues to drink.

The physician prescribes Mr. Williams oxycodone hydrochloride with acetaminophen (Percocet), which controls his pain if he takes 4 or 5 per day. He goes to an alcohol detoxification center and stops drinking. He continues to require pancreatic enzyme replacement with meals and has no further problems. He gets a job as a construction worker and works 40 to 60 hours per week. He keeps his appointments at 2-month intervals to get his medicine refilled and shows no progression of disease. Approximately 1 year later, still sober, Mr. Williams calls his physician to say he is out of pain medicine, although his last refill was just 2 weeks earlier. He says he now requires 10 to 15 pills per day to control his pain, but they just do not seem to be working anymore. He denies nausea, vomiting, steatorrhea, or any other problems. He comes to the office for a physical examination, which is unremarkable.

Is this patient getting addicted to the pain medicine?

Although this is a definite possibility, the physician must first search for a pathologic reason for the increased pain. This patient has remained abstinent for more than 1 year and was managed for a long period on a stable dose of pain medication; now he has a sudden increase in his analgesic requirement. One possibility is that he has begun drinking again. This information may be sought by speaking with family members or friends or with random toxicology screening. If there is nothing to suggest a relapse, further diagnostic tests should be done.

How should Mr. Williams be worked up at this point? (Algorithm 18.2)

As always, it is prudent to begin with a thorough history and physical examination. Are the character and location of this pain the same as with his previous pancreatitis? Does he have an abdominal mass or unexplained weight loss? Is there any evidence to suggest other diagnoses, such as peptic ulcer disease, reflux esophagitis, biliary disease, or tumor? If the findings suggest progressive pancreatitis, further evaluation of the pancreas is indicated. Abdominal CT is helpful to assess the size of the gland and the main pancreatic duct, the CBD, any pseudocyst or abscess, and any intrinsic or extrinsic mass or adenopathy. MRCP or ERCP will assess the pancreatic duct for strictures or other abnormality.

Mr. Williams's laboratory tests are normal. Abdominal CT shows pancreatic calcifications and a dilated pancreatic duct. The CBD is normal. No gallstones are seen. No masses or adenopathy are seen, and there is no edema of the pancreas. There is no ascites or fluid around the pancreas. ERCP shows multiple pancreatic ductal strictures with dilation of the intervening segments of the duct, the so-called chain of lakes.

What causes strictures of the pancreatic duct?

They may be caused by tumor or more commonly by recurrent bouts of pancreatitis with resultant scarring. If only a single stricture is seen, especially with no history of pancreatitis, brush cytology of the duct should be done during ERCP, and CT or MRCP should be performed to rule out an extrinsic mass.

What is the treatment for a stricture of the pancreatic duct?

If a tumor is suspected, surgical resection is indicated when technically feasible. Dilation and stenting of a malignant stricture for inoperable patients may provide symptomatic relief, although the patient will require stent changes. For benign strictures, management depends on symptoms. If the patient has minimal or no pain, expectant management is preferred. If, as in this case, the patient has progressive pain while abstinent and compliant with medical therapy, consider surgery.

What is the surgery for benign strictures?

Therapy is aimed at relieving the obstruction of the duct. If there is a single stricture in the body or tail of the gland, a distal pancreatectomy is curative. A Puestow procedure is performed for multiple strictures. The pancreatic duct is identified, then opened along its length to obliterate all strictures. Some advocate the removal of any pancreatic duct stones. A Roux-en-Y pancreatojejunostomy is then formed to drain the pancreas. This relieves pain in selected patients; however, those who continue to imbibe or who have idiopathic pancreatitis do not have such good results. Surgery is therefore reserved for compliant, good-risk patients who understand that the procedure may or may not result in permanent or even temporary pain relief (Table 18.5).

TABLE 18.5.

PAIN RELIEF AFTER SURGERY FOR CHRONIC PANCREATITIS

Average Procedure	Good + Fair (%)	Poor (%)	Follow-up (Yrs)
Longitudinal pancreaticojejunostomy	81.0	19.0	5.7
Short pancreaticojejunostomy	35.0	65.0	8.0
Short pancreaticogastrostomy	83.0	17.0	4.0
Caudal pancreaticojejunostomy	34.0	66.0	5.7
Total pancreatectomy	72.5	27.5	5.8
Pancreaticoduodenectomy	82.0	18.0	4.7
Duodenal preservation and local resection	88.0	12.0	2.7
Distal pancreatectomy			
Less 80%	85.0	15.0	5.8
Greater 80%	65.0	35.0	6.5

From Cameron J. Current Surgical Therapy. 5th ed. St. Louis, Mo: Mosby–Year Book; 1995:443, with permission.

Are there any other options?

Pancreatic duct stents may be placed via ERCP and may provide temporary relief for patients who are not candidates for surgery. These stents occlude and thus require repeated ERCP for stent changes, usually at 2-month intervals. Another option for patients who have persistent pain or who are not candidates for pancreatic surgery is celiac ganglionectomy or percutaneous nerve blocks, although results are variable. The only other option is to prescribe stronger analgesics, but be aware of potential for abuse.

The patient undergoes a successful Puestow procedure (pancreatojejunostomy) and recovers uneventfully. Within 2 weeks, he no longer requires any pain medication, although he still takes enzyme replacement. He has a friend who was recently diagnosed with unresectable pancreatic cancer after being told for years he had pancreatitis. He wants to be sure he does not have cancer too.

How can this patient be reassured that he does not have cancer?

There is a higher incidence of pancreatic cancer in patients with previous pancreatitis than in the general population, but this risk is still very low. The physician can explain that no evidence of tumor is seen, but frequent follow-up may help detect a mass if it develops. Most masses seen on CT in patients with pancreatitis are acute inflammation, but a new mass discovered without acute increase in pain should be evaluated for possible tumor.

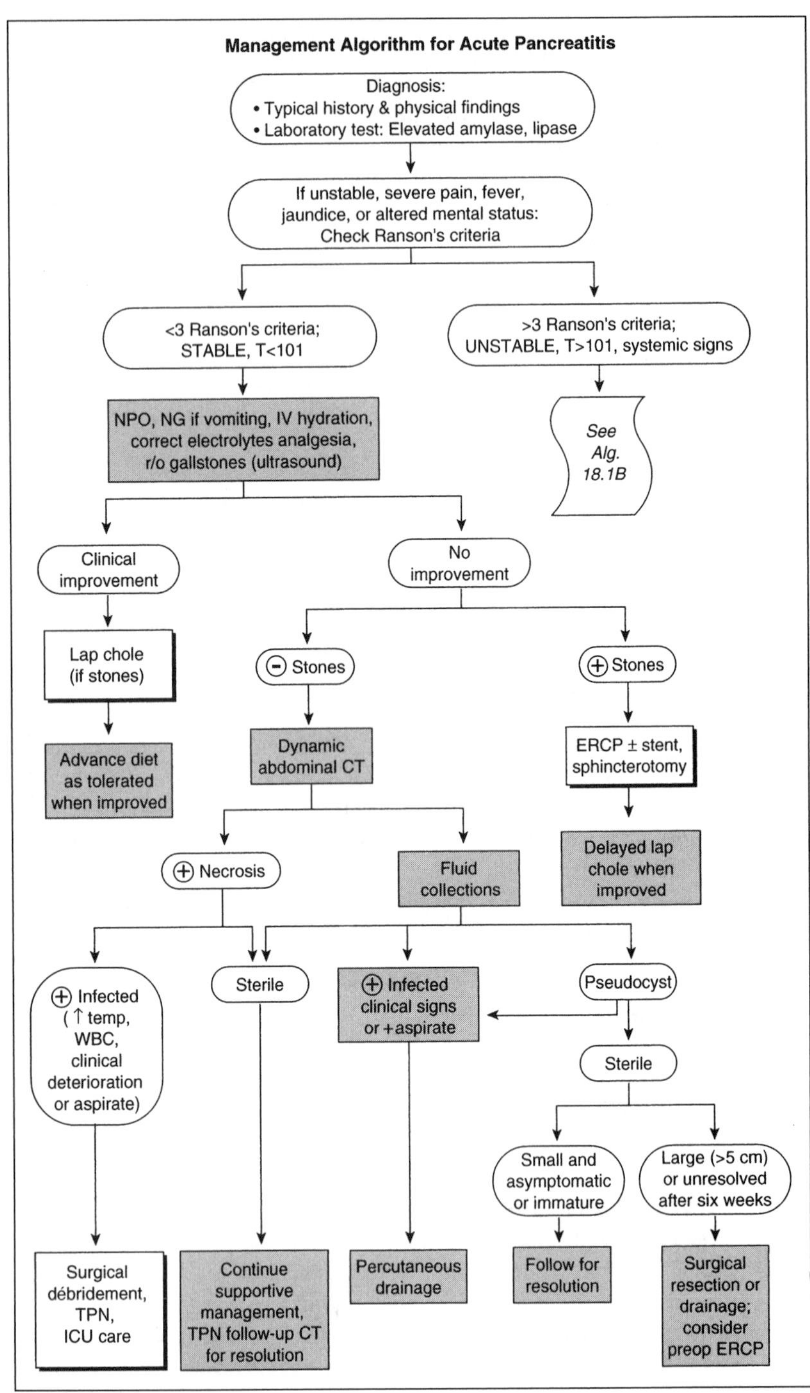

Algorithm 18.1A.

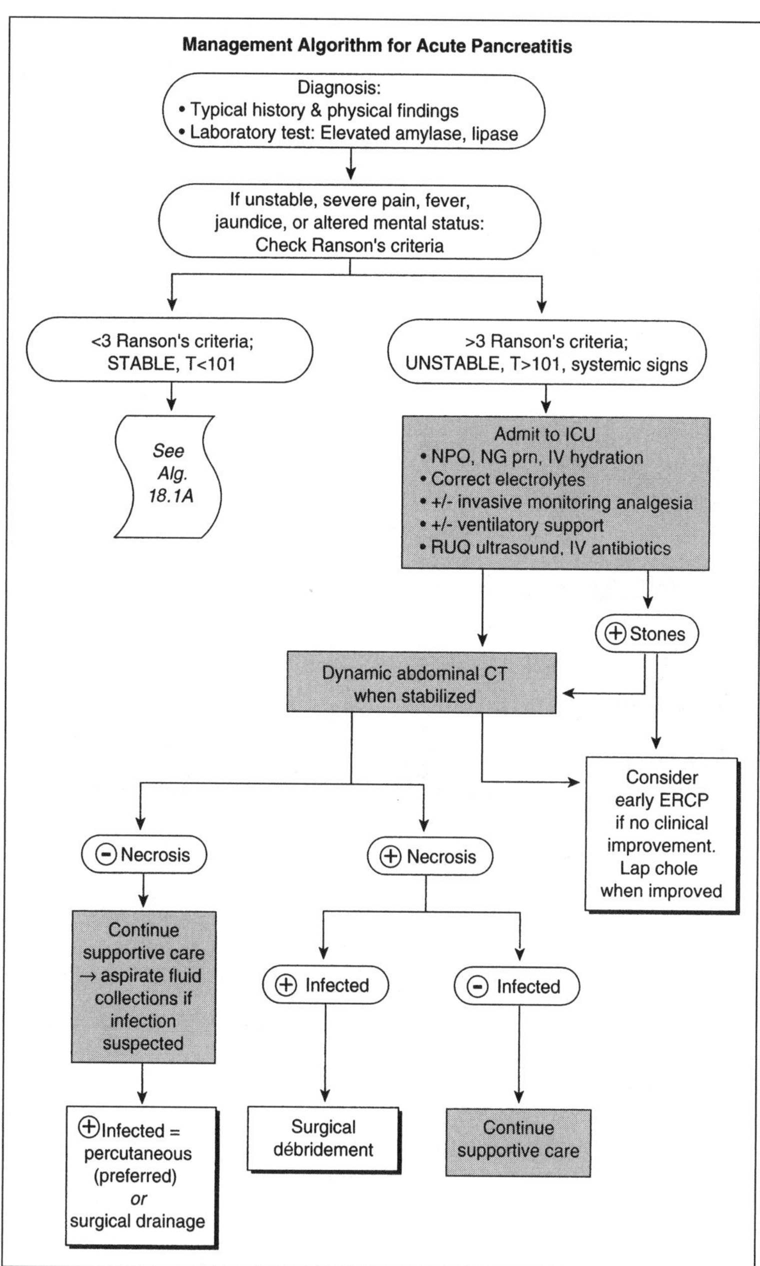
Management Algorithm for Acute Pancreatitis
Diagnosis:
• Typical history & physical findings
• Laboratory test: Elevated amylase, lipase
If unstable, severe pain, fever, jaundice, or altered mental status: Check Ranson's criteria
<3 Ranson's criteria; STABLE, T<101
See Alg. 18.1A
>3 Ranson's criteria; UNSTABLE, T>101, systemic signs
Admit to ICU
• NPO, NG prn, IV hydration
• Correct electrolytes
• +/- invasive monitoring analgesia
• +/- ventilatory support
• RUQ ultrasound, IV antibiotics
⊕ Stones
Dynamic abdominal CT when stabilized
Consider early ERCP if no clinical improvement. Lap chole when improved
⊖ Necrosis
⊕ Necrosis
Continue supportive care → aspirate fluid collections if infection suspected
⊕ Infected
⊖ Infected
⊕Infected = percutaneous (preferred) or surgical drainage
Surgical débridement
Continue supportive care

Algorithm 18.1B.

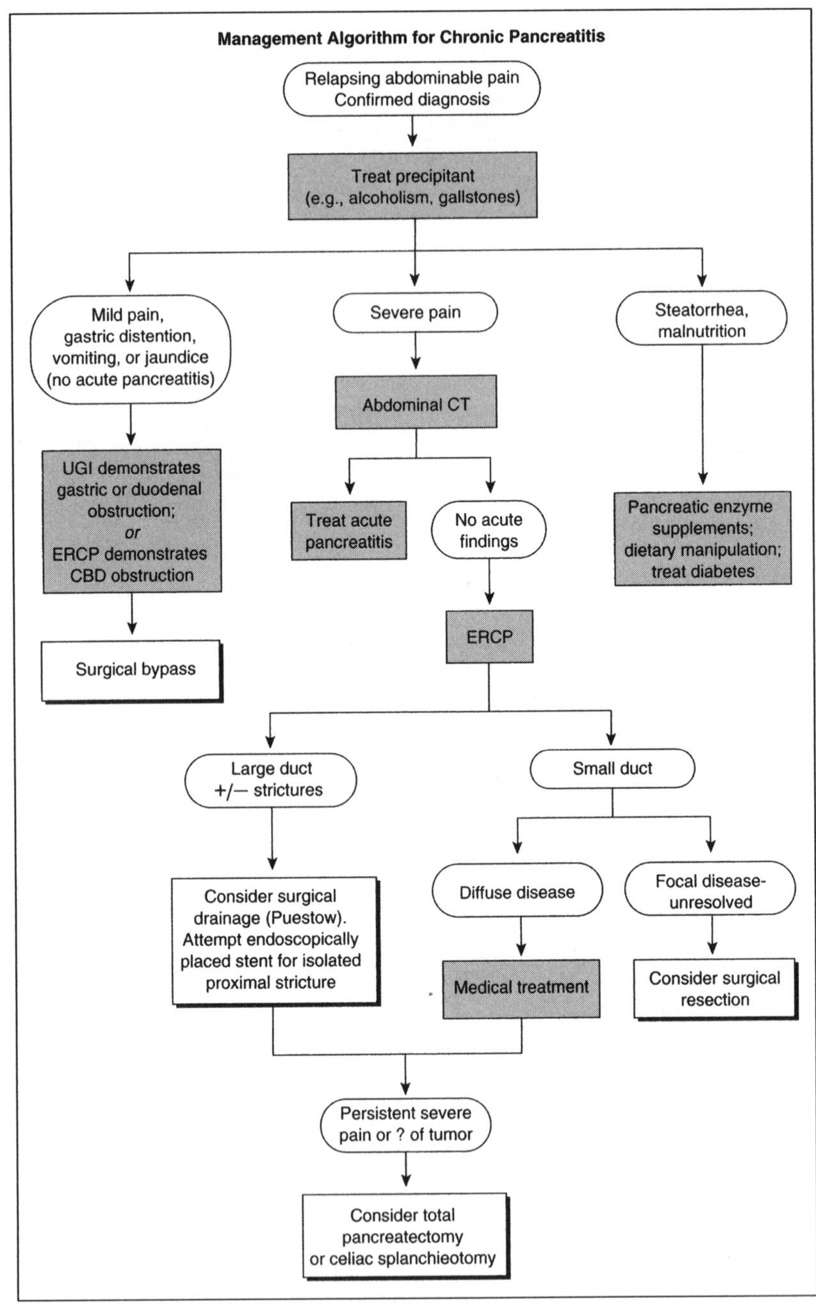
Management Algorithm for Chronic Pancreatitis
Relapsing abdominable pain
Confirmed diagnosis
Treat precipitant
(e.g., alcoholism, gallstones)
Mild pain,
gastric distention,
vomiting, or jaundice
(no acute pancreatitis)
Severe pain
Steatorrhea,
malnutrition
UGI demonstrates
gastric or duodenal
obstruction;
or
ERCP demonstrates
CBD obstruction
Abdominal CT
Treat acute
pancreatitis
No acute
findings
Pancreatic enzyme
supplements;
dietary manipulation;
treat diabetes
Surgical bypass
ERCP
Large duct
+/— strictures
Small duct
Diffuse disease
Focal disease-
unresolved
Consider surgical
drainage (Puestow).
Attempt endoscopically
placed stent for isolated
proximal stricture
Medical treatment
Consider surgical
resection
Persistent severe
pain or ? of tumor
Consider total
pancreatectomy
or celiac splanchieotomy

Algorithm 18.2.

REFERENCES

1. Beger HG, Rau B, Mayer J, Pralle U. Natural course of acute pancreatitis. World J Surg. 1997;21:130–135.
2. Steinberg W, Tenner S. Acute pancreatitis. N Engl J Med. 1994;330:1198.
3. Ranson JHC, Rifkind KM, Roses DF, et al. Prognostic signs and the role of operative management in acute pancreatitis. Surg Gynecol Obstet. 1974;139:69.
4. Wassef W, Zfass A. Gallstone pancreatitis: an update. Gastroenterologist. 1996;4:70–75.
5. Pederzoli P, Bassi C, Vesentini S, et al. A randomized multicenter clinical trial of antibiotic prophylaxis of septic complications in acute necrotizing pancreatitis with imipenem. Surg Gynecol Obstet. 1993;176:480.
6. Lang EK, Paolini RM, Pittmeyer A. The efficacy of palliative and definitive percutaneous versus surgical drainage of pancreatic abscesses and pseudocysts: a prospective study of 85 patients. South Med J. 1991;84:55.
7. Bradley EL III. Fifteen year experience with open drainage for infected pancreatic necrosis. Surg Gynecol Obstet. 1993;177:215–222.
8. Sheung-Taf F. Early treatment of acute biliary pancreatitis by endoscopic papillotomy. N Engl J Med. 1993;328:228–232.
9. Neoptolemos JP, Carr-Locke DL, London NJ, et al. Controlled trial of urgent endoscopic retrograde cholangiography and endoscopic sphincterotomy versus conservative treatment for acute pancreatitis due to gallstones. Lancet. 1988;2:979.
10. Sherman S, Lehman GA. ERCP and endoscopic sphincterotomy-induced pancreatitis. Pancreas. 1991;6:350.
11. Soto JA. Magnetic resonance cholangiography: comparison with ERCP. Gastroenterology. 1996;110:589–597.
12. Yeo CJ, Bastidas JA, Lynch-Nyhan A, et al. The natural history of pancreatic pseudocysts documented by computed tomography. Surg Gynecol Obstet. 1990;170:411.
13. Ridgeway MG, Stabile BE. Surgical management and treatment of pancreatic fistulas. Surg Clin North Am. 1996;76:1159–1173.
14. Parekh D, Segal I. Pancreatic ascites and effusion: risk factors for failure of conservative therapy and the role of octreotide. Arch Surg. 1992;127:707.
15. Steer ML, Waxman I, Freedman S. Chronic pancreatitis. N Engl J Med. 1995;332:1482.

CHAPTER

19

PANCREAS CANCER

Todd M. Tuttle

Mr. Brown is a 59-year-old man whose barber noticed that his skin was yellow. Mr. Brown has also noticed a 10-pound weight loss, dark urine, and pale stools. Other than jaundice and icterus, his physical examination is normal. Pertinent laboratory findings include total bilirubin, 13.1; serum glutamic-oxaloacetic transaminase (SGOT), 60; serum glutamate pyruvate transaminase (SGPT), 67; alkaline phosphatase, 336; hemoglobin, 11.8; white blood cell count, 9.9; platelet count, 124,000; and international normalized ratio (INR), 1.8.

What is the differential diagnosis of jaundice?

The list is extensive, and it includes hepatitis, cirrhosis, hemolysis, enzyme deficiencies (e.g., Gilbert syndrome), drugs, sclerosing cholangitis, primary biliary cirrhosis, benign bile duct stricture (usually pancreatitis), choledocholithiasis, and periampullary tumors.

What are the four periampullary tumors?

1. Head of pancreas (most common)
2. Duodenum
3. Distal common bile duct
4. Ampulla of Vater

The exact origin of periampullary tumors is often difficult to determine using preoperative imaging studies.

Why is the INR elevated?

Mr. Brown has decreased absorption of vitamin K secondary to biliary obstruction and the lack of bile salts for uptake of this fat-soluble vitamin. The INR should be corrected with parental vitamin K before any surgical procedure.

What imaging tests should be performed?

Both ultrasonography (US) and abdominal computed tomography (CT) will identify bile ductal dilation, a finding that distinguishes obstructive (choledocholithiasis, benign stricture, or periampullary tumors) from nonobstructive jaundice. US is recommended if choledocholithiasis is suspected (young patient age, intermittent abdominal pain). CT is recommended if cancer is suspected (old patient age, weight loss).

Mr. Brown's CT demonstrates bile duct and pancreatic duct dilation ("double-duct sign") and a 3-cm mass in the head of the pancreas.

What are the signs and symptoms of pancreatic cancer?

The most common symptoms of pancreatic cancer are abdominal pain, weight loss, jaundice, fatigue, back pain, anorexia, nausea, and vomiting. Glucose intolerance is present in most patients with pancreatic cancer. Patients with cancers of the head of the pancreas frequently notice jaundice and usually have less advanced cancers. In contrast, patients with cancers of the pancreas body and tail usually do not develop jaundice and almost always have advanced cancers.

What causes pancreatic cancer?

Cancer of the pancreas remains a significant health problem in the United States and is the fourth leading cause of cancer-related death for both men and women. Approximately 30% of pancreatic cancer cases are related to cigarette smoking. The risk of developing pancreatic cancer increases with age. Although a few early studies suggested that coffee and excessive alcohol consumption could be risk factors, more recent studies have failed to demonstrate a risk. Diets high in meats, cholesterol, and nitrosamines may increase the risk. Several studies have suggested that diabetics have an increased risk. Some studies have reported an association between chronic pancreatitis and pancreatic cancer.

Familial predisposition is associated with 5% to 8% of all pancreatic cancer cases. Several hereditary conditions predispose individuals to pancreatic neoplasms. These syndromes include von Hippel-Lindau syndrome, hereditary nonpolyposis colon cancer, multiple endocrine neoplasia I, ataxia-telangiectasia, and familial atypical mole melanoma syndrome.

What further tests should be performed to determine Mr. Brown's treatment?

The two major goals of preoperative staging are (a) to identify metastases and (b) to determine whether the tumor is locally resectable with negative margins. Patients do not benefit from surgery if metastases are present or if the tumor cannot be completely removed with tumor-free margins. Thus, pretreatment imaging should identify patients who will not benefit from exploratory laparotomy. Only 10% to 15% of all patients with pancreatic cancer have resectable tumors.

After complete history and physical examination, abdominal CT is the single most important staging tool. CT identifies pancreatic masses, determines operability, and identifies metastases. Magnetic resonance imaging may provide similar information, but surgeons and radiologists have more experience with CT. Endoscopic retrograde cholangiopancreatography (ERCP) should not be performed for diagnostic purposes. Magnetic resonance cholangiopancreatography is a noninvasive test that provides equivalent information. ERCP may be useful for stent placement to palliate biliary obstruction for patients who are not candidates for surgical resection. Endoscopic US is a useful test that can identify small pancreatic masses not visible on CT. Endoscopic US also provides important information regarding tumor involvement of the superior mesenteric artery and vein. All patients should also have a chest radiograph.

What factors exclude patients from definitive surgery?

Exclusion criteria for resection include (a) extrapancreatic disease (usually liver or peritoneal metastases), (b) tumor involvement of the superior mesenteric artery, and (c) occlusion of the superior mesenteric vein or portal vein.

Mr. Brown is told that he probably has a localized and potentially resectable pancreatic cancer. Should a biopsy be performed before surgery?

Diagnostic needle biopsy of pancreatic masses can be successfully and safely performed with either CT or endoscopic US guidance. Despite early concerns, preoperative needle biopsy rarely results in seeding or peritoneal metastases. A patient with a resectable pancreatic mass and a double-duct sign generally does not require a preoperative needle biopsy. If preoperative chemoradiation is recommended for patients with borderline resectable tumors, needle biopsy is required before beginning treatment. Finally, some patients may desire tissue confirmation of malignancy before proceeding with surgery.

Mr. Brown decides to undergo surgical resection. What procedure should be performed?

After induction of general anesthesia, staging laparoscopy is performed before laparotomy. Laparoscopy can identify unsuspected peritoneal or hepatic metastases in approximately 10% of patients. These patients can be spared the side effects of a major abdominal incision and proceed with systemic therapy.

The Whipple operation is the only potentially curative treatment for pancreatic cancer. The resection has six separate steps (Fig. 19.1):

1. **Cattell-Braasch maneuver:** the right colon is mobilized, exposing the superior mesenteric vein.
2. **Kocher maneuver:** the lateral attachments of the duodenum are divided and the duodenum and head of pancreas are mobilized.
3. **Portal dissection:** the common hepatic duct is divided and the gastroduodenal artery is ligated and divided.

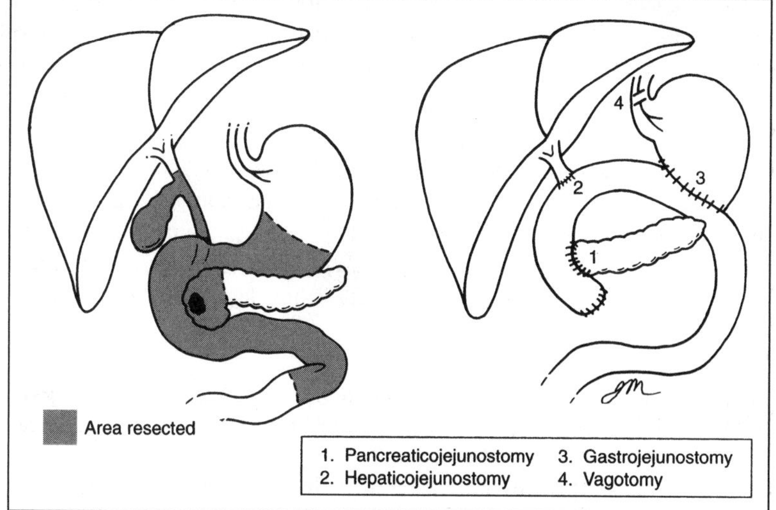

Figure 19.1. The classic Whipple procedure.

4. **Distal stomach:** the distal stomach is divided.
5. **Proximal jejunum:** the proximal jejunum is divided.
6. **Pancreas dissection:** the neck of the pancreas is divided and the uncinate process is dissected off the superior mesenteric vein and artery.

The reconstruction has three separate steps:

1. Pancreaticojejunostomy anastomosis
2. Hepaticojejunostomy anastomosis
3. Gastrojejunostomy anastomosis

What is a pylorus-preserving Whipple?

Instead of removing the distal stomach, the surgeon divides the duodenum just distal to the pylorus. The duodenum is anastomosed to the jejunum to complete the reconstruction. Proponents of the pylorus-preserving Whipple argue that the operation provides improved nutritional outcomes. Proponents of the classic Whipple contend that pylorus preservation can yield higher recurrence rates. In fact, there are no apparent differences in complications, weight gain, gastric emptying, or survival between the two operations.

If the tumor abuts or focally invades the superior mesenteric or portal vein, should the surgeon perform a Whipple?

Isolated tumor involvement of the superior mesenteric or portal vein is not considered an absolute contraindication for resection. The venous complex can be safely removed with the pancreatic tumor. Venous reconstruction is frequently completed with an internal jugular vein interposition graft. The morbidity, mortality, and long-term survival are similar to that of patients without venous involvement. In contrast, tumor involvement of the superior mesenteric artery remains a contraindication.

What complications can occur after Whipple operation?

The major postoperative complications include anastomotic leak (pancreatic, bile duct, or gastric reconstruction), bleeding, abscess, pneumonia, deep venous thrombosis, and delayed gastric emptying. With advances in operative techniques, anesthesia, and critical care, mortality rate is now less than 2% after Whipple operation.

Mr. Brown has an uneventful postoperative recovery and is discharged home from the hospital 8 days after surgery. What is the 5-year survival after resection for pancreatic cancer?

The 5-year survival is only about 15% after the Whipple operation for pancreas cancer. Favorable prognostic factors include tumor-free margins, small tumor size (less than 2 cm), negative lymph nodes, and lower tumor grade. Most 5-year survivors ultimately die of recurrent pancreatic cancer; thus, few patients with pancreatic cancer are cured. The survival of patients with other periampullary cancers (ampulla of Vater, duodenum, distal common bile duct) is significantly better.

Can long-term survival be improved with a more radical operation?

The so-called extended Whipple includes the classic resection plus removal of celiac, superior mesenteric, hepatic, renal, inferior mesenteric, aortic, and renal lymph nodes. Prospective randomized trials have failed to demonstrate a survival benefit for the extended Whipple operation.

Can long-term survival be improved with adjuvant therapy?

Chemoradiation has been shown to improve survival after surgery for pancreatic cancer. In the Gastrointestinal Tumor Study Group Trial, patients were randomized to surgery alone versus surgery plus postoperative chemoradiation therapy. Median survival was significantly improved with postoperative treatment. A nonrandomized trial from Johns Hopkins demonstrated similar findings. However, Neoptolemos et al. recently reported the results of a prospective randomized trial that demonstrated no benefit from postoperative radiation and a significant benefit from postoperative chemotherapy (11). Although the data are conflicting, either chemoradiation or chemotherapy alone should be considered for most patients with resectable pancreatic cancer.

Some treatment centers administer chemoradiation therapy before surgery. Preoperative chemoradiation offers several potential benefits. More patients are likely to receive all treatment modalities. Chemoradiation is more effective on oxygenated tissue as compared with postoperative tissue. Restaging after preoperative chemoradiation will identify metastases in 25% of patients, thus avoiding nontherapeutic surgery in those patients. Pancreatic leak rates are lower after preoperative chemoradiation. However, no survival advantage of preoperative treatment over postoperative treatment has been demonstrated.

Is palliative surgery useful for patients with unresectable (due to metastases or vascular invasion) pancreatic cancer?

Patients with unresectable pancreatic cancer suffer from biliary obstruction (jaundice and pruritus), gastric outlet obstruction (nausea, vomiting, and inability to eat), and celiac plexus invasion (back pain). If preoperative imaging studies demonstrate an inoperable tumor, then nonsurgical palliation is preferred. Biliary obstruction can be relieved by endoscopic placement of metal biliary stents. Likewise, gastric outlet obstruction can be palliated by endoscopic duodenal stents. Pain relief can be accomplished with analgesic drug therapy, radiation therapy, systemic chemotherapy, intrathecal pumps, and percutaneous celiac plexus blocks.

Still, some patients undergo laparotomy and are found to have unresectable pancreatic tumors despite appropriate preoperative imaging studies. Surgical palliation should be considered for these patients because the primary morbidity of surgery is the incision. Hepaticojejunostomy (jaundice), gastrojejunostomy (gastric outlet obstruction), and chemical splanchnicectomy with alcohol (pain) can relieve and prevent symptoms with little additional morbidity.

What treatment, if any, should be given to patients with metastatic adenocarcinoma of the pancreas?

The median survival of patients with metastatic pancreatic cancer is 3 to 6 months. In recent years, systemic administration of gemcitabine has replaced 5-fluorouracil as the standard treatment for patients with advanced pancreas cancer. Gemcitabine treatment improves overall survival and quality of life for these patients.

How are cystic pancreatic neoplasms distinguished from pancreatic pseudocysts?

Cystic pancreatic neoplasms are a distinct entity from pancreatic pseudocysts. Detailed medical history, physical examination, laboratory tests, and imaging procedures can usually establish the diagnosis (Table 19.1). The two main types of cystic pancreatic neoplasms are serous cystadenoma and mucinous cystadenoma. Serous cystadenoma are benign and have a characteristic starburst central scar on CT. These tumors are associated with von Hippel-Lindau syndrome. Appropriate management is observation. Surgical resection is reserved for tumors that are large and symptomatic or if diagnosis is unclear. In contrast, mucinous

TABLE 19.1.

DISTINGUISHING PANCREATIC PSEUDOCYST FROM CYSTIC NEOPLASM

Characteristic	Pseudocyst	Cystic Neoplasm
Age	Younger	Older
Gender	Male > Female	Female > Male
History	Pancreatitis	No pancreatitis
Amylase	Elevated	Normal
CT	No septations	Septations
	Inflammation	No inflammation
	Unilocular	Multilocular
ERCP/MRCP	Ductal communication	No ductal communication
Cyst Aspiration	No tumor cells	Tumor cells
	High amylase	Normal amylase
	Normal CEA	Elevated CEA
	Normal 19-9	Elevated 19-9

CEA, carcinoembryonic antigen; CT, computed tomography; ERCP, endoscopic retrograde cholangiopancreatography; MRCP, Magnetic resonance cholangiopancreatography.

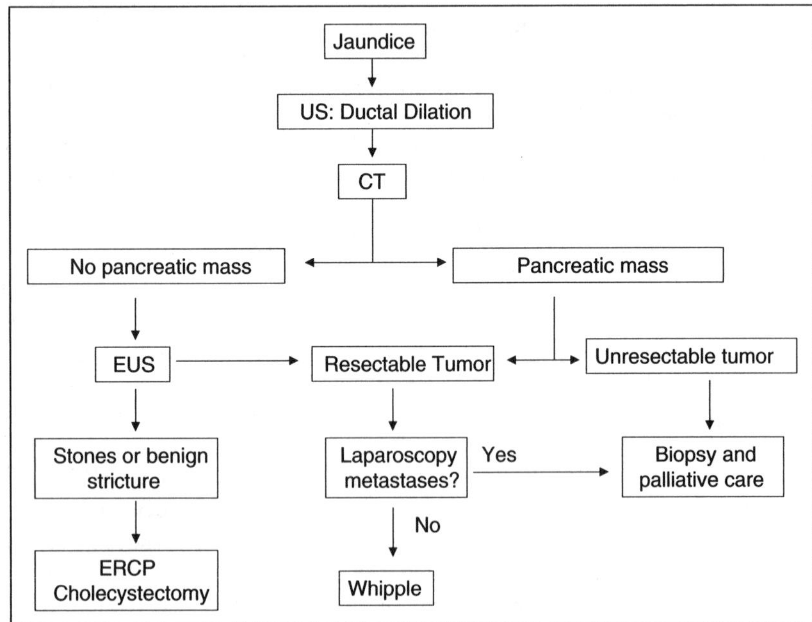

Algorithm 19.1.

cystadenoma should be considered either malignant (mucinous cystadenocarcinoma) or premalignant. These tumors should be removed: Whipple, distal pancreatectomy, or total pancreatectomy (if required to achieve negative margins).

What are intraductal papillary mucinous neoplasms (IPMN)?
IPMNs are a group of rare tumors that arise from either the main pancreatic duct or a side branch. Patients usually present with abdominal pain. Abdominal CT usually demonstrates a dilated pancreatic duct; ERCP frequently demonstrates a dilated ampulla and intraductal mucin or tumor. These tumors should be considered malignant or premalignant and surgery is the treatment of choice.

RECOMMENDED READINGS

Pedrazzoli S, DiCarlo V, Dionigi R, et al. Standard versus extended lymphadenectomy associated with pancreatoduodenectomy in the surgical treatment of adenocarcinoma of the head of the pancreas: a multicenter, prospective, randomized study. Lymphadenectomy Study Group. Ann Surg. 1998;228: 508–517.

Yeo CJ, Abrams RA, Grochow LB, et al. Pancreaticoduodenectomy for pancreatic adenocarcinoma: postoperative adjuvant chemoradiation improves survival. A prospective, single-institution experience. Ann Surg. 1997;225:621–633.

Gastrointestinal Tumor Study Group. Further evidence of effective adjuvant combined radiation and chemotherapy following curative resection of pancreatic cancer. Cancer. 1987;59:2006–2010.

Raut CP, Grau AM, Staerkel GA, et al. Diagnostic accuracy of endoscopic ultrasound-guided fine-needle aspiration in patients with presumed pancreatic cancer. J Gastrointest Surg. 2003;7:118–126.

Lillemoe KD, Cameron JL, Kaufman HS, et al. Chemical splanchnicectomy in patients with unresectable pancreatic cancer. A prospective randomized trial. Ann Surg. 1993;217:447–455.

Cameron JL, Pitt HA, Yeo CJ, et al. One hundred and forty-five consecutive pancreaticoduodenectomies without mortality. Ann Surg. 1993;217:430–435.

Fuhrman GM, Charnsangavej C, Abbruzzese JL, et al. Thin-section contrast-enhanced computed tomography accurately predicts the resectability of malignant pancreatic neoplasms. Am J Surg. 1994;167:104–111.

Mosca F, Giulianotti PC, Balestracci T, et al. Long-term survival in pancreatic cancer: pylorus-preserving versus Whipple pancreatoduodenectomy. Surgery. 1997;122:553–566.

Cusack JC Jr, Fuhrman GM, Lee JE, et al. Managing unsuspected tumor invasion of the superior mesenteric-portal venous confluence during pancreaticoduodenectomy. Am J Surg. 1994;168:352–354.

Compagno J, Oertel JE. Mucinous cystic neoplasms of the pancreas with overt and latent malignancy (cystadenocarcinoma and cystadenoma). A clinicopathologic study of 41 cases. Am J Clin Pathol. 1978;69:573–580.

Neoptolemos JP, Stocken DD, Friess H, et al. European Study Group for Pancreatic Cancer. A randomized trial of chemoradiotherapy and chemotherapy after resection of pancreatic cancer. N Engl J Med. 2004;350:1200–1210.

Silverman DT, Dunn JA, Hoover RN, et al. Cigarette smoking and pancreas cancer: a case-control study based on direct interviews. J Natl Cancer Inst. 1994;86:1510–1516.

Kulke MH. Recent developments in the pharmacological treatment of advanced pancreatic cancer. Expert Opin Investig Drugs. 2003;12:983–992.

CHAPTER

20

INGUINAL HERNIAS

Mohammad K. Jamal and Eric J. DeMaria

Mr. Jones is a 72-year-old man who presented to the emergency department with complaints of abdominal pain, nausea, vomiting, and poor appetite during the preceding 2 days. His last bowel movement was 3 days ago. His medical history was significant for recently diagnosed hypertension, myocardial infarction 4 years ago, and a stab wound to the abdomen. When questioned about the stab wound, he indicated that an exploratory laparotomy with small-bowel resection was performed. He smoked one to two packs of cigarettes a day for 50 years but quit just this year. His medications include occasional nifedipine, nitroglycerin, and occasional antibiotics for seasonal bronchitis.

A physical examination reveals the following vital signs: temperature, 37.2°C; blood pressure, 140/85 mm Hg; pulse, 100 beats per minute; and respiratory rate, 24 breaths per minute. The head and neck examination produces normal findings, the chest examination reveals mild wheezes in both lower lung fields, and cardiovascular examination shows mild tachycardia. Mr. Jones is moderately obese, and his abdomen is distended and diffusely tender. There is no guarding or rebound detected. A few high-pitched bowel sounds are discernible. The prostate gland is slightly enlarged and firm and has no irregularities. The stool examination reveals traces of occult blood. Pedal pulses are intact.

What is the working diagnosis on the basis of these findings?
Bowel obstruction is the likely diagnosis.

What further tests confirm the diagnosis?
Tests that can confirm this diagnosis are discussed in Chapter 10.

A radiographic series for diagnosis of acute abdominal pain is ordered along with blood tests. Radiographs of the abdomen reveal multiple

loops of small bowel with air and fluid levels; the colon is free of gas. The chest radiograph does not show free air under the diaphragm but does indicate some mild streaking in both lower lung fields. The following are results of laboratory tests: sodium, 145 mEq per L; chloride, 95 mEq per L; potassium, 3.2 mEq per L; bicarbonate, 17 mEq per L; hematocrit, 48%; amylase, 50 mIU per mL; and white blood cell count, 14,000 per mL with 10% bands. Urinalysis is unremarkable except for a specific gravity of 1.035. The electrocardiogram shows sinus tachycardia without signs of ischemia.

Mr. Jones is admitted to the surgical service. A nasogastric tube is inserted, and normal saline with potassium replacement is administered intravenously after the urine output is confirmed. He is allowed nothing by mouth. Repeat radiographs are ordered for the next day. The admitting diagnosis is small-bowel obstruction, most likely the result of adhesions arising from the previous abdominal exploration. During the admitting physical examination, a firm, painful swelling is noted in Mr. Jones's right groin, midway between the testicle and the symphysis pubis. The penis, testicles, and scrotum are otherwise normal, as is the skin over the mass.

What is the diagnosis?

The patient has an incarcerated inguinal hernia that is causing small-bowel obstruction. There is a possibility of strangulated bowel.

What are the most common causes of small-bowel obstruction?

In patients of all ages, the most common cause of small-bowel obstruction is adhesive bands, followed by groin hernias and small-bowel tumors. These three conditions account for 80% of bowel obstructions. Groin hernia is the leading cause in children, and diverticulitis and colorectal carcinoma are the common causes in the elderly. Incisional and groin hernias are easily detected during a physical examination and must be sought in all cases of bowel obstruction.

What are other significant history and laboratory findings?

Smoking and chronic bronchitis may predispose patients to development of groin hernias because of frequent coughing and straining. Smokers may actually develop a defect in collagen that increases the risk of both new and recurrent herniation. Occult blood in the stool may indicate a problem with the bowel mucosa. The occult blood may be explained by a tumor or ischemic necrosis from strangulation. Although in the past all patients with hernias were evaluated for large-bowel tumors because hernia was believed to result from increased intraabdominal pressure from the narrowed bowel lumen, the association between hernia and large-bowel tumors has never been proven.

What is a hernia?

A hernia is a defect in a wall through which contents normally contained by that wall may protrude. In a groin hernia, abdominal contents may protrude through a congenital defect. This is best exemplified by an indirect hernia, in which abdominal contents protrude through an enlarged internal ring and a patent processus vaginalis. Groin hernias may also develop over time because of thinning of the abdominal wall itself. For example, a direct inguinal hernia results when the transversalis fascia (the inguinal floor in the region of Hesselbach's triangle) has thinned, allowing abdominal contents to protrude. A hernia typically has three components: (a) neck, (b) body (or sac), and (c) contents.

What are some of the etiologic factors contributing to the development of groin hernias?

Groin hernias are generally related to congenital variations in the inguinal anatomy and the fatigue of the abdominal wall supporting structures over time, "the chronic stress and injury theory." Furthermore, the presence of a patent processus vaginalis has been considered the *sine qua non* of indirect inguinal hernias. Several conditions that increase intraabdominal pressure (e.g., obesity, ascites, constipation, chronic obstructive pulmonary disease, urinary retention, pregnancy) may contribute to the development of abdominal wall hernias.

What are the symptoms of a hernia?

A hernia is often asymptomatic and can be found only on physical examination when the patient is asked to strain or cough, actions that force abdominal contents through the defect. Patients who have large defects may have abdominal contents in the sac at all times but may have no symptoms. Some patients complain of a dull ache or intermittent pain and notice periodic bulging. Small defects can produce a constricting ring around protruding contents and when swelling increases, can become very painful and lead to ischemia. The hernia contents occasionally become necrotic.

What are some of the important anatomic landmarks to be considered when examining a patient with groin hernia?

The important anatomic landmarks in the groin can be remembered as boundaries of a canal and triangle.

The femoral canal is the site of occurrence of a *femoral hernia* and is bounded by the external iliac vein laterally, inguinal ligament superiorly, Cooper's ligament posteriorly, and iliopubic tract medially.

The Hesselbach triangle is the site of a *direct inguinal hernia* and is bounded by the inferior epigastric artery, inguinal ligament, and the rectus sheath. Direct inguinal hernias are typically located medial to whereas indirect inguinal hernias are lateral to the inferior epigastric vessels.

How should a patient with a hernia be examined?

The patient should be standing, if possible, facing the seated examiner. Often, the protruding bulge can be seen above or below the inguinal ligament, which passes between the anterior superior iliac spine and the symphysis pubis. The internal ring lies midway along this line. Femoral hernias are usually felt below this line, but a large bulge may appear to be above the line.

If the hernia is not readily apparent, the examiner should ask the patient to indicate where the bulge was. Palpation of the inguinal canal while the patient strains may reproduce the bulge. The physician can best produce a Valsalva effect by asking the patient to bear down as during a bowel movement. Using the index finger of the gloved hand, the physician should invaginate the upper scrotal skin and follow the testicular cord (vessels and vas deferens) up into the canal. Attention must be directed at palpating the inguinal floor and the external inguinal ring. Indirect hernias may be felt protruding through this ring, and a weak floor can sometimes be palpated lateral to this ring. When both protrusions are felt simultaneously, the hernia is called a *pantaloon type.*

Can the three types of hernia (direct, indirect, and femoral) be accurately differentiated during a physical examination?

Femoral hernias are differentiated from inguinal hernias on physical examination because the bulge of a femoral hernia is below the inguinal ligament and medial to the femoral pulsation. However, reliable differentiation between a direct and an indirect inguinal hernia can be done only at surgery because the distinction is based on the relation of the epigastric vessels to the defect. Direct hernias lie medial to these vessels, whereas indirect hernias originate lateral to the vessels. The location of the hernia in relation to the epigastric vessels and the size of the opening are important determinants of the type of repair needed and the propensity for recurrence.

The size of the hernia orifice is classified as follows

Grade I: less than 1.5 cm
Grade II: 1.5 to 3 cm
Grade III: more than 3 cm

The average size of the examining fingertip is approximately 1.5 cm.

Where are the most common sites of hernias?

Indirect inguinal hernias are the most common type of abdominal hernias in both genders and account for 75% of all cases. Men are five times more likely to develop an indirect inguinal hernia. These are more prone to incarcerate and strangulate than direct hernias (Fig. 20.1).

Direct inguinal hernias are the second most common abdominal wall hernias and are produced by a weakness in the floor of the inguinal canal.

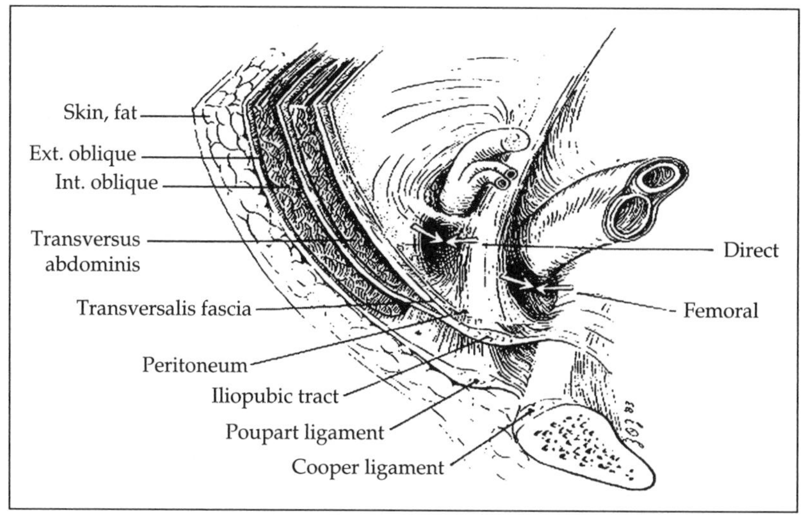

Figure 20.1. Muscular support of the abdominal wall in relation to the development of direct, indirect, and femoral hernia. (From Nyhus LM. lliopubic tract repair of inguinal and femoral hernia: the posterior (pre-peritoneal) approach. In Nyhus LM, Baker RJ, eds. Mastery of Surgery. 2nd ed. Boston, Mass: Little, Brown and Company; 1992:1853, with permission.)

These are usually seen in older, active patients and generally do not have a tight neck with less chances of incarceration. Most recurrent inguinal hernias are of the direct type.

Femoral hernias, although less common than inguinal hernias, tend to be more common in women (33% of all groin hernias). These are generally difficult to diagnose and can be detected as a bulge in the lower groin or upper medial thigh. These may sometimes require a computed tomography scan or ultrasound for diagnosis.

A **sliding hernia** is an advanced indirect inguinal hernia in which a portion of the posterior wall is made up of the urinary bladder, ovary, cecum, or sigmoid colon.

Umbilical hernias are ventral, occurring in the anterior abdominal wall, excluding the groin.

Epigastric hernias occur in the midline of the abdomen, above the umbilicus.

Spigelian hernias, which are unusual, occur along the lateral border of the rectus muscle below the umbilicus, at its junction with the linea semilunaris.

Other less frequent types include lumbar, obturator, sciatic, congenital diaphragmatic, incisional, and hiatal hernias, and gastroschisis and omphaloceles.

What is an incarcerated hernia?

A hernia is considered incarcerated or irreducible when the sac contents cannot be pushed back through the hernia ring into the cavity from which it protruded. Strangulation occurs when the incarcerated contents lose their blood supply and tissue necrosis sets in. A hernia is considered reducible if its contents can be pushed back into the abdominal cavity, in which case there is no risk of strangulation.

What is a Richter's hernia?

A Richter's hernia typically has less than the full circumference of the bowel wall becoming entrapped, hence usually presenting without bowel obstruction.

Which intraabdominal organ is incarcerated most frequently within the inguinal canal?

The omentum is the most frequently incarcerated structure. The large or small bowel or a woman's ovary may also be involved. Herniation of ovaries is especially common in newborn girls. In rare cases, the appendix protrudes into the inguinal canal, which leads to obstruction of the appendix and acute appendicitis within the hernia sac. Treatment consists of appendectomy and hernia repair. In a sliding hernia, the bowel wall or bladder forms one wall of the hernia. In a Littre hernia involving the Meckel's diverticulum, strangulation usually occurs early without evidence of bowel obstruction. Treatment involves Meckel's diverticulectomy and herniorrhaphy.

What are the complications of incarceration?

Incarceration may lead to swelling of the sac contents against a tight hernia ring. A loop of bowel that has been incarcerated can present as an acute bowel obstruction. Strangulation occurs when a reduction in blood flow to the incarcerated contents leads to tissue ischemia and ultimately to necrosis. A strangulated bowel may rupture and cause peritonitis, sepsis, and even death.

Are small hernias less likely to incarcerate than large ones?

Contents that have herniated through a small ring are more prone to constriction, swelling, and strangulation than if the ring is large.

When should an incarcerated hernia be repaired?

An incarcerated hernia is a surgical emergency and should be repaired as soon as the diagnosis is made. Delaying surgery can result in strangulation, tissue necrosis, infection, and sepsis. These complications are associated with high morbidity and mortality. Tissue necrosis not only makes hernia repair more difficult because of swelling but also is associated with higher rates of infection and recurrence. In addition, ischemic tissue may preclude the use of prosthetic materials to repair the hernia defect, which can further increase the recurrence rate.

When should a reducible hernia be repaired?

All hernias are susceptible to incarceration and strangulation and should therefore be repaired when discovered. Hernias do not disappear and almost always enlarge over time. The rates of complications and recurrence are higher after surgical repair of incarcerated or strangulated hernias than after elective repair.

Mr. Jones is taken to the operating room for exploration of the groin, reduction of the hernia, and repair of the defect. At surgery, a loop of small bowel is found in a large indirect hernia sac. The bowel is thickened and hyperemic, but it softens and assumes its normal color when the constricting ring is cut.

Which body layers must be traversed for entry into the inguinal canal and the peritoneal cavity?

The skin, subcutaneous tissue, Scarpa's fascia, external oblique fascia (which makes up the external inguinal ring), and external oblique aponeurosis (which is contiguous with the inguinal ligament) are anatomic layers that must be crossed to enter the inguinal canal. To gain entry to the abdominal cavity the internal oblique muscle, transversus abdominis muscle, transversalis fascia, properitoneal fat, and finally the peritoneum must be traversed. The spermatic cord lies over the transversalis fascia, beneath the external oblique aponeurosis. The cord enters the abdomen laterally through the transversalis fascia (internal ring), forming the floor of the inguinal canal.

What are the important structures that constitute the spermatic cord?

The structures can be easily remembered as part of three broad groups: vessels, nerves, and lymphatics. The vessels include the testicular and cremasteric artery, the artery of the ductus deferens, and the pampiniform venous plexus. The nerves include the sympathetic nerve fibers on arteries, the sympathetic and parasympathetic nerve fibers on the ductus deferens, and the genital branch of the genitofemoral nerve supplying the cremaster muscle. Lymphatic vessels draining the testis and closely associated structures empty into lumbar lymph nodes. The ilio-inguinal nerve lies outside the spermatic cord and must be isolated and preserved during inguinal herniorrhaphy.

What are the surgical options if the bowel is strangulated and nonviable?

The strangulated loop of bowel must be resected if it appears nonviable. A primary anastomosis can be performed for small-bowel involvement, and both resection and anastomosis can be carried out through the original incision. If the colon is to be resected, a proximal diverting colostomy must be performed. These procedures require a separate incision, and the floor of the inguinal canal may have to be opened to obtain proper exposure.

What is the intraoperative procedure if the hernia's contents cannot be reduced?

The hernia opening is made larger by incising the floor of the inguinal canal through the constricting internal ring.

Mr. Jones's hernia is reduced with high ligation of the hernia sac. When palpated through the sac before closure, the floor of the inguinal canal feels lax, and there is a grade II opening (1.5 to 3 cm).

How can a direct hernia defect such as Mr. Jones's be repaired?

Several options are available for repair of a defect in the floor of the inguinal canal. Mr. Jones has a pantaloon hernia; that is, his hernia has both direct and indirect components. The direct portion is defined by the lax fascia found medial to the epigastric vessels, whereas the indirect component is indicated by the ligated sac, which is lateral to the epigastric vessels. Tension-free repair is the guiding principle in any hernia operation. Because of the dual nature of Mr. Jones's hernia, an appropriate repair can include a mesh plug inserted into the indirect defect and an onlay mesh that covers the inguinal floor for repair of the direct defect. This mesh can be sutured circumferentially and without tension. Mesh such as Marlex sticks to the tissues. Ultimately, tissue grows into the patch and permanently secures it in place. Most surgeons sew at least one edge of the mesh to the inguinal ligament or to the *iliopubic tract,* the fascia that appears as a yellow layer of tissue lying just below and medially to the inguinal ligament. Some surgeons also tack the mesh to the aponeurotic layer just under the external oblique. This type of repair, in which a mesh onlay is used, is known as *Lichtenstein repair* (Fig. 20.2).

Which other procedures can be used to repair hernias?

Shouldice repair, in which the patient's own tissues are used. The transversalis fascia is opened from the pubic bone into the internal ring; any thinned redundant tissue (the direct hernia) is removed; and the tissues are sewn, imbricating in four layers, to form a new floor for the inguinal canal.

McVay repair, in which the transversalis fascia and conjoint tendon are used. The tendon is sewn to the deeper Cooper's ligament medially, with a transition area over the femoral vessels as the repair progresses laterally onto the inguinal ligament. Interrupted sutures are used in the McVay repair, and care must be taken not to injure the femoral vein or artery. This procedure can also be used to close the femoral canal for treatment of femoral hernias.

Bassini repair, in which the transversalis fascia and conjoint tendon are used as in the McVay procedure, but sewn to Poupart's ligament (inguinal ligament) from the pubic tubercle medially to the internal ring laterally.

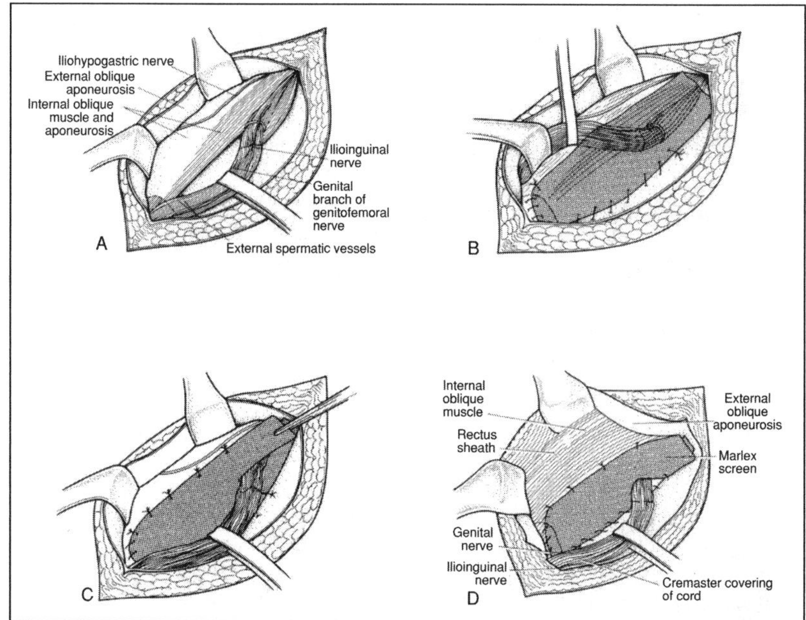

Figure 20.2. Lichtenstein tension-free repair. **A:** Spermatic cord with its cremasteric covering, inguinal nerve, external spermatic vessels, and genital nerve is raised and the cremasteric fibers are cut transversely or longitudinally at the level of the internal ring. **B:** Spermatic cord is placed in between the two tails of the mesh. **C:** Crossing of the two tails. **D:** The lower edges of the two tails are sutured to the inguinal ligament for creation of a new internal ring made of mesh. In Fischer JE, Baker RJ, eds. Mastery of Surgery. 4th ed. Philadelphia, Pa: Lippincott, Williams & Wilkins; 2001:1970–1972, with permission.)

If a bowel resection with or without an anastomosis is required, avoid repair with a foreign body mesh plug or patch. Instead, use a Shouldice, McVay, or Bassini repair. Unlike repairs that use mesh plugs or patches, hernia repairs performed with only native tissue are more likely to develop tension, hence recurrence.

Can hernias be repaired laparoscopically?

Although some surgeons repair groin hernias exclusively with laparoscopic techniques, Mr. Jones's situation is not one in which the laparoscope would be an advantage. Laparoscopic herniorrhaphy is advantageous for uncomplicated recurrent hernia or bilateral hernias. Laparoscopic herniorrhaphy involves two techniques both aimed at properitoneal repair of the hernia: TEPP (totally extra

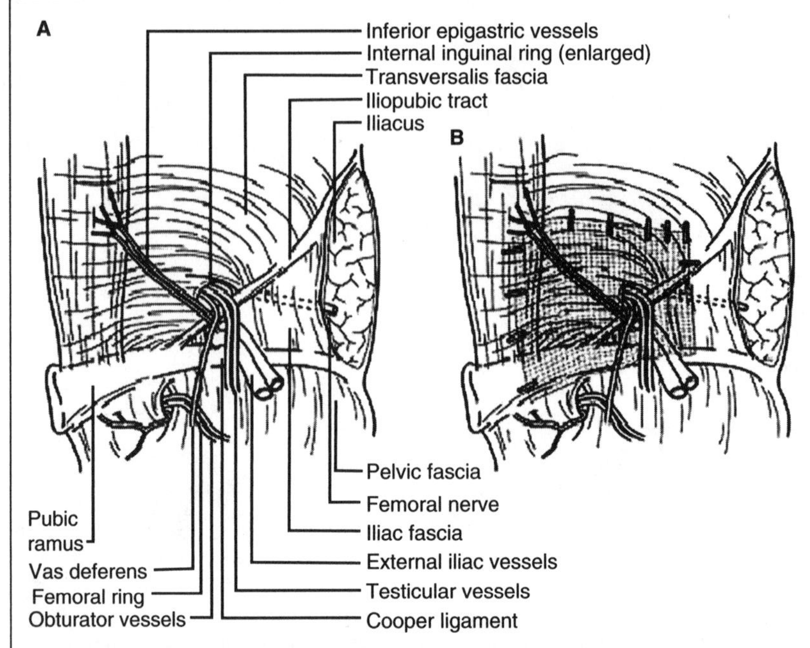

Figure 20.3. Laparoscopic herniorrhaphy: mesh placement in a TEPP repair. **A:** Important anatomical landmarks including the inferior epigastric vessels, spermatic cord, and the iliac vessels. **B:** Final position of the mesh after TEPP repair. In Eubanks WS. Hernias, Townsend C: Sabiston's Textbook of Surgery. 16th ed. Philadelphia, Pa: WB Saunders; 2001, with permission.)

pre-peritoneal) and TAPP (transabdominal pre-peritoneal). Both techniques use a mesh over the deep inguinal ring and the floor of the canal in the properitoneal position (Fig 20.3).

Should antibiotics be given to patients undergoing hernia repair?

High infection rates are associated with the following:

- Patient more than 70 years old
- Use of a drain
- Repair of incarcerated hernia
- Repair of recurrent hernia
- Surgery lasting longer than 90 minutes

Use of a foreign body such as mesh in a repair is believed to increase the risk of infection because significantly fewer bacteria can cause infection when a foreign body is present. Parenteral antibiotics have no advantage unless they are administered preoperatively, and, if used, they should target only skin organisms. With a patient such as Mr. Jones, parenteral antibiotics are necessary because he is over age 70, he has incarcerated bowel in the hernia, and mesh is used for the repair.

Mr. Jones has an uncomplicated hernia repair. No bowel is resected, and a mesh plug with onlay patch is used to repair the defects. His small-bowel obstruction rapidly resolves, and he is eating on the third postoperative day.

What is the most serious postoperative complication of hernia repair?

The use of a foreign body in the wound makes infection a serious potential complication. Infection prolongs treatment and may require removal of the mesh. Other complications after an inguinal hernia repair include hematomas, hydroceles, dysejaculation, testicular atrophy, and neuralgias from nerve entrapment.

How is an infection in a groin incision treated?

The wound must be opened and antibiotics administered intravenously if mesh was used and not initially removed. Otherwise, simple drainage of the infection is the most important treatment. After the wound is opened, care includes removing necrotic tissue, providing a moist, occlusive wound environment, and allowing secondary closure (granulation and wound contraction). Use of a calcium alginate wound packing after removal of necrotic tissue is a good way to allow moist wound healing with dressing changes daily. The alginate absorbs wound exudate and prevents wound maceration while providing a moist healing environment. After it is hydrated, the alginate dressing can easily be removed because it does not adhere to tissue.

What is the recurrence rate after inguinal herniorrhaphy, and what are the risk factors?

Recurrences within 2 to 3 years of operation are the result of poor technique. Examples of technical error include inadequate dissection of an indirect sac, poor choice of suture (e.g., using braided absorbable suture), excessive tissue tension in the repair, and infection. Late recurrences are usually caused by collagen or fascial degradation, producing a new hernia. This type of recurrence is found around an old hernia in patients in whom a localized herniorrhaphy was used to repair a direct floor defect. Recurrence rates after the classic Shouldice herniorrhaphy have been reported to be less than 1% when the surgery was performed by experienced surgeons. The McVay (Cooper's ligament) repair is reported to have a recurrence rate of 3.5%, whereas the Bassini repair has a recurrence rate of 5%. Comparable recurrence rates are claimed with the mesh plug onlay techniques. Advocates of the tension-free mesh technique report low recurrence rates even in inexperienced hands, generally as low as 0.5%.

A week after his operation, Mr. Jones is examined and is found to have a swollen, painful right scrotum, with the testicle high in the scrotal sac. His hernia incision has healed and is not painful or swollen.

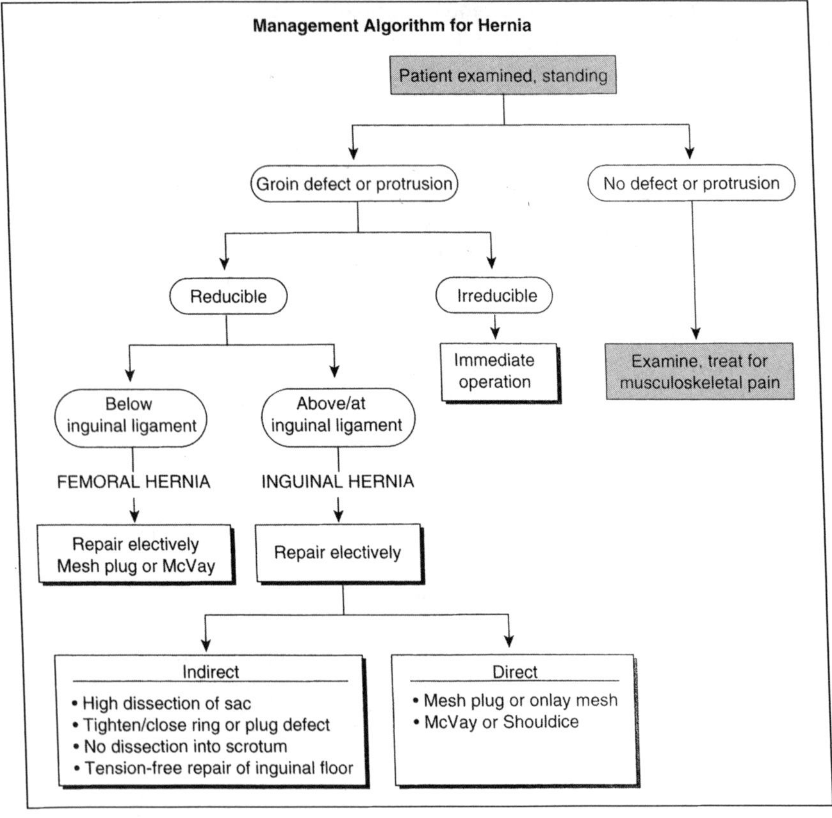

Algorithm 20.1.

What is the problem and how can it be treated?

Mr. Jones has ischemic orchitis, a condition that may ultimately result in testicular atrophy. Ischemic orchitis can be prevented by limiting the dissection around the spermatic cord. Limited dissection prevents injury to the delicate testicular veins and the pampiniform plexus. Therapy consists of symptomatic care. Analgesics and anti-inflammatory medications can alleviate the symptoms.

RECOMMENDED READINGS

Nyhus LM, Condon RE, eds. Hernia. 4th ed. Philadelphia, PA: JB Lippincott Co; 1995.

Soper NJ, Bendavid R, Arregui ME, eds. Problems in General Surgery: Problems in the Management of Inguinal Hernias. Part 1, vol 12, no. 1. Philadelphia, Pa: Lippincott–Raven Publishers; 1995.

Soper NJ, Bendavid R, Arregui ME, eds. Problems in General Surgery: Problems in the

Management of Inguinal Hernias. Part 2, vol 12, no. 2. Philadelphia, Pa: Lippincott-Raven Publishers; 1995.

Lichtenstein IL, Shulman AG, Amid PK, et al. The tension-free hernioplasty. Am J Surg. 1989;157:188–193.

Eubanks WS. Hernias. In: Townsend C. Sabiston's Textbook of Surgery. 16th ed. Philadelphia, Pa: WB Saunders; 2001.

Nyhus LM, Baker RJ. Surgery of Hernia, Mastery of Surgery. 4th ed. Philadelphia, Pa: Lippincott Williams & Wilkins; 2001.

Amid PK, Shulman AG, Lichtenstein IL. Critical scrutiny of the open "tension free" hernioplasty. Am J Surg. 1993;165:369–375.

Amid PK, Shulman AG, Lichtenstein IL. Open, tension-free repair of inguinal hernias: the Lichtenstein technique. Eur J Surg. 1996;162:447–453.

Contemporary Surgery. Symposium: Operative Repair of Inguinal Hernias. Part 1. Torrance, CA: Bobit; 1997:387–397.

Contemporary Surgery. Symposium: Operative Repair of Inguinal Hernia. Part 2. Torrance, CA: Bobit Publishing, 1998:61–72.

CHAPTER

21

CAROTID ARTERY DISEASE

Gregory K. Albaugh and Mark M. Levy

Mr. Wilson was referred after his primary care physician detected a bruit in his left neck on routine physical examination. He is 64 years old and smoked 1 pack of cigarettes daily until 17 years ago, when he quit smoking. He occasionally drinks alcohol. He has hypertension and hypertriglyceridemia. He takes atenolol 50 mg once a day and a statin agent for his cholesterol.

What is a bruit and what causes it?

A bruit is an abnormal sound auscultated over a vessel; it is typically rumbling in character. The bruit represents noise generated from turbulent blood flow within the vessel. Normally, blood flows through a vessel in laminar fashion. When there are luminal irregularities in the vessel, the blood flow becomes turbulent, generating audible sound energy referred to as a *bruit*. If the turbulence becomes more severe, it generates a palpable mechanical disturbance referred to as a *thrill*.

What is the chance that this bruit is associated with a high-grade carotid artery stenosis?

The chance that a bruit reflects significant stenosis is not high. Even with cerebrovascular symptoms, a bruit alone is insufficient to predict high-grade stenosis (1). Transmitted heart sounds may be auscultated in the neck. Other turbulent flow heard in the neck may be from the external carotid artery or, more rarely, from the thyroid in some cases of hyperthyroidism. It remains important to listen for carotid bruits nevertheless, because they may be indicative of carotid stenosis and guide further diagnostic workup. Both the presence of a bruit and advancing age have been demonstrated to be predictive factors for eventual transient ischemic attacks (TIAs) and cerebrovascular accidents (CVAs). Bruits may be most predictive for TIA or CVA in older diabetic female patients (2).

What symptoms would you ask about to determine if Mr. Wilson is having symptoms associated with his carotid disease?

Classic symptoms of carotid disease are those associated with TIAs or CVAs, namely focal sided motor or sensory loss, or aphasia. In addition, *amaurosis fugax*, meaning temporary monocular blindness and frequently described as a window-shade drawing down over one eye, is a characteristic symptom associated with embolization from a carotid lesion to the ophthalmic artery. In contrast to these localizing symptoms, more global nonlateralizing symptoms such as headache, presyncope, and confusion are not characteristically associated with carotid disease.

What is a TIA?

TIA: a reversible neurologic deficit lasting fewer than 24 hours. TIAs are frequently the consequence of emboli from the extracranial carotid system or the heart.

Acute CVA: a neurologic deficit that lasts longer than 24 hours

RIND (reversible ischemic neurologic deficit): a syndrome lasting between 24 and 72 hours. This term has fallen out of favor due to evidence that, although the neurologic deficit improves, areas of infarction can be demonstrated.

Crescendo TIAs: a syndrome of serial TIAs occurring over days to weeks, representing an ominous prodrome to frank stroke

Which diagnostic test should be ordered to evaluate the bruit?

Duplex ultrasound (US) is the primary diagnostic modality used to evaluate carotid stenosis. The duplex scan is composed of two components.

The first component is the two-dimensional B-mode black and white image that represents a cross-sectional shadow of the body part examined. The B-mode image can show the vessel calcification and homogeneity compared with the heterogeneity of the carotid plaque. In addition, the B-mode can be used to offer a preliminary estimate of the degree of stenosis observed in the carotid bulb or proximal internal carotid artery.

The second component of the duplex examination is the Doppler evaluation of blood flow traversing through the carotid artery itself. According to the Doppler frequency shift principal, sound energy of a given emitted frequency is reflected off of moving red cells and then received back on an US probe. By measuring differences between emitted and received sound frequencies and taking into account angles of insonation, the speed of blood traversing through a particular carotid segment may be accurately estimated. These flow velocities then can be correlated to either normal vessel diameters or vessel stenosis; the latter is generally associated with remarkable increases in associated blood velocity.

What other tests are available to study the carotid arteries?
Magnetic resonance arteriography (MRA) is increasingly performed to demonstrate the arterial anatomy of the carotid system. As a noninvasive study, like duplex, it offers negligible risk to the patient. Unlike carotid duplex examinations, however, its visual window includes the innominate artery and intrathoracic carotid segments. It also visualizes the carotid artery cephalad to the midcervical segment most easily visualized by duplex examination. Magnetic resonance imaging may depict the intracranial arteries including the circle of Willis, and standard tomographic imaging can rule out aneurysm or another mass lesion. Although many vascular surgeons do not consider MRA to be accurate enough as the sole evaluation modality on which to base surgery, many use it together with duplex US, when these studies offer consistent results.

Although carotid duplex US may best demonstrate carotid arterial flow physiology, contrast angiography, an invasive procedure, remains the gold standard in characterizing the corresponding anatomy. Contrast arteriography provides thorough evaluation not only of the midcervical carotid artery (like the duplex examination provides) but also of the aortic arch, the innominate artery, the intrathoracic carotid artery, the intracranial carotid, and the cerebral circulation itself. Conventional contrast arteriography has an associated risk of stroke and femoral access complications; therefore, it is not always performed before endarterectomy, particularly in facilities where the noninvasive imaging has a documented accuracy.

Mr. Wilson has a history of smoking, hypertension, and hypertriglyceridemia. What medications would be potentially helpful in lowering his risk of stroke or myocardial infarction (MI)?
Among the primary risk factors for CVA, hypertension, cigarette smoking, diabetes, and hypercholesterolemia are four that can potentially be modified with lifestyle or medical management. Mr. Wilson, although no longer smoking, has hypertension and hyperlipidemia. The use of beta-blockers and diuretics to treat hypertension has been shown to decrease the risk of stroke and myocardial events (3). In addition to a beta-blocker, this patient is also appropriately treated with a statin agent. Patients treated with statin agents demonstrated a 46% reduction in CVA risk in a meta analysis (4).

Due to these factors, Mr. Wilson is at increased risk for CVA and MI. Antiplatelet therapy has been shown to decrease adverse outcomes such as CVA and MI (5,6). Antiplatelet therapy consists of many different medications. The most commonly used agent is aspirin. Lipid-lowering agents such as lovastatin have shown benefit in controlling progression of disease (7). Control with beta-blockers decreases cardiac work and blood pressure. Angiotensin-converting enzyme inhibitors have also shown reduction in CVA, MI, and major cerebrovascular events in these patients (8). Most survival benefits from medical therapy in these patients are related to the reduced risk of cardiac ischemic events and cerebrovascular events.

Because Mr. Wilson's carotid stenosis is presently considered asymptomatic, what is an accepted threshold at which to intervene beyond best medical management?

If the duplex scan demonstrate 80% to 99% stenosis and the individual surgeon's operative stroke and death rates are low, then the asymptomatic patient may be offered carotid endarterectomy (CEA). Patients who present with greater than 60% stenosis on contrast arteriography were shown to suffer fewer fatal and nonfatal strokes over a 5-year period if CEA was performed according to the Asymptomatic Carotid Atherosclerosis Study (ACAS) trial (9).

It is generally accepted that a lesion that, on duplex US, is shown to be 80% to 99% stenotic will be at least 60% stenotic on contrast angiography. Lesions that fall short of these guidelines are commonly treated more conservatively with serial follow-up duplex US and antiplatelet therapy. (See Algorithm 21.1)

What is the acceptable upper limit of morbidity and mortality when performing this operation?

The American Heart Association Stroke Council's published acceptable upper limit of morbidity and mortality in asymptomatic patients undergoing CEA is 3%. If the indication for CEA is TIA, the operative morbidity and mortality upper limit is 5%, and if the indication is prior CVA the limit is 7% (10). Those institutions involved in the ACAS trial had an aggregate operative morbidity and mortality rate of 1.5%.

Mr. Stevens presents to the emergency department with right arm weakness that lasted approximately 2 hours and is now starting to resolve. He also has a history of hypertension and had a small MI 4 years ago. He is 68 years old and is a current 1 pack per day smoker.

What is Mr. Stevens' diagnosis?

In the scenario presented, Mr. Stevens has had a TIA. A TIA is a temporary focal neurologic deficit that lasts fewer than 24 hours. TIAs occur most commonly as a consequence of carotid disease; however, they can occur as emboli from a cardiac source. Focal emboli to the ophthalmic artery (the first intracranial branch of the internal carotid artery) cause a transient loss of vision or blurring of vision in the ipsilateral eye, which is termed *amaurosis fugax*.

What should be the initial study performed in the emergency department?

When patients present to the emergency department with a neurologic deficit, a computed tomographic (CT) scan of the head is done to rule out an intracranial hemorrhage or mass. Due to the radiographic appearance of acute extravascular blood in the head, a noncontrast study should be done.

What pharmacologic therapy should be initiated if the study is negative?
Depending on the duration of the symptoms, patients with acute CVAs may be candidates for thrombolytic therapy. If the duration of symptoms is less than 3 hours, a time-sensitive process is initiated, including head CT, to rule out an intracranial hemorrhage. Then the patient may be given a dose of the thrombolytic of choice.

There is evidence against using heparin infusion in patients who are having embolic TIAs while experiencing atrial fibrillation. Adding heparin is also contraindicated if there is evidence of hemorrhagic stroke. If the stroke involves more than 30% of the hemisphere, then heparinization should be delayed for 5 to 14 days. In three randomized trials, heparin failed to show any benefit in outcome of ischemic stroke. Aspirin, however, has shown some benefit in reducing embolic events in patients who present with embolic stroke (11).

Which imaging modality is appropriate for preoperative workup?
In most patients, the modality used for both screening and diagnosis is carotid duplex US. This modality can depict plaque morphology as described earlier. By comparing duplex scanning velocities with angiographic findings, institutions are better able to standardize their procedures, thus allowing more accurate estimation of carotid stenosis within a specific institution.

Why are physicians using less angiography than they used to for patients with carotid disease?
The North American Symptomatic Carotid Endarterectomy Trial (NASCET) and the ACAS trials' morbidity for the surgery group included a 1.2% incidence of CVA caused by the neuroarteriogram alone. With improvement of duplex scanning technology and institutional correlation of duplex data and angiogram, velocity-based estimates of stenosis are generated. Duplex is noninvasive, is relatively inexpensive, requires no radiation exposure, adds no additional risk of CVA, and is reproducible. Many vascular surgeons will perform CEA based on duplex data alone.

Mr. Stevens has had a TIA. Under what circumstances should he be offered a CEA?
If the patient has US evidence of stenosis greater than 70% and either TIA or minor ipsilateral CVA, then by following the NASCET recommendations, this patient should undergo CEA. This will decrease the risk of fatal and nonfatal stroke from 24% to 7% over an 18-month period. Data supporting endarterectomy for symptomatic moderate stenoses (50% to 69%) are less powerful, albeit

statistically significant (12). For lesions that are symptomatic and 30% to 49% stenotic, endarterectomy has not demonstrated any benefit over best medical management (13).

Mr. Stevens goes to the operating room to have a left CEA under general anesthesia. An incision is made over the anterior aspect of the sternocleidomastoid (SCM) muscle and the platysma muscle is divided. The SCM is reflected laterally to expose the carotid sheath.

What structures are inside the carotid sheath?
The structures in the carotid sheath are the carotid artery, the internal jugular vein, and the vagus nerve (CNX). Injury to the vagus nerve can cause hoarseness because this is the origin of the recurrent laryngeal nerve on that side. The patient will have a paralyzed vocal cord on the ipsilateral side if this nerve is injured.

What structures drape over the bifurcation of the carotid artery?
Superficially, the facial vein drapes across the bifurcation and is a good landmark to find it. Another structure near the bifurcation is the hypoglossal nerve (CNXII). Injury to this nerve by division or by traction will cause ipsilateral deviation of the tongue that may be permanent or temporary. This will lead to tongue dysfunction and will interfere with speaking and chewing. The ansa hypoglossal is a branch of the hypoglossal nerve, which innervates the strap muscles of the neck. Medial branches can be divided to allow exposure with little sequela.

What are the extracranial branches of the internal carotid artery?
This is a trick question. There are no extracranial branches of the internal carotid artery. The first branch of the internal carotid artery is the ophthalmic artery.

What carotid branches are dissected out during an endarterectomy?
The common carotid artery is usually dissected out first. This provides the proximal control important in vascular surgery. The distal vessels routinely isolated are the internal carotid, external carotid, and superior thyroid artery.

Why is heparin given?
Heparin is given to avoid thrombus formation in the artery when the artery is clamped.

What is the sequence in which the clamps are placed on the arteries?
The internal carotid is clamped first. This is done to avoid embolization from the common carotid when clamping. The other arteries are clamped next. When unclamping, the internal carotid is unclamped last to allow any debris from the endarterectomy to be flushed up the external carotid artery.

What nerves can be injured?

The most common nerve injured is the vagus nerve. This manifests as hoarseness, which usually is self-limiting. The most dramatic and second most common nerve injury is to the hypoglossal nerve. Tongue deviation to the ipsilateral nerve is dramatic and usually self-limiting. Traction injuries to the marginal mandibular branch of the facial nerve can lead to an ipsilateral lip droop on the side of the surgery.

What is performed during a standard CEA?

After clamping the carotid vessels above and below the bifurcation stenosis, the vessel is opened. The surgeon observes some separation of the vessel wall like the layers of an onion. An endarterectomy plane is created using a spatula-type instrument called an *elevator.* The plaque will shell out from the artery. The proximal end is divided with scissors. The plaque is lifted toward the head and pulled out of the superior thyroid and external carotid. The critical step is allowing the distal end of the internal carotid plaque to taper down before it detaches. Leaving a flap at the distal endpoint is the biggest concern at this time. Various steps are taken to either avoid this or repair it. All the adherent debris is removed and the vessel is washed multiple times to ensure a clean surface. Depending on surgeon preference, the vessel will be closed with or without a patch. The rationale for a patch is to decrease the incidence of restenosis after CEA.

What is a shunt and why is it used?

A shunt is a plastic tube that allows the surgeon to maintain blood flow to the brain while the vessel is opened. There are multiple types of shunts and surgeons use whichever one they are most comfortable with. There are several different approaches to shunt use. Some vascular surgeons routinely use shunts; others use them selectively based on varied criteria (electroencephalogram changes, neurologic changes under local anesthesia, stump pressure measurements), whereas others never use shunts. Depending on the individual patient, anesthesia modality used, special monitoring available, and surgeon preference, a shunt may be placed to maintain blood flow as described earlier.

What are the most common postoperative complications of CEA?

The most dramatic and severe complication of CEA is CVA. The individual surgeon's stroke rate in normal-risk patients undergoing CEA should be less than 3%. Many vascular surgeons have an operative stroke rate of less than 1%. The stroke and death rate of CEA is somewhat higher in the 30-day postoperative period. Most of the deaths are due to underlying cardiac disease that most of these patients have concurrently. Some extremely high-risk patients have a 7% to 12% stroke and death rate in some studies. More common complications include cranial nerve injury and hematoma. A large hematoma may cause airway obstruction from extrinsic compression on the trachea. If such postoperative airway obstruction occurs, opening the incision can be lifesaving.

Does carotid stenosis recur?

Yes, the restenosis rate after CEA ranges from 1% to 21% in long-term follow-up. This is more common in women with small arteries (14,15). Some of this stenosis may be avoided by closing the carotid artery with a patch. Despite routine use of patch angioplasty, some restenosis will occur. The lesions that form are usually from neointimal hyperplasia and have a low incidence of embolization. There can, however, be recurrence of atherosclerosis that can progress to critical stenosis. In this case, a "re-do" CEA can be done, but the incidence of nerve injury is increased and the upper limit of acceptable operative morbidity and mortality with this operation is 10%.

Mrs. Jones is a 78-year-old woman who presents to your clinic for CEA. She had a previous MI, which left her with an ejection fraction of 25%. She is still smoking and has been hospitalized with congestive heart failure twice this year. Her duplex US shows a 90% carotid artery stenosis bilaterally, and she had an episode of right hand weakness and aphasia. The last time she had general anesthesia she developed ventilator-dependent respiratory failure. She shows you the healing tracheostomy scar on the midline neck.

With 90% stenosis bilaterally, which artery is symptomatic and which carotid lesion would you address first?

The patient describes aphasia and right arm paresthesia. The brain centers that control speech (e.g., Broca's area) are usually located in the left hemisphere, particularly in right-handed patients. The right-sided body weakness also represents a left cerebral hemispheric symptom, which again indicates that the left carotid lesion is, in fact, symptomatic. With bilateral disease of the internal carotid arteries, the symptomatic or left carotid stenosis in this patient should be addressed first.

Beyond best medical management, is CEA the only treatment for carotid stenosis?

No. There has been recent progress with carotid angioplasty and stenting (CAS). Although earlier series with CAS demonstrated significant cerebrovascular morbidity (16), technological device-related improvements continue. The procedure involves carefully passing a wire and then an angioplasty balloon across the carotid stenosis under fluoroscopic guidance. The balloon is then inflated to dilate the stenotic plaque. In most instances, the stenotic lesion is stented open with a variety of investigational devices. During the angioplasty procedure, fractured plaque

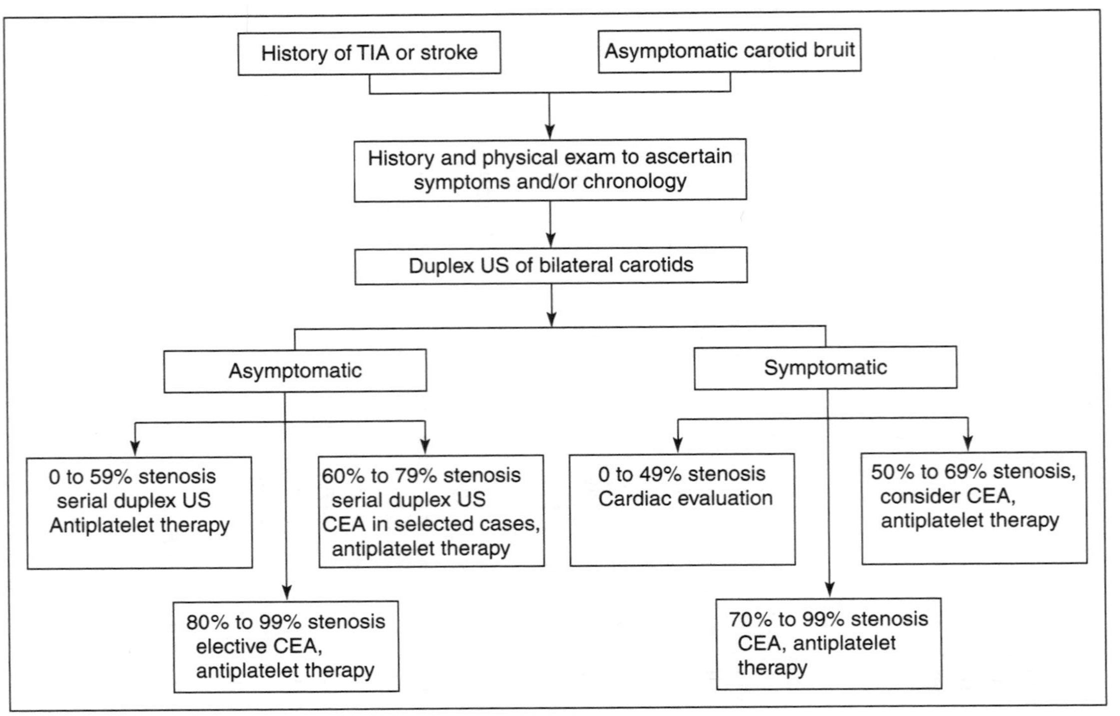

Algorithm 21.1.

segments may embolize to the brain. In addition, in the process of plaque fracture, subendothelial collagen is exposed. Circulating platelets may potentially attach here and aggregate in the carotid artery. Subsequent vessel thrombosis or distal brain embolization are the proposed mechanisms for TIA or CVA following CAS.

Are there any new advancements in CAS that may decrease its morbidity?

Yes, newer technology has made this procedure potentially safer. Small devices placed distal to the carotid lesion have been introduced. These devices are either occlusion balloons or umbrella-like filters and are employed to catch the debris created by carotid angioplasty. The early results are promising for those patients who are at high risk for CEA but who have significant carotid disease (17).

Are there any instances in which CAS is preferred?

CAS may be most useful in patients who experience restenosis after CEA and patients who have carotid stenosis after receiving radiation therapy following radical neck dissection for head and neck malignancy. In addition, CAS is potentially helpful in treating patients with fibromuscular dysplasia. The lesions in these patients are located in the media of the artery. Traditionally, these lesions were dilated with progressively larger dilators through a carotid arteriotomy. These lesions now can be dilated by using newer endovascular techniques, thus avoiding a formal operation.

REFERENCES

1. Sauve JS, Thorpe KE, Sackett DL, et al. Can bruits distinguish high-grade from moderate symptomatic carotid stenosis? The North American Symptomatic Carotid Endarterectomy Trial. Ann Intern Med. 1994;120:633–637.
2. Davis BR, Vogt T, Frost PH, et al. Risk factors for stroke and type of stroke in persons with isolated systolic hypertension. Systolic Hypertension in the Elderly Program Cooperative Research Group. Stroke. 1998;29:1333–1340.
3. Collins R, Peto R, MacMahon S, et al. Blood pressure, stroke, and coronary heart disease. II. Short-term reductions in blood pressure: overview of randomized drug trials in their epidemiological context. Lancet. 1990;335:827–838.
4. Byrington RP, Jukema JW, Salonen JT, et al. Reduction in cardiovascular events during pravastatin therapy: pooled analysis of clinical events of the pravastatin atherosclerosis intervention group. Circulation. 1995;92:2419–2425.
5. Weber E. Randomized trial of prophylactic daily aspirin in British male doctors. BMJ. 1988;296:1193.
6. Antiplatelet Trialists' Collaboration. Collaborative overview of randomized trials of antiplatelet therapy. I. Prevention of death, myocardial infarction, and stroke by prolonged antiplatelet therapy in various categories of patients. BMJ. 1994;308:81–106.
7. The Scandinavian simvastatin survival study (4S). Randomized trial of cholesterol lowering in 4444 patients with coronary heart disease. Lancet. 1994;334: 1383–1389.

8. Neal B, MacMahon S, Chapman N. Blood Pressure Lowering Treatment Trialists' Collaboration. Effects of ACE inhibitors, calcium antagonists, and other blood pressure-lowering drugs: results of prospectively designed overviews of randomized trials. Blood Pressure Lowering Treatment Trialists' Collaboration. Lancet. 2000;356:1955–1964.
9. Endarterectomy for asymptomatic carotid artery stenosis. Executive Committee for the Asymptomatic Carotid Atherosclerosis Study. JAMA. 1995;273:141.
10. Moore WS, Barnett HJM, Beebe HG, et al. Guidelines for carotid endarterectomy—a multidisciplinary consensus statement from the Ad Hoc Committee, American Heart Association. Circulation. 1995;91:566.
11. Hart RG, Palacio S, Pearce LA. Atrial fibrillation, stroke, and acute antithrombotic therapy: analysis of randomized clinical trials. Stroke. 2002;33:2722–2727.
12. Barnett HJ, Taylor DW, Eliasziw M, et al. Benefit of carotid endarterectomy in patients with symptomatic moderate or severe stenosis, for the North American Symptomatic Carotid Endarterectomy Trial Collaborators. N Engl J Med. 1998;339:1415–1425.
13. Beneficial effect of carotid endarterectomy in symptomatic patients with high grade carotid stenosis. North American Symptomatic Carotid Endarterectomy Trial Collaborators. N Engl J Med. 1991;325:445.
14. Eikelboom BC, Ackerstaff RG, Hoeneveld H, et al. Benefits of carotid patching: a randomized study. J Vasc Surg. 1988;7:240–247.
15. Hertzer NR, Beven EG, O'Hara PJ, et al. A prospective study of vein patch angioplasty during carotid endarterectomy. Three-year results for 801 patients and 917 operations. Ann Surg. 1987;206:628–635.
16. Roubin GS, New G, Iyer SS, et al. Immediate and late clinical outcomes of carotid artery stenting in patients with symptomatic and asymptomatic carotid artery stenosis: a 5-year prospective analysis. Circulation. 2001;103:532–537.
17. Fox DJ, Moran CJ, Cross DT, et al. Long-term outcome after angioplasty for symptomatic extracranial carotid stenosis in poor surgical candidates. Stroke. 2002;33:2877–2880.

CHAPTER

ABDOMINAL AORTIC ANEURYSM

Jerry Holleman

Mark Anderson is a 65-year-old retired Army officer who was in good health until 2 years ago, when a routine physical examination revealed a pulsatile, nontender upper midline abdominal mass.

What is the differential diagnosis of a pulsatile abdominal mass?

Not every pulsatile mass is an aneurysm, although abnormal dilation of the aorta or one of its branch vessels (hepatic, splenic, superior mesenteric, renal, or iliac arteries) should be high on the list of possible diagnoses. A cystic or solid intraperitoneal or abdominal wall mass may also have referred aortic pulsations. A cystic mass in the small bowel mesentery, an inflammatory or neoplastic lesion in the colon, and a mass in the lesser sac related to previous pancreatitis may all have a presentation similar to Mr. Anderson's, especially if the patient is thin.

What is an aneurysm?

An *aneurysm* is a fixed, or permanent, enlargement of an artery to twice the normal diameter. True aneurysms have all three layers present, whereas false aneurysms or pseudoaneurysms have disruption of one or more of the walls of the artery. The normal abdominal aorta averages 1.5 to 2.5 cm in diameter, depending on the age and gender of the person (1).

What causes abdominal aortic aneurysms (AAAs)?

Atherosclerosis is the cause of AAAs in approximately 95% of patients (2). The atherosclerotic process creates an intrinsic weakness in the arterial wall that leads to progressive dilation over time. Genetic factors also play a role in AAAs. The incidence of AAA in first-degree relatives of patients with AAA is approximately 25% (3). Less common causes of AAAs include trauma, syphilis, mycotic infection, congenital defects, Marfan's syndrome, inflammation, and pregnancy.

Aneurysms associated with reconstructive arterial surgery are being reported with increasing frequency (4).

How common are AAAs?

AAAs are the most common of the atherosclerotic aneurysms, estimated to occur in as many as 2% of the elderly population in Western countries. Their incidence is increasing steadily, and they are the aneurysms most commonly diagnosed by physicians (5).

Mr. Anderson undergoes an abdominal ultrasound (US) examination, which reveals a 3.5-cm AAA. No further studies are performed, and he is monitored with serial US examinations.

Why is the size of an aneurysm important, and how does it guide surgical treatment?

Rupture of an aortic aneurysm ranks 10th as the cause of death in men older than 55 years (6). Other complications of aneurysm include thrombosis, embolization, dissection, and obstruction of or erosion into an adjacent organ. Arterial wall tension, hence rupture risk, can be approximated by the law of La Place, in which tension is proportional to the product of the pressure and the radius ($t = p \times r$).

The risk of rupture increases considerably with aneurysm size. For an aneurysm less than 4 cm in diameter, the risk of rupture is generally thought to be negligible, although it can occur. Aneurysms 4.0 to 5.5 cm in diameter have a 0.5% to 1.0% annual risk of rupture, whereas those 6 to 7 cm in diameter have a 6.6% annual risk of rupture. Aneurysms 7.0 cm or greater have 19% annual rupture risk (7). Elective repair should be considered in most patients with an aneurysm 5.5 cm or larger.

How should a patient such as Mr. Anderson be managed?

A patient with a 3.5-cm aneurysm should be observed for symptoms and any evidence of growth. A 6-month follow-up US examination is routine. If the aneurysm is stable, yearly follow-up is recommended. Any indication of growth should prompt more frequent follow-up—for example, every 3 months.

What is the best radiologic technique for monitoring an aneurysm?

There are essentially two options for surveillance: computed tomography (CT) and US. Magnetic resonance imaging is not cost-effective. CT is also helpful for evaluating other intraabdominal lesions. Both CT and US are noninvasive, but in most centers, US is accurate and cost-effective. Regardless of the test chosen, the same test must be used for follow-up examinations. Aortography and magnetic resonance angiography (MRA) are not used for surveillance; they are discussed later.

Mr. Anderson is reevaluated 1 year later, at which time the abdominal US examination shows that the maximal transverse diameter of the AAA is 3.7 cm and that it extends to the common iliac arteries bilaterally.

What is the average annual rate of growth of an AAA?

US studies show that expansion rates vary from 2 to 8 mm per year, with an average of 4 mm annually (3). Traditional belief was that almost all aneurysms expand over time (8). However, it is now clear that some aneurysms show very little growth over a long period of follow-up, whereas others grow rapidly over a relatively short period (9). Individuals may often experience a staccato growth pattern in which periods of growth are followed by periods of stability. Certain risk factors, such as hypertension and chronic obstructive lung disease, are associated with rapidly growing aneurysms (10).

Mr. Anderson is scheduled for a repeat examination in 6 months, but he is lost to follow-up. He returns to the clinic 2 years later, at which time a follow-up abdominal US examination reveals enlargement of the aneurysm to 5.5 cm. Mr. Anderson is referred to surgery for further evaluation and elective surgical repair of his AAA.

Mr. Anderson does not have abdominal pain or tenderness, low back pain, extremity pain, hematuria, melena, or bloody stools. He has had no recent illness and has no history of angina, congestive heart failure, or cerebrovascular disease. He had a transurethral retrograde prostatectomy for benign prostatic hypertrophy 12 years ago. A physical examination shows Mr. Anderson appearing normal and in no apparent distress. His vital signs are blood pressure, 130/75 mm Hg; pulse, 78 beats per minute; respiratory rate, 18 breaths per minute; and temperature, 36.9°C.

The only abnormal finding on physical examination is a large immobile pulsatile mass palpated in the midepigastrium just above the umbilicus. The mass is not tender, and there is no audible bruit. The stools are guaiac negative. The laboratory data are hematocrit, 41%; leukocyte count, 7200 per mL; platelet count 284,000 per mL; blood urea nitrogen, 33 mg per dL; creatinine 1.1 mg per dL; electrolytes, normal; and coagulation tests, normal. The electrocardiogram and chest radiograph are normal. Plain abdominal radiographs show a calcified aortic wall with infrarenal aneurysmal dilation to approximately 4.5 cm.

What is the most frequent presentation of an AAA?

AAAs are more common in men than in women by a ratio of 4:1, and they occur mainly in the sixth or seventh decade of life (3). In 75% of patients, the aneurysm is asymptomatic at the time of diagnosis. AAAs are most commonly diagnosed on routine physical examination or on imaging studies obtained for other reasons. With US, an increasing number of smaller aneurysms are being detected (11). When symptoms are present, the most common complaint is vague abdominal and back pain, which may be caused by expansion or rupture of the aneurysm. The pain frequently begins in the epigastrium and penetrates to the back. Tenderness on direct palpation of the aneurysm and flank pain are other signs of rupture. On rare occasions, patients have flank pain from ureteral obstruction or gastrointestinal bleeding from a primary aortoenteric fistula. Ureteral obstruction should raise suspicion of an inflammatory aneurysm (12).

What are the important findings from a physical examination?

The physical examination is diagnostic in many cases. A large pulsatile immobile mass in the epigastrium is the most frequent finding. Because the bifurcation of the aorta is at the level of the umbilicus, the mass is usually at or above this level. Tenderness may be present on palpation, and a bruit may be found on auscultation of the abdomen. Distal pulses of the lower extremities may be diminished. Unfortunately, many aneurysms are not detected on physical examination, particularly in obese patients. In one study, only 15% of aneurysms in obese patients were diagnosed on physical examination and only 33% were palpable when the diagnosis was known (13).

What is the natural history of AAAs?

The natural history of AAAs was described by Estes in 1950, before the advent of surgical repair (14). Of 102 patients with AAAs, only 67% were alive 1 year after diagnosis, 49% at 3 years, and 19% at 5 years. Rupture of the AAA caused the death of 63% of these patients. In a 1972 report on 156 patients who had been rejected for surgical repair, Szilagyi et al. (15) showed that among patients with aneurysms bigger than 6 cm, 43% died of aneurysm rupture and 37% died of myocardial infarction; among patients with aneurysms smaller than 6 cm, 36% died of myocardial infarction and 31% died of rupture.

What are the guidelines for recommending repair of an aneurysm?

Treatment must be individualized, but the natural history of the condition provides general guidelines. Patients with an AAA larger than 6 cm should be considered for elective repair unless they have severe uncorrectable coronary artery disease (CAD) or severe chronic obstructive pulmonary disease (COPD). Most patients with an aneurysm that is 5.5 to 6 cm and no active CAD or COPD should also be considered for elective repair. The treatment of aneurysms smaller than 5 cm is controversial and probably should be rarely performed.

What is the appropriate preoperative radiologic workup for an aneurysm?

The preoperative radiologic workup includes finding answers to the following questions:

1. What is the maximum diameter of the aneurysm?
2. Are there complicating features such as renal artery involvement, iliac artery occlusive disease, mesenteric artery occlusive disease, juxtarenal or suprarenal involvement?
3. Is the patient likely to be a candidate for stent graft repair?

Helical CT scan with thin cuts and 3-dimensional reconstructions, with and without contrast, is an excellent initial imaging study and will answer most of these questions (16–18).

Angiography as a subsequent examination is often useful in the presence of the following:

- History of difficult hypertension
- Renal insufficiency
- Intermittent claudication
- Diminished femoral pulses
- Verification of measurements in planning for stent graft repair
- Clarification of anatomy if a stent graft is being considered

MRA is also accurate at delineating AAA. It compares well with CT and aortography, especially with 3-dimensional reconstruction (19). The definition and accuracy of spiral CT and MRA depend on the ability to reconstruct images after they are acquired.

What is an aortic stent graft and how does it prevent aneurysm rupture?

An *aortic stent graft* is a device composed of a scaffold of metal stents attached to a fabric graft introduced into the aorta with the aid of catheters and guidewires. When the stent graft is properly deployed in the aorta, it attaches to the wall of the normal aorta above and below the aneurysm so that pressurized blood remains inside the stent graft rather than in the aneurysm.

What are the advantages and disadvantages of open repair versus stent graft repair?

Open repair has a longer track record, with clinical experience dating to the 1950s, and it has proven to be an effective, safe, and durable procedure.

Disadvantages of open repair are listed:

- It is more of a physiologic assault on an individual than a stent graft repair.
- Recuperation takes much longer.
- Patients with significant comorbidities such as CAD and pulmonary disease may have a higher mortality rate.

Advantages of stent graft repair are listed:

- It requires a much shorter recuperation.

- Patients experience less discomfort.
- There are possibly lower mortality rates in patients with serious comorbid conditions.

Who should have an open repair and who should have a stent graft repair?

Most patients 65 years old or younger who are in otherwise good health are probably best served by having an open repair because the long-term durability of stent graft repair is unclear. Additionally, patients who have unfavorable anatomy, such as a short or angulated neck or tortuous, small, or calcified iliac arteries, are best treated with an open procedure. A stent graft repair best serves patients who are elderly, who have significant cardiac or pulmonary disease, or who have had previous abdominal surgery. Patients who fall between these extremes, have moderately unfavorable anatomy for stent grafting, and have moderately severe medical illnesses require careful judgment. Participation by these patients in decision-making is essential.

What is an endoleak?

Endoleak: a leak of pressured blood in the aneurysm sac

Type 1 endoleak: a leak at the attachment site of the aneurysm, either at the upper end of the stent graft in the aorta proximal to the aneurysm or at the lower end of the stent graft at the attachment sites within the iliac arteries

Type 2 endoleak: a leak of collaterals, such as the inferior mesenteric artery (IMA) or lumbar arteries, into the aneurysm sac

Type 3 endoleak: a junctional leak that occurs between components of the graft, usually from distortion of the graft following remodeling of the aorta

Type 4 endoleak: a fabric leak that is usually the result of heparinized blood leaking through the thin fabric or the stent graft; Type 4 endoleaks usually resolve spontaneously with reversal of heparin

How is the stent graft repair performed?

Both common femoral arteries are exposed through bilateral groin incisions. A flush angiography catheter is inserted into the aorta on one side, and a stiff guidewire is inserted up the other side. Angiographic images are acquired to define the anatomy, particularly the renal arteries, and the graft is deployed just below the renal arteries.

The currently available stent grafts are called *modular* and consist of at least two components. The main body of the stent graft lands in the aorta proximal to the aneurysm below both renal arteries and in the iliac artery distal to the aneurysm on one side. The other iliac limb is advanced up from the other femoral artery. Angiograms are taken throughout the course of the procedure to ensure that the renal arteries are not covered and that the hypogastric arteries are not inadvertently covered. Small extension pieces may be needed to complete the procedure. After all of the components are in place, an aortogram is performed to look for endoleaks and to verify good perfusion of the kidneys and the lower extremities.

What is the appropriate cardiac workup before repair of an AAA?

Because atherosclerosis is a systemic disease and because repair of an AAA is a major surgical procedure, patients require careful cardiac evaluation to recognize concomitant CAD. For patients with significant risk factors for CAD or a history of angina or myocardial infarction, nuclear stress imaging is useful. If stress imaging is positive for reversible ischemia, coronary angiography and subsequent revascularization (either percutaneously or surgically) may be indicated. If stress imaging shows no evidence of reversible ischemia, proceed with aneurysm repair. Of note, adverse cardiac events are significantly reduced with perioperative beta blockade.

Before admission, digital subtraction aortography is performed on Mr. Anderson to confirm the infrarenal aneurysm with extension to the level of the common iliac arteries. This study also shows significant peripheral vascular disease involving the superficial femoral arteries bilaterally, with two-vessel runoff in the right lower extremity and single-vessel runoff in the left lower extremity. Extensive bilateral lower extremity collateral vessels are also noted.

What is the typical location of AAAs?

More than 95% of these aneurysms arise below the renal vessels (3). Approximately 66% extend inferiorly to involve the common iliac vessels (2). Rarely do they extend far enough to involve the internal iliac vessels.

Are prophylactic perioperative antibiotics indicated in patients undergoing repair of an aneurysm?

The infection rate without prophylactic antibiotic coverage approaches 7% and is reduced to about 1% with the use of antibiotics (20). Therefore, prophylactic antibiotics are indicated.

Mr. Anderson undergoes open surgery the next day. Dissection is performed through a midline abdominal incision, down to and around the aorta. A fusiform aneurysm approximately 5.5 cm in diameter is noted. After aortic cross-clamping, an uncomplicated repair of the aneurysm is performed using a woven polyester (Dacron) bifurcating graft.

What precautions should be taken during repair of an AAA?

Cardiovascular monitoring and management are of utmost importance. A Swan-Ganz catheter is inserted before the operation to help maintain fluid balance and monitor pressure. A radial arterial line is placed for accurate blood pressure monitoring. Renal function must be monitored closely, and a Foley catheter is essential. Mannitol is occasionally administered to minimize the risk of renal failure during aortic cross-clamping.

What are the physiologic consequences of cross-clamping the aorta?

An acute interruption of the distal aortic flow increases afterload on the heart and decreases cardiac output. The systemic vascular resistance proximal to the cross-clamp also increases. A sudden decrease of blood flow to the lower extremity leads to lactate acidosis and a decreased venous return from the lower extremity. Administer heparin before aortic cross-clamping to prevent arterial thrombosis.

What is the physiologic response after the aortic cross-clamp is released?

A sudden release of the cross-clamp sharply reduces the aortic blood pressure. In addition, there is a sudden increase of lactate-containing venous blood from the lower extremities. Particular attention must be given to acidosis, hypovolemia, and electrolyte abnormalities after the aorta is unclamped (3). Any fluid and bicarbonate should therefore be administered before the aortic cross-clamp is released.

What is a meandering mesenteric artery, and why is it significant for AAA surgery?

In patients with atherosclerosis of the abdominal aorta, either the superior mesenteric artery (SMA) or the IMA may be occluded at its origin, requiring collateral vessels to supply the area of deficit. The meandering mesenteric artery is a large and tortuous collateral artery coursing from a branch of the SMA, the middle colic artery, to a branch of the IMA, the left colic artery, and is visible at the center of the abdomen on a preoperative angiogram in 25% of patients with AAA (21). (The meandering mesenteric artery, also called the *arc of Riolan,* is a separate entity from the marginal artery of Drummond.)

The IMA is the only major vessel usually involved in the aortic aneurysm. This vessel supplies blood to the left colon and rectosigmoid region of the bowel. It can be ligated without consequence during surgery on the AAA in most patients because of the rich collateral circulation from the superior mesenteric system. However, in patients with a meandering mesenteric artery visible on an angiogram arising as a result of previous SMA occlusion and a retrograde collateral flow from the IMA, inadvertent ligation of the IMA during surgery leads to severe mesenteric ischemia. In that case, preservation of the IMA during surgery is critical. If interruption of the IMA is unavoidable, reimplantation of the IMA onto the aortic graft may be necessary to avoid bowel ischemia. Measurement of mesenteric arterial stump pressure may be useful in identifying patients at risk for postoperative ischemic colitis (22).

What is the significance of a bloody bowel movement after aneurysm surgery?

A bloody bowel movement (or any bowel movement within the first few days after surgery) should raise the suspicion for colon ischemia. Perform prompt flexible sigmoidoscopy. If mild to moderate colon ischemia, as manifest by erythematous mucosa or patchy exudate, is present, the patient is given broad-spectrum antibiotics and undergoes serial flexible sigmoidoscopy examinations. If there are findings suggestive of transmural necrosis, immediate reoperation is indicated, with resection of the involved segment of colon.

In an open repair, is the aneurysm removed?

The aneurysm is not removed. The anterior wall and thrombus are resected, with the posterior wall kept intact and undissected. The wall is then wrapped around the prosthetic graft and is reapproximated anteriorly by separating the graft from surrounding structures to prevent formation of aortoenteric or aortocaval fistulas.

Who performed the first successful repair of an AAA?

Dubost performed the first successful repair of an AAA in Paris in 1951. His repair included reconstruction of the aorta with an aortic homograft (23).

Mr. Anderson remains hemodynamically stable throughout the rest of his surgery and is admitted to the surgical intensive care unit.

What is the prognosis after elective repair of an AAA?

The operative and postoperative results of elective open surgical repair of AAAs have improved in recent years. Most centers report an operative mortality of 1% to 5% after elective repair of these aneurysms (3). Furthermore, long-term survival reported by Debakey is 84% at 1 year, 72% at 3 years, and 58% at 5 years (24). Most of the deaths were associated with continued atherosclerosis of the coronary, renal, and cerebrovascular vessels. With successful repair of an aneurysm, the prognosis for a patient such as Mr. Anderson is very good. The long-term success of stent graft repairs is not known at this time because the currently available devices have been available for fewer than 10 years. What is known is that there is a 0.5% to 1.0% incidence of late rupture following aortic stent graft repair, and there is a 10% to 15% incidence of secondary procedures following stent graft repair (25).

What is the prognosis after emergency repair of an AAA?

The operative mortality for emergency repair of a ruptured AAA is approximately 50% at most centers (26). Death is usually from massive intraoperative hemorrhage, cardiopulmonary complications, or acute postoperative renal failure.

Which potential postoperative complications should be discussed with the patient when obtaining consent for surgery?

Postoperative complications after repair of an AAA are common in both elective and emergency cases. The following is a list of some of these complications and their relative frequencies (3,4). When obtaining consent, discuss these problems with the patient.

Pulmonary atelectasis is seen in all patients to some degree and may lead to pneumonia in severe cases.

Acute renal failure occurs in approximately 2.5% of elective surgery and in more than 20% of cases of rupture. Mortality in these patients approaches 90%.

Abdominal distention arising from paralytic ileus occurs in most cases of intraperitoneal approach. This usually self-limited process requires nasogastric decompression until bowel function returns.

Embolization of thrombi to the lower extremities leads to acute ischemia in as many as 7% of patients. Treatment depends on the nature and extent of the obstruction and the ischemic tissues.

Bleeding may occur from the anastomosis site or through the interstices of the graft and mandates reexploration in some patients. Rupture of the suture line is rare but may occur with erosion into surrounding viscera. Emergency reoperation may be required in this situation.

Infection of the graft occurs in approximately 1% of patients in most studies. This requires removal of the graft material and ligation of the aorta below the renal vessels. Flow to the lower extremities is reestablished with an axillary-bifemoral graft. Treatment with appropriate antibiotics is essential.

False aneurysms may develop at the suture lines and may produce pain and a pulsatile mass. Diagnosis is by aortography. Reoperation with revision of the aortic repair may be indicated to reduce the risk of spontaneous rupture.

Cardiac arrhythmias are common and are usually caused by underlying CAD with myocardial ischemia. Aggressively treat arrhythmias to maintain hemodynamic stability.

Bowel ischemia is rare but may result from ligation of the IMA and inadequate collateral flow. Bowel movements within 48 hours of surgery should raise suspicion of colonic ischemia.

Sexual dysfunction in men is characterized by retrograde ejaculation in as much as 66% of patients and impotence in as much as 30% of patients. This results from disturbance or ligation of the sympathetic nerve plexus as it crosses the aortic bifurcation. Take care to avoid these nerves during surgical manipulation of the aorta to reduce the risk of these complications.

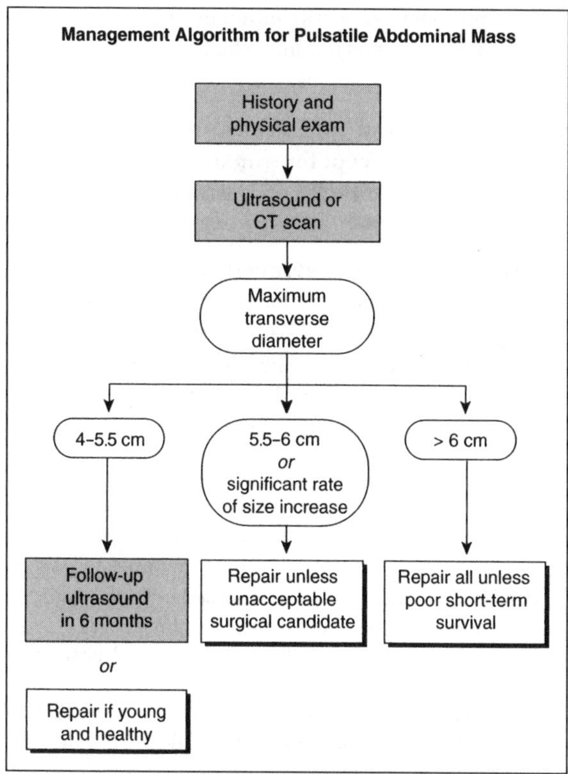

Algorithm 22.1.

Spinal cord ischemia is a rare complication characterized by an anterior spinal artery syndrome. In most cases, it is caused by hypotension or prolonged intraoperative ischemia. Some cases of spinal cord ischemia result from thrombosis or embolism.

Endoleak is a leak involving a stent graft in which pressurized blood leaks from the graft and continues to pressurize the aneurysm sac.

What is the artery of Adamkiewicz, and what is its significance in surgery for AAA?

Blood supply to the spinal cord is provided by the posterior spinal artery on the dorsal side and the anterior spinal artery on the ventral side. The posterior spinal artery is well collateralized through the entire length of the spinal cord, but the anterior spinal artery depends on a key collateral system from the aorta to supply the distal anterior spinal cord. This collateral artery, the artery of Adamkiewicz, arises from the aorta at the level of T8 to L2 in 85% of cases (it may occur as low as L4) (27) and is vulnerable to disruption during surgical dissection around the aorta or during aortic cross-clamping, which can lead to anterior spinal cord ischemia.

Mr. Anderson is transferred to the ward on postoperative day 2. His recovery is unremarkable except for transient ileus and mild pulmonary atelectasis. He is discharged home on postoperative day 10.

Should routine US screening be performed for AAA?

Among persons aged 55 and older who have a first-degree relative with an AAA, men have an approximately 20% to 25% risk of AAA and women have an approximately 6% risk (2). Screening on the basis of age alone is not cost-effective (25); however, patients who have a first-degree relative with an AAA should have a screening US examination at age 50 to 55 years.

REFERENCES

1. Ouriel K, Green RM, Donayre C, et al. An evaluation of new methods of expressing aortic aneurysm size: relationship to rupture. J Vasc Surg. 1992;15:12.
2. Crisler C, Bahnson HT. Aneurysms of the aorta. In: Ravitch MM, ed. Current Problems in Surgery. St. Louis, Mo: Mosby–Year Book; 1989.
3. Johanson K, Koepsell T. Familial tendency for abdominal aortic aneurysms. JAMA. 1986;256:1934.
4. Rutherford RB. Infrarenal aortic aneurysms. In: Rutherford RB, ed. Vascular Surgery. 4th ed, vol 2. Philadelphia, Pa: WB Saunders; 1994:1032–1060.
5. Green RM, Ouriel K. Peripheral arterial disease. In: Schwartz SI, ed. Principles of Surgery. 6th ed. New York, NY: McGraw Hill; 1994:925–987.
6. Department of Health and Human Services. Vital Statistics of the United States, 2: Mortality, Part A. Washington, DC: US Government Printing Office; 1987.Pub PHS 87–1101.
7. UK Small Aneurysm Trial Participants. Mortality results for randomized controlled trial of early elective surgery or ultrasonographic surveillance for small abdominal aortic aneurysms. Lancet. 1998;1649.
8. Darling RC, Messina CR, Brewster DC, et al. Autopsy study of unoperated abdominal aortic aneurysm. Circulation. 1977;56(Suppl 2):II–161.
9. Cronenwett JL, Sargent SK, Wall MH, et al. Variables that affect the expansion rate and outcome of small abdominal aortic aneurysms. J Vasc Surg. 1990;11:260.
10. Sterpetti AV, Cavallaro A, Cavallaro N, et al. Factors influencing the rupture of abdominal aortic aneurysms. Surg Obstet Gynecol. 1991;173:175.
11. Bickerstaff LK, Hollier LH, Van Peenan HJ. Abdominal aortic aneurysms: the changing natural history. J Vasc Surg. 1984;1:6.
12. Goldstone J, Malone JM, Moore WS. Inflammatory aneurysms of the aorta. Surgery. 1978;83:425.
13. Cherru A, Clagoff GP, Valentine RJ, Viyess SI, Rossi PJ. Role of physical examination in detection of abdominal aortic aneurysms surgery. 1995;4: 454–7.

14. Estes JE Jr. Abdominal aortic aneurysm: a study of one hundred and two cases. Circulation. 1950;2:258.
15. Szilagyi DE, Elliott JP, Smith RF. Clinical fate of the patient with asymptomatic aortic aneurysm and unfit for surgical treatment. Arch Surg. 1972;104:600.
16. Pillari G, Chang JB, Zito J, et al. Computed tomography of abdominal aortic aneurysm. Arch Surg. 1988;123:727.
17. Todd GJ, Nowygrod R, Benvensity A. The accuracy of CT scanning in the diagnosis of abdominal and thoracoabdominal aortic aneurysms. J Vasc Surg. 1991;13:302.
18. Fillinger MF. Utility of Spiral CT in the Preoperative Evaluation of Patients with Abdominal Aortic Aneurysms: Advances in Vascular Surgery. Vol 5. St. Louis, Mo: Mosby–Year Book; 1997:115–131.
19. Pavone P, Di Cesare E, Di Renzi P. Abdominal aortic aneurysm evaluation: comparison of US, CT MRI, and aortography. Magn Reson Imaging. 1990;8:199.
20. Thompson JE, Hollier LH, Patman RD, et al. Surgical management of abdominal aortic aneurysms: factors influencing mortality and morbidity: a 20 year experience. Ann Surg. 1975;181:654.
21. Ernst CB. Prevention of intestinal ischemia following abdominal aortic reconstruction. Surgery. 1983;93:102–106.
22. Ernst CB, Hagihara PF, Daugherty ME, et al. Inferior mesenteric artery stump pressure: a reliable index for safe IMA ligation during abdominal aorta aneurysmectomy. Ann Surg. 1978;187:641.
23. Dubost C, Allary M, Oeconomos N. Resection of an abdominal aortic aneurysm: reestablishment of the continuity by a preserved human arterial graft, with results after five months. Arch Surg. 1952;64:405.
24. Debakey ME, Crawford ES, Cooley DA, et al. Aneurysm of abdominal aorta: analysis of results of graft replacement therapy one to eleven years after operation. Ann Surg. 1964;160:622.
25. Zarins CK, Bloch DA, Crabtree T, et al. Aneurysm enlargement following endovascular aneurysm repair: AneuRx clinical trial. J Vasc Surg. 2004;39:1.
26. Lawrence MS, Crosby VG, Ehrenhart JL. Ruptured abdominal aortic aneurysm. Ann Thorac Surg. 1966;2:159.
27. Ferguson LR, Bergan JJ, Conn J Jr, et al. Spinal ischemia following abdominal aortic surgery. Ann Surg. 1975;181:267–272.

CHAPTER

23

ADRENAL TUMORS

Ronald Merrell

Ms. Lucas is a 78-year-old African American woman. She is a retired university professor who had an episode of ureterolithiasis several months ago for the first time in her life. She was evaluated for residual stones and renal pathology by computed tomography (CT) scan and a 5-cm left adrenal mass was identified. Ms. Lucas has been hypertensive for many years and is well controlled with an angiotensin-receptor antagonist. She is referred to you for consideration of the adrenal mass.

What is the significance of an asymptomatic adrenal mass?

The generous application of CT discloses a great deal of unsuspected and usually innocuous masses. Adrenal masses are identified in 0.06% of the general population; although most are of no significance, the chance finding of a silent but significant adrenal tumor must be seized by evaluation.

What is the differential diagnosis of an incidental adrenal mass discovered by CT scan?

The adrenal gland is a common site for metastatic disease, and this diagnosis should be strongly entertained in patients with bilateral masses or a history of cancer. Primary tumors of the adrenal cortex include adenomas, carcinomas, and myelolipomas. They may be functional with excess hormonal status or without function. The adrenal medulla may develop neuroblastoma, neuroganglioma, or (in adults) pheochromocytoma. Pheochromocytoma may be malignant or benign.

How is an incidental adrenal mass evaluated?

The first test is to rule out pheochromocytoma even if the patient has no clinical manifestations of catecholamine excess. Testing also should include cortical hormone testing for cortisol. If the tumor has no endocrine activity and there is a suspicion of metastatic disease, a CT-guided needle biopsy may clarify the situation.

How is an incidental adrenal tumor treated?

If the tumor has no endocrine activity and is less than 3 cm in diameter, the patient may be followed with repeat CT at 6 months and again at 1 year. If endocrine activity is discovered, resection is indicated. Tumors smaller than 3 cm are quite unlikely to represent malignant disease, and expectant management is safe. For tumors larger than 5 cm, resection is the treatment of choice, regardless of secretory status. The probability of malignancy climbs into the clearly finite range of some 10%, and expectant management is not reasonable. If the tumor is between 3 and 5 cm, there is not a clear answer as to the best management, and the next steps must be considered in light of the patient's informed consent and overall health management.

What are the anatomic and functional characteristics of the adrenal glands?

The adrenal glands lie above the kidney on either side and represent a composite of mesodermal cortex that envelops the medulla, which derives from the neural crest sympathogonia. The cortex has three layers:

1. The most superficial layer is the *zona glomerulosa,* which synthesizes the steroid mineralocorticoid hormone aldosterone upon stimulation by angiotensin II. This synthesis is possible because of the phenotypic expression of 18-hydrozylase.
2. Below the zona glomerulosa, the *zona fasciculate* synthesizes glucocorticoids.
3. The inner layer synthesizes the androgen dehydroepiandrosterone (DHEA).

The zona fasciculata and reticulata are controlled by adrenocorticotrophic hormone (ACTH) in the pituitary-adrenal axis.

What supplies blood to the adrenal glands?

The superior adrenal artery is a branch of the inferior phrenic artery; the middle adrenal artery arises directly from the aorta; and the inferior adrenal artery branches from the renal artery. Venous drainage on the right is directly into the vena cava, and this vein can be treacherously short. Venous drainage on the left is into the renal vein.

Ms. Lucas tells you she has no endocrine symptoms and her blood pressure has been stable for many years. She only switched to the angiotensin receptor antagonist in order to avoid diuretics. However, she had a left mastectomy and axillary node dissection 20 years ago for infiltrating ductal carcinoma. She has been followed diligently and has consistently

had a reassuring report with regard to physical examination and chest radiograph. Your testing begins with urinary catecholamine and metanephrine determination, which is normal. Her urinary cortisol levels are also normal.

What is the next step in her management?

Even though the history of breast cancer is distant, CT-guided needle biopsy of the adrenal gland is appropriate. Needle biopsy is not particularly useful to distinguish benign from malignant adrenal tumors, and needle biopsy of a pheochromocytoma is dangerous in that a catastrophic release of catecholamine may occur. Needle biopsy should probably be reserved for cases of possible metastatic disease.

Ms. Lucas has a needle biopsy after CT-guided needle biopsy to rule out pheochromocytoma and adrenal cortical cells are recovered.

What is the treatment for an adrenal cortical tumor 5 cm or larger that has no endocrine function?

Adrenalectomy is strongly recommended if this is consistent with overall patient management. A tumor of 5 cm may be resected by laparoscopy or laparotomy or through a retroperitoneal approach. Laparoscopy becomes problematic when the gland is large and when the tumor is malignant with uncertain invasion of surrounding tissue. The recommendation of laparotomy to explore has lost impetus, and advanced imaging techniques such as spiral CT, even with tumors that have a strong likelihood of bilaterally such as pheochromocytoma, have come into favor. The posterior approach offers no advantage over laparoscopy, which may become the preferred operation for all small adrenal tumors.

At operation, a benign adrenal adenoma is removed by laparoscopy.

What further treatment is needed?

Follow the laparoscopy with physical examination and CT every 2 years. The histology of adrenal cortical tumors is not sufficiently precise to absolutely differentiate between cortical adenomas and carcinoma. Occasionally, only malignant behavior such as local or distant metastasis declares a tumor to be a cancer.

Ms. O'Brien is a 38-year-old white woman who is referred after her cousin recently had a pheochromocytoma removed and advised her relatives of the importance of family screening. She is in good health and has no hypertension, weight loss, hyperglycemias, or anxiety. In recent months, she has had menstrual irregularity and hot flashes; she attributed these symptoms to early menopause, which is not unusual in her family. On examination she is a healthy woman with no positive physical findings.

What is the importance of evaluation for potential family members with pheochromocytoma?

Some 10% of patients with pheochromocytoma have a familial variant, and the most common is multiple endocrine neoplasia type II (MEN-II), an autosomal dominant condition characterized genetically by mutation of the RET gene on chromosome 10. The clinical manifestations include pheochromocytoma, medullary carcinoma of the thyroid, and primary hyperparathyroidism. The endocrine conditions are usually metachronous, and the first condition appears in no particular order in the third or fourth decade of life. Family screening is simply done by checking urinary catecholamines.

Ms. O'Brien has a modest increase in urinary epinephrine. She had a CT scan several months earlier for back pain, which subsequently resolved without intervention. The referring physician had the scan reviewed and the radiologist, in retrospect, identified a 1-cm left adrenal mass.

What are the diagnostic possibilities here?

When urinary catecholamines are not compelling but just barely abnormal, plasma catecholamines may be more sensitive, especially if drawn while the patient is blocked with clonidine. This blockade eliminates physiologic elevation of catecholamines associated with anxiety. The 1-cm tumor, which was missed earlier, may be spurious. In this patient, clonidine suppression clearly identified elevated catecholamines in the plasma.

Ms. O'Brien is suspected to have MEN-II. What testing is appropriate for the other elements of this syndrome?

Certainly serum calcium and parathyroid hormone can determine the presence of primary hyperparathyroidism. Ms. O'Brien had no masses in the neck, and a normal serum thyrocalcitonin was reassuring with regard to medullary carcinoma of the thyroid. This determination can be made much more sensitive by provoking calcitonin with glucagon, which is not a normal secretagogue for calcitonin but causes a marked release from malignant parafollicular or C cells in the thyroid.

In familial pheochromocytoma, when the adrenal tumor is contemporaneous with either hyperparathyroidism or medullary cancer, which lesion should be treated first?

The pheochromocytoma is the most dangerous member of this trio and should always be the priority in planning treatment.

Pheochromocytoma is familial in 10% of patients. What are the other attributes of pheochromocytoma that have a probability of 10%?

The tumors are extraadrenal in 10% of patients and may be bilateral, malignant, or found in children with a similar incidence of 10%. Bilaterally is much more common in children and patients with familial pheochromocytoma. The contralateral tumor should be detectable by CT.

What is the treatment for this patient with a small pheochromocytoma?
This tumor should be resected. The operation can be very hazardous with regard to the anesthetic. Most anesthetic agents are associated with catecholamine release and disastrous discharge of catecholamine from a pheochromocytoma in the course of an anesthetic may be fatal. The drastic excisions of catecholamines must be blocked in their actions by alpha-adrenergic antagonists. Phenoxybenzamine has greater action on $alpha_1$ receptors and is widely used for preoperative preparation. Prazosin is also a selective $alpha_1$ antagonist. If the alpha blockade leads to a tachycardia, beta blockade with propranolol is necessary.

The alpha blockade is accomplished over a number of weeks with oral dosing. The endpoint is not complete blockade, which would be associated with an incapacitating orthostatic problem. The blockade will release a tonic constriction of the capacitance venous system and an expansion of the intravascular volume. This is compensated by taking in ample fluids and will be marked by a drop of the hematocrit of 3% to 6% points over 2 to 3 weeks. Red cell mass does not expand in this time frame and the dilutional effect on the hematocrit is excellent proof that the block is in place and that anesthesia may be safely applied.

Are there unique intraoperative considerations during resection of pheochromocytoma?
Aside from the anatomic consideration for the adrenal gland, there are several points. Excessive manipulation of the tumor will lead to a dramatic rise in systemic catecholamines. Remember that the alpha blockade is relative and not absolute. There is probably no other operation in which the dialogue between surgeon and anesthesiologist is more important. The adrenergic situation is dynamic to say the least. It is advisable to divide the adrenal vein early to end the excess catecholamine release with tumor manipulation. When this happens there may be profound hypotension. Remember the alpha blockade was in balance with excess catecholamines and when the brief half-life of these potent vasoactive agents has passed, the patient almost always has a sudden relaxation of the arterial and venous circulation and a need for an abundant infusion of saline. In addition, since a patient with chronic elevation of catecholamines has a cardiomyopathy, which is reversible, the surgeon and anesthesiologist may be surprised by a poorly performing left ventricle that cannot accommodate rapidly to the sudden fluid shifts.

Some 10% of pheochromocytomas are malignant. How is this determined and what are the implications?
The histology may not give the proper answer because malignant pheochromocytomas may have very bland microscopic features. Subsequent metastasis is the real answer. Even benign pheochromocytomas may implant in the retroperitoneum

if the capsule is breached and cells spilled. This phenomenon is important to the laparoscopic surgeon, and an open procedure may be performed in order to avoid a devastating local recurrence with benign disease. The malignant pheochromocytoma has a 5-year survival of a little less that 50%, whereas the benign lesion is associated with essentially normal life expectancy.

Ms. O'Brien had a laparoscopic adrenalectomy. The tumor was indeed a very small pheochromocytoma. The postoperative recovery was uneventful and the hot flashes disappeared and normal menstrual pattern resumed. Therefore, the patient's complaint was due to paroxysm and menstrual irregularity often seen in pheochromocytoma.

How should she be followed?

She should have an annual catecholamine check and annual assessment of calcium and thyrocalcitonin. She should be examined every 6 months to probe for suspicious history of recurrence or the appearance of another of the triad of MEN-II. The other family members should be notified that there are now two members with probable MEN-II. Genetic testing for RET mutation and genetic counseling should be considered.

Mr. Hampton is a 38-year-old African American computer engineer who has enjoyed good health and a vigorous lifestyle until about 5 months ago when he began to lose exercise tolerance because of fatigue. His slow decline culminated in an ambulance trip to an emergency department where he was arousable but essentially unable to move in response to pain or command. His wife reported that he could not get up from bed after retiring in utter fatigue early the evening before.

His vital signs showed a blood pressure of 150/100 mm Hg. The only other abnormal findings were areflexia and almost no muscular strength. His evaluation included measurement of serum electrolytes, and his potassium was 1.7 mEq per L. A diagnosis of primary hyperaldosteronism was strongly suspected. He responded to a potassium infusion over the next several days with full recovery of his strength and he was discharged on spironolactone.

What are the diagnostic steps to confirm the diagnosis?

Primary hyperaldosteronism is distinguished from the vastly more common secondary hyperaldosteronism by the patient having an elevated aldosterone level in the face of a low plasma renin. Secondary hyperaldosteronism is seen in edematous states when renin rises and aldosterone release is a secondary effect. In primary hyperaldosteronism, the adrenal cortex without stimulation releases excess aldosterone without any extraadrenal stimulation. The adrenal pathology includes bilateral hyperplasia and adenoma. These two conditions can generally be distinguished by spiral CT.

The spiral CT showed a 1.6-cm adrenal mass on Mr. Hampton's right side. Should any other tests be considered?

Spiral CT is usually sufficient. The average aldosteronoma is only 1.5 cm in diameter and uniformly benign. Aldosterone excess may also be associated with adrenal cortical carcinomas. These tumors average over 12 cm in diameter at the time of diagnosis, and there is little diagnostic debate.

When the tumors are extremely small or unapparent, the patient could have bilateral hyperplasia. This condition is *not* treated by bilateral adrenalectomy. The operation leads to addisonian problems such that the treatment may be worse than the disease. Furthermore, bilateral disease is rarely associated with dangerous hypokalemia, and the hypertension can be treated in ways other than adrenalectomy. As a final condemnation of bilateral adrenalectomy, it is well known that the hypertension is usually not relieved by adrenalectomy. Adenomas may be so small as to elude identification on CT. Therefore, when the tumors are extremely small and may represent only an exaggeration of hyperplasia more prominent on one side than the other or when there is no mass seen in the adrenal but the adenoma may be too small to detect, bilateral adrenal vein cannulation and sampling can sort things out. If the adrenal vein sample is tested for both cortisol and aldosterone and compared to vena cava, a high cortisol level confirms placement of the catheter in the adrenal vein. If a true adrenal venous vein sample shows strong lateralization, that side harbors an adenoma and resection can be recommended.

What surgical treatment is recommended?

Unilateral adrenalectomy can be done by transperitoneal laparotomy or laparoscopy or through a posterior approach. These small tumors are almost ideal for laparoscopy, although conversion to an open procedure may be necessary. Many patients with significant comorbidities have been treated with spironolactone for years without particular difficulty and even those with less than ideal responses to medical management have been deemed too ill for laparotomy. Introduction of laparoscopic adrenalectomy in 1993 has caused many internists to rethink the operative approach for higher risk patients. Thus many patients previously refused surgical treatment are now coming to a safer less morbid operation.

Mr. Hampton had an uneventful right laparoscopic adrenalectomy. Six months later he has a normal serum potassium but a blood pressure of 140/98 mm Hg.

What are the diagnostic considerations?

Nearly a quarter of patients treated for aldosteronoma will still be mildly hypertensive a year after operation. Hypertension does not imply residual disease; in fact, recurrence of aldosteronoma is not expected.

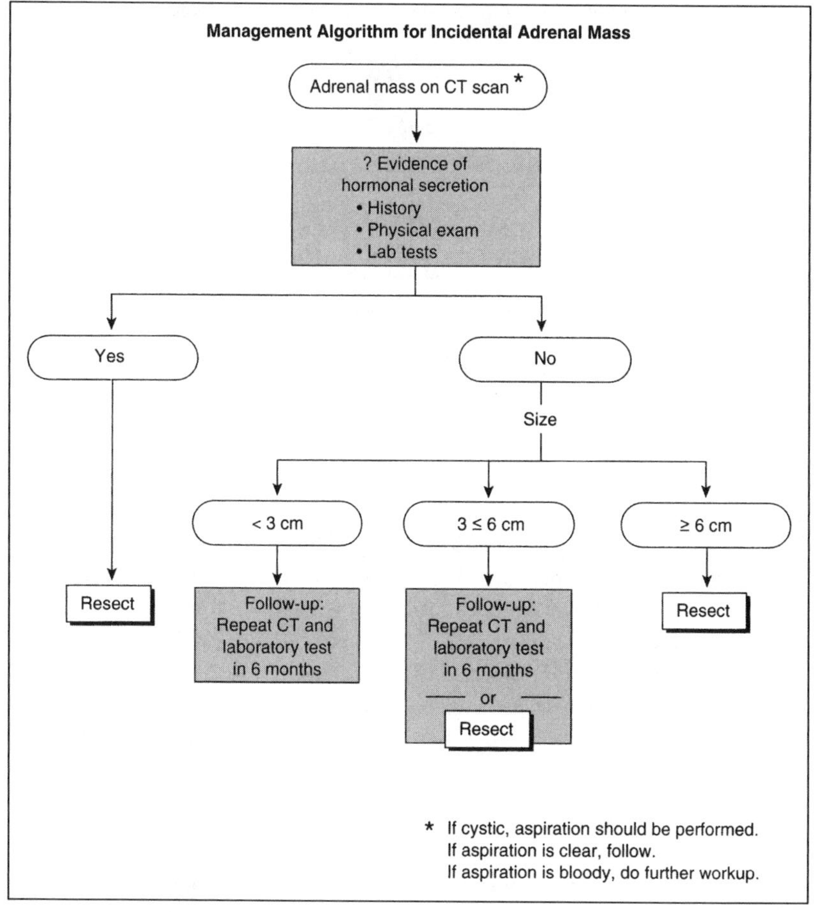

Algorithm 23.1.

RECOMMENDED READINGS

De Jong SA. What's new in general surgery: endocrine. J Am Coll Surg. 2003;197:434–443.

Bentrem DJ, Pappas SG, Ahuja Y, et al. Contemporary surgical management of pheochromocytoma. Am J Surg. 2002;184:621–624.

Cheah WK, Clark OH, Horn JK, et al. Laparoscopic adrenalectomy for pheochromocytoma. World J Surg. 2002;25:1048–1051.

Kebebew E, Siperstein AE, Clark OH, et al. Results of laparoscopic adrenalectomy for suspected and unsuspected malignant adrenal neoplasms. Arch Surg. 2002;137:948–953.

Henry JF, Sebag F, Iacobone M, et al. Results of laparoscopic adrenalectomy for large and potentially malignant tumors. World J Surg. 2002;26:1043–1047.

CHAPTER

24

CORONARY ARTERY DISEASE

Cornelius Dyke

Mr. Sternbergh is a 62-year-old salesman who presents to the emergency room with chest pain that began 2 hours earlier. He has had occasional episodes of epigastric discomfort over the last several months that he has attributed to indigestion. He describes the feeling as a heaviness that occurs in the middle of his chest and that spreads to his neck and throat. He denies back pain, arm pain, or nausea. Although he has a rather sedentary lifestyle, the pain usually occurs when he walks uphill to his office, or occasionally after meals. He also has noticed that stress from work will bring on the symptoms. Mr. Sternbergh smokes cigarettes at work and when he feels stressed. He has never been told he has diabetes. He is being treated for hypertension and dyslipidemia.

What are the major risk factors for coronary artery disease (CAD)?

Tobacco use, dyslipidemia, hypertension, and diabetes are the major modifiable risk factors for atherosclerosis, which can manifest itself in the coronary circulation, the cerebral circulation, or the peripheral circulation. Not surprising, there is considerable overlap in the involved vascular bed, such that approximately 10% of patients suffer from atherosclerotic occlusive disease affecting all three systems and over 25% of patients have two or more vascular beds involved.

What are the current recommendations for target goals for the treatment of hypertension and dyslipidemia?

The targets for both blood pressure control and lipid levels are evolving, and the trend for both is "lower is better." Current recommendations from the Joint National Committee on Hypertension 7 define the blood pressure readings as follows:

Normal: 120/80 mm Hg
Prehypertension (an abnormal pathophysiologic state): 121 to 139/81 to 89 mm Hg
Stage I hypertension: 140/90 mm Hg

The National Cholesterol Education Program Adult Treatment Panel III (NCEP ATP III) guidelines for cholesterol management state a low-density lipoprotein (LDL) level of less than 100 mg per dL is optimal and 130 to 159 mg per dl is borderline. A total cholesterol level of less than 200 mg per dL is desirable. A high-density lipoprotein (HDL) level of less than 40 mg per dL is recognized as an independent risk factor for CAD. Many lipid specialists state that more aggressive LDL lowering to below 70 mg per dL results in even greater reduction of risk.

Although these targets may change and become even more stringent, it is important to realize that a large number of patients fail to reach their targets, leaving significant room for improvement in the prevention of atherosclerotic disease.

What is your diagnosis of Mr. Sternbergh's condition?

Mr. Sternbergh is suffering from angina pectoris. Usually substernal or centered in the left chest, the feeling has been described as crushing, pressure, or heaviness, occasionally radiating to the neck, left shoulder, or left arm. Typical anginal symptoms come on slowly, reach maximal intensity within minutes, and reside with rest and nitrates within minutes. Noncardiac causes of chest pain should be considered in patients with a sharp or stabbing pain, pain that lasts seconds only, or pain associated with specific movements of the arms or shoulders. Changes in position or posture usually do not affect anginal chest pain. It is important to note, however, that symptoms of breathlessness, fatigue, belching, or epigastric discomfort may also represent anginal equivalents. Also, some patients (e.g., diabetics) may be asymptomatic. The New York Heart Association Functional Classification of angina pectoris is useful to quantitate and compare anginal symptoms (Table 24.1).

Name other causes of chest pain that may mimic angina.

The differential diagnosis of chest pain includes esophageal disorders, biliary disease, costochondritis, musculoskeletal pain or cervical radiculopathy, pericarditis, pulmonary hypertension, pulmonary embolism, and acute aortic dissection. Acute myocardial infarction (MI) must be excluded in any patient with a prolonged episode of chest pain.

What causes angina?

Angina is caused by *myocardial ischemia,* a mismatch between myocardial oxygen supply and demand. Typical angina is caused by an increase in myocardial oxygen demand brought about by physical activity. Patients with *stable angina* have fixed obstructive lesions in their coronary arteries and impaired vasodilatory

TABLE 24.1.

NEW YORK HEART ASSOCIATION FUNCTIONAL CLASSIFICATION OF ANGINA PECTORIS

Class	Activity Level
I	No limitations in physical activity. Ordinary activity does not precipitate symptoms.
II	Slight limitation in physical activity. Comfortable at rest. Ordinary activity may precipitate anginal symptoms.
III	Marked limitation in physical activity. Comfortable at rest. Less than ordinary activity precipitates anginal symptoms.
IV	Severe limitation in physical activity. Symptoms occur even at rest. Any activity exacerbates anginal symptoms.

capabilities. When the demands placed on the myocardium exceed the threshold at which the coronary arteries can supply oxygenated blood (due to the fixed obstruction), myocardial ischemia occurs and symptoms develop.

What are the determinants of myocardial oxygen consumption?

Myocardial oxygen consumption is determined by the tension developed within the wall of the heart, the contractile state of the heart, the heart rate, and the energy costs of maintaining the integrity of the myocardial cells. Heart rate is of particular importance because conditions that increase heart rate, such as exercise, stress, hyperthyroidism, and sepsis, significantly increase myocardial oxygen consumption.

What is unstable angina?

Unstable angina and acute MI are two manifestations of acute ischemic syndromes distinct from stable angina. An anginal pattern of increasing intensity or frequency is considered unstable and puts the patient at risk for acute MI. Unstable angina occurs when existing atherosclerotic plaques rupture, exposing the thrombogenic subendothelial layer. This results in localized platelet activation and thrombin generation. The localized clot may lyse, resulting in an unstable angina pattern or non–ST elevation MI, or it may progress to completely occlude the artery, causing an ST-elevation MI. The change from a stable to an unstable anginal pattern is important to recognize because medical therapy directed at inhibition of platelet function and coagulation can reduce the risk of acute MI. Although warfarin is ineffective in preventing MI in patients with acute coronary syndromes, platelet inhibition with aspirin or the more potent inhibitor clopidogrel significantly reduces the risk of MI.

Mr. Sternbergh is admitted to the emergency department. He is hypertensive and diaphoretic. An electrocardiogram demonstrates ST depression in the inferior leads. Cardiac enzymes are drawn. He is placed on oxygen, given 325 mg of aspirin, and treated with intravenous labetalol and unfractionated heparin. His blood pressure normalizes and his pain goes away. He is admitted to the hospital with a diagnosis of acute coronary syndrome and subsequently is diagnosed with a non-ST elevation MI. He remains pain free and is scheduled for cardiac catheterization.

What is the difference between an ST elevation MI and a non-ST elevation MI?

ST elevation MI represents complete occlusion of the coronary artery resulting in a transmural MI. Therapy for ST elevation MI relies on immediate reperfusion strategies, either with percutaneous coronary intervention (PCI) or with thrombolytic drugs. PCI has been demonstrated to be a superior reperfusion strategy both in terms of safety and efficacy, but it requires immediate, 24/7 catheter laboratory availability.

Non–ST elevation MI implies partial occlusion at the site of plaque rupture with ongoing thrombosis and localized lysis of the clot. Medical therapy with antiplatelet drugs and thrombin inhibitors is effective. Cardiac catheterization to assess coronary anatomy is indicated after stabilization.

Complete algorithms for the care of patients with ST elevation MI and non–ST elevation MI are beyond the scope of this chapter but are readily available.

The next day, Mr. Sternbergh undergoes elective cardiac catheterization.

Describe the anatomy of the coronary arteries.

The first branches off the aorta are the right and left coronary arteries. The left coronary artery (or left main artery) quickly branches into two large vessels, the left anterior descending artery and the circumflex artery. The left anterior descending artery and its diagonal branches supply the anterolateral left ventricular wall as well as the interventricular septum. The obtuse marginal branches of the circumflex artery supply the posterolateral wall of the left ventricle. The right coronary artery and its branches supply the right ventricular free wall and, in 85% to 90% of patients, provide blood to the posterior left ventricular wall and posterior septum through the posterior descending artery. The origin of the posterior descending artery determines the *dominance* of the coronary circulation: 10% to 15% of the population have a left dominant coronary circulation in which the posterior descending artery arises from the circumflex system.

An understanding of the blood supply of several vital cardiac structures is important. The artery to the sinus node usually arises from the right coronary artery but in up to 40% of patients it may arise from the left system. The atrioventricular node is usually supplied by a branch of the right coronary artery. The anterolateral papillary muscle of the left ventricle is usually supplied by branches of the left anterior descending artery, whereas the posteromedial papillary muscle may arise from either the right or left systems, depending on which is dominant.

Mr. Sternbergh's catheterization reveals a 90% stenotic lesion of the proximal right coronary artery and a 50% lesion in the proximal left anterior descending artery. The first obtuse marginal of the circumflex has a 20% to 30% stenosis. Left ventricular function is normal.

Which lesions are hemodynamically significant?

To restrict flow, a 75% reduction in luminal area is required; because coronary arteriograms are displayed in cross-section, this translates into a 50% reduction in cross-sectional area and therefore a stenosis of greater than 50% is generally considered to be significant. Determination of the severity of stenosis is relatively subjective and, in general, coronary angiography tends to underestimate lesion severity.

Are stenoses of less than 50% physiologically significant?

Yes. The vulnerability to rupture of atherosclerotic plaque is not related to the degree of luminal obstruction. Plaque rupture and subsequent MI can occur wherever there is atherosclerotic plaque. The vast majority of MIs, in fact, occur in vessels with less than 50% luminal stenosis, highlighting the importance of plaque stabilization and antithrombotic therapies in the prevention of acute coronary syndromes.

What are the treatment options?

Patients with atherosclerotic coronary disease may be successfully treated with medications, percutaneous angioplasty, or coronary artery bypass surgery, depending on the severity of the disease and the overall health of the patient. Patients with significant symptomatology and one- or two-vessel coronary disease with suitable coronary angiographic morphology are usually considered for percutaneous revascularization. Consensus American Heart Association/American College of Cardiology guidelines for coronary artery bypass grafting (CABG) have been published (1).

Patients with left main CAD, two-vessel disease involving the proximal left anterior descending coronary artery, multivessel coronary disease, and significant left ventricular dysfunction represent classes of patients in whom CABG provides long-term benefit. Additionally, patients with diabetes are a special category in whom surgical intervention may have greater long-term survival benefit. Elective coronary revascularization may also be necessary in patients who develop restenosis after multiple PCIs. Emergent coronary artery bypass surgery for acute angioplasty failures occurs rarely in this era of intracoronary stenting (less than 0.5% of PCIs).

Are there any randomized trials comparing angioplasty with CABG?

Oh yes. Revascularization for ischemic heart disease is one of the most intensely studied therapies for any disease. Several large, randomized trials from the 1970s compared angioplasty with coronary artery bypass, including the Veterans Administration cooperative study (2), the CASS study (3), and the European Cooperative study (4). Although these trials were important and highlighted several important lessons (e.g., the importance of surgery for multivessel and left main disease), dramatic changes in practice patterns and advancement in surgical- and catheter-based techniques have occurred since these trials were enrolling patients. Advances include the now ubiquitous use of the internal mammary artery (IMA) as a conduit, as well as the use of intracoronary stenting and pharmacologic support for percutaneous interventions. These caveats must be considered even in the interpretation of recent trials.

Many trials comparing coronary artery bypass with angioplasty were reported in the 1990s. In a follow-up of the CASS trial, 15 years after originally receiving angioplasty, 70% of patients had undergone CABG. Higher-risk patients had significantly better survival after surgery. The Bypass Angioplasty Revascularization Investigation (BARI) trialists in 1996 found an equivalent 5-year survival in patients after CABG and angioplasty; however, angioplasty patients required more frequent revascularizations. Additionally, patients with diabetes had a significantly improved survival with CABG than with angioplasty. In the Coronary Angioplasty versus Bypass Revascularization Investigation (CABRI) trial, patients after surgery had fewer anginal symptoms and were on fewer medications than patients after percutaneous transluminal coronary angioplasty (PTCA). In the EAST trial, patients had equivalent survival at 3 years (5). A meta-analysis of multiple randomized trials demonstrates a long-term survival advantage for patients at the highest risk (6). As the risk level reduces, advantages of surgical therapy decrease. It is important to note, however, that important technological advances (intracoronary stenting, drug-eluting stents, statin use, better anticoagulants) make this a continually changing environment.

In summary, long-term survival in low-risk patients with multivessel CAD is probably equivalent after percutaneous intervention or coronary bypass surgery. In higher-risk subgroups (e.g., patients with diabetes and with impaired left ventricular function), however, survival after surgical revascularization is superior. Additionally, most data demonstrate a need for multiple procedures after percutaneous intervention, as well as an increased incidence of anginal symptoms and need for anti-anginal medications. Cost implications are difficult to quantify. These and other issues remain the focus of intense study.

Mr. Sternbergh underwent successful percutaneous revascularization with angioplasty and intracoronary stenting of the right coronary artery. He recovered uneventfully. Five months later he returns to his cardiologist with recurrence of his chest pain. Evaluation and recatheterization demonstrate that the right coronary artery has restenosed with a 90% lesion within the midportion of the stent. The left anterior descending artery is approximately 70% stenosed. The first obtuse marginal branch of the left circumflex artery has a 50% to 60% stenosis. His left ventricular function is still normal.

What is restenosis?

Restenosis occurs in approximately 30% of patients after balloon angioplasty. Intracoronary stenting was a major advance in percutaneous coronary interventions in the 1990s, dramatically reducing the rate of acute vessel closure. Hyperplasia within the indwelling stent, however, may occur 3 to 6 months after placement of the stent and represents a pathophysiologic healing response at the site of the intervention. The disruption of the endothelial layer and injury to the subendothelial tissues that occurs with angioplasty promotes a strong wound healing response; intimal hyperplasia and fibroblast proliferation occur and result in a fixed, obstructive lesion within the stent. Patients typically present with recurrent, stable angina. The pathogenesis of restenosis and methods for its prevention are the subject of intense investigation.

What is a drug-eluting stent?

In an attempt to abolish the hyperplastic growth response at the site of stent implantation, stents have been impregnated with drugs that inhibit cellular proliferation. The first drug-eluting stent to reach the market was impregnated with the immunosuppressant sirolimus. A second drug-eluting stent using the antineoplastic drug paclitaxel has more recently received Food and Drug Administration approval. Both significantly reduce restenosis rates compared with bare metal stents. Other stent–drug combinations are under study. Although drug-eluting stents reduce restenosis, their impact on survival is unclear.

What are Mr. Sternbergh's treatment options now?

Again, the choice for revascularization is between a percutaneous and a surgical method. Repeat angioplasty of one or more vessels is frequently successful, with a similar incidence of restenosis. CABG should be considered more strongly now than previously, as Mr. Sternbergh has two severely stenotic lesions (including a severe left anterior descending coronary artery stenosis) with an additional lesser but still hemodynamically significant lesion (OM1). The choice of therapy should be thoroughly discussed with the patient.

What are the risks of CABG?

Kirklin demonstrated that the risk of death after coronary bypass surgery is time-related; the hazard function for death has an early phase (perioperative), a middle and constant phase (from 2 to 3 months to about 6 years), and a late, rising phase (beyond 6 years). The early risk of death relates to problems that occur during and immediately after surgery, such as stroke, perioperative MI, wound complications, bleeding, or technical problems during surgery. After recovery from operation, the risk of death is rather low and does not begin to rise again for 5 to 6 years as native coronary disease progresses and vein grafts become stenotic.

What are risk factors for morbidity and mortality after CABG?

Preoperative low ejection fraction; acute MI; cardiogenic shock; advanced age; female gender; and significant comorbid conditions such as transient ischemic attacks, stroke, renal dysfunction, and severe obstructive pulmonary disease all increase surgical risks. This is not to say that these risk factors are prohibitive, as many of these patients will derive the greatest benefit from surgical revascularization compared to medical therapy.

You note that among Mr. Sternbergh's medications he is taking clopidogrel and aspirin. You ask him to continue his aspirin and stop the clopidogrel and schedule him for elective CABG.

How does clopidogrel affect the timing of Mr. Sternbergh's surgery?

Clopidogrel is an oral theinopyridine inhibitor that reduces the risk of MI and stroke in patients at risk. Clopidogrel inhibits the adenosine diphosphate–mediated pathway for platelet activation, and its effects last for the lifetime of the platelet. Clopidogrel has been demonstrated to increase the risk of bleeding and transfusion in patients undergoing CABG. For patients with acute coronary syndromes, the increased risk of bleeding must be weighed against the risk of ischemic complications by delaying surgery. A 5-day washout period is recommended when the risks are not prohibitive. Interestingly, data are accumulating that clopidogrel used postoperatively may significantly improve graft patency and long-term outcomes after CABG.

Mr. Sternbergh asks if he will have a beating heart operation or one that uses the pump. He read on the Internet that beating heart surgery is safer.

Which surgery will you use?

Off-pump (or beating heart) CABG has significantly increased in frequency since the late 1990s. Off-pump bypass surgery uses various cardiac stabilizers to stabilize the beating heart while the coronary anastomosis is performed. All of the coronary arteries may be approached by various techniques. The rationale for off-pump surgery lies in the avoidance of cardiopulmonary bypass, which stimulates the inflammatory system, is a potent generator of thrombin, requires intensive anticoagulation, and requires manipulation of the ascending aorta. Avoidance of cardiopulmonary bypass is thought to decrease capillary leak after surgery, reduce neurologic complications after surgery, and reduce blood loss and the need for transfusions. Currently, approximately 25% of patients undergoing CABG are done with off-pump techniques. Whether results of off-pump CABG are superior to conventional CABG that uses cardiopulmonary bypass is controversial. Despite its theoretic appeal, it is difficult to demonstrate lower stroke rates, improved outcomes, or reduced hospital stay with off-pump surgery. This remains a rapidly evolving area of cardiac surgery.

After discussing the pros and cons of off-pump surgery, Mr. Sternbergh says he will agree with whichever technique you recommend. He is at relatively low risk for neurologic complications; therefore, you decide to use cardiopulmonary bypass during surgery.

Are there advances in on-pump surgery?

Yes. Making cardiopulmonary bypass safer is another area of intense investigation. Aprotinin, a serine protease inhibitor used intraoperatively, reduces fibrinolysis, improves platelet function, and reduces the systemic inflammatory response of cardiopulmonary bypass. Other drugs in late stage development reduce perioperative MI, down regulate the inflammatory response, improve graft patency, and reduce bleeding during bypass. Additionally, the bypass circuits are evolving. On-pump surgery is also an area of rapid change.

At the time of Mr. Sternbergh's operation, an arterial pressure line, a central venous catheter, and a transesophageal echocardiography are used for intraoperative monitoring. Before aortic cannulation, an epiaortic echocardiographic probe is used to assess the ascending aorta for atherosclerotic plaque. Cardiopulmonary bypass is used. The IMA is anastomosed to the left anterior descending coronary artery and reversed saphenous vein grafts are placed to the posterior descending branch of the right coronary artery and the obtuse marginal branch of the circumflex artery. His intraoperative course is unremarkable and he is transferred to the cardiac surgery intensive care unit (ICU) in good condition.

How is echocardiography used in the operating room?

The role of intraoperative echocardiography has expanded significantly and in many institutions is a routine component of intraoperative monitoring. Transesophageal echocardiography allows real-time visualization of the four cardiac chambers and allows assessment of ventricular loading condition, contractility, and regional wall motion. Epiaortic ultrasonography is the most effective way to visualize plaque within the ascending aorta and is an important component of strategies to minimize stroke and neurologic complications.

Why is the IMA the preferred conduit for revascularization?

Use of the IMA as a conduit improves both short- and long-term survival, reduces the incidence of perioperative MI, and dramatically reduces the need for subsequent revascularization. Patency of the IMA–left anterior descending coronary artery graft is 95%+ at 15 years, compared with a 50% patency rate for saphenous vein grafts at 10 years. The left internal artery to left anterior descending coronary artery bypass is used in virtually all patients, and there are few contraindications for its use.

What makes the IMA such a good conduit?

The IMA is a branch of the subclavian artery. Anatomically, the IMA has a well-formed internal elastic membrane, a very thin media with few smooth muscle cells, and a highly metabolic and active endothelium. Atherosclerosis of the IMA is virtually nonexistent. The IMA is quite reactive, with the ability to vasodilate to accommodate the metabolic needs of the tissue it is perfusing. Occasionally, patients may have a proximal subclavian stenosis that precludes its use as a pedicled graft.

There are two IMAs (right and left). Should they both be used for bypass?

Perhaps. Although it has not been demonstrated that use of bilateral IMA grafting results in improved survival over unilateral IMA grafting, there is intuitive appeal to the use of both IMAs as conduits. Use of bilateral IMAs has a down side, however, as the sternum is significantly devascularized after harvest of the right and left IMAs. This may predispose to serious infectious complications in certain patient groups, such as diabetic or obese patients. Other arterial grafts that may be considered for grafting include the right gastroepiploic artery, the radial arteries, and the inferior epigastric arteries. Whether these other conduits will match the superiority of the IMA is unclear.

What is cardioplegia?

Cardioplegic solutions arrest the heart in diastole, allowing the surgeon to operate within a still, bloodless field. By reducing all mechanical activity, myocardial oxygen consumption is reduced to basal levels. There is tremendous variety in the particular solutions, mode of delivery, temperature, and timing of delivery of cardioplegia. Using a high concentration of potassium (15 to 30 mEq per L) to induce depolarized arrest is a unifying concept. Cardioplegia may be crystalloid or blood based and may contain additives such as Kreb's cycle substrates or buffers. Cardioplegia may be delivered antegrade, through the aortic root of the cross-clamped aorta or down completed vein grafts, or in a retrograde fashion through a catheter placed within the coronary sinus. Most centers use cold cardioplegia to cool the heart to 12°C, although tepid or warm cardioplegia may be used as well. Note that some surgeons use techniques of fibrillatory arrest without cardioplegia delivery with good results. Using standard techniques of myocardial protection, cross-clamp times of over 2 hours or more can be well tolerated.

Mr. Sternbergh is noted to put out 300 mL of blood from his mediastinal chest tubes in his first hour in the ICU. He remains hemodynamically stable, although he appears mildly hypovolemic.

What conditions contribute to excessive bleeding after cardiopulmonary bypass?

Bleeding requiring reoperation occurs in approximately 1% of patients after CABG, although this incidence is higher in patients with reoperations, those with endocarditis, and those requiring hypothermic circulatory arrest. Multiple factors are causative. The potential for surgical bleeding is significant and requires strict attention to technical detail. Hypothermia, excess heparin, and platelet dysfunction after bypass all contribute to varying degrees of coagulopathy. Coagulation factor deficits are not usually problematic due to the innate redundancy of the coagulation cascade.

Are there any pharmacologic agents that can reduce bleeding after cardiopulmonary bypass?

Aprotinin (Trasylol) is a serine protease inhibitor first studied as an anti-inflammatory agent that has been demonstrated to be effective in reducing mediastinal bleeding after cardiopulmonary bypass. Aprotinin reduces the platelet dysfunction seen after cardiopulmonary bypass and inhibits kallikrein activation and subsequent fibrinolysis (perhaps through its action on protein C, a naturally circulating fibrinolytic). Aprotinin also reduces the inflammatory response after cardiopulmonary bypass. Some surgeons reserve aprotinin for patients at risk for excessive bleeding (e.g., patients undergoing reoperations, patients who have endocarditis, Jehovah's Witnesses), whereas others use it routinely. Other agents such as tranexamic acid and epsilon-aminocaproic acid (Amicar) are also used as adjuncts to hemostasis.

What are the indications for reexploration?

Chest tube output of 400 mL for the first hour or persistent bleeding of several hundred milliliters per hour for several hours should prompt the surgeon to consider reexploration. Cardiac tamponade and hemodynamic instability are the inevitable result of significant mediastinal bleeding and are best avoided by early, rather that late, reexploration.

Mr. Sternbergh's bleeding subsides gradually with warming and platelet transfusion. He remains hemodynamically stable, is extubated uneventfully, and is transferred from the ICU on the first postoperative day.

What are his chances for developing recurrent angina or MI?

Several recent trials have demonstrated an 85–90% event-free survival five years after coronary bypass grafting (5). Atherosclerosis is a relentless disease however; progression of native CAD distal to the bypass grafts, or the development of atherosclerotic plaques within saphenous bypass grafts may result in the recurrence of symptoms. Patency rates of saphenous vein grafts was thought to be approximately 50% at 10 years, though it is likely the patency rates are higher in the current era of statin therapy and more aggressive antiplatelet therapy. As mentioned above, use of the IMA–left anterior descending bypass graft positively affects survival in all groups of patients.

Mr. Sternbergh recovers well and is transferred from the ICU to a monitored bed. On postoperative day 3 his heart rate suddenly increases to 130 beats per minute and he is slightly short of breath.

What is the likely cardiac rhythm?

Atrial fibrillation with a rapid ventricular response is the likely rhythm, occurring in up to 30% of patients after cardiac surgery. The etiology is unclear but may involve the significant fluid shifts that occur after bypass and their effects on atrial stretch receptors. Atrial fibrillation is less common after off-pump surgery.

The initial treatment for atrial fibrillation is focused on slowing the ventricular rate; digoxin and diltiazem are frequently used. Amiodarone has become the preferred agent for pharmacologic cardioversion, especially in patients with impaired ventricular function. The class IA antiarrhythmics (procainamide or quinidine) are also used, although less frequently. Anticoagulation and cardioversion are required in refractory cases. Prevention of atrial fibrillation after cardiac surgery is an important and unsolved issue.

Mr. Sternbergh is treated with diltiazem and converts into a normal sinus rhythm. The rest of his recovery is uneventful and he is discharged home on postoperative day 5.

Atherosclerosis is a chronic, systemic disease; what can Mr. Sternbergh do to prevent recurrence of his angina?

Cessation of smoking is the number one preventative step patients can take to improve their long-term survival and avoid recurrence of symptoms. Statin therapy for risk reduction is imperative. Antiplatelet therapy with aspirin and clopidogrel also reduce subsequent cardiac events. Cardiac rehabilitation programs are useful to help patients initiate and maintain positive lifestyle changes such as weight loss and regular exercise.

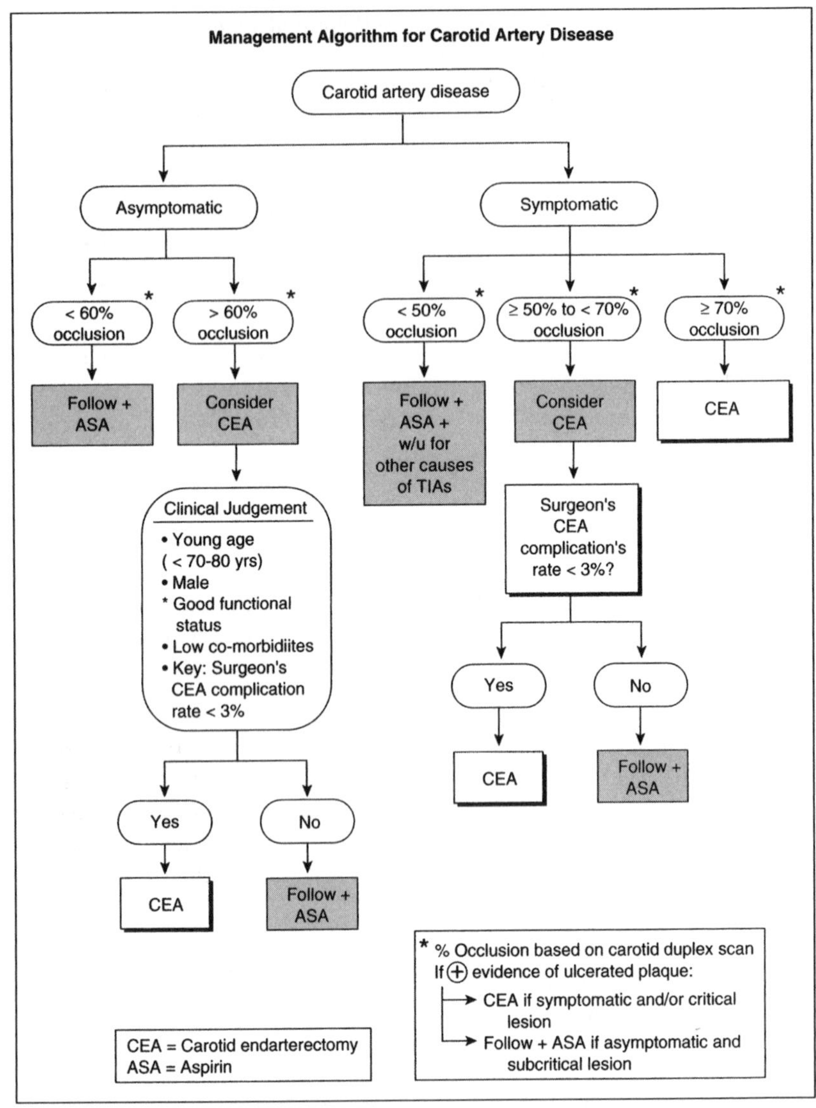

Algorithm 24.1.

REFERENCES

1. Anonymous. Comparison of coronary bypass surgery with angioplasty in patients with multivessel disease. The Bypass Angioplasty Revascularization Investigation (BARI) Investigators. N Eng J Med. 1996;335:217–225.
2. Davis KB, Chaitman B, Ryan T, Bittner V, Kennedy JW. Comparison of 15 year survival for men and women after initial medical or surgical treatment for coronary

artery disease: A CASS registry study. J American Coll Cardiol 1995;25:1000–1009.

3. European Surgery Study Group: Long Term Results of a Prospective, Randomized Study of Coronary Artery Bypass Surgery in Stable Angina Pectoris. Lancet 1982;2:1173.
4. Anonymous. First year results of CABRI (Coronary Angioplasty versus Bypass Revascularization Investigation). Lancet 1995;346:1179–1184.
5. Loop FD, Lytle BW, Cosgrove DM, et al. Influence of the internal mammary artery on 10-year survival and other cardiac events. N Engl J Med 1986;314:1–6.
6. Pocock SJ, Henderson RA, Seed P, Treasure T, Hampton JR. Quality of life, employment status, and anginal symptoms after coronary angioplasty or bypass surgery. Three year follow up in the Randomized Intervention Treatment of Angina (RITA). Circulation. 1996;94:135–142.

CHAPTER

25

VALVULAR HEART DISEASE

James S. Gammie

AORTIC STENOSIS

Stanley Osis is a 75-year-old man with no significant medical history. While mowing his lawn, he suffers a brief syncopal event. He is taken to the local emergency department and evaluated. A careful review of systems is unrevealing. On physical examination, his heart rate is 80 beats per minute and regular. Auscultation reveals a harsh crescendo-decrescendo systolic murmur that is best heard in the right second intercostal space and along the left sternal border. The murmur radiates to both carotid arteries. His peripheral pulse has a delayed upstroke and low volume (pulsus parvus et tardus). The lungs are clear, and the examination is otherwise normal. The electrocardiogram (ECG) shows normal sinus rhythm and left ventricular hypertrophy. The chest radiograph shows mild left ventricular enlargement.

What is the most likely diagnosis?

On the basis of the characteristic murmur on physical examination, the most likely diagnosis is a syncopal event caused by severe aortic stenosis.

Mr. Osis is admitted to the hospital for 24 hours. Continuous ECG monitoring shows no evidence of arrhythmia. Serial creatine phosphokinase levels are normal. Carotid Doppler studies show only mild stenosis of the left internal carotid artery. A two-dimensional transthoracic echocardiogram reveals concentric left ventricular hypertrophy with severe aortic stenosis. The calculated aortic valve area is 0.7 cm^2. Mitral valve function is normal, and the ejection fraction is estimated to be 60%.

What are the three most common causes of aortic stenosis, and what is the most likely cause in this patient?

The following are the three most common causes of aortic stenosis:

Degenerative (senile) calcific aortic stenosis: the most common cause of aortic stenosis in patients undergoing aortic valve replacement. It is characterized by immobilization of the aortic valve cusps by dense deposits of calcium. The calcium prevents normal opening of the valve during systole. Degenerative aortic stenosis is seen most commonly in patients over age 65.

Congenital bicuspid aortic valve: affects as many as 2% of infants at birth. Although a bicuspid valve usually does not cause symptoms early in life, it does generate turbulent flow that ultimately leads to fibrosis of the leaflets and to valvular stenosis. Patients with congenital bicuspid aortic valves usually develop symptoms in their 50s and 60s. Congenital bicuspid aortic valve is the most common cause of aortic stenosis in patients under 65 years of age.

Rheumatic aortic stenosis: usually occurs in a previously normal valve. It is characterized by commissural fusion (attachment of the valve cusps to each other in the clefts between the cusps). Some aortic regurgitation is common in patients with rheumatic aortic stenosis, and the mitral valve is almost always diseased.

What are the three cardinal symptoms of aortic stenosis, and what is the pathophysiology of each?

Angina, syncope, and congestive heart failure (CHF) are the three cardinal symptoms of aortic stenosis. Progressive obstruction to left ventricular outflow by the stenotic valve causes compensatory concentric left ventricular hypertrophy. This permits maintenance of cardiac output despite a significant obstruction. The hypertrophied left ventricle can maintain a large pressure gradient across the valve without a decrease in cardiac output, left ventricular dilation, or symptoms.

Angina: occurs in two thirds of patients with critical aortic stenosis and in 50% of patients it is associated with coronary artery disease (CAD). Angina is typically associated with exertion. In patients without CAD, angina results from an imbalance in myocardial oxygen supply and demand. Oxygen demand increases as a result of the increased left ventricular mass and wall tension, and myocardial blood flow is compromised by compression of intramyocardial coronary arteries.

Syncope: a result of inadequate cerebral perfusion. Syncope normally occurs during exertion, when arterial blood pressure decreases as a result of systemic vasodilation in the presence of a fixed cardiac output.

Left ventricular failure: caused by increased left ventricular filling pressures. As the ventricle progressively hypertrophies to compensate for the aortic valvular obstruction, it becomes less compliant (stiffer), and left ventricular filling pressures increase. In turn, elevated left ventricular filling pressure is transmitted to the left atrium and the pulmonary capillary bed, which results in clinical symptoms of left ventricular failure, including dyspnea with exertion, paroxysmal nocturnal dyspnea, and orthopnea. Synchronized left atrial contraction is especially important for filling of the thickened, noncompliant ventricle in aortic stenosis. The onset of atrial fibrillation and loss of this atrial kick can lead to significant hemodynamic and clinical deterioration in patients with advanced aortic stenosis.

What is the natural history of aortic stenosis, and what is the characteristic time interval between onset of each of the cardinal symptoms and death?

Patients with severe aortic stenosis can remain hemodynamically compensated for years. However, the onset of symptoms is an ominous event that portends a poor prognosis. Once patients develop angina or syncope, the average survival is 2 to 3 years. Average survival with CHF is 1.5 years. The characteristic natural history of this disease (prolonged compensated survival in the absence of symptoms, with rapid deterioration and dismal survival after the onset of symptoms) was defined by Ross and Braunwald (1) in a classic article in 1968 (Fig. 25.1). Death is rare

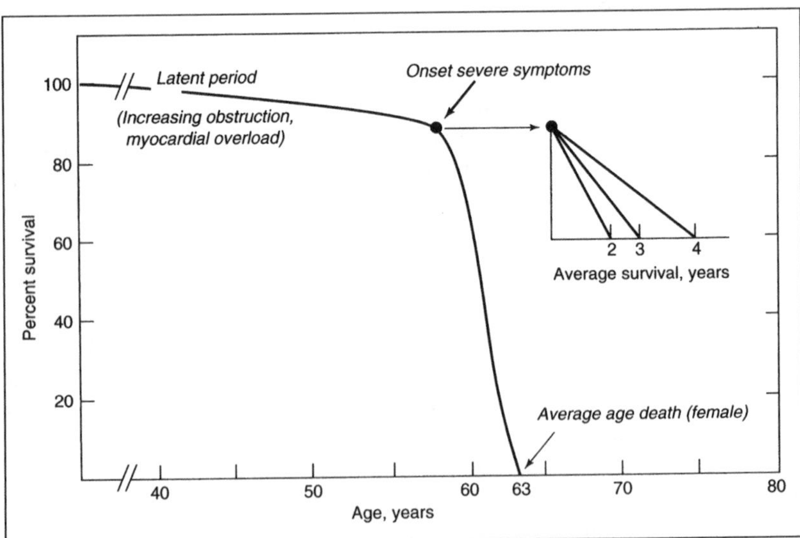

Figure 25.1. Natural history of patients with aortic stenosis. (From Ross J, Braunwald E. Aortic stenosis. Circulation. 1968;38[Suppl 5]:V61–67, with permission.)

among patients who have aortic stenosis but do not display symptoms. Thus, the indication for operation in a patient with severe aortic stenosis is the development of symptoms.

What is the next step in the workup for patients with aortic stenosis?

Cardiac catheterization is mandatory to assess the coronary anatomy. Significant CAD is common among patients with aortic stenosis, and these patients require coronary artery bypass grafting at the time of aortic valve replacement. Cardiac catheterization allows simultaneous measurement of pressure within the left ventricle and in the proximal aorta. Measurement of the pressure gradient across the aortic valve allows precise determination of aortic valve area. Catheterization also allows estimation of left ventricular function and rules out coexisting valvular heart lesions.

What is the Gorlin formula?

Developed by Richard Gorlin and his father at Peter Bent Brigham Hospital in Boston, this formula allows accurate calculation of the aortic valve area on the basis of hemodynamic data obtained during cardiac catheterization (2):

$$AVA = \frac{CO/(SEP \times HR)}{C \times \sqrt{\Delta P}}$$

where AVA is the aortic valve area (cm^2), CO is the cardiac output in liters per minute, SEP is the systolic ejection period in seconds per beat, HR is the heart rate, C is a constant, and (P) is the pressure gradient across the aortic valve. The normal aortic valve area is 3 to 4 cm^2. Symptoms generally do not develop until aortic valve area is less than 1 cm^2.

Are there any medical alternatives to aortic valve replacement?

There are no medical alternatives to aortic valve replacement. In percutaneous balloon aortic valvuloplasty, the stenotic aortic valve is dilated with a balloon. Patients generally have a reduction of peak transvalvular gradient of about 50% and an increase in valve area of 0.5 to 1 cm^2. However, 50% to 75% of patients develop restenosis within 9 months, and the 1-year mortality is 30% (3). Thus, aortic valvuloplasty should be considered only a palliative procedure applicable to patients who are not candidates for aortic valve replacement.

Mr. Osis is scheduled for elective aortic valve replacement. After a detailed discussion of the risks and benefits of surgery, he agrees to proceed.

Do patients undergoing valve surgery need any special preoperative preparation?

All patients planning to have elective heart valve surgery should undergo a careful dental examination. Severely diseased teeth (abscess, periodontal disease) should be extracted before operation to remove a source of sepsis. Other possible sources of sepsis, such as urinary tract infections, respiratory infections, or septic processes within the gastrointestinal tract should be identified and treated before operation. Prosthetic heart valves are particularly susceptible to bacterial seeding in the first few months after surgery. Prosthetic valve endocarditis has a very high (50% to 70%) mortality rate.

What are the ideal characteristics of a valve substitute?

An ideal replacement valve would have hemodynamic characteristics similar to those of native human cardiac valves, which are characterized by minimal transvalvular gradients during forward flow and freedom from regurgitation during closure. The perfect valve would be nonthrombogenic and durable, completely free of structural degeneration, resistant to infection, nondestructive to blood elements, readily available, and low in cost. Such a valve substitute has yet to be created.

What are the different types of replacement aortic valves? What factors guide the choice of a valve?

The two main categories of replacement valves are mechanical prostheses and bioprostheses. In special cases, homograft aortic valves may be used.

Bioprostheses. The most commonly used bioprostheses are stented tissue valves. They consist of a round cloth sewing ring (used to suture the valve in place) and metal struts that support the three tissue leaflets. The leaflets are made from glutaraldehyde-fixed bovine pericardium or porcine valve leaflets. Stentless bioprostheses are made from a glutaraldehyde-fixed porcine aortic root (the aortic valve and the proximal ascending aorta). Durability is similar to stented tissue valves. Stentless valves are less obstructive than stented tissue valves (they have a larger effective orifice area), but stentless valves are somewhat more time-consuming to insert. Bioprostheses have the advantage of not requiring chronic anticoagulation. This benefit is offset by a limited valve lifespan, 15 to 17 years, in the aortic position. Bioprostheses last longest in older patients; therefore, they are commonly implanted in patients older than 65 years of age and in patients with a life expectancy of less than 15 years. Bioprostheses have a gradual failure mode, such that reoperation can be performed on an elective basis.

Mechanical prostheses. The most commonly implanted mechanical prosthesis is a bileaflet tilting disc valve made of pyrolytic carbon. Mechanical prostheses have excellent long-term durability, but this advantage is offset by the requirement for long-term anticoagulation with warfarin (Coumadin). This results in a 1% to 2% rate of anticoagulant-related hemorrhage per patient-year and 0.2% annual mortality. Women of childbearing age should not receive a mechanical valve because warfarin is teratogenic. In general, mechanical valves should be implanted in patients without contraindications to anticoagulation who have a life expectancy longer than 15 years and who are not intending to bear children. Both bioprosthetic and mechanical valves carry a risk of thromboembolism of 1% to 2% per year. Older patients, whose risk of anticoagulation is greater and who have a life expectancy of less than 15 years, generally benefit from a bioprosthetic valve. Most surgeons would probably recommend a bioprosthetic valve for Mr. Osis.

Mr. Osis undergoes uncomplicated aortic valve replacement. A 25-mm bioprosthesis is inserted in the aortic position. He is extubated 4 hours after surgery and is discharged home on postoperative day 4.

What are the key technical considerations in aortic valve replacement?
After cardiopulmonary bypass is established and the heart has been arrested, the aorta is opened and the diseased valve is exposed. The valve leaflets are excised, and calcium deposits are removed. Great care must be taken to remove all loose debris to avoid a stroke. A valve of appropriate size is chosen and sutured in place.

What postoperative complications are unique to aortic valve replacement surgery?
The conduction system passes inferiorly and close to the aortic annulus near the junction of the right coronary and noncoronary valve leaflets (Fig. 25.2). Sutures placed too deep at this location can produce temporary or permanent postoperative heart block. Heart block that requires a permanent pacemaker occurs in about 1% of cases.

What is the average mortality for an aortic valve replacement?
Mortality averages 3% to 5%.

What is the long-term prognosis after aortic valve replacement?
The 5-year survival after aortic valve replacement is 75%, and the 10-year survival is 60%.

How should anticoagulation be managed in the early postoperative period? What is the target international normalized ratio (INR) for patients with artificial heart valves?
Most patients are given intravenous heparin starting 24 to 48 hours after operation. Warfarin is also administered, and heparin is stopped when the INR is therapeutic, which is 2.5 for prosthetic heart valves (4). Anticoagulation in patients who have received bioprosthetic valves usually consists of warfarin for 3 months after the operation and aspirin only thereafter, although some surgeons administer only aspirin after surgery. Mechanical valves require lifelong anticoagulation.

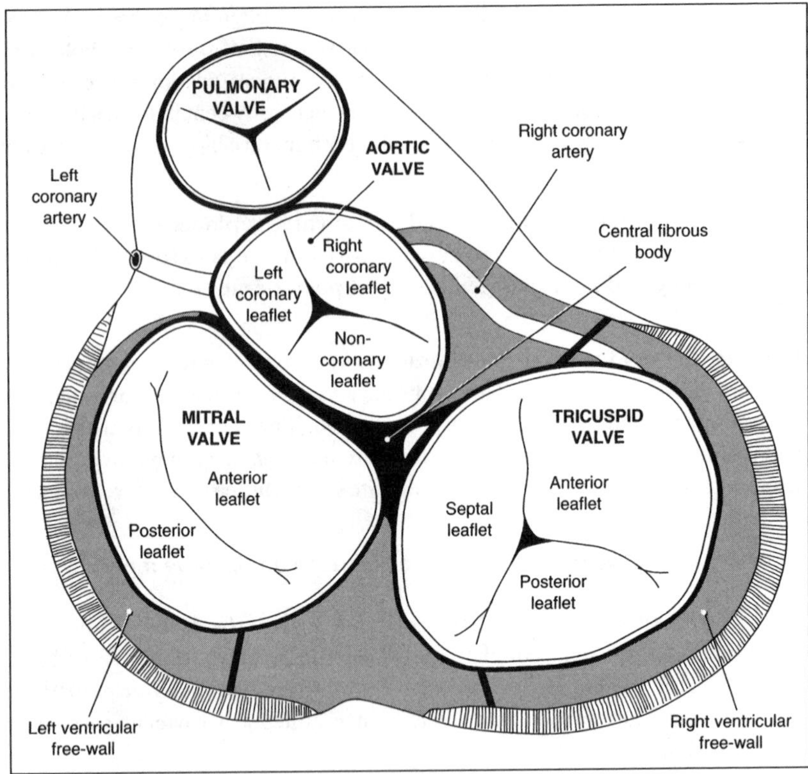

Figure 25.2. Anatomy of the aortic valve. (From Khonsari S. Cardiac Surgery: Safeguards and Pitfalls in Operative Technique. 2nd ed. Philadelphia, Pa: Lippincott–Raven; 1997, with permission.)

When can a patient resume normal activities after aortic valve replacement surgery?

Light work can generally be resumed 4 to 6 weeks after operation; heavy work, such as lawn mowing, can be resumed 3 to 4 months after operation.

AORTIC REGURGITATION

Fred Smith is a 54-year-old peanut farmer who is referred by his family physician because of an abnormal chest radiograph, which was obtained because of a recent fever and cough. Although there is no evidence of pneumonia or pulmonary disease on radiograph, the physician thought the ascending aortic silhouette looked abnormal. Mr. Smith says he has

no symptoms, and his cough has resolved. He works up to 10 hours daily on his farm and has not noted any decrease in his exercise tolerance or activity level. On physical examination, he appears in general good health. His blood pressure is 160/60 mm Hg with a heart rate of 84 beats per minute. His pulses are prominent and brisk. On auscultation, a diastolic murmur is audible, at the beginning of diastole. No systolic or carotid murmurs are appreciated, and no third or fourth heart sounds are heard. The rest of his examination is unremarkable.

What is the significance of Mr. Smith's blood pressure?

The *pulse pressure* (defined as the systolic–diastolic blood pressure) is abnormally wide, suggesting an incompetent aortic valve. This suggestion is supported by the diastolic murmur and the bounding, or water hammer, pulses. Systolic hypertension is also common.

What other pertinent findings (or lack of findings) should be elucidated from the patient's history and physical examination?

The patient should be carefully evaluated for symptoms of CHF. Patients with aortic regurgitation are asymptomatic for long periods; however, when symptoms do occur, dyspnea on exertion, orthopnea, and paroxysmal nocturnal dyspnea are common. Angina may occur even with normal coronary arteries. Onset of symptoms is a significant turning point for patients with aortic regurgitation, and it should prompt physicians and patients to seek consultation with a cardiac surgeon.

Why are the pulses bounding?

The pulse characteristics of aortic regurgitation reflect the abrupt filling of the arterial tree with the increased volume at end-diastole and the abrupt decrease in the systolic pressure due to the incompetent aortic valve. In end-stage aortic regurgitation, water hammer pulses may not be present because ventricular systolic function decreases and end-diastolic pressure increases (less regurgitant flow into the left ventricle as the pressure differential across the valve decreases).

What is an Austin-Flint murmur?

Using a stethoscope, skilled practitioners can distinguish subtle differences in the diastolic murmurs associated with aortic regurgitation. The murmur of aortic insufficiency is early in diastole and trails off in late diastole except in severe aortic insufficiency, in which the diastolic murmur may be holodiastolic. The diastolic murmur is best heard along the left and right sternal borders. The *Austin-Flint murmur,* a mid-diastolic murmur best heard at the apex, is a result of turbulence caused by the regurgitant stream of blood hitting the anterior leaflet of the mitral valve. It may be distinguished from a mitral stenosis murmur by the absence of an opening snap and loud S_1 (heard with mitral stenosis).

What are the common causes of aortic regurgitation?

Rheumatic valve disease with leaflet retraction used to be the most common cause of aortic regurgitation, but as rheumatic disease becomes less common in the United States, *annuloaortic ectasia* (dilation of the aortic root) has become the most common cause of aortic valve incompetence. The cause of the aortic root dilation is idiopathic in the vast majority of patients, although Marfan's syndrome is an important cause in a subset of these patients. Acute causes of aortic valve incompetence include Stanford type A aortic dissection and acute infective endocarditis.

How does an incompetent aortic valve affect loading conditions within the heart?

Severe acute aortic regurgitation causes volume overload of the left ventricle that is poorly tolerated and requires urgent surgical intervention. Chronic aortic regurgitation, however, produces both volume and pressure overload upon the heart. End-diastolic volume is increased, raising systolic pressure as well. Over time, the heart dilates to maintain normal systolic function and to compensate for the increased regurgitant volume. Left ventricular hypertrophy occurs to normalize left ventricular wall stress. These compensatory mechanisms work well, providing a normal cardiac output and keeping the patient asymptomatic for years. However, continued aortic valve incompetence tests the limits of these compensatory changes; eventually, left ventricular end-diastolic pressure increases, left ventricular systolic wall stress increases, and systolic and diastolic impairment ensues. At this point, symptoms occur. If treated (e.g., restoring valvular competence), these changes do not progress and, if corrected early enough, may regress. Untreated aortic regurgitation results in continued and worsening symptoms, irreversible myocardial damage, and death.

What is the natural history of mild to moderate aortic regurgitation?

Patients with mild to moderate aortic regurgitation have a 90% 10-year survival rate. Once symptoms develop, however, mean survival is only 2 years.

Is medical therapy effective treatment for aortic regurgitation?

Medications do not address the underlying problem of the leaky valve. Aortic valve replacement is required to stop the volume overload and break the vicious cycle of ventricular dilation, hypertrophy, and failure.

When is aortic valve replacement indicated for aortic regurgitation?

Timing of valve replacement is critical. It depends on the balance of two competing risks: the risks of valve replacement surgery combined with the morbidity of a prosthetic valve versus the risk of further left ventricular damage due to continued valvular incompetence. It is generally agreed that truly asymptomatic patients with normal ventricular function should be observed. Symptomatic patients with moderate to severe aortic regurgitation should undergo surgery to avoid irreversible left ventricular damage and to alter the natural history of rapidly progressive CHF. Treatment of asymptomatic patients who are beginning to show evidence of left ventricular impairment is controversial. Most surgeons and cardiologists agree that objective evidence of progressive left ventricular dysfunction is an indication for aortic valve replacement and signifies the end of the effective compensatory period.

What objective tests are useful in assessing the need for aortic valve replacement with aortic regurgitation?

Echocardiography is the most useful tool. Two critical echocardiographic criteria are the left ventricular end-systolic dimension and the ejection fraction. A left ventricular end-systolic dimension larger than 55 mm and an ejection fraction below 55% signify the beginning of left ventricular failure and the near-onset of symptoms. Surgery should be considered at this point (5).

Radionuclide scanning and cardiac catheterization also provide useful information.

How is the ascending aorta managed in patients with annuloaortic ectasia?

If the aorta is smaller than 4.5 to 5.0 cm, it does not need repair, and valve replacement only may be performed. In patients *without* Marfan's syndrome, an ascending aorta larger than 4.5 to 5.0 cm is an indication for repair at the time of valve replacement to prevent progressive dilation and rupture.

Mr. Smith undergoes an echocardiogram and chest computed tomography to assess his heart and ascending aorta. His ventricular function is normal, with a 65% ejection fraction and a left ventricular end-systolic diameter of 4.1 cm. His aortic valve leaflets appear normal, but the annulus is enlarged and the degree of regurgitation is estimated to be moderate. The ascending aorta has a diameter of 3.8 cm. Mr. Smith is advised to return to his cardiologist every 6 months for examination.

MITRAL STENOSIS

Lydia Neal is a 55-year-old woman who complains to her family physician of increasing shortness of breath, which she has noticed for several months. She works at home, and she has become increasingly fatigued and out of breath while doing her housework as well as when she is on her feet for long periods while shopping. This is a relatively new problem because she does not recall feeling breathless the previous summer. She has never been hospitalized, and her only medication is an oral hypoglycemic agent for non–insulin-dependent diabetes. She has no chest

pain, hemoptysis, fevers, stroke, weight fluctuations, or pulmonary disease. She does not smoke.

On physical examination, Mrs. Neal appears healthy, is in no distress, and has normal vital signs. Her heart rate is regular. Her head and neck examination reveals no carotid bruits, and there is a prominent jugular venous pulsation. Her lungs are clear. On cardiac auscultation, the first heart sound is loud, and the second is split normally. A soft diastolic murmur is heard. The examiner carefully listens for an opening snap but is unsure whether one is present or not. Her pulse is normal, as is the rest of her physical examination.

What are the symptoms of mitral stenosis?

Dyspnea, the classic symptom of mitral stenosis, is caused by obstruction of blood flow from the left atrium to the left ventricle by the stenotic valve. The resultant increase in left atrial pressure is transmitted to the pulmonary venous circulation and causes pulmonary congestion and dyspnea. Fatigue is a common symptom of mitral stenosis and is caused by low cardiac output and the inability to augment cardiac output with exertion. Thromboembolic events, especially stroke, may be the presenting symptom. Before the advent of anticoagulant therapy and surgical treatment, thromboembolic events were a major cause of death in patients with mitral stenosis, nearly always occurring in patients who had developed atrial fibrillation. With current therapy, this complication is much less common.

What are the classic signs of mitral stenosis?

A prominent *a* wave in the jugular venous pulse reflects the increased transmitted force of atrial contraction in patients with mitral stenosis who are in normal sinus rhythm. Patients in atrial fibrillation do not have a detectable *a* wave. The first heart sound is usually prominent and the second heart sound is normally split, at least until the development of severe pulmonary hypertension, when only a single S_2 is audible. An opening snap due to the sudden tensing of the subvalvular chordae may be heard if the leaflets are pliable. The classic diastolic murmur of mitral stenosis is low and rumbling and is a reflection of the pressure gradient across the mitral valve orifice. As the mitral valve becomes more stenotic, the murmur lengthens and consumes more of diastole. The murmur is relatively low pitched because the pressure gradients across the mitral valve are relatively low (e.g., compared with the high-pitched and high-pressure gradients of aortic stenosis). Maneuvers that reduce flow across the valve (e.g., Valsalva) reduce the intensity of the murmur.

What is the most common cause of mitral stenosis?

Rheumatic fever is the only known cause of mitral stenosis, although only 50% of patients will give a history of rheumatic fever. Patients with a history of rheumatic fever develop symptoms after a latency period that may last 20 to 25 years. Once symptoms develop, the disease progresses quickly; patients may develop severe disability in a few years. Left atrial myxoma may cause many of the signs and symptoms of mitral stenosis because of obstruction of the mitral valve orifice.

According to the New York Heart Association (NYHA) classification (see Table 24.1 in chapter 24), what functional class is Mrs. Neal in?

Although unavoidably subjective and not strict, the NYHA classification is a convenient, universal, and quick way to categorize symptoms. Mrs. Neal is fatigued with exercise and therefore falls into NYHA class II.

As an outpatient, Mrs. Neal has a normal chest radiograph and an ECG that demonstrates normal sinus rhythm without ischemia. A transthoracic echocardiogram shows moderate left atrial enlargement and normal left ventricular size and function. No thrombus is visible within the left atrium. Pulmonary artery pressure is estimated to be 35/20 mm Hg. The mitral valve leaflets are noted to be thickened, with limited excursion. Calcification is minimal. The mitral valve area (MVA) is calculated to be 1.4 cm^2, with a transvalvular gradient of 8 mm Hg.

What is the normal MVA?

The normal MVA is 4 to 6 cm^2 with no pressure gradient across the valve during diastole. Stenosis of the valve must be significant for any hemodynamic consequence; the MVA must decrease to less than 2 cm^2 (mild mitral stenosis) before left atrial pressure begins to increase. As the MVA decreases, the pressure gradient across the valve increases, so that with critical mitral stenosis (MVA less than 1 cm^2), the gradient approaches 20 mm Hg.

What are the hemodynamics of significant mitral stenosis?

As the MVA decreases into the severe and critical range, left atrial pressure rises, creating a pressure gradient across the valve. The elevated left atrial pressure is transmitted retrograde into the pulmonary veins and capillaries, increasing the hydrostatic pressure within the pulmonary circulation. Pulmonary edema and hemoptysis may result. Pathologic changes within the pulmonary arteriolar tree may be seen with long-standing severe mitral stenosis. Right-sided abnormalities, such as right ventricular dysfunction and tricuspid valvular disease, may result.

Why is the development of atrial fibrillation in patients with mitral stenosis a significant event?

In patients with mitral stenosis in normal sinus rhythm, left atrial contraction augments the transvalvular pressure gradient by approximately 30%, helping to maintain cardiac output in the normal range. The development of atrial fibrillation may be manifested by symptoms of CHF because this atrial boost to left ventricular filling is suddenly lost.

Why does exercise or exertion exacerbate symptoms?

Exercise demands an increase in flow across the valve (cardiac output) to keep up with the metabolic demands of the body. Laws of fluid dynamics dictate that at any orifice size, the gradient across the orifice is a function of the square of the transvalvular flow rate (6). Doubling the flow rate (increasing the cardiac output) quadruples the pressure gradient across the valve; this dramatic increase in left atrial pressure is transmitted to the lungs, resulting in dyspnea on exertion.

Mrs. Neal is in NYHA functional class II and has echocardiographic evidence of mild to moderate mitral stenosis. How should she be treated?

Although Mrs. Neal has recently developed symptoms and her mitral valve is stenotic, the natural history of patients with mild to moderate mitral stenosis is quite good. Patients may survive for years before the inevitable deterioration in symptoms begins; that is, the 10-year survival rate for patients with mitral stenosis and NYHA class I or II symptoms is approximately 85%. Patients with more severe symptoms (NYHA classes III and IV) have 5-year survival rates that are much worse (40% and 15%, respectively). Therefore, Mrs. Neal should be treated medically and closely followed.

Mrs. Neal is started on furosemide and digoxin and, on follow-up several weeks later, she says she feels better. She does well for the next 2 years, but at that time returns to her physician complaining that she cannot do as much as she used to. She gets short of breath in the grocery store and has to take a break while doing her laundry. A repeat echocardiogram at this time demonstrates that her MVA is 0.9 cm^2, with a transvalvular gradient at rest of 12 mm Hg.

What are the indications for mitral valve replacement or repair?

In general, surgery is recommended for patients who are significantly symptomatic (NYHA class III or IV) with severe mitral stenosis (MVA less than 1 cm^2). Patients who have had a thromboembolic event should also be considered for surgery because the risk of recurrent thromboembolism from the left atrium is high.

Are there any alternatives to surgical repair or replacement of the mitral valve?

Percutaneous balloon mitral valvotomy is a catheter-based technique for performing mitral commissurotomy. In selected patients, balloon valvotomy can double the effective mitral orifice and halve the gradient. The major benefit of balloon valvotomy is the avoidance of median sternotomy and cardiopulmonary bypass; this can be especially useful in patients for whom surgery poses a high risk. Echocardiographic scores help identify patients in whom balloon valvotomy is most effective: younger patients with minimal valvular calcification, good leaflet morphology (not much leaflet chordal thickening), and minimal mitral regurgitation may benefit from balloon valvotomy. Significant mitral regurgitation, unacceptable echocardiographic score, and known left atrial thrombus discourage balloon valvotomy.

What are the surgical options for the treatment of mitral stenosis?

Closed mitral commissurotomy was initially performed in 1923 and successfully applied by Harken and Bailey in 1948. Closed mitral commissurotomy is accomplished without cardiopulmonary bypass. It consists of inserting a finger through a hole in the left atrium to separate the fused commissures. In some cases, a mechanical dilator is introduced via the apex of the left ventricle to assist with commissurotomy. Closed mitral commissurotomy is particularly effective for patients with minimal valvular calcification, absent mitral regurgitation, and no left atrial thrombus. The requirement for reoperation averages 50% at 10 years. The development of safe and effective techniques for cardiopulmonary bypass has permitted direct vision of the valve during open mitral commissurotomy. Closed mitral commissurotomy is still commonly used in developing nations, where access to cardiopulmonary bypass is limited.

Open mitral commissurotomy is performed via a median sternotomy: the heart is arrested and the left atrium is opened and examined for thrombus. The left atrial appendage is oversewn to prevent formation of further thrombi. The fused commissures are divided with a scalpel to within 2 mm of the annulus, and the underlying subvalvular apparatus (the chordae tendinea and the papillary muscles) are inspected. Areas of fusion of the chordae or papillary muscles are incised. The operative risk of open mitral commissurotomy is less than 1%, and the incidence of reoperation for recurrent mitral stenosis is 10% to 20% at 10 years.

Mitral valve replacement is required when the degree of disease of the mitral valve or subvalvular apparatus makes mitral valve repair impossible. The choice between a bioprosthetic and a mechanical replacement valve is dictated by similar considerations for aortic valve replacement (discussed earlier). If possible, the posterior leaflet and chordae of the mitral valve are preserved during mitral valve replacement; the posterior leaflet is folded between the sewing ring of the valve and the annulus. Preservation of this structure improves postoperative ventricular function and long-term survival.

Describe the surgical anatomy of the mitral valve. What key structures surrounding the mitral valve are at risk for injury during operation, and where are they?

The mitral valve is the doorway to the left ventricle. It consists of two leaflets, the anterior and posterior, which are anchored by the circumferential mitral annulus.

The anterior leaflet is attached to the anterior third of the annulus, whereas the posterior leaflet is anchored to the remaining two thirds of the annulus. Prolapse of the mitral valve into the left atrium during systole is prevented by the subvalvular apparatus, which consists of the chordae tendineae, the papillary muscles, and the left ventricle. The chordae are anchored to the papillary muscles, which in turn arise from the left ventricle. Key structures surrounding the mitral valve include the left circumflex coronary artery, the coronary sinus, the atrioventricular node, and the noncoronary leaflet of the aortic valve.

Mrs. Neal successfully undergoes open mitral commissurotomy. Findings at operation include fused commissures that are easily incised and several fused chordae that are similarly incised. She is discharged from the hospital on postoperative day 4. At follow-up examination, she is symptom free (NYHA class I) and has resumed normal activities. A follow-up echocardiogram demonstrates a mitral valve of 3 cm^2 and no evidence of mitral regurgitation. Ventricular function is normal.

Should Mrs. Neal take an anticoagulant?

No. After valve repair, only patients with atrial fibrillation or with a preoperative history of a thromboembolic event require anticoagulation.

MITRAL REGURGITATION

James Hovis is a 54-year-old National Park ranger with a 4-month history of progressive shortness of breath. He notes that he is becoming increasingly fatigued at work, especially walking up hills. He has no chest, back, or arm pain and says that 6 months ago he was completely asymptomatic. He does not smoke and takes no medications. He has a family history of heart disease. Pertinent findings on physical examination include a holosystolic murmur best heard at the apex of the heart and radiating to the axilla. It is high pitched, with little respiratory variation. His lungs are clear to auscultation. The remainder of his examination is unremarkable. An ECG demonstrates atrial fibrillation and no evidence of ischemic injury. The chest radiograph demonstrates clear lungs and a slightly enlarged cardiac silhouette. No significant annular calcification is present.

What is the working diagnosis?

Mr. Hovis's symptoms and cardiac examination suggest mitral valve regurgitation. Mr. Hovis has had some degree of mitral regurgitation for many years. The character of the murmur helps differentiate it from aortic stenosis, which is harsher, radiates to the neck rather than the axilla, and is associated with a diminished upstroke of the central pulses.

Is this a chronic or acute process?

It is likely that Mr. Hovis's mitral regurgitation is chronic. The atrial fibrillation suggests that the mitral regurgitation is long-standing and has led to left atrial distention and fibrillation. Acute mitral regurgitation is usually associated with a normal left atrial size, increased pulmonary artery pressures, and sometimes flash pulmonary edema. Important causes of acute mitral regurgitation that may be elicited from the history and physical examination include bacterial endocarditis (with ruptured chordae tendineae) and ischemic heart disease resulting in papillary muscle dysfunction or rupture.

What should be the next diagnostic test?

Echocardiography is a powerful tool for examining valvular heart disease and is useful in determining the causation and hemodynamic consequences of mitral regurgitation. It is also useful in evaluating the other heart valves and left ventricular function.

What important anatomic features of the mitral valve should be assessed?

The mitral annulus, leaflets, and subvalvular apparatus (chordae tendineae and papillary muscles) may all contribute to mitral regurgitation. The normal mitral annulus is approximately 4 cm^2, but any disease process causing left ventricular dilation may cause annular dilation. Annular dilation reduces the coapting surface area of the anterior and posterior leaflets and may result in a central jet of regurgitation. It is also critical to assess the degree of annular calcification, particularly in the elderly. Severe mitral annular calcification may preclude valve repair or replacement. Causes of chordal rupture include degenerative valve disease, endocarditis, rheumatic disease, and ischemic heart disease. Posterior chordae rupture more frequently and may result in a flail leaflet segment, causing an eccentric regurgitant jet; this anatomic detail is detectable with echocardiography. A ruptured papillary muscle head produces a similar regurgitant picture. Leaflet abnormalities causing valve retraction or thickening may occur with rheumatic heart disease (although stenosis is more common), systemic lupus erythematosus, and healed endocarditis.

Mr. Hovis has an echocardiogram, which shows a dilated mitral annulus, a flail segment of the posterior leaflet with an eccentric regurgitant jet tracking posteriorly along the left atrial wall. The left atrium is dilated, and there is no significant calcification of the valve or subvalvular apparatus. The degree of regurgitation is severe. His left ventricular function is normal.

Why is Mr. Hovis short of breath and easily fatigable?

Left atrial compliance and effective forward cardiac output are two principal factors that determine symptoms in patients with mitral regurgitation. When mitral regurgitation has sudden onset, the normally small atrium is loaded with a large regurgitant volume, and the left atrial pressure may increase dramatically. Pulmonary congestion and hypertension may result, with sudden shortness of breath or flash pulmonary edema. With chronic mitral regurgitation, the left atrium enlarges with time, sometimes to quite massive dimensions, allowing large volumes of regurgitant flow to enter the left atrium with little change in pressure (increased compliance). This is one reason patients may tolerate mitral regurgitation for years without symptoms.

Mitral regurgitation places an increased volume load on the heart. In addition to the forward cardiac output across the aortic valve, a significant portion of the stroke volume is regurgitant and enters the left atrium. To maintain cardiac output, end-diastolic volume increases, and the heart dilates progressively, which over time exacerbates the regurgitation (hence the saying "mitral regurgitation begets more mitral regurgitation"). However, because the left ventricle is unloaded, left ventricular wall tension does not increase or increases very slowly, which is another reason why patients tolerate significant degrees of mitral regurgitation for years without symptoms. Eventually, however, these compensatory mechanisms are exhausted; exercise intolerance and easy fatigability occur because the left ventricle cannot maintain an adequate cardiac output to meet the systemic demands of exercise. Hence, exertional dyspnea occurs.

What medical management of patients with mitral regurgitation is available?

Diuretics are important because they reduce pulmonary artery pressure and reduce stroke volume, hence left ventricular dimension. This allows improved leaflet coaptation and can significantly reduce the degree of mitral regurgitation.

What are the indications for operation for patients with severe mitral regurgitation?

There are several important indications for operation for patients with mitral regurgitation. The presence of symptoms mandates surgical repair or replacement of the valve: symptoms can be relieved with surgery, and progressive left ventricular dysfunction can be prevented or in some cases reversed. Asymptomatic patients with evidence of *left ventricular dysfunction* (defined as an ejection fraction less than 60%, end-systolic diameter larger than 45 mm) should undergo surgical correction of mitral regurgitation because further delay results in a poor outcome after surgery. Although patients without symptoms and normal left ventricular function may not appear to warrant surgery, there are strong data to support an aggressive early operative approach. If the mitral valve is repairable, most surgeons would recommend surgery to prevent long-term mortality. Such patients have a risk of sudden death of approximately 4% per year.

Should Mr. Hovis have his valve surgically repaired or replaced?

Definitive treatment requires surgical replacement or repair of the flail segment. Patients with symptoms or patients whose ventricle is progressively dilating on serial echocardiographic examinations are candidates for surgery.

What is the difference between mitral valve repair and mitral valve replacement?

Standard therapy for mitral valve disease for decades has been mitral valve replacement with a prosthesis. Although this approach results in a competent valve, the morbidity of a prosthetic valve is significant (e.g., bleeding, degeneration of a bioprosthesis requiring a reoperation, stroke, prosthetic valve endocarditis). In the 1980s, Dr. Alain Carpentier introduced and popularized techniques to repair the native valve. The advantages of mitral valve repair are clear: repair avoids the need for long-term anticoagulation, the risk of stroke and endocarditis are extremely low, operative mortality is lower (1% to 2 % for mitral valve repair versus 6% for mitral valve replacement), and valve repair is durable, with durability of greater than 95% 20 years after surgery.

How should Mr. Hovis's valve be repaired?

Using cardiopulmonary bypass and cardioplegia, the left atrium is entered and the valve carefully inspected. If the valve is reparable, a variety of techniques can be employed to effect a repair. These include insertion of a circular cloth covered ring (an annuloplasty ring) around the valve to restore coaptation of the valve leaflets, resection of a portion of the diseased leaflet, reconstruction of broken or elongated chords with Gore-Tex suture, and incision of the commissures to enlarge the mitral valve orifice. In this patient's case, the flail segment of the posterior leaflet is excised and the edges reapproximated. An annuloplasty ring is sewn to the annulus (taking care not to reduce the annular size excessively), and the valve is tested. Transesophageal echocardiography is critical to assess valve function in the operating room after weaning from cardiopulmonary bypass.

What incision will be required for Mr. Hovis's valve repair surgery?

Traditionally, mitral valve surgery has been performed through a median sternotomy. A newer approach that is rapidly gaining acceptance is *minimally invasive videoscopic mitral valve repair*. Using a videoscope for visualization of the valve, the repair is performed through a 2-inch incision in the middle of the right chest. Patients undergoing minimally invasive videoscopic mitral valve repair can return to work within a few weeks (as compared with 2 to 3 months with a sternotomy) and require fewer blood transfusions.

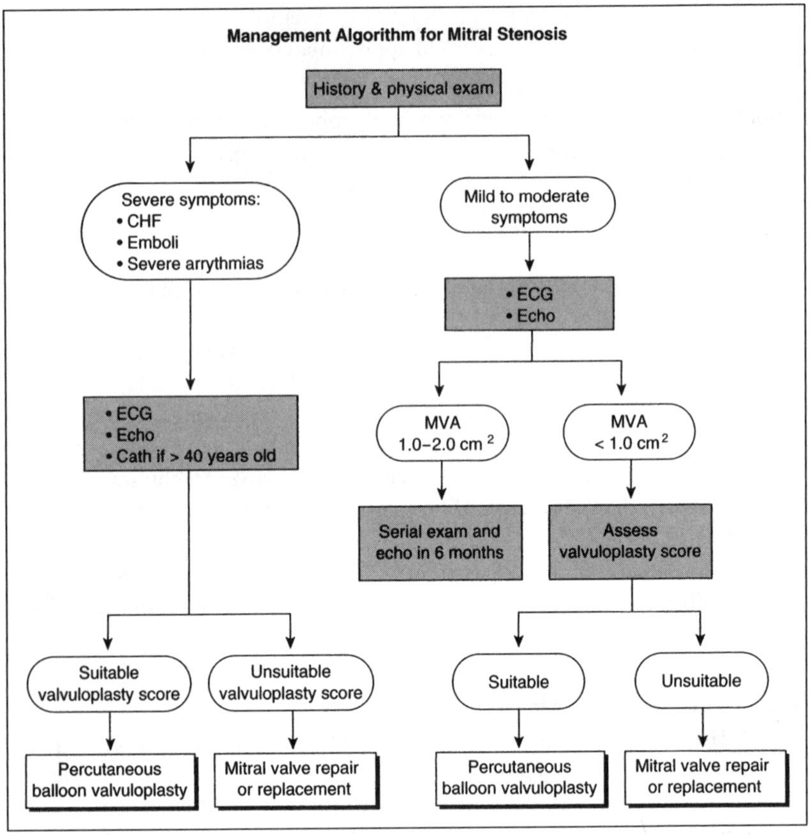

Management Algorithm for Mitral Stenosis

History & physical exam

- Severe symptoms:
  - CHF
  - Emboli
  - Severe arrythmias
  - → • ECG • Echo • Cath if > 40 years old
    - Suitable valvuloplasty score → Percutaneous balloon valvuloplasty
    - Unsuitable valvuloplasty score → Mitral valve repair or replacement
- Mild to moderate symptoms → • ECG • Echo
  - MVA 1.0–2.0 cm ^{2} → Serial exam and echo in 6 months
  - MVA < 1.0 cm ^{2} → Assess valvuloplasty score
    - Suitable → Percutaneous balloon valvuloplasty
    - Unsuitable → Mitral valve repair or replacement

Algorithm 25.1A.

What is the MAZE procedure?

The MAZE procedure is a surgical cure for atrial fibrillation. Atrial fibrillation is a macro-reentry arrhythmia and requires a critical mass of atrial tissue to be maintained. (Atrial fibrillation is uncommon in small animals whereas it is common in large animals.) The MAZE procedure involves division of the right and left atria into smaller segments, such that atrial fibrillation cannot be sustained. It was introduced in 1987 by Dr. James Cox and involved cutting and suturing large segments of the atria. Normal sinus rhythm is restored in 90% to 95% of patients undergoing the MAZE procedure. New technologies, such as cryotherapy, now allow the MAZE procedure to be performed quickly, without cutting and sewing, and have equivalent success rates to the traditional MAZE procedure. Mr. Hovis should have a concomitant MAZE procedure to cure his atrial fibrillation. This approach will avoid the need for long-term anticoagulation therapy.

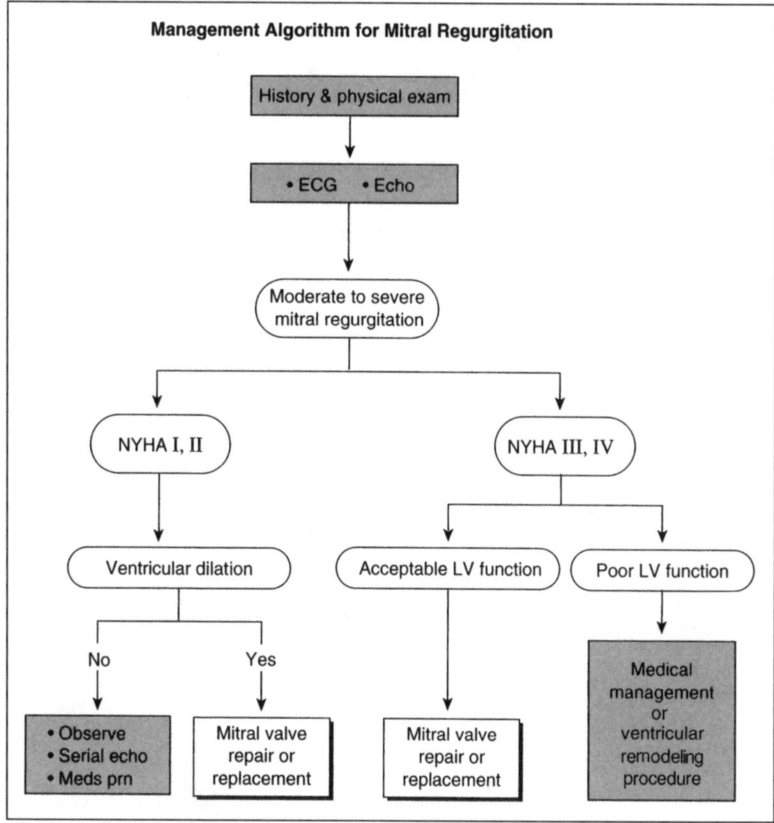

Algorithm 25.1B.

Mr. Hovis undergoes successful mitral valve repair with a MAZE procedure and recovers uneventfully. After a 6-week recuperative period, he returns to work.

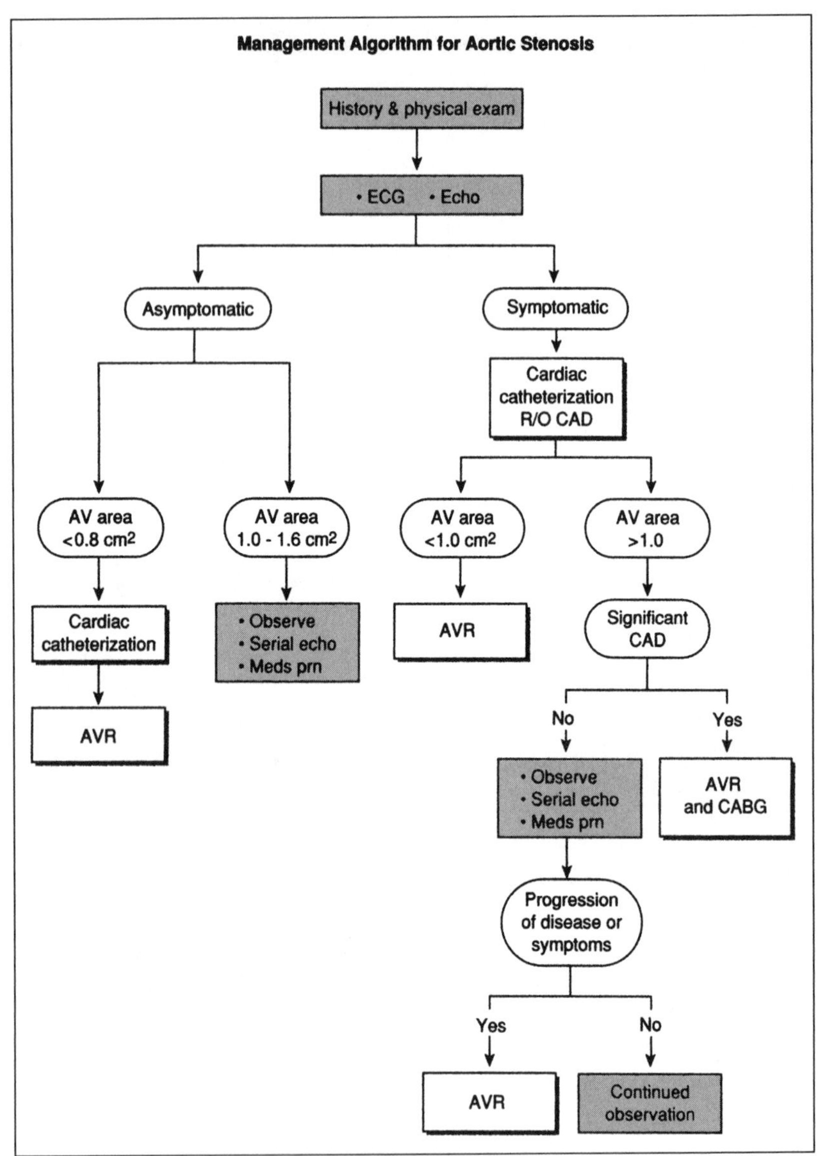

Algorithm 25.1C.

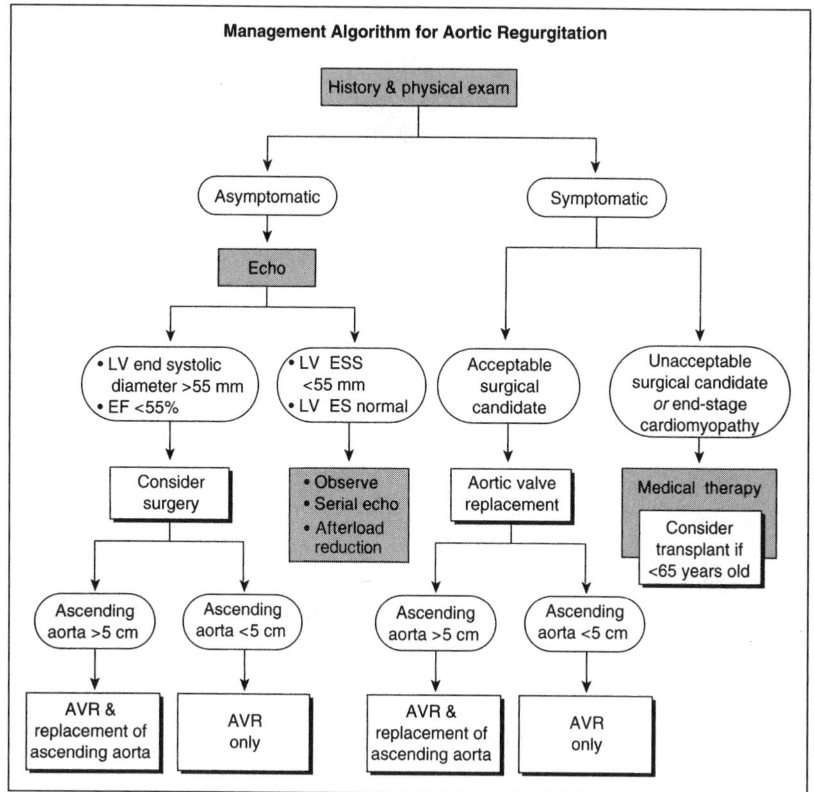

Algorithm 25.1D.

REFERENCES

1. Ross J Jr, Braunwald E. Aortic stenosis. Circulation. 1968;38(Suppl 5):V61–67.
2. Gorlin R, Gorlin G. Hydraulic formula for calculation of area of stenotic mitral valve, other cardiac values and central circulatory shunts. Am Heart J. 1951;41:1.
3. Desnoyers MR, Isner JM, Pandian NG, et al. Clinical and noninvasive hemodynamic results after balloon angioplasty for aortic stenosis. Am J Cardiol. 1988;62:1078–1084.
4. Stein PD, Alpert JS, Copeland J, et al. Antithrombotic therapy in patients with mechanical and biological prosthetic heart valves. Chest. 1995:108:371s–379s.
5. ACC/AHA Guidelines for the management of patients with valvular heart disease: a report of the American College of Cardiology/American Heart Association Task Force on Practice Guidelines. J Am Coll Cardiol. 1998;32:1486–1588.
6. Olsean KH. The natural history of 271 patients with mitral stenosis under medical treatment. Br Heart J. 1962;24:349–357.

CHAPTER

26

LUNG CANCER

Pasquale Ferraro and André Duranceau

Derek Ferguson is a 59-year-old auto mechanic who is admitted to the hospital with a fever, persistent cough, and blood-streaked sputum. He was treated by his family doctor with oral antibiotics for an episode of acute bronchitis 2 weeks ago. He has a 40-pack-year smoking history and his medical history is significant for non–insulin-dependent diabetes mellitus and peptic ulcer disease. Over the years, he has had several episodes of what he calls bronchitis. He is mildly short of breath on exertion but denies any chest pain or wheezing. His weight is stable and he maintains an active 40-hour work week.

What are the possible diagnoses based on this history?

The differential diagnosis at this point includes community-acquired pneumonia, acute bronchitis, exacerbated chronic bronchitis, and lung cancer.

Is fever a common finding with lung cancer?

Fever, which affects only 10% of patients with lung cancer, is usually associated with postobstructive atelectasis or pneumonia. An abscess can develop in a tumor cavity, but this is rare.

What are the clinical manifestations of lung cancer?

More than 90% of patients with lung cancer have symptoms (pulmonary, metastatic, systemic, or paraneoplastic) at the time of diagnosis. Bronchopulmonary symptoms, including coughing, dyspnea, chest pain, and hemoptysis, are found in up to 80% of patients. Some 30% of patients have metastatic disease at presentation, and the usual symptoms are those associated with central nervous system (CNS), bone, or liver metastases. Although common, adrenal gland metastases are rarely symptomatic. Systemic symptoms such as malaise, weight loss, and anorexia are found in 34% of patients. Paraneoplastic syndromes (found in 2% of patients) secondary to lung cancer are among the most varied in clinical presentation. The different types of syndromes include endocrine (hypercalcemia, Cushing's syndrome, syndrome of inappropriate antidiuretic hormone secretion, gynecomastia), neurologic (encephalopathy, peripheral neuropathy, polymyositis, Eaton-Lambert syndrome), skeletal (clubbing, pulmonary hypertrophic osteoarthropathy), cutaneous (acanthosis nigricans), and hematologic disorders. Only 5% of patients with lung cancer are asymptomatic at the time of diagnosis (1,2).

On physical examination, Mr. Ferguson appears healthy. He is mildly overweight and shows no signs of respiratory distress. His heart rate, blood pressure, and respiratory rate are normal, and his temperature is 38°C. There is no clubbing, and the head and neck examination shows no suspicious lymph nodes. Chest auscultation reveals some crackles over the left lung; the right lung is clear; heart sounds are normal; and the liver is not tender.

Which tests are ordered initially?

Blood tests should include a complete blood count and electrolyte, blood urea nitrogen, and creatinine levels. A chest radiograph and electrocardiogram (ECG) should be ordered as well.

The results of the initial blood tests and ECG are normal. The chest radiograph shows a 4-cm mass in the left upper lung and a clear right lung field.

What is the differential diagnosis on the basis of these findings?

1. Inflammatory or infectious conditions such as abscess, granuloma, tuberculosis, fungal infection, or pneumonia
2. Neoplastic disorders, including benign lung tumors and malignant tumors (primary lung cancers and secondary or metastatic lesions)
3. Congenital lesions
4. Traumatic lesions

What are other pertinent findings on a simple chest radiograph in a patient suspected of having lung cancer?

Important radiologic findings include a mass with irregular borders, no calcifications, a pleural effusion, an elevated diaphragm, a widened mediastinum, and contralateral nodules. Areas of pneumonitis often surround central tumors with an endobronchial component. When possible, comparison with older radiographs is essential to establish the evolving nature of a nodule or mass.

Which radiologic features characterize a benign lesion in a patient with a solitary pulmonary nodule?

Features of a benign nodule include a smooth border, homogenous appearance, fat within lesion, calcifications in a benign pattern (central, laminated, or diffuse), and stable size over 2 years (3).

What is the likelihood that a radiologically detected mass in a patient such as Mr. Ferguson is cancer?

In a 59-year-old man with a history of heavy smoking and a newly discovered 4-cm mass, the likelihood is greater than 90% that the lesion is a bronchogenic carcinoma. Generally, in the adult population, any new pulmonary nodule carries a 50% risk of being a malignancy if the patient has a significant smoking history (1).

What is the incidence of lung cancer in the United States?

The estimated total number of new cases in 2004 is 173,770, and the estimated number of lung cancer deaths is 160,440. The probability of developing lung cancer is 1 in 12 for men and 1 in 19 for women (4).

What factors have been linked to the development of lung cancer?

Tobacco smoking is undoubtedly the most important causative factor in lung cancer. The lung cancer mortality is 20- to 70-fold higher in smokers than in nonsmokers. Although generally believed to be an important factor, air pollution independent of tobacco use increases the risk of lung cancer only slightly. Exposure to uranium, asbestos, arsenic, nickel, chromium, or beryllium carries proven occupational risk. Certain organic compounds (aromatic hydrocarbons, chlormethyl ether, and isopropyl oils) have also been implicated. The association of dietary factors with lung cancer is less convincing. The consumption of vegetables or fruits containing beta-carotene is considered to be protective, whereas dietary animal fat is believed to promote the development of lung cancer (5).

What additional workup does a patient with probable lung cancer require?

Additional workup is needed to (a) confirm the diagnosis, (b) establish the extent and resectability of the lesion, and (c) assess operability.

How is the diagnosis of lung cancer confirmed?

The diagnosis may be confirmed with sputum cytology, bronchoscopy, or transthoracic needle biopsy. Histologic confirmation may be obtained with a more invasive procedure, such as cervical mediastinoscopy, scalene node biopsy, thoracoscopy, or exploratory thoracotomy.

What is the yield from and the importance of these different diagnostic tests?

Sputum cytology is the most useful test for central hilar lesions, endobronchial tumors, and squamous cell carcinoma, with an overall diagnostic yield of 82%

when three early morning specimens are analyzed; with peripheral tumors, the yield is 40% to 50%. The overall rate of false-positive results with sputum cytology is 1% to 3% (6). Bronchoscopy is diagnostic in 25% to 50% of patients with small cell or squamous cell carcinoma. Additional analysis of brushings and washings increases the yield to 90% (2). Bronchoscopy also provides information on tumor location and extent that helps in staging the tumor, and it helps identify a synchronous cancer in another lobe or in the contralateral lung in 1% to 2% of patients. A transthoracic needle biopsy should not be performed as part of the routine workup for lung cancer because the results seldom affect management, it has no value in the staging process, and the procedure is associated with a 30% risk of pneumothorax. Furthermore, the rate of false-negative findings can be as high as 15% to 25% (7). Transthoracic needle biopsy should be limited to patients with a clinically unresectable lesion, to high-risk patients who are inoperable for medical reasons, and to patients who refuse surgery.

How are patients assessed for operability?

Determination of operability necessitates a cardiac workup in patients with symptoms of heart disease, a significant medical history, or risk factors for coronary artery disease. Pulmonary function tests, exercise tolerance, and overall performance status must be assessed in all patients. Renal function and presence of other major systemic diseases also should be evaluated in selected patients.

How is lung cancer classified and staged?

The TNM staging classification is based on a number of specific criteria with respect to the tumor (T) (size, site, local invasion, associated atelectasis), the lymph nodes (N) (hilar, mediastinal, or extrathoracic nodes; ipsilateral or contralateral nodes), and the presence of distant metastases (M). The TNM classification is shown in Table 26.1. The staging of lung tumors according to the TNM classification is shown in Table 26.2.

Why is the TNM classification important?

The TNM system serves several purposes, such as selecting the most appropriate therapy, establishing the prognosis, and permitting the comparison of data and results.

How are the extent of the lesion and its resectability evaluated?

Bronchoscopy and computed tomography (CT) of the chest are the best techniques for evaluating the local and regional extent of lung cancer. A bronchoscopic finding that suggests unresectability is invasion of the trachea or main carina. On CT of the chest, indications of unresectability include bulky N2 disease (metastatic ipsilateral mediastinal adenopathy), N3 disease (contralateral mediastinal or extrathoracic metastatic adenopathy), or any T4 lesion (invasion of the heart, great vessels, esophagus, trachea, or vertebral body).

TABLE 26.1.

TNM CLASSIFICATION FOR LUNG CANCER

Primary Tumor (T)

T0	No evidence of primary tumor
TIS	Carcinoma in situ
T1	Tumor 3 cm or smaller, not involving the visceral pleura and not invading proximal to the lobar bronchus
T2	Tumor larger than 3 cm; tumor with invasion of visceral pleura or extending into mainstem bronchus but more than 2 cm from carina; or tumor with lobar atelectasis
T3	Tumor of any size with invasion of parietal pleura, chest wall, pericardium, mediastinal pleura, or diaphragm; tumor in mainstem bronchus within 2 cm of carina but not involving carina; tumor with atelectasis of entire lung; or superior sulcus (Pancoast) tumor
T4	Tumor of any size with invasion of mediastinum, heart, great vessels, esophagus, vertebral body, trachea, or carina; or tumor with malignant pleural effusion

Nodal Involvement (N)

N0	No metastases to regional lymph nodes
N1	Metastases to peribronchial or ipsilateral hilar lymph nodes
N2	Metastases to ipsilateral mediastinal lymph nodes
N3	Metastases to contralateral hilar or mediastinal lymph nodes or to extrathoracic lymph nodes (scalene or supraclavicular)

Distant Metastases (M)

M0	No known distant metastases
M1	Distant metastases present

Which tests are included in the workup for metastatic disease?

Blood tests consist of liver function tests and determination of the serum calcium level. CT of the chest includes imaging of the liver and adrenal glands, both frequent sites of lung metastases. Unsuspected metastases have been found in the liver or adrenal glands in 3% to 7% of patients (8,9). A bone scan and head CT is obtained in selected cases and in all symptomatic patients.

What is the role of positron-emission tomography (PET) scanning in patients with suspected lung cancer?

PET scanning can be used to characterize pulmonary nodules as malignant or benign, to stage lung cancer both locoregionally and systemically, and to help assess response to treatment in a neoadjuvant or adjuvant setting.

TABLE 26.2.

STAGING OF LUNG CANCER WITH TNM CLASSIFICATION

Stage	Classification
IA	T1, N0, M0
IB	T2, N0, M0
IIA	T1, N1, M0
IIB	T2, N1, M0, T3, N0, M0
IIIA	T3, N1, M0; T1, N2, M0; T2, N2, M0; T3, N2, M0
IIIB	T4, any N, M0; any T, N3, M0
IV	Any T; any N; M1

What types of malignant tumors may yield false-negative results with a PET scan?

Bronchoalveolar carcinomas and carcinoid tumors typically have a low metabolic activity and thus a reduced level of FDG accumulation, resulting in a negative PET scan. Also, tumors less than 1 cm in diameter are generally not visualized with PET imaging.

What are the most frequent sites of metastases from a lung cancer?

In descending order of occurrence, the most frequent sites are the mediastinal lymph nodes, the contralateral lung, the adrenal glands, the liver, the brain or CNS, and the bones.

Mr. Ferguson's blood tests, including liver enzymes, are normal. CT shows a 4-cm mass in the anterior segment of the left upper lobe. The hilar or mediastinal nodes are not enlarged, there is no pleural effusion, and the left lower lobe and the right lung appear normal. Both the liver and the adrenal glands are free of metastases. Bronchoscopy shows a large, friable, irregular mass in the left upper lobe bronchus 2 cm from its origin on the left main stem bronchus. Biopsy of the lesion reveals a squamous cell carcinoma.

What is the clinical stage of Mr. Ferguson's disease?

According to the TNM classification, the tumor is T2, N0, M0. It is stage IB.

How are malignant tumors of the lung classified histologically?

The histologic classification of lung tumors is presented in Table 26.3.

Which are the most common metastatic tumors to the lung?

The most common tumors responsible for lung metastases are breast, prostate, kidney, and colon tumors; soft tissue sarcoma; and thyroid carcinoma.

TABLE 26.3.

HISTOLOGIC CLASSIFICATION OF MALIGNANT LUNG TUMORS

Primary Malignant Tumors

- Bronchogenic carcinoma
  - Squamous cell carcinoma (spindle cell, exophytic endobronchial)
  - Adenocarcinoma (acinar, papillary, bronchoalveolar)
  - Large cell carcinoma (giant cell, clear cell, neuroendocrine)
  - Small cell carcinoma (oat cell, intermediate, mixed)
  - Adenosquamous carcinoma
  - Bronchial gland carcinoma (carcinoid tumors, adenoid cystic, mucoepidermoid)
- Nonbronchogenic carcinoma
  - Sarcoma
  - Lymphoma
  - Melanoma
  - Pulmonary blastoma

Secondary Malignant Tumors

- Metastatic lesions from primary tumors outside the lung

What is the incidence of the different types of bronchogenic carcinomas?

The frequencies of the different types of bronchogenic carcinomas are as follows (10):

- Adenocarcinoma (the most common type), 40% to 45%
- Squamous cell carcinoma, 30% to 35%
- Large cell carcinoma, 5% to 15%
- Small cell carcinoma, 20% to 25%

What are some important characteristics of each of the four types of bronchogenic carcinoma?

Squamous cell carcinoma. This was once the most frequent type of bronchogenic carcinoma but now accounts for approximately one third of cases. Typically located in major bronchi (lobar or first segmental bronchus), it is often perihilar, slow growing, and large when diagnosed. Central necrosis with cavitation is possible, and distant metastases occur late in the evolution.

Adenocarcinoma. Adenocarcinoma is the most common type of lung cancer. Most lesions arise from peripheral bronchial branches rather than from major bronchi and present initially as solitary nodules less than 3 cm in diameter. Endobronchial central adenocarcinomas are much less common. Spread to hilar and mediastinal nodes occurs readily, and 20% of patients with this tumor have distant metastases at the time of diagnosis. A subtype known as *bronchoalveolar* *carcinoma* presents as multicentered nodules or as a diffuse infiltrate with air bronchograms. Although local recurrences after surgery are common with bronchoalveolar carcinomas, these tumors have a more favorable prognosis.

Large cell carcinoma. Large cell carcinoma is a peripheral lesion in 60% of patients, and two thirds of these tumors are larger than 4 cm. Some 10% of patients have metastatic mediastinal adenopathy at the time of diagnosis. These poorly differentiated carcinomas are believed by some experts to be anaplastic adenocarcinomas.

Small cell carcinoma. Small cell carcinoma accounts for 20% to 25% of bronchogenic cancers. These tumors arise in major bronchi and are generally central. Half of patients have metastatic hilar and mediastinal adenopathy. Subtypes include oat cell, intermediate cell, and combined oat cell carcinomas. Features of squamous cell carcinoma or glandular differentiation are common (1,2,10).

After the clinical stage and histology of the tumor have been determined, how is preoperative pulmonary functional status assessed?

All patients undergoing a thoracotomy must have pulmonary function tests (PFTs) (spirometry and diffusing capacity for carbon monoxide [DLCO]) to establish the extent of resection (wedge, lobectomy, or pneumonectomy) that will be tolerated. Selected patients may require more advanced testing, including arterial blood gas (ABG) analysis, quantitative ventilation/perfusion ($\dot{V}/\dot{Q}$) scanning, and exercise testing to determine maximal oxygen consumption ($\dot{V}O_2$ max). The $\dot{V}/\dot{Q}$ scan allows calculation of the amount of functional residual lung tissue after a resection by establishing the percentage of blood flow to each segment before the surgery. Echocardiogram and right heart catheterization with pulmonary artery measurements may be indicated in the rare patient with clinical signs of pulmonary hypertension or right ventricular failure.

What PFT values constitute an acceptable operative risk for pneumonectomy?

Risk associated with pneumonectomy is considered acceptable if preoperative forced expiratory volume in 1 second (FEV_1) is greater than 60% (2 L), the maximal voluntary ventilation is greater than 50%, and DLCO is more than 60%; or if predicted postoperative values are FEV_1 higher than 40% and DLCO higher than 40%. Most patients with a preoperative FEV_1 of more than 40% tolerate lobectomy well (11,12).

How does the VO_2 max help in assessing operability?

A patient whose predicted postoperative FEV_1 is less than 30% to 40% should undergo formal exercise testing and a desaturation study. The VO_2 max alone has been used as an independent predictor of postoperative morbidity. A VO_2 max greater than 15 to 20 mL per kg per minute is generally associated with low mortality and acceptable operative risk, whereas a V_{O_2} max less than 10 mL per kg per minute contraindicates any resection other than a biopsy or wedge (12,13).

Mr. Ferguson's PFTs show an FEV_1 of 1.5 L (50%), maximum voluntary ventilation (MVV) of 45%, and DLCO of 40%. The PFT results prompt ABG analysis and quantitative $\dot{V}/\dot{Q}$ scanning. The ABG determinations on room air are normal, and the $\dot{V}/\dot{Q}$ scan shows 57% of the perfusion to the right lung and 43% to the left lung with an equal distribution to the left upper and left lower lobe. V_{O_2} max measurement reveals oxygen consumption of 12 mL per kg per minute.

What is the appropriate resection for a patient with these pulmonary test results?

The patient can tolerate a wedge resection, segmentectomy, or lobectomy. A pneumonectomy would probably be associated with poor postoperative pulmonary function and should not be carried out.

Should a cervical mediastinoscopy be performed in a case such as Mr. Ferguson's?

Before the advent of CT, mediastinoscopy was performed as a staging procedure in all patients with lung cancer. However, the routine use of mediastinoscopy is associated with a positive yield of 30% to 35% for central lesions and only 5% for peripheral tumors. Metastases are rarely detected with nodes that are smaller than 1 cm on the chest CT (in only 2% to 7% of patients). However, with nodes larger than 1 cm, mediastinoscopy reveals metastases in 60% to 80% of patients (14–16). Mr. Ferguson's CT shows no nodes larger than 1 cm; he should probably not undergo a mediastinoscopy before thoracotomy.

In what circumstances is a mediastinoscopy recommended?

Mediastinoscopy is recommended in patients with (a) nodes larger than 1 cm in the paratracheal region, (b) nodes larger than 1.5 cm in the subcarinal area, (c) large hilar masses, (d) chest wall involvement, (e) recurrent lung cancer before surgery, or (f) bilateral lesions. Mediastinoscopy may also be used to exclude small cell lung cancer.

Mr. Ferguson is taken to the operating room and a left posterolateral thoracotomy is performed. Exploration shows no signs of metastatic disease. A standard lobectomy with a mediastinal nodal dissection is carried out. The left lower lobe is free of nodules and masses.

Why is it important to do frozen section analysis during the procedure?

The resection margins must be verified by pathologic analysis to be free of tumor, and any suspicious nodules in the remaining lobe must be sampled for biopsy. Also, the status of the hilar and interlobar nodes should be established, and whether there is N2 disease must be determined during the procedure because this may influence the type and extent of resection.

What should be done if a pleural effusion is discovered at the time of thoracotomy?

If pleural effusion is present, metastatic seeding of the parietal pleura must be ruled out. A malignant effusion is classified as a T4 tumor (stage IIIB) and contraindicates resection. If the pleura appears normal, a sample should be sent for immediate cytologic examination. Lung cancer patients may have an inflammatory effusion (transudate), which does not preclude a pulmonary resection. Despite an extensive preoperative workup, 2% to 5% of patients are found at the time of thoracotomy to have unresectable lesions (1,2).

The final pathologic examination shows that Mr. Ferguson's tumor is a moderately differentiated squamous cell carcinoma with metastases to two peribronchial lymph nodes (T2, N1, M0, stage IIB). Resection margins on the bronchus are free of tumor.

Is a lobectomy optimal therapy for Mr. Ferguson's lung cancer?

For a stage II non–small cell lung cancer, a complete surgical resection with negative margins is sufficient treatment. Although the incidence of local or regional recurrences is reduced with postoperative radiation therapy, survival is not improved. Trials with neoadjuvant chemotherapy and radiation therapy are under way. Adjuvant therapy after a complete resection is not recommended (17–19).

What are the survival rates for patients with stage I and stage II disease, and what are some prognostic factors?

Stage I (T1, N0 and T2, N0) tumors are associated with a 5-year survival rate of 60% to 80%. Lesions less than 3 cm in diameter have a significantly better prognosis than do larger T2 lesions. Adjuvant therapy is not recommended for patients after a complete resection. Recurrences, mainly distant metastases, are found in 20% of patients. Stage II (T1, N1; T2, N1; and T3, N0) lung cancers are associated with a 40% 5-year survival rate. Prognostic factors include size of the tumor, histology (squamous cell carcinoma has a more favorable prognosis than does adenocarcinoma), and the number of N1 nodes. The location of the tumor and invasion of the visceral pleura do not affect survival. The sites of recurrence appear to depend on tumor histology. Squamous cell carcinomas recur locally, whereas adenocarcinomas have a tendency to recur at distant sites (20–22).

What is recommended therapy for stage IIIA cancers, especially for N2 disease?

For locally advanced stage IIIA lesions (T3, N1), the mainstay of therapy is complete surgical resection with a mediastinal node dissection. Peripheral tumors with chest wall involvement should be resected en bloc. Prognostic factors with T3 tumors include complete resectability, extent of chest wall invasion, and any regional lymph node metastases. The 5-year survival rate varies from 20% to 40% (23–25).

The management of N2 disease remains controversial. Symptomatic N2 disease with rare exceptions is considered unresectable. Median survival in these patients varies from 6 to 12 months. Asymptomatic patients with bulky N2 disease as determined by CT or bronchoscopy also have a poor prognosis, with a 10% 5-year survival rate (26). A number of trials to evaluate the role of neoadjuvant chemotherapy and radiation therapy are under way (27–31). Surgery alone is not recommended in this situation. Patients in whom N2 disease is discovered at mediastinoscopy are an interesting subset of patients with stage IIIA disease. Generally, 80% of such patients have unresectable tumors. However, prognostic factors (e.g., number of nodes, number of nodal stations, location of nodes, and extracapsular extension) have been identified, and surgery may therefore be indicated in selected patients.

In patients with micrometastases, aortopulmonary window involvement, or metastasis limited to one node in whom the tumor is completely resected, 5-year survival rates of 15% to 20% have been reported. Overall, the prognosis remains poor, and neoadjuvant therapy in combination with surgery should be recommended for most patients (32,33). Patients with unsuspected but completely resectable N2 disease discovered at thoracotomy have a more favorable outcome. Prognostic factors include the number of nodes, number of nodal stations, location of nodes, and any extracapsular invasion. The tumor status also influences survival. A 5-year survival rate of 20% to 30% has been reported in selected patients after a complete resection (34–36). T1, N2 lesions are associated with survival as high as 45%, and a rate of 10% has been reported with larger T3, N2 lesions. Postoperative radiation therapy for N2 disease discovered at thoracotomy seems beneficial in patients at high risk for local recurrence and in patients with an incomplete resection (37).

How should stage IIIB tumors be managed?

With stage IIIB disease (T4 or N3 lesions), therapy is limited, prognosis is poor, and patients should be considered inoperable (20,21). Neoadjuvant therapy is being studied and may be favorable (30). Within this subgroup, a T4 lesion invading the superior vena cava with negative mediastinal nodes may be considered resectable in selected patients. Unfortunately, local recurrences ultimately develop in most patients even after a complete resection (22).

Mr. Ferguson's immediate postoperative course is uneventful. Chest tubes are removed on the fourth postoperative day. He is comfortable, walking, and mildly short of breath on exertion. A chest radiograph

shows a well-reexpanded left lower lobe with a small residual pleural effusion. However, on the day before his discharge, he suddenly becomes markedly short of breath as he is getting out of bed. His vital signs are heart rate, 110 beats per minute; blood pressure, 160/85 mm Hg; respiratory rate, 24 breaths per minute; and O_2 saturation, 88% on room air. Both lung fields are relatively clear on auscultation.

What is the most likely diagnosis, and what measures should be taken?

The most likely diagnosis is a pulmonary embolus or pneumothorax. Included in the differential diagnosis are atelectasis, aspiration pneumonia, and acute myocardial infarction. Supplemental oxygen should be administered to maintain saturation at more than 92%, a peripheral intravenous line should be inserted, and blood tests, ABG measurements, chest radiographs, and ECG should be ordered.

With a 50% oxygen facemask, Mr. Ferguson's respiratory rate decreases to 18 breaths per minute and oxygen saturation increases to 94%. The ECG and chest radiographic findings are normal. ABG testing shows a pH of 7.31, partial pressure of carbon dioxide of 34 mm Hg, partial pressure of oxygen of 68 mm Hg, and bicarbonate level of 24.

How should the patient be managed?

The most probable diagnosis is a pulmonary embolus. If the patient has no contraindications, heparin should be started and a $\dot{V}/\dot{Q}$ scan should be ordered to confirm the diagnosis. Monitoring in an intensive care unit may be necessary if the patient becomes hemodynamically unstable or develops progressive hypoxemia. Although pulmonary emboli are relatively uncommon after thoracic surgery (fewer than 2% of patients), they are associated with a mortality that may be as high as 50% (38).

Mr. Ferguson's $\dot{V}/\dot{Q}$ scan shows perfusion defects in both left and right lower lobes, suggesting a high probability of pulmonary emboli. He remains clinically stable, with only mild hypoxemia and no signs of right ventricular failure. A Doppler ultrasound study of his lower extremities does not reveal any signs of deep venous thrombosis. He is eventually discharged home 10 days after the incident and is treated with oral anticoagulation for 6 months.

What are the morbidity and mortality after pulmonary resection for lung cancer?

Major complications occur in 10% of patients with stage I and II disease. A complication rate of 20% is reported in patients who require an extended resection for locally advanced tumors (stage III). Mortality after lobectomy and

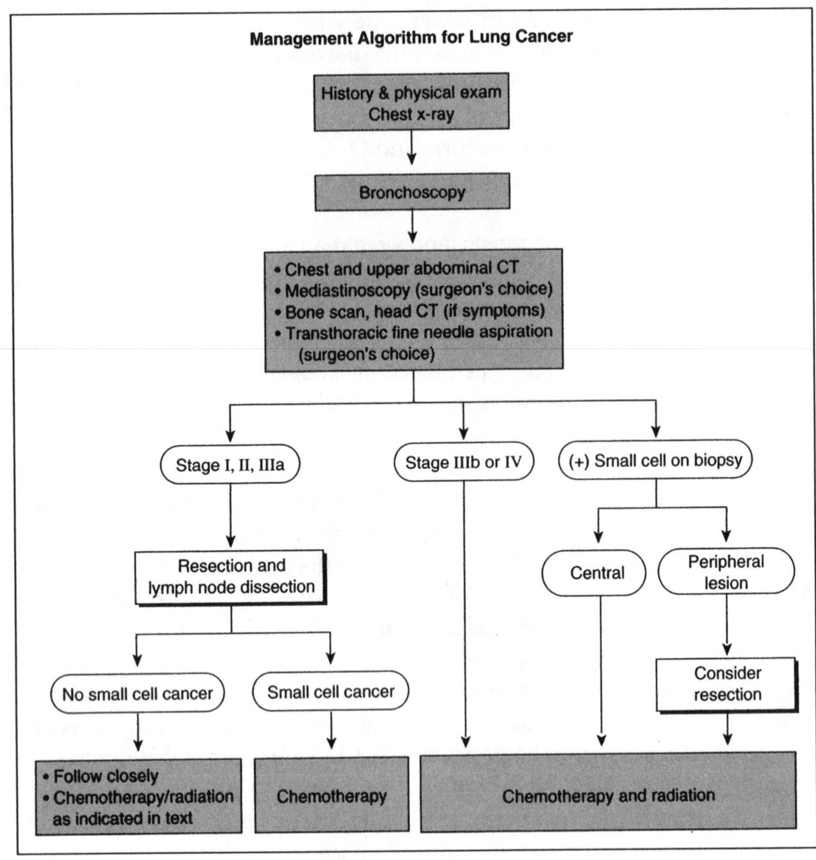

Algorithm 26.1.

pneumonectomy is 1% to 2% and 4% to 7%, respectively. Risk factors for postoperative complications include age over 70 years, restricted pulmonary reserve, and the need for pneumonectomy (39,40).

REFERENCES

1. Shields TW. Presentation, diagnosis, and staging of bronchial carcinoma and the asymptomatic solitary pulmonary nodule. In: Shields TW, ed. General Thoracic Surgery. 4th ed. Philadelphia, Pa: Williams & Wilkins; 1994:1122–1154.
2. Maddaus M, Ginsberg RJ. Lung cancer: diagnosis and staging. In: Pearson FG, ed. Thoracic Surgery. New York, NY: Churchill Livingstone; 1995:671–690.
3. Khouri NF, Meziane MA, Zerhouni EA, et al. The solitary pulmonary nodule: assessment, diagnosis and management. Chest. 1987;91:128–133.
4. American Cancer Society. Cancer Statistics 2004.

5. Miller AB. Lung cancer: epidemiology. In: Pearson FG, ed. Thoracic Surgery. New York, NY: Churchill Livingstone; 1995:648–661.
6. Ng A, Horak GC. Factors significant to the diagnostic accuracy of lung cytology in bronchial washings and sputum samples. Acta Cytol. 1983;27:397.
7. Wescott JL. Direct percutaneous needle aspiration of localized pulmonary lesions: results in 422 patients. Radiology. 1980;137:31.
8. Lewis JW, et al. Can computed tomography of the chest stage lung cancer: yes or no? Ann Thorac Surg. 1990;49:591.
9. Pagani JJ. Non–small cell lung carcinoma adrenal metastases: computed tomography and percutaneous needle biopsy in their diagnosis. Cancer. 1984;53:1058.
10. Zaman MB. Lung cancer: pathology. In: Pearson FG, ed. Thoracic Surgery. New York, NY: Churchill Livingstone; 1995:661–670.
11. Arroglia AC, Buzaid AC, Mattay RA. Which patients can safely undergo lung resection? J Respir Dis. 1991;12:1080.
12. Epstein SK, Faling JL, Daly B, et al. Predicting complications after pulmonary resection: preoperative exercise testing vs a multi-factorial cardiopulmonary risk index. Chest. 1993;104:694.
13. Bechard D, Wetstein L. Assessment of exercise oxygen consumption as preoperative criterion for lung resection. Ann Thorac Surg. 1987;44:344.
14. Luke WP, Pearson FG, Todd TRJ, et al. Prospective evaluation of mediastinoscopy for assessment of carcinoma of the lung. J Thorac Cardiovasc Surg. 1986;91:53–56.
15. Gross BH, Glazer GM, Orringer MB, et al. Bronchogenic carcinoma metastatic to normal sized lymph nodes: frequency and significance. Radiology. 1988;166:71–74.
16. Backer CL, Shields TW, Lockhart CG, et al. Selective preoperative evaluation for possible N_2 disease in carcinoma of the lung. J Thorac Cardiovasc Surg. 1987;93:337–343.
17. Martini N, Burt ME, Bains MS, et al. Survival after resection in stage II non–small cell lung cancer. Ann Thorac Surg. 1992;54:460.
18. Holmes EC, Gail M. Surgical adjuvant therapy for stage II and stage III adenocarcinoma and large cell undifferentiated carcinoma. J Clin Oncol. 1986;4:710–715.
19. Lung Cancer Study Group. Effects of postoperative mediastinal radiation on completely resected stage II and stage III epidermoid cancer of the lung. N Engl J Med. 1986;315:1377–1381.
20. Mountain CF. Value of the new TNM staging system for lung cancer. Chest. 1989;96:47S.
21. Naruke T, et al. Prognosis and survival in resected lung carcinoma based on the new international staging system. J Thorac Cardiovasc Surg. 1988;96:440.
22. Martini N, Ginsberg RJ. Lung cancer: surgical management. In: Pearson FG, ed. Thoracic Surgery. New York, NY: Churchill Livingstone; 1995:690–705.
23. McCaughan BC, Martini N, Bains MS, et al. Chest wall invasion of carcinoma of the lung: therapeutic and prognostic implications. J Thorac Cardiovasc Surg. 1985;89:836.
24. Piehler JM, Pairolero PC, Weeland LH, et al. Bronchogenic carcinoma with chest wall invasion: factors affecting survival following en-bloc resection. Ann Thorac Surg 1982;34:684.

25. Allen MS, Mathisen DJ, Grillo HC, et al. Bronchogenic carcinoma with chest wall invasion. Ann Thorac Surg. 1991;51:948–951.
26. Shields TW. The significance of ipsilateral mediastinal lymph node metastasis (N_2 disease) in non–small cell carcinoma of the lung. J Thorac Cardiovasc Surg. 1990;99:48–53.
27. Faber LP, Kittle CF, Warren WH, et al. Preoperative chemotherapy and irradiation for stage III non–small cell lung cancer. Ann Thorac Surg. 1989;47:669–677.
28. Weiden PL, Piantadosi S, The Lung Cancer Study Group. Preoperative chemotherapy and radiation therapy in stage III non–small cell lung cancer: a phase II study of the Lung Cancer Study Group. J Natl Cancer Inst. 1991;83:266–272.
29. Burkes RL, Ginsberg RJ, Shepherd F, et al. Induction chemotherapy with mitomycin, vindesine and cisplatin for stage III unresectable non–small cell lung cancer: results of the Toronto phase II trial. J Clin Oncol. 1992;10:580–586.
30. Rusch VW, Albain KS, Crowley JJ, et al. Surgical resection of stage IIIA and stage IIIB non–small cell lung cancer after concurrent induction chemoradiotherapy: a Southwest Oncology Group trial. J Thorac Cardiovasc Surg. 1993;105:97–106.
31. Martini N, Kris MG, Flehinger BJ, et al. Preoperative chemotherapy for stage IIIA (N_2) lung cancer: the Sloan Kettering experience with 136 patients. Ann Thorac Surg. 1993;55:1365–1374.
32. Roth JA, Fossella F, Komaki R, et al. A randomized trial comparing perioperative chemotherapy and surgery with surgery alone in resectable stage IIIA non–small cell lung cancer. J Natl Cancer Inst. 1994;86:673–680.
33. Rosell R, Gomez-Codina J, Camps C, et al. A randomized trial comparing preoperative chemotherapy plus surgery with surgery alone in patients with non–small cell lung cancer. N Engl J Med. 1994;330:153–158.
34. Martini N, Flehinger BJ. The role of surgery in N2 lung cancer. Surg Clin North Am. 1987;67:1037.
35. Naruke T, Goya T, Tsuchuya R, et al. The importance of surgery to non–small cell carcinoma of the lung with mediastinal lymph node metastasis. Ann Thorac Surg. 1988;46:603.
36. Patterson GA, Piazza D, Pearson FG, et al. Significance of metastatic disease to subaortic lymph nodes. Ann Thorac Surg. 1987;43:155.
37. Swayer TE, Bonner JA, Gould PM, et al. Effectiveness of postoperative irradiation in stage IIIA non–small cell lung cancer according to regression tree analyses of recurrence risks. Ann Thorac Surg. 1997;64:1402–1408.
38. Tedder M, Anstadt MP, Tedder SD, et al. Current morbidity, mortality and survival after bronchoplastic procedures for malignancy. Ann Thorac Surg. 1992;54:387.
39. Ginsberg RJ, Hill LD, Eagan RT, et al. Modern thirty-day operative mortality for surgical resections in lung cancer. J Thorac Cardiovasc Surg. 1983;86:498.
40. Deslauriers J, Ginsberg RJ, Dubois P, et al. Current operative morbidity associated with elective surgical resection for lung cancer. Can J Surg. 1989;32:335.

CHAPTER

27

SURGERY FOR CHRONIC OBSTRUCTIVE PULMONARY DISORDER

Pasquale Ferraro and André Duranceau

Jerry Robinson, a retired 52-year-old postal worker, goes to his local hospital's emergency department for shortness of breath. Mr. Robinson states that while lifting boxes in his garage, he suddenly felt an intense pain over his right chest and began breathing heavily. He says he has never had this type of pain before in his life, and he describes it as worsening with deep breathing. His medical history is significant only for hypertension and a cholecystectomy. He admits to having smoked two packs of cigarettes a day since age 20 years, but he has not smoked a single cigarette during the past 18 months. He denies any chest pain, coughing, or hemoptysis before this episode. He has been short of breath on mild exertion (dyspnea scale, 2.75) for a number of years, and he has used bronchodilators occasionally for what he calls a wheezing problem. The patient has no drug allergies, and his medication includes a calcium channel blocker for high blood pressure.

What is the most likely diagnosis in Mr. Robinson's case?

The most likely diagnosis with this history is spontaneous pneumothorax. The differential diagnosis at this point includes pulmonary embolus, acute bronchospasm, myocardial infarction, and less probably, dissecting aortic aneurysm.

On physical examination, Mr. Robinson is agitated, diaphoretic, and tachypneic. He is conscious, well oriented, and not cyanotic. His vital signs are as follows: heart rate, 112 beats per minute, regular sinus; blood pressure, 168/94 mm Hg; respiratory rate, 24 breaths per minute; temperature, 37.3°C; and oxygen saturation, 90% on room air. His jugulars are not distended, his heart sounds are normal, and chest auscultation reveals decreased breath sounds diffusely, no wheezing, and increased

resonance on percussion over his right chest. Examination of his abdomen and lower extremities is unremarkable.

What should be included in Mr. Robinson's initial workup?

The workup on admission should consist of a complete blood count, electrolytes, blood urea nitrogen and creatinine levels, cardiac enzymes, a chest radiograph, and an electrocardiogram (ECG).

Mr. Robinson's blood work, cardiac enzymes, and ECG are within normal limits. The chest radiograph shows a 3-cm pneumothorax starting at the apex of his chest cavity and extending down to his diaphragm. There is no cardiomegaly, and the left lung appears to be normal.

How should the patient be managed at this point?

The chest radiograph confirms the diagnosis suggested by the history and physical examination. A 3-cm pneumothorax in a symptomatic patient necessitates drainage. Supplemental oxygen should be administered to maintain an oxygen saturation above 92%, and a peripheral intravenous line should be started. Information about Mr. Robinson's arterial blood gases is not useful at this point because it does not add any pertinent information and only delays the necessary procedure.

What type of pneumothorax is presented in this case?

This is a secondary spontaneous pneumothorax because it occurs in a patient who probably has an underlying pulmonary disorder: chronic obstructive pulmonary disease (COPD). Primary spontaneous (or idiopathic) pneumothoraces occur in young, healthy persons with no underlying pulmonary disease. The general classification of pneumothoraces is given in Table 27.1.

What clinical features are associated with a primary spontaneous pneumothorax?

Primary spontaneous pneumothoraces occur with an incidence of 6 to 7 per 100,000 men and 1 to 2 per 100,000 women in North America (1). The rupture of a small subpleural bleb within the visceral pleura allows air to escape into the pleural cavity, where it accumulates and collapses the lung. These pneumothoraces are most prevalent in young adults; 85% of patients are younger than 40 years of age. Typically, the patient is a tall, slim 20- to 25-year-old man with a smoking history. Without definite therapy, the recurrence rate is high, estimated at 25% after a first episode, 40% to 50% after a second episode, and more than 60% after a third episode (2,3).

What is the pathophysiology of subpleural blebs?

The formation of subpleural blebs results from the rupture of apical alveoli. The gradient between the intrabronchial and intrapleural pressures is greater at the

TABLE 27.1.

CLASSIFICATION OF PNEUMOTHORACES

Etiology	Mechanism
Spontaneous pneumothorax	Primary (idiopathic) Secondary
Traumatic	Blunt chest injury Penetrating chest injury
Iatrogenic	Thoracentesis Central vein catheterization Mechanical ventilation
Neonatal	
Catamenial	
Diagnostic	

lung apices, creating more tension on the walls of the apical alveoli, which leads to their overexpansion and eventual rupture. Once the alveolus ruptures, gas escapes and dissects peripherally along the lobular septa and collects as blebs beneath the visceral pleura. These blebs are generally found at the lung apex, in the superior segment of the lower lobes, and along the fissures. By definition, they are smaller than 2 cm in diameter.

What alterations of pulmonary physiology are caused by pneumothoraces?
A pneumothorax causes a reduction in pulmonary volumes, lung compliance, and diffusing capacity. Blood shunting through a lung that is poorly ventilated creates a ventilation/perfusion ($\dot{V}/\dot{Q}$) mismatch, and hypoxemia results.

How are secondary spontaneous pneumothoraces defined?
Secondary spontaneous pneumothoraces accompany underlying pulmonary disease. They account for only 20% of spontaneous pneumothoraces overall (80% are primary or idiopathic) and most often are associated with COPD. The mean age of patients is older than 50 years, and as pulmonary functions are compromised, they are more commonly symptomatic (4).

What other diseases are associated with secondary spontaneous pneumothoraces?
Other pulmonary disorders include cystic fibrosis, bullous disease, interstitial diseases (e.g., idiopathic pulmonary fibrosis, sarcoidosis, eosinophilic granuloma), and infectious processes (e.g., pneumonia, tuberculosis, abscesses). Neoplasms, whether primary or metastatic, also may cause a pneumothorax, but this is rare.

Mr. Robinson is seen by the general surgeon on call that day in the emergency department. After reviewing the history, physical examination, and chest radiograph findings, the surgeon proceeds with a tube thoracostomy of the right chest.

What size chest tube should be inserted and where?

The size of a chest tube depends on what type of substance is being drained from the pleural cavity. Generally, a size 20-French chest tube is sufficient for pneumothorax. When draining blood, pus, or thick fluid, a large-bore tube (size 28 to 36 French) is recommended. The chest tube for a pneumothorax is inserted in the fifth intercostal space on the midaxillary or anterior axillary line, and it is directed toward the apex of the pleural cavity. A chest tube for an apical pneumothorax also may be inserted through the anterior chest wall in the second intercostal space on the midclavicular line. A pleural effusion is drained with a chest tube in the fifth or sixth intercostal space directed posteriorly and inferiorly (5).

Once inserted, should the chest tube have suction?

Suction on a chest tube is used to ensure optimal drainage of the pleural cavity. Suction is required for pneumothorax when chest radiograph does not show the lung to be completely expanded after tube thoracostomy or if there is a large air leak. Once the lung is completely expanded, suction should be reduced to a minimum or stopped to help seal the air leak.

The chest radiograph taken after Mr. Robinson's chest tube is inserted shows adequate tube placement and a small residual 8-mm pneumothorax at the apex of the right lung field. A moderate-sized air leak from the tube is also shown. The chest tube is placed under water seal drainage, and 20 cm of negative pressure is applied. The patient is admitted to the hospital, and a daily chest radiograph is ordered.

Is chest tube drainage required for all patients with a pneumothorax, and if not, what are the criteria for conservative management?

All patients with a symptomatic pneumothorax need drainage. Some patients who meet specific criteria may be treated with observation alone. These criteria include no symptoms, a pneumothorax less than 20% or 2 cm, and a young and reliable patient (i.e., primary spontaneous pneumothorax). Patients with secondary pneumothorax have much less pulmonary reserve and thus are at higher risk for complications or even death if the pneumothorax progresses rapidly. Conservative management is possible in 15% to 20% of patients overall (2,6).

When pneumothorax is treated conservatively, how long does resolution take?

The rate of resorption of air from the pleural cavity is estimated to be 1.25% of the volume of the pneumothorax per 24 hours (50 to 70 mL per day) or the equivalent of 1 mm a day. A 2-cm pneumothorax takes up to 3 weeks to resolve completely.

What types of drainage procedures are available?

A spontaneous pneumothorax may be drained by simple needle aspiration using a 16- to 18-gauge needle catheter and a three-way stopcock. However, this procedure is associated with a 50% to 70% failure rate and thus is rarely used (4). Drainage of the pleural space may be obtained with any of a variety of small-caliber catheters (10 to 16 French) to which suction usually can be applied. Although less traumatic on insertion and more comfortable for the patients, these small-bore tubes easily become clogged with fibrin and blood clots. Conventional tube drainage with a 20- to 24-French chest tube remains the gold standard because it is safe, effective, and reproducible and is associated with an 80% to 90% success rate in the management of spontaneous pneumothorax (7).

What is a Heimlich valve, and when is its use indicated?

The Heimlich valve is a one-way flutter valve that is connected to the end of a chest tube, eliminating the need for an underwater seal drainage bottle or suction. The valve is designed to let air out of the pleural cavity in the presence of an air leak (8). The valve is ideally suited for outpatient management of uncomplicated spontaneous pneumothorax and for persistent air leaks. It is recommended only for patients whose lungs are fully reexpanded and for reliable patients with adequate pulmonary function. Regular chest radiographs and follow-up are necessary. The chest tube is removed once the air leak has resolved.

What complications are associated with spontaneous pneumothoraces?

Complications include pleural effusion (15%), persistent air leak (10%), tension pneumothorax (5%), hemothorax (3%), pneumomediastinum (2%), and empyema (less than 1%).

How does a hemothorax secondary to a pneumothorax occur?

When a pneumothorax occurs suddenly, adhesions between the parietal and visceral pleura may tear as the lung collapses. These adhesions may contain blood vessels, so when they are torn, bleeding results. Avulsion of a subclavian vein also has been reported in association with a spontaneous pneumothorax. When the hemorrhage is massive or continuous, an exploratory thoracotomy is indicated.

Mr. Robinson's air leak persists for 5 days and eventually seals spontaneously. The chest radiograph shows a well-expanded lung. The chest tube is removed uneventfully, and the patient is discharged from the hospital. Then, 2 weeks after returning home, Mr. Robinson once again develops acute-onset shortness of breath with right-sided chest pain. He is rushed to the hospital, where an emergency department chest

radiograph shows complete collapse of his right lung secondary to a pneumothorax. A chest tube is rapidly inserted by the thoracic surgery resident on call. The patient's shortness of breath markedly improves shortly after the chest tube is placed. Mr. Robinson is admitted to the hospital, and his chest tube is set on 20 cm of suction.

How should Mr. Robinson's problem now be managed?

The patient's spontaneous pneumothorax is managed the same as the first episode. At this point, surgical therapy must be considered.

What are the indications for surgery in patients with primary and secondary spontaneous pneumothoraces?

- Second episode of ipsilateral pneumothorax
- Previous contralateral pneumothorax
- Air leak persisting longer than 7 to 10 days
- Massive air leak preventing adequate lung expansion
- Bilateral simultaneous pneumothorax
- Complications of a pneumothorax (e.g., hemothorax, empyema)
- Indications specific to the underlying pulmonary disorder

Is this patient's occupation an important consideration?

Some occupations carry an inherent risk of pneumothorax. Airline pilots and scuba divers are managed more aggressively, and surgery is considered after a first episode. Patients who live far from medical centers also are managed surgically after an initial episode of spontaneous pneumothorax (4).

What are the objectives of surgical therapy?

The foremost objective of surgery for spontaneous pneumothorax is preventing recurrences. Other objectives include ensuring complete expansion of the lung, treating complications, and managing bronchopleural fistulas.

How are these objectives met?

Surgery for spontaneous pneumothorax consists of resecting the bullous disease at the lung apices (apical bullectomy) and obliterating the pleural space. The pleural space can be obliterated in a number of ways, including parietal pleurectomy (subtotal versus total), mechanical pleurodesis (abrasion), and chemical pleurodesis (e.g., tetracycline, bleomycin, talc, hypertonic glucose) (9,10).

What type of surgical approach is recommended?

Although the operation can be carried out through a standard posterolateral thoracotomy, most surgeons prefer a miniaxillary thoracotomy in the third intercostal space or video-assisted thoracoscopic surgery (VATS) (11–13).

Although Mr. Robinson is doing fine clinically with only a minimal amount of dyspnea at rest and a completely expanded lung on the chest radiograph, his air leak persists for 8 days. Considering that this is his second episode of pneumothorax and his air leak did not seal spontaneously, the patient is seen in consultation by a thoracic surgeon. The surgeon and Mr. Robinson agree that an operation is in his best interest.

What preoperative workup should Mr. Robinson have?

Although this type of operation is not considered major, patients with secondary spontaneous pneumothoraces must be thoroughly screened before surgery. Operability is assessed, and a cardiac evaluation is done when indicated. From a pulmonary standpoint, a baseline study of pulmonary function tests (PFTs) should be obtained in all patients with COPD. Chest computed tomography (CT) also is recommended because patients with a history of heavy smoking are at risk for developing a malignancy. CT also may help direct the intervention if areas of bullous disease are found away from the lung apices.

Mr. Robinson's CT shows a 2.5-cm anterior pneumothorax on the right, mild emphysematous changes in both lung fields, no distinct bullae, and no suspicious-looking lesions. His PFTs are as follows: forced expiratory volume in 1 second (FEV_1), 1.5 (38% of predicted); forced vital capacity (FVC), 2.4 (60%); FEV_1/FVC, 62%; and carbon monoxide diffusion in the lung (DLCO), 54%. His workup is otherwise unremarkable.

What type of intervention is best suited for Mr. Robinson?

Although a number of options are available, a VATS approach is best because it allows a thorough inspection of the lung. If specific areas of blebs are found, they should be resected with a stapler. A subtotal pleurectomy or pleural abrasion is performed in most cases. Some surgeons recommend chemical pleurodesis at the time of surgery for secondary spontaneous pneumothoraces. Generally, one chest tube is left in the pleural cavity.

What are the advantages of pleurectomy over pleural abrasion?

The pleurectomy is believed to create a more intense inflammatory reaction and thus better obliteration of the pleural cavity. However, it is associated with a major complication rate of 10% (e.g., hemothorax, fibrothorax, Horner's syndrome) and makes subsequent thoracotomy for unrelated disease more difficult. Pleural abrasion is simpler, more effective, and safer (3% complication rate) (14,15).

What are the results of surgery for spontaneous pneumothorax?

The standard procedure, consisting of an apical bullectomy with a pleurectomy or pleural abrasion, is highly effective and associated with morbidity below 10% and a mortality rate of 1% to 2%. The postoperative morbidity and mortality may be significantly higher in patients with COPD. The rate of recurrent pneumothoraces after surgery is reported by many surgeons as 1% to 2% for primary spontaneous pneumothorax and 5% to 6% for the secondary type (7,9–11).

Mr. Robinson's air leak persists for 2 more days. He is finally taken to the operating room, where he undergoes a VATS apical bullectomy and a subtotal pleurectomy. His chest tube, which shows a minimal air leak on the first postoperative day, is removed 3 days later. He is discharged from the hospital after an uneventful postoperative course. Mr. Robinson recovers well from his surgery, and on follow-up visits his radiograph shows a well-expanded lung with no signs of a pneumothorax.

Over the years, however, the patient's dyspnea continues to progress, and he now requires inhaled bronchodilators on a regular basis. On two occasions in the past 10 months, he is hospitalized for acute bronchitis and receives antibiotic therapy. He is becoming short of breath even at rest and is no longer able to attend to his regular activities.

How is Mr. Robinson's clinical course described?

Mr. Robinson's evolution is typical of long-standing COPD. Most patients require regular bronchodilators and oral steroids as their dyspnea progresses with time, and hospitalizations for episodes of exacerbated chronic bronchitis become more frequent. More than 50% of patients with end-stage disease become oxygen dependent (16).

What form of COPD is most frequent?

The most frequent type of COPD is emphysema, which affects an estimated 2 million Americans.

How is emphysema defined?

Emphysema is a condition of the lung characterized by abnormal and permanent enlargement of air spaces distal to the terminal bronchioles accompanied by destruction of their walls and without obvious fibrosis (17).

How is emphysema classified morphologically?

Three subtypes of emphysema have been described: centriacinar, or centrilobular; panacinar, or panlobular; and paraseptal. *Centriacinar emphysema* develops in the proximal portion of the acinus and is associated with inflammatory destruction of the respiratory bronchioles. This form of emphysema is most common in the upper lung fields and is secondary to tobacco smoking. In *panacinar emphysema*, all portions of the acinus are uniformly destroyed. It diffuses throughout the lung. It has been associated with deficiencies in α_1-antitrypsin. *Paraseptal emphysema* results from disruption of subpleural alveoli with the secondary formation of blebs and bullae. These lesions usually are found along the apical segments of the lung and along the fissures, and they are responsible for most episodes of spontaneous pneumothorax (18).

What radiologic features are found on chest radiographs in patients with emphysema?

Common findings include hyperinflation of the lungs, depression or flattening of the diaphragm, vascular deficiency in the parenchyma, bullae, increased intercostal space, increased anteroposterior diameter of the chest, and vertical position of the heart.

What are typical PFT values in a patient with advanced COPD?

PFTs show airflow obstruction (FEV_1 less than 35%), marked thoracic hyperinflation (total lung capacity [TLC] greater than 120%; residual volume [RV] greater than 200%), and altered alveolar gas exchange (DLCO less than 50%).

What is the pathophysiology of respiratory failure in patients with emphysema?

The mechanisms are airflow obstruction, dead space ventilation, compression of normal parenchyma, increase in pulmonary vascular resistance, and respiratory muscle and diaphragmatic dysfunction.

Why does airflow obstruction occur in the emphysematous lung?

In the normal lung, the small bronchi and bronchioles depend on the radial traction forces of the surrounding parenchyma to remain open during expiration. Emphysema destroys the lung tissue and decreases its elastic recoil properties, which in turn causes the small airways to collapse on expiration. Cartilage atrophy in emphysema may render the small bronchi vulnerable to expiratory collapse, also producing airflow obstruction, air trapping, and hyperinflation (19).

What are the objectives of surgery for emphysema?

The primary objective is to improve lung and thoracic function, hence decrease dyspnea, increase exercise tolerance, and improve the quality of life.

What types of surgery can treat emphysema?

Operations for emphysema date to the early 1900s. They include a variety of techniques, most of which are no longer in use. Procedures were developed for the chest wall (costochondrectomy), the diaphragm, the pleura, the nervous system (lung denervation), and the major airways (tracheoplasty). Surgery on the lung itself consists of excision or plication of bullae in patients with bullous lung disease, and volume reduction for patients with diffuse emphysema (20).

What are the objectives of lung volume reduction surgery (LVRS)?

The goals of LVRS for diffuse emphysema are to improve the elastic recoil properties of the lung, correct the chest wall mechanics and respiratory muscle dysfunction, resect the part of the lung with the most important $\dot{V}/\dot{Q}$ mismatch, and improve hemodynamics by decreasing the pulmonary vascular resistance and afterload to the right ventricle.

What patients are candidates for LVRS?

The inclusion and exclusion criteria are given in Table 27.2.

How is LVRS done?

LVRS consists of a unilateral or bilateral lung resection (stapling device versus laser technique) using a standard thoracotomy approach, a median sternotomy, or VATS. The "functionless" areas of the lung are identified with one-lung ventilation (the emphysematous lung remains hyperinflated). With a stapler, the lung is resected beginning on the anterior surface of the upper lobe, moving toward the apex, and then around and toward the diaphragm. This creates a continuous U-shaped line of excision on the periphery of the lung. A buttress of bovine pericardium is usually applied to the staple line. A pleural tent is developed, and two chests tubes are left in each pleural cavity.

How much lung is resected?

The exact amount is difficult to define, but generally 20% to 30% of the lung volume on each side is resected.

TABLE 27.2.

SELECTION CRITERIA FOR LUNG VOLUME REDUCTION SURGERY

Inclusion Criteria	Exclusion Criteria
Diagnosis of emphysema	Age >80 years
Disabling dyspnea (grade 3–4/4)	Tobacco use within last 6 months
FEV_1 <35%	Pulmonary hypertension (systolic >45; mean >35)
Residual volume >200%	Resting CO_2 >55 mm Hg
Total lung capacity >120%	Marked obesity or cachexia
Hyperinflated lungs on chest radiograph	Unstable coronary artery disease
Regional heterogeneity of lung perfusion	Dependence on ventilator
Potential for preoperative rehabilitation	Underlying bronchiectasis or chronic bronchitis

FEV_1, forced expiratory volume in 1 second.

What are the results and clinical outcome of LVRS for diffuse emphysema?

The outcome of LVRS varies according to the surgical approach used. Results with a VATS-laser technique show only modest improvement. Reports have documented a mean FEV_1 increase of 13% to 18%, a decrease in RV of 11% to 14%, an improvement in the partial pressure of arterial oxygen (PaO_2) of 2 to 4 mm Hg, and cessation of oxygen therapy in only 16% of patients. Reports indicate that using a bilateral stapling technique by median sternotomy, surgeons increased FEV_1 by 49% to 96%, decreased RV by 28% to 30%, improved PaO_2 by 8 mm Hg, and eliminated supplemental oxygen therapy in 70% of patients.

Results with a bilateral VATS stapling technique are comparable with those of the median sternotomy approach (21–26). In a large nationwide randomized trial comparing LVRS and medical therapy for severe emphysema (National Emphysema Treatment Trial), no clear survival advantage was found with surgery in the overall group of patients. LVRS did increase exercise capacity in most patients and improved survival in some well-selected candidates (27).

What are the long-term benefits of LVRS?

Although many studies have confirmed the short-term benefits of LVRS in selected patients, data are sparse regarding long-term results. It generally is believed that over time lung function deteriorates, and the initial benefits of LVRS may be lost.

What are the complication rates associated with LVRS?

The major complication rate ranges from 10% to 40%, and the rate of mortality is reported as 3% to 17%. Air leaks requiring chest tubes for more than 5 days postoperatively are found in 30% to 48% of patients. Pneumonia has been documented in 9% to 22% of patients and respiratory failure in 2% to 13% (24,26,27).

Mr. Robinson, now 58 years old, is severely handicapped by emphysema. He is being followed by a pneumologist who regularly repeats his workup. His PFTs now show FEV_1, 28%; RV, 270%; TLC, 180%; DL_{CO}, 30%; PaO_2 on room air, 51 mm Hg; and PCO_2, 50 mm Hg. After a long discussion with his physician regarding the possibility of LVRS, he decides to go ahead with the preoperative workup. Unfortunately, Mr. Robinson's cardiac evaluation shows moderate right ventricular dysfunction on echocardiogram, and pulmonary hypertension (pulmonary artery pressure is 65/40 mm Hg) is found during his right heart catheterization. These findings rule out LVRS for Mr. Robinson. However, he remains hopeful that a solution for his problem can be found and insists on seeing a lung transplant surgeon.

TABLE 27.3.

SELECTION CRITERIA FOR LUNG TRANSPLANTATION

General Criteria	Specific Criteria
Progressive and disabling pulmonary disease	Functional class 3–4/4 (NYHA)
Poor quality of life	Age <55–65 years
No effective medical therapy	Potential for rehabilitation
Life expectancy without transplantation <12–24 months	Psychosocial stability
	No tobacco use >6 months
	No systemic disease (e.g., renal, cardiac, hepatic)

NYHA, New York Heart Association.

What are the most common indications for lung transplantation?

Lung transplantation is indicated for a variety of diseases. These include COPD (50% to 55% of cases), infections, diseases such as cystic fibrosis (10% to 15%), interstitial lung disease (15% to 20%), and pulmonary vascular disease (5% to 10%) (28).

What are the selection criteria for candidates for lung transplantation?

Selection criteria usually are classified as general and specific (Table 27.3).

What generally are accepted as contraindications to lung transplantation?

Contraindications to lung transplantation include cachexia, ventilator dependency, other end-organ dysfunction, symptomatic osteoporosis, history of malignancy, and alcoholism or drug addiction. Some of these criteria vary from one institution to another and according to the underlying pulmonary disease (29).

When should lung transplantation be considered for a patient with emphysema?

The ultimate goals of lung transplantation are to prolong the patient's life and improve the quality of life. A successful transplantation improves a patient's quality of life in more than 85% of cases. Exercise tolerance usually is markedly increased, and supplemental oxygen therapy is discontinued in more than 90% of patients. However, improving survival is more controversial in patients with COPD. Other disease entities have specific guidelines on the indication and timing of the transplantation based on survival data. Emphysema often evolves very slowly over several years when treated with supplemental oxygen, even with end-stage disease (i.e., FEV_1 less than 30%). In this group of patients, 2-year survival rates of 60% to 80% have been reported (30,31). It generally is accepted that transplantation prolongs the life of COPD patients whose FEV_1 reaches 20%. Patients in the 25% FEV_1 range who have deteriorated rapidly over a short period or who require regular hospitalizations also live longer after transplantation.

What type of transplantation should be performed in a patient with COPD?

A single-lung transplant is sufficient for most patients from a functional standpoint. A double-lung transplant is considered for emphysema patients younger than 40 years with α_1-antitrypsin deficiencies and for patients with end-stage disease who develop bronchiectasis and have recurrent infections (32). More recently, as data seem to show a survival benefit with double-lung transplants on long-term follow-up, some centers now recommend the procedure in most emphysema patients (28).

How often is cardiopulmonary bypass required for transplants in these patients?

Bypass is required for fewer than 4% to 5% of patients with COPD. Patients who do not tolerate one-lung ventilation or who have right ventricular failure and pulmonary hypertension are at increased risk for requiring cardiopulmonary bypass during the transplantation.

What are the functional results of lung transplantation for COPD?

A number of factors influence the early and long-term functional results after a single- or double-lung transplantation. These factors include native lung disease, overall cardiac function, operative factors (e.g., incisional pain, chest wall restriction, pleural complications), and posttransplant complications. In double-lung transplant recipients, 12 months after the operation the FEV_1 reaches 78% of the predicted value, the DLCO is 76%, and the PaO_2 is within the normal range. After a single-lung transplant, the FEV_1 is found to be in the 50% range for COPD patients and 79% for patients with pulmonary fibrosis, and the DLCO is 60%. In these patients, the PaO_2 is normal, but the alveolar-arterial gradient remains wide. Overall, study of the functional status using the New York Heart Association (NYHA) grades shows 70% of patients class I and 21% class 2 (33).

What are the causes of early and late mortality and overall survival?

In the early postoperative period (up to 30 days), the most frequent cause of death is nonspecific graft failure followed by infection. In the intermediate time (31 days to 1 year), infection is the most common cause of death. After 1 year, bronchiolitis obliterans is responsible for the greatest number of deaths. The operative mortality for a lung transplantation ranges from 5% to 10%. The 1- and 5-year actuarial survival rates are 70% and 50%, respectively. Results

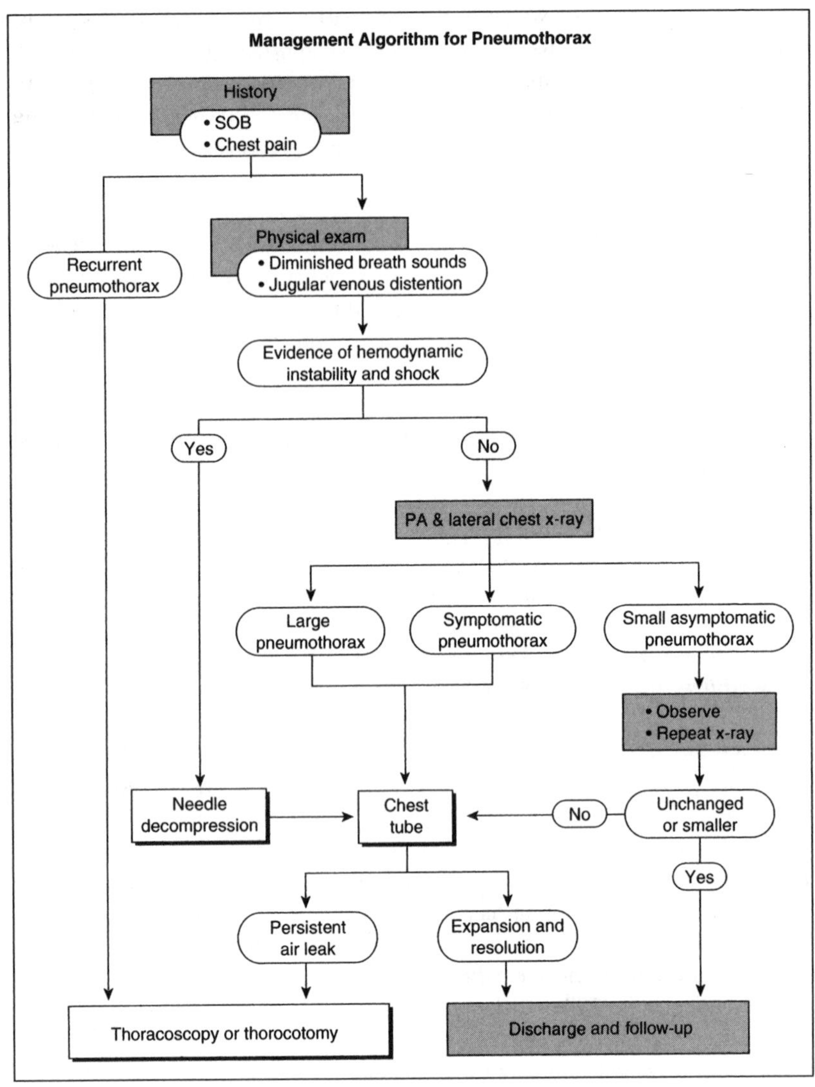

Algorithm 27.1.

in patients with emphysema are significantly better, with 1- and 5-year survival rates of 80% and 60%, respectively. In COPD patients, the outcome seems to be superior when a double-lung transplant is performed (28).

Mr. Robinson is seen and evaluated by representatives of the lung transplant program in his city. He is considered a candidate for transplant

and undergoes the full workup. He now requires oxygen 24 hours a day, and his functional status has reached NYHA class 4. To his great relief, no specific contraindications to a lung transplantation are found. Mr. Robinson's name is placed on the patient waiting list for a single-lung transplant. He is told that patients with his blood type, B, have a mean waiting time of 12 to 18 months.

REFERENCES

1. Melton LJ, Hepper NG, Orford KP. Incidence of spontaneous pneumothorax in Olmstead County, Minnesota: 1950–1974. Am Rev Respir Dis. 1979;120:1379–1382.
2. Getz S, Beasley W. Spontaneous pneumothorax. Am J Surg. 1983;145:823–827.
3. Gobbell WG, Rhea WG, Nelson IA, et al. Spontaneous pneumothorax. J Thorac Cardiovasc Surg. 1963;46:331–345.
4. Beauchamp G. Spontaneous pneumothorax and pneumomediastinum. In: Pearson FG, ed. *Thoracic Surgery.* New York, NY: Churchill Livingstone; 1995: 1037–1054.
5. Miller KS, Sahn SA. Chest tubes: indications, technique, management, and complications. Chest. 1987;91:258–264.
6. O'Rourke J, Yee E. Civilian spontaneous pneumothorax. Chest. 1989;96:1302–1306.
7. Ferraro P, Beauchamp G, Lord F, et al. Spontaneous primary and secondary pneumothorax: a 10-year study of management alternatives. Can J Surg. 1994;37:197–202.
8. Heimlich HJ. Valve drainage of the pleural cavity. Dis Chest. 1968;53:282.
9. Singh SV. The surgical treatment of spontaneous pneumothorax by parietal pleurectomy. Scand J Thorac Cardiovasc Surg. 1982;16:75–80.
10. Weeden D, Smith GH. Surgical experience in the management of spontaneous pneumothorax. Thorax. 1983;38:737–743.
11. Deslauriers J, Beaulieu M, Despres JP, et al. Transaxillary pleurectomy for treatment of spontaneous pneumothorax. Ann Thorac Surg. 1980;30:569–574.
12. Cannon WB, Vierra MA, Cannon A. Thoracoscopy for spontaneous pneumothorax. Ann Thorac Surg. 1993;56:686–687.
13. Hazelrigg SR, Landreneau RJ, Mack M, et al. Thoracoscopic stapled resection for spontaneous pneumothorax. J Thorac Cardiovasc Surg. 1993;105:389–393.
14. Gaensler EA. Parietal pleurectomy for recurrent spontaneous pneumothorax. Surg Gynecol Obstet. 1956;102:293–308.
15. Clagget OT. The management of spontaneous pneumothorax. J Thorac Cardiovasc Surg. 1968;55:761–762.
16. Maltais F, Bourbeau J. Medical management of emphysema. Chest Surg Clin North Am. 1995;5:673–689.
17. American Thoracic Society. Chronic bronchitis, asthma, and pulmonary emphysema. Am Rev Respir Dis. 1968;85:762–768.
18. Deslauriers J, Leblanc P. Bullous and bleb diseases of the lung. In: Shields TW, ed. *General Thoracic Surgery.* 4th ed. Philadelphia, Pa: Williams & Wilkins; 1994:907–929.

19. Celli BR. Pathophysiology of chronic obstructive pulmonary disease. Chest Surg Clin North Am. 1995;5:623–634.
20. Deslauriers J. A perspective on the role of surgery in chronic obstructive lung disease. Chest Surg Clin North Am. 1995;5:575–602.
21. Hazelrigg S, Boley T, Henkle J, et al. Thoracoscopic laser bullectomy: a prospective study with 3-month results. J Thorac Cardiovasc Surg. 1996;112:319.
22. Little AG, Swain JA, Nino JJ, et al. Reduction pneumoplasty for emphysema: early results. Ann Surg. 1995;222:365–374.
23. McKenna RJ, Brenner M, Gelb AF, et al. A randomized prospective trial of stapled reduction versus laser bullectomy for diffuse emphysema. J Thorac Cardiovasc Surg. 1996;111:317–322.
24. Cooper JD, Patterson GA, Sundaresan RS, et al. Results of 150 consecutive bilateral lung volume reduction procedures in patients with severe emphysema. J Thorac Cardiovasc Surg. 1996;112:1319.
25. Keenan RJ, Sciurba FC, Landreneau RJ, et al. Superiority of bilateral versus unilateral thoracoscopic approaches to lung reduction surgery. Am J Respir Crit Care Med. 1996;153:A268.
26. Martinez FJ, Flaherty KR, Iannettoni M. Patient selection for lung volume reduction surgery. Chest Surg Clin N Am. 2003;13:669–685.
27. Fishman A, Martinez F, Naunheim K, et al. National Emphysema Treatment Trial Research Group. A randomized trial comparing lung-volume-reduction-surgery and medical therapy for severe emphysema. N Engl J Med. 2003;348:2059–2073.
28. Trulock EP, Edwards LB, Taylor DO, et al. The Registry of the International Society for Heart and Lung Transplantation: twentieth official adult lung and heart-lung transplant report—2003. J Heart Lung Transplant. 2003;22:625–635.
29. Smith CM. Patient selection, evaluation, and preoperative management for lung transplant candidates. Clin Chest Med. 1997;18:183–197.
30. Anthonisen NR, Wright EC, Hodgkin JE, et al. Prognosis in chronic obstructive pulmonary disease. Am Rev Respir Dis. 1986;133:14–20.
31. Nocturnal Oxygen Therapy Trial Group. Continuous or nocturnal oxygen therapy in hypoxemic chronic obstructive pulmonary disease: a clinical trial. Ann Intern Med. 1980;93:391–398.
32. Patterson GA. Indication for unilateral, bilateral, heart-lung and lobar transplant procedures. Clin Chest Med. 1997;18:225–230.
33. Williams TJ, Snell GI. Early and long-term functional outcomes in unilateral, bilateral, and living-related transplant recipients. Clin Chest Med. 1997;18:245–257.

CHAPTER 28

MELANOMA

William P. Reed

Dennis O'Shea is a 45-year-old executive who undergoes a shave biopsy of a mole on the upper part of his right back. He has always had numerous moles scattered over his back and chest but never paid them much attention until his wife noted that one had become somewhat larger than the rest. The pathology report on tissue submitted at the time of the shave biopsy shows a tan to dark brown piece of skin measuring 9 × 5 mm. Microscopic examination shows a benign Spitz nevus extending to the margins of the specimen. Considering the benign nature of the lesion, he is advised that no further therapy is warranted at this time. He seeks a second opinion because several members of his family have died of cancer, and he is concerned that this may be an early sign of malignancy. During physical examination, Mr. O'Shea appears to be a healthy, tanned white man with sandy hair and blue eyes. His vital signs are normal. His lungs are clear. The heart sounds are normal, with no murmurs. His abdomen shows no scars or masses. There is no lymphadenopathy. There is a recent scar over the right scapula that is slightly reddened, with a suggestion of darker pigmentation at the medial margin. He has freckles on the tops of his shoulders and numerous benign-appearing moles scattered over his torso and extremities.

Given this presentation, what is the initial clinical impression?

Any change in a mole or pigmented lesion should be assumed to be malignant melanoma until proven otherwise.

Doesn't the diagnosis of a Spitz nevus prove that this is not a melanoma?

The Spitz nevus has many features in common with melanoma (1–3). Often, the distinction is made on the basis of microscopic features at the depths of the lesion or on the basis of the clinical features. The Spitz nevus tends to be less than

6 mm in diameter, symmetric, and uniform in color, with a progressively benign appearance of cells on histologic examination (maturation) as the deepest margin of the lesion is approached. In contrast, melanoma presents with the distinct features of *a*symmetry, *b*order irregularity, *c*olor variegation, and *d*iameter greater than 6 mm (the so-called ABCDs of melanoma). Histologic examination of the lesion shows invasion at the deepest portion.

What is the origin of melanoma?

Melanoma develops from melanocytes, which are pigment-producing cells derived from the neural crest that migrate during fetal development into the skin, eye, central nervous system, and mucous membranes. The most common site of melanoma is the skin, but these tumors can develop in any tissue that contains melanocytes. This cancer comprises 3% to 4% of malignancies, with 55,000 new cases each year in the United States (4). From the 1930s to the mid-1980s, there was a rapid rise in the incidence of this disease, doubling every 10 years (5). Epidemiologic studies from 1995 suggested that the incidence was leveling off in susceptible populations. Perhaps this reflects better attention to preventive measures as the causation becomes clearer (6).

What is the cause of melanoma?

The direct cause is unknown, but there is considerable evidence to suggest that ultraviolet light is the principal carcinogen. Susceptible people are those with pale complexions and reddish hair who are most prone to skin injury upon exposure to sunlight. An inverse relationship between latitude and incidence of disease has been noted for such people both in Australia and in North America. Melanoma most commonly occurs on the skin that is left uncovered, such as the back and chest in men and the arms and legs in women.

Is there a gender or race predilection for malignant melanoma? Do these groups differ in prognosis?

A survey of more than 8,500 malignant melanoma patients revealed a slight predominance in men (52%) over women (48%) with regard to the total number of cases reported (7). With regard to race, 98% of this group were white. In general, women tend to have a longer survival time than men. In blacks, malignant melanoma tends to occur on the palms of the hands, the soles of the feet, or beneath the nail plate; it tends to exhibit an aggressive growth pattern and early metastasis with a poor overall prognosis. The 5-year survival in the black population has been estimated to be as low as 23% (8).

Is there a difference between genders in the anatomic location of malignant melanoma? Does the location of pigmented lesions offer any prognostic information?

Different patterns of sun exposure lead to a significant difference between men and women with respect to body location of melanoma. Men tend to have more lesions on their trunks, whereas women have more extremity lesions, particularly on the lower limbs. Melanomas in women tend to be thinner, with less tendency to ulcerate. It is unknown whether this is an inherent feature of the location or is due to easier detectability. As a result, regional lymph node involvement and distant metastases occur less often in women than in men. Therefore, men with a predominance of trunk lesions have a relatively poor prognosis, whereas women with a predominance of extremity lesions have a relatively good prognosis (5).

Are there any precursor lesions of melanoma?

Yes. The dysplastic nevus syndrome is familial and is believed to be a precursor of malignant melanoma. This syndrome follows a familial pattern and is characterized by a large number of irregularly shaped nevi on the trunk. Those with dysplastic nevus syndrome are believed to have a cumulative lifetime risk of melanoma approaching 100% (9). Giant congenital nevi in children are believed to be premalignant, with a risk of malignancy reported to be as high as 40%.

What specific changes in nevi indicate the need for biopsy?

Any change in size, shape, or color of a nevus, as well as any itching, ulceration, or bleeding, suggests that biopsy should be considered. Changes in size and shape occur in approximately 70% of melanomas. The change in color is usually toward increasing pigmentation; however, amelanotic melanomas do exist. In addition, pigment may fade in some areas (regression) while deepening in others. Ulceration and bleeding are late signs that usually indicate deeply invasive disease (10).

What are the histologic types of cutaneous melanoma? Which have the overall best prognosis and worst prognosis? Which is the most common type?

The histologic types of melanoma and their approximate incidences are as follows: superficial spreading (70%), lentigo maligna (5%), acral lentiginous (10%), and nodular (15%). Both lentigo maligna and superficial spreading melanomas have a relatively good prognosis if they are diagnosed early. These types of melanoma have a predominant horizontal growth pattern such that the melanocytes proliferate superficially along the epidermal–dermal junction and only later become locally invasive. For patients with these types of melanoma, changes in size, shape, or color can be detected while the tumor is locally noninvasive.

Acral lentiginous tumors, which develop on the palms and soles or beneath the nails, also have a prominent horizontal growth component, but they are a bit more invasive than the superficial types. These lesions, which are more common in African Americans (70% of melanomas) and Asians, present late and carry a worse prognosis. Nodular melanoma develops early deep invasion and tends to metastasize early. This type of melanoma most often presents as a uniform pigmented nodule, but 5% will be amelanotic.

Nodular melanoma carries the worst prognosis.

What is the difference between an incisional and excisional biopsy?

An incisional biopsy entails removal of only a portion of the lesion. The size of the incision varies, but the specimen must be large enough to permit an adequate diagnosis. It is best to include the most raised area of the lesion to allow adequate microstaging. An excisional biopsy entails removal of the entire lesion, leaving only normal tissue at the excised wound edge.

Should an incisional or excisional biopsy be performed?

When possible, an excisional biopsy is performed. In some areas, such as the face or scalp, excision may not be cosmetically acceptable until a diagnosis of malignancy is established. Incisional biopsy is used in these cases for initial histologic examination. Incisional biopsy may also be appropriate for large lesions where grafting will be needed for closure.

Punch biopsy can provide a full-thickness sample without the need for suture closure. These biopsies are obtained from the thickest area of the lesion. It is not necessary to obtain normal surrounding skin. Superficial skin biopsy by shaving should *never* be used when melanoma is the suspected diagnosis because this technique may not provide a specimen that is deep enough to extend into the tumor proper. Not only will the diagnosis be missed in such cases, but the partial removal of the upper layers of tumor may interfere with microstaging on subsequent excision.

Why is an excisional biopsy preferable?

An excisional biopsy is preferable because it provides the pathologist with the entire lesion. This allows the deepest extent of the tumor to be determined for microstaging purposes (discussed later). Sometimes, an incisional biopsy permits only a histologic diagnosis and not an accurate determination of the depth of invasion. In addition, excision with adequate margins may obviate further intervention when a thin melanoma or preinvasive lesion is encountered. When an incisional or punch biopsy is used, it should be obtained from the most raised portion of the lesion. This will provide the greatest chance of determining depth of invasion, which in turn determines the ideal margins for excision. When the clinical appearance leaves little doubt about the diagnosis, punch biopsy allows histologic confirmation and staging with minimal disruption of lymphatics for later nodal mapping by lymphoscintigraphy.

Mr. O'Shea notes some itching in addition to the change in size and shape of his mole. When he scratches the mole, occasionally it bleeds.

What should the next step be in the management of Mr. O'Shea's mole?

The remaining lesion should be excised.

Biopsy results show a melanoma invasive into the reticular dermis. The thickness of the lesion is 0.95 mm. The melanoma is on the epidermal surface in some areas, suggesting ulceration.

How are melanomas staged clinically? What is Mr. O'Shea's stage?
Melanoma is staged as follows (11); see also Table 28.1:

Stage I: local to the upper (superficial) dermis
Stage II: local to the lower (deep) dermis or subcutaneous tissues
Stage III: regional metastases, either to lymph nodes or to intralymphatic spaces (satellitosis or in-transit metastases)
Stage IV: distant metastases are present

TABLE 28.1.

STAGE GROUPINGS FOR CUTANEOUS MELANOMA

	Clinical Staging			Pathologic Staging		
	T	*N*	*M*	*T*	*N*	*M*
0	Tis	N0	M0	Tis	N0	M0
IA	T1a	N0	M0	T1a	N0	M0
IB	T1b	N0	M0	T1b	N0	M0
	T2a	N0	M0	T2a	N0	M0
IIA	T2b	N0	M0	T2b	N0	M0
	T3a	N0	M0	T3a	N0	M0
IIB	T3b	N0	M0	T3b	N0	M0
	T4a	N0	M0	T4a	N0	M0
IIC	T4b	N0	M0	T4b	N0	M0
III	Any T	N1	M0			
		N2				
		N3				
IIIA				T1-4a	N1a	M0
				T1-4a	N2a	M0
IIIB				T1-4b	N1a	M0
				T1-4b	N2a	M0
				T1-4a	N1b	M0
				T1-4a	N2b	M0
				T1-4a/b	N2c	M0
IIIC				T1-4b	N1b	M0
				T1-4b	N2b	M0
				Any T	N3	M0
IV	Any T	Any N	Any M1	Any T	Any N	Any M1

The information provided indicates that Mr. O'Shea's tumor is at least stage Ib because the deeper dermis is involved. Nothing is known regarding regional nodes or distant metastatic sites at this point. The thinness of his tumor (less than 1.0 mm) would ordinarily place him in the stage Ia category, but the prior shave biopsy has removed the upper portion of the tumor, making the Clark's level a more reliable measure of invasion in this instance (discussed next). Ulceration also has the effect of increasing the stage by one level.

What is the microstaging used for melanoma?

The two systems commonly used are the level of skin invasion (Clark's level) and tumor thickness (Breslow's). Both are now incorporated as measures of tumor in the tumor, node, metastasis (TNM) classification system (Table 28.2). Clark's level is based on the anatomic depth of skin to which the tumor invades (12). The levels are as follows:

I: Confined to the dermal–epidermal junction
II: Invading the papillary dermis only
III: Extending to the junction of the papillary and reticular dermis
IV: Invading the reticular dermis
V: Extending into subcutaneous tissues

Breslow's microstaging uses an ocular micrometer to measure the thickness of the lesion in millimeters below the granular layer of the epidermis (13). Originally, four levels were found to correlate with increasingly poor prognosis: tumor up to 0.75 mm thick; tumor thicker than 0.75 and up to 1.5 mm thick; tumor thicker than 1.5 and up to 4 mm thick; and tumor thicker than 4 mm. More recently, the even integers of 1.0, 2.0, and 4.0 mm have been found to provide better thresholds for prognosis than those proposed by Breslow (14).

Is one microstaging system more accurate in predicting survival than the other?

The tumor thickness (Breslow) is a more accurate predictor of survival than is Clark's level of invasion. In studies in which survival was correlated to both tumor thickness and level of invasion, it was found that within each Clark's level, there was a wide variation in Breslow thickness and in the associated 5-year survival rates. At various Clark's levels, comparable Breslow measurements were associated with similar 5-year survival rates when matched to thickness. Thus, Breslow thickness is a more consistent prognostic indicator (14,15).

Thickness can be altered by inappropriate removal of the upper portion of a tumor through shave biopsy, however. Under these circumstances, Clark's levels may indicate the true stage when a discrepancy between the two levels is found. The current American Joint Committee on Cancer (AJCC) manual considers Clark's level to be an independent predictor of outcome only for thin (T1) lesions. Tumors

TABLE 28.2.

MELANOMA TNM CLASSIFICATION

T Classification	Characteristics
Tis	Melanoma in situ, not invasive (Clark's level I)
T1	Tumor ≤1.0 mm thick
	a. Without ulceration and Clark's level II/III
	b. With ulceration and Clark's level IV/V
T2	Tumor >1.0 mm but not >2.0 mm thick
	a. Without ulceration
	b. With ulceration
T3	Tumor >2.0 mm but not >4.0 mm thick
	a. Without ulceration
	b. With ulceration
T4	Tumor >4.0 mm thick
	a. Without ulceration
	b. With ulceration
N Classification	
N0	No regional nodal involvement
N1	One lymph node involved
	a. Micrometastases
	b. Macrometastases
N2	2–3 lymph nodes involved
	a. Micrometastases
	b. Macrometastases
	c. Intransit disease without positive nodes
N3	4 or more nodes involved
M Classification	
M0	No systemic metastases
M1	Any systemic metastases
	a. Distant skin, soft tissues or nodes
	b. Pulmonary metastases
	c. All other visceral metastases

less than or equal to 1.0 mm are classified as T1a if they are not ulcerated and do not extend into the reticular dermis (Clark's level II or III). When ulceration is present or the tumor extends to Clark's level IV or V, thin lesions are classified as T1b. The 10-year survival for T1b lesions is lower than that of T1a lesions, approaching that of T2a tumors (greater than 1.0 mm to 2 mm thickness without ulceration) (Fig. 28.1).

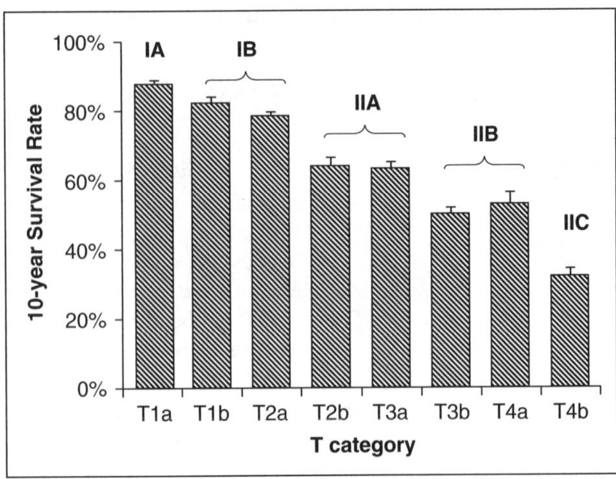

Figure 28.1. Ten-year survival rates comparing the different T categories and the stage groupings for stages I and II melanoma. Note that the groupings upstage patients with melanoma ulceration with the next level T substage of patients with thicker, nonulcerated melanomas.

What is the primary treatment of melanoma? What constitutes an adequate margin for these tumors?

Local melanoma can be cured by excision alone. Three prospective studies established that 2-cm margins are adequate to treat melanomas up to 4 mm thick (16–19). Even narrower margins are adequate for thinner melanomas, as established by a prospective World Health Organization (WHO) study (17).

Current recommendations are that in situ tumors (Clark's level I) be excised with 0.5-cm margins, melanomas less than 1 mm thick be excised with 1-cm margins, and melanomas 1 to 4 mm thick be excised with 2-cm margins. For lesions 1 to 2 mm thick, the WHO study shows the overall survival to be the same whether 1- or 3-cm margins are used. Because there was a slightly higher level of local relapse with the narrower margins, it is safer to use 2-cm margins whenever possible for such tumors, reserving 1-cm margins for situations in which a local flap or skin graft would be required for closure (20). Margins wider than 2 cm may be appropriate for tumors that extend deeper than 4 mm, but distant metastases rather than local recurrence usually determine outcome for such lesion.

Should the underlying fascia be removed with the specimen?

There is no evidence that removal of the muscular fascia improves local control or long-term survival. Unless the tumor extends to the fascia, there is no reason to include it in the resection.

Should clinically negative regional lymph nodes be removed at the time of initial local excision?

Elective lymph node dissection (ELND), or the dissection of clinically uninvolved nodes, has been investigated as a means of removing microscopic deposits in nodes before they progress to distant disease. The rationale for this procedure is based on the observation that patients with microscopic nodal deposits at the time of node dissection have better survival rates (50%) than patients with gross nodal involvement (15%) (20). Several retrospective studies also have shown improved survival when ELND is added to local excision for 1- to 4-mm-thick tumors. Two prospective randomized surgical trials have failed to confirm a survival benefit for ELND, however (21,22). The most recent trial, the Intergroup Melanoma Surgical Trial, did show that ELND was beneficial for certain subgroups—namely, patients who were 60 years of age or younger with 1- to 2-mm-thick tumors that had not ulcerated. For patients with these characteristics, ELND appears to improve survival by 10% at 5 years ($P < .005$) (23). For other patients, ELND actually may lower survival.

Are there any drawbacks to ELND?

Expected complications after axillary dissection include wound infections (11%), wound separation (3.5%), and lymphedema (3%). The resulting disability may add 21 to 30 days to the time lost from work for surgical treatment of melanoma. For inguinal node dissection, complications occur in as many as 50% of patients, including wound infections (21%), wound separation (20%), and lymphedema (21%) (23).

Mr. O'Shea is a 45-year-old man with an intermediate-thickness nonulcerated melanoma of the upper back.

Which nodal basins are dissected to provide him with the benefits of ELND?

Lesions of the upper back may metastasize to the cervical or axillary nodal basin. If the lesion is near the midline, either side or both sides may drain the primary site. To determine which basin is most likely to contain nodal metastases, preoperative lymphatic mapping (i.e., lymphoscintigraphy) should be carried out by injecting ^{99}Tc-labeled sulfur colloid in the subcuticular space around the tumor and scanning the patient to determine the nodal basins draining the tumor-bearing area.

Is there any way to limit the complications of dissection in the patients who have uninvolved nodes?

Studies have now shown that lymphatic mapping by tumor injection of ^{99}Tc–sulfa colloid and isosulfan blue (Lymphazurin 1%), a vital blue dye, to identify the first draining node (sentinel node) allows a limited sampling to replace full node dissection in patients without nodal metastasis. Negative nodal status by sentinel node biopsy (SNB) has been shown to be the single most important predictor of disease-free survival next to Breslow depth (24). Lymphatic mapping with SNB provides a more accurate means of assessing nodal status than elective node dissection, which is targeted to an assumed nodal basin of involvement and may actually miss the true site of metastases. It also allows the complications of full nodal dissection to be limited to those patients with proven nodal metastases. For those patients whose sentinel nodes are free of metastases, disease-free survivals in excess of 85% at 3 years can be anticipated.

Who should undergo SNB?

Once depth of invasion exceeds 1 mm or involves Clark's level IV or V, or ulceration is present (T1b), the rate of positive SNB reaches 5% and justifies examining the nodal status. For T1a lesions, 10-year survival rates approach 90% with excision alone.

Suppose Mr. O'Shea had a 2- to 3-cm firm node palpated in his right axilla. Is there any reason to perform an axillary dissection, considering the poor prognosis of stage III disease?

Once nodes are clinically involved, it is standard practice to remove them. Surgical removal is still the most effective treatment for regional nodal metastases. Survival rates as high as 40% at 10 years can be achieved with node dissection alone when only one node is affected. With two to four positive nodes, survival drops to 26%; with five or more positive nodes, survival drops to less than 10% (25).

Are effective adjuvant treatments available to patients with positive nodes?

Until recently, no systemic therapy had shown a significant survival advantage for patients with melanoma. Recombinant interferon (IFN-α_{2b}) has been shown to improve the survival of node-positive stage III patients when given at maximally tolerated intravenous and subcutaneous doses for 1 year after node dissection (26).

Mr. O'Shea undergoes wide excision of his melanoma and an axillary node dissection. He accepts interferon treatment postoperatively but gives up after the first month because of toxicity. Six months later, he has progressive symptoms of crampy abdominal pain. Physical examination is unremarkable except for heme-positive stool on rectal examination.

What is the diagnosis?

Along with the usual causes of gastrointestinal blood loss, metastatic melanoma in the small bowel must be considered. This is a common site for metastatic disease. Other common sites are the liver, lungs, brain, skin, and bone.

Is there a role for surgery in the treatment of metastatic disease? Is systemic therapy effective?

With rare exceptions, resection of metastatic disease is palliative. Patients may benefit from resection of metastatic lesions that are symptomatic if their overall condition warrants intervention. Gastrointestinal metastases that produce obstruction or significant hemorrhage fit into this category. Long survivals, up to 20 years, have occasionally resulted from removal of a solitary gastric or intestinal metastasis. Survival after resection of brain metastases combined with radiation also appears better than survival after radiation alone. A number of nonsurgical approaches to widespread disease, including chemotherapy, immunotherapy, and irradiation, have provided only temporary and inconsistent results.

Suppose Mr. O'Shea's melanoma was deeper than 4 mm and just above his left knee on the anterior thigh. Does this location suggest any additional therapeutic modality?

Patients with advanced extremity lesions may be candidates for regional hyperthermic perfusion. This treatment entails tourniquet isolation of the extremity and cannulation of the vessels supplying the affected limb. Chemotherapeutic agents (usually melphalan) are infused at temperatures up to 40°C for at least 1 hour through an extracorporeal membrane oxygenation system. A large number of patients have received this treatment; however, no unifying criteria for treatment have been established, which makes it difficult to draw conclusions. At best, it may be fair to say that local chemotherapy results in local or regional control for a limited amount of time.

Are there noncutaneous forms of melanoma?

Yes, primary melanomas of the mucous membranes occur mainly in the head and neck region and in the vulva or vagina. A study of 47 patients older than 27 years indicates that head and neck tumors are the most common (43%), followed by the vulva (30%) and vagina (15%). Other sites include the anorectum (6%) and the esophagus (2%). The overall 5-year survival rate of these patients was less than 25% (27–29).

How does melanoma of the anorectum typically present?

Unfortunately, anorectal melanoma usually presents with rectal bleeding, which is a sign of advanced and locally invasive disease.

What is the general prognosis of patients with anorectal melanoma?

Because of the occult nature of anorectal melanoma, it may go undetected, resulting in locally advanced invasive disease. Abdominoperineal resection has been attempted with poor survival rates, less than 10%, at 5 years. Fortunately, this form of melanoma is rare, accounting for fewer than 1% of all primary melanomas.

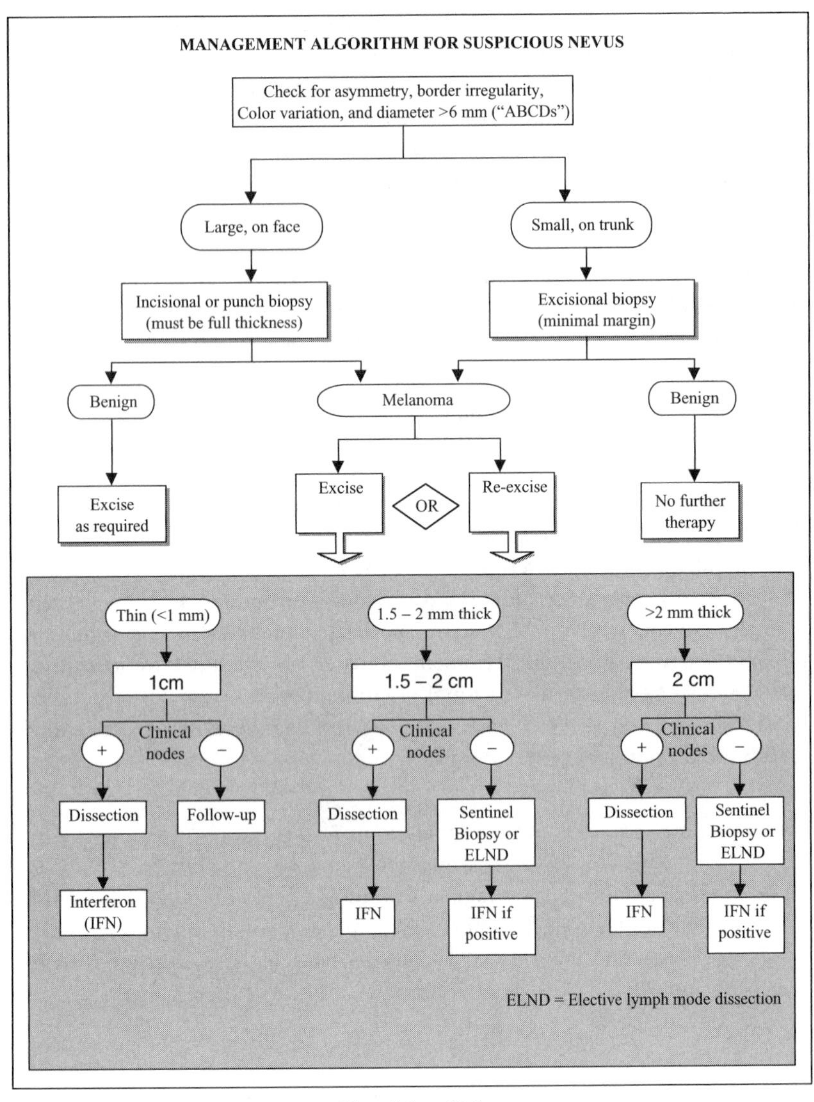

Algorithm 28.1.

Should a patient with a history of melanoma receive an ophthalmologic evaluation?

Yes. Both primary and metastatic ocular melanomas have been described. These lesions usually arise from the choroidal layer, and as with cutaneous melanoma, if they are recognized and treated early, the prognosis is relatively good.

Thorough workup of Mr. O'Shea did not reveal any metastatic melanoma, and his abdominal symptoms resolved without intervention. He is discharged with a follow-up appointment 1 month later.

REFERENCES

1. Reed RJ, Ichinose H, Clark WH, et al. Common and uncommon melanocytic nevi and borderline melanomas. Semin Oncol. 1975;2:119–147.
2. Weedon D, Little JH. Spindle and epithelioid cell nevi in children and adults: a review of 211 cases of the Spitz nevus. Cancer. 1977;40:217–225.
3. Paniago-Pereira C, Maize JC, Ackerman AB. Nevus of large spindle and/or epithelioid cells (Spitz's nevus). Arch Dermatol. 1978;144:1811–1823.
4. Jemal A, Tiwari RC, Murray T, et al. Cancer statistics, 2004. CA Cancer J Clin. 2004;54:8–29.
5. Balch CM, Soong SJ, Multon GW, et al. Changing trends in cutaneous melanoma over a quarter century in Alabama, USA, and New South Wales, Australia. Cancer. 1983;52:1748–1753.
6. Korsary CL, Ries LAG, Miller BA, et al. SEER Cancer Statistics Review, 1973–1992. Tables and graphs. Bethesda, Md: National Cancer Institute; 1995 [abstract].NIH Pub 96–2789.
7. Balch CM, Soong SJ, Shaw HM, et al. An analysis of prognostic factors in 8500 patients with cutaneous melanoma. In: Balch CM, Houghton AN, Milton GW, et al., eds. Cutaneous Melanoma. 2nd ed. Philadelphia, Pa: JB Lippincott Co; 1992:165–187.
8. Balch CM, et al. Management of cutaneous melanoma in the United States. Surg Gynecol Obstet. 1984;158:311–318.
9. Greene MH, Clark WH, Tucker MA, et al. Acquired precursors of cutaneous malignant melanoma. The familial dysplastic nevus syndrome. N Engl J Med. 1985;312:91–97.
10. Langley RGB, Fitzpatrick TB, Sober AJ. Clinical characteristics. In: Balch CM, Houghton AN, Sober AJ, et al., eds. Cutaneous Melanoma. 3rd ed. St. Louis, Mo: Quality Medical; 1998:82–101.
11. Balch CM, Buzaid AC, Soong S-J, et al., eds. Final version of the American Joint Committee on Cancer staging system for cutaneous melanoma. J Clin Oncol. 2001;19:3635–3648.
12. Clark W Jr, From L, Bernardino E, et al. The histogenesis and biologic behavior of primary human malignant melanomas of the skin. Cancer Res. 1969;29:705–727.
13. Breslow A. Thickness, cross-sectional areas and depth of invasion in the prognosis of cutaneous melanoma. Ann Surg. 1970;172:902–908.
14. Balch CM, Soong S-J, Gershenwald JE, et al. Prognostic factors analysis of 17,600 melanoma patients: validation of the American Joint Committee on Cancer melanoma staging system. J Clin Oncol. 2001;19:3622–3634.
15. Vollmer RT. Malignant melanoma: a multivariate analysis of prognostic factors. Pathol Annu. 1989;24:383–407.
16. Veronesi U, Cascinelli N. Narrow excision (1 cm margin): a safe procedure for thin cutaneous melanoma. Arch Surg. 1991;126:438–441.

17. French Cooperative Group. In: Balch CM, Houghton AN, Sober AJ, et al., eds. Cutaneous Melanoma. 3rd ed. St. Louis, Mo: Quality Medical; 1998:143.
18. Balch CM, Urist MM, Karakousis CP, et al. Efficacy of 2 cm surgical margins for intermediate-thickness melanomas (1–4 mm): results of a multi-institutional randomized surgical trial. Ann Surg. 1993;218:262–267.
19. Karakousis CP, Balch CM, Urist MM, et al. Local recurrence in malignant melanoma: long-term results of the multi-institutional randomized surgical trial. Ann Surg Oncol. 1996;3:446–452.
20. Reintgen DS, Albertini J, Miliotes G, et al. The accurate staging and modern day treatment of malignant melanoma. Cancer Res Ther Control. 1995;4:183.
21. Veronesi U, Adamus J, Bandiera DC, et al. Inefficacy of immediate node dissection in stage I melanoma of the limbs. N Engl J Med. 1997;297:627–630.
22. Sim FH, Taylor WF, Pritchard DJ, et al. Lymphadenectomy in the management of stage I malignant melanoma: a prospective randomized study. Mayo Clin Proc. 1986;61:697–705.
23. Balch CM, Soong SJ, Bartolucci AA, et al. Efficacy of an elective regional lymph node dissection of 1 to 4 mm thick melanomas for patients 60 years of age and younger. Ann Surg. 1996;224:255–263.
24. Gersheuwald JE, Thompson W, Mansfield PF, et al. Multi-institutional melanoma lymphatic mapping experience: the prognostic value of sentinel node status in 612 stage I or II melanoma patients. J Clin Oncol. 1999;17:976–983.
25. Balch CM, Soong SJ, Murad TM, et al. A multifactorial analysis of melanoma: III. Prognostic factors in melanomas with lymph nodes metastases (stage II). Ann Surg. 1981;193:377–388.
26. Kirkwood J, Strawderman MH, Ernstoff MS, et al. Interferon alfa-2b adjuvant therapy of high-risk resected cutaneous melanoma. Eastern Cooperative Oncology Group Trial EST 1684. J Clin Oncol. 1996;14:7–17.
27. Iversen K, Robins RE. Mucosal malignant melanomas. Am J Surg. 1980;139:660–664.
28. Manola J, Alkins M, Ibrahim J, Kirkwood J. Prognostic factors in metastatic melanoma: a pooled analysis of Eastern Cooperative Oncology Group trials. J Clin Oncol. 2000;18:3782–3793.
29. Balch CM, Soong S-J, Atkins MB, et al. An evidince-based staging system for cutaneous melanoma. CA Cancer Clin. 2004;54:131–149.

CHAPTER

29

BURN INJURY

Dennis Gore

You are the physician working in a rural emergency room when a child arrives by Emergency Medical Service (EMS). The paramedics tell you that 8-year-old Donny McMaster was playing near an electrical transformer when a loud spark was heard and the child was knocked about 10 yards. His shirt was on fire but his friends extinguished it by rolling him on the ground.

What is the initial priority in the care of Donny?

As in all trauma, immediately assess the ABCs (*a*irway, *b*reathing, and *c*irculation) Airway compromise is common with severe burn and electrical injuries, usually associated with edematous occlusion of the upper airway as appropriate fluid resuscitation is given. Likewise, breathing may be compromised from either detriment in mental obtundation or a constrictive burn eschar circumscribing the chest with an impedance to thoracic excursion and ventilation.

Circulatory arrest is frequent following electrical injury and is apparently associated with the abnormal electrical conduction through the heart and subsequent cardiac arrhythmias. Circulation is also compromised until fluid resuscitation can replenish and then maintain plasma lost from the extensive edema within the injured tissue. Therefore, establishing intravenous (IV) access is an important early step in the management of a burn patient.

An index to the adequacy of fluid resuscitation, the Foley catheter is essential for monitoring. Other monitors, such as pulse oximetry and electrocardiography (ECG), are important (1). Furthermore, removal of all clothing and jewelry and a thorough inspection to assess the extent of wounding and to look for other injuries is important.

On initial assessment, Donny's airway was patent, his respiratory rate was 24 breaths per minute and comfortable, his pulse was 110 beats per minute, and his blood pressure was 108/64 mm Hg. He had a deep white burn about the size of a quarter on the lateral aspect of his left hand and another wound on his right knee. The skin on his chest, neck, face, and left arm was erythematous with patches of blisters.

What is the significance of the deep burns on the hand and knee?
These small but deep wounds are most likely the entrance and exit sites for the high-voltage electrical current. The extent of injury associated with the electrical current is often deceptive because the overlying skin appears normal. Bone, however, has a high resistance to electrical conductivity, and thus a tremendous amount of heat is generated around the bone, which damages adjacent muscle.

What is the fluid formula for the resuscitation of Donny?
There is no fluid formula for electrical injuries. As noted earlier, the extent of tissue damage is not readily apparent. The best management is to promptly place a Foley catheter and closely monitor the urine output, adjusting the rate of fluid infusion to maintaining an adequate urine output of no less than 0.5 mL per kg body weight per hour.

Since placement of the Foley catheter 40 minutes ago, there has been only 5 mL of dark tea-colored urine despite 3 L of normal saline given to this 33-kg child.

What is the significance of the dark urine?
Damaged muscle releases myoglobin. If the damaged muscle remains compartmentalized, the myoglobin enters the circulation. This myoglobin coagulates within the glomeruli and renal tubules, precipitating renal dysfunction and possibly failure (2). Initial management advocates infusion of large quantities of crystalloid. In cases in which urine output is unresponsive to fluid administration, mannitol and sodium bicarbonate may also be helpful in maintaining renal tubular patency. Loop diuretics are contraindicated because they may diminish renal tubular perfusion and may exacerbate precipitation of myoglobin. One concern is that any renal dysfunction may impede the excretion of the large quantity of fluids given. Therefore, monitoring of central venous pressure is often helpful.

One hour after Donny's arrival in the emergency room, his left, burned forearm is now tight and pulses at the wrist are no longer palpable.

What is the significance of this finding and what procedure is urgently required?
Edema is obligatory in damaged tissue. The electrical current and heat generated from the conduction through bone has damaged the muscle. The muscle is

confined within a fascial compartment, thereby limiting the edematous expansion of the muscle. As the pressure within this muscle compartment rises, first venous and then arterial perfusion diminishes. This could lead quickly to a nonviable extremity. The appropriate emergency procedure is a fasciotomy, in which incisions are made through the skin and the fascia of each muscle compartment (3). The muscle then bulges out through the fascial incision, lowering the compartment pressure with a return of perfusion to the extremity.

This rural county 40-bed hospital is ill-equipped to handle this severe injury.

What are some of the appropriate management steps to safely transfer Donny to an established burn facility?

As in the initial care, assurance of the ABCs of Trauma is essential for the safe transport of a patient to a designated trauma facility (4). If there is any concern about airway patency and breathing, intubation and ventilatory support are appropriate. To maintain circulation, sew into place two large-bore IVs. Adhesive tape does not stay well on sloughing, blistered, and burned skin, whereas suturing the IVs is a reliable way to secure placement. Two IVs are recommended as a precaution because at least one IV frequently fails.

The Foley catheter is also important because it allows ongoing monitoring, and the transport personnel can be instructed to adjust fluids to maintain the appropriate urine output. Immediately addressing the wound is not a priority concern. But because burn patients often lose their ability to thermally regulate, they can become very cold. It is imperative that a warm environment be ensured by using multiple warm blankets, by engaging a Bair-Hugger warming system, or by simply increasing the ambient temperature in the helicopter or ambulance to very hot. Also, frequent communication between the transferring and receiving physicians and the transport team is also important.

You are the resident physician in charge of the Burn Unit when EMS arrives with Jerry Folino, a 60-year-old man who was found unconscious on the bedroom floor during a house fire. He was intubated on the scene and arrives with pulse oximetry of 88%.

What are the priorities in care?

As with all initial trauma evaluations, follow the ABCs. Although this scenario notes that the patient was intubated, endotracheal tubes can be either placed poorly or dislodged en route. Because airway patency is the highest priority, make sure that the endotracheal tube is placed properly. This can be readily accomplished by either auscultation of the chest during insufflation or confirmation of the presence of end tidal CO_2 in the expired breath.

After airway patency is secured, the next priority is breathing. This also can be quickly assessed by auscultation of the chest. Disparity of breath sounds between sides of the chest can be explained by poor endotracheal tube placement into a main stem, bronchus, pneumothorax, hemothorax, or aspiration of a foreign body.

The third priority is circulation. This is most readily monitored by blood pressure, heart rate, palpation of the pulse, and pulse oximetry. For burn victims, massive volumes of IV fluids are sometimes needed to maintain blood volume and support circulation.

How much fluid should be given to Mr. Folino?

Work in the 1950s and 1960s led to the development of formulas to estimate the volume of fluid needed for adequate resuscitation. One of the more widely used formulas still commonly applied today is the Parkland formula (5). This formula estimates the need for fluids for the first 24 hours following the injury. The basic component of the Parkland formula is as follows:

4 mL × kg body weight ×
% total body surface area burn including both second- and third-degree burns

Half of this volume of fluid is given over the first 8 hours post-burn and the rest is given over the next 16 hours. The recommended solution is Ringer's lactate. Thus, to apply this fluid formula you need to know the time since the injury, the patient's general weight, and the percentage of body surface area with second- and third-degree burns.

Mr. Folino weighs approximately 70 kg and has burns to his head, both arms, anterior torso, and entire right leg. Burns to his head are erythematous, blistering, and tender to touch. Burns to his arms, torso, and leg are thick, white, rubbery in texture, and look fairly insensate.

How do you calculate the percentage of burned body area surface?

A quick and easy rule for estimating the percentage of the body surface area burn is the rule of 9s. This formula allocates percentages as follows:

9% of the body surface area for the head
9% for each arm
2 × 9 for the anterior torso
2 × 9 for the posterior torso
2 × 9 for each leg

The percentage of total body surface burned on Mr. Folino is 9% for the head, 18% for both arms, 18% for the anterior torso, and 18% for the right leg; this equals a 63% total body surface area burn.

How can you tell the depth of burn?

First-degree burns are erythematous and tender yet there are no blisters (6). This burn depth is analogous to sunburn and heals readily in 3 to 4 days. Because the endothelial integrity remains intact, extraneous fluid losses are minimal.

Second-degree burns typically blister and are very painful. Because viable epidermis remains along the skin appendages and because hair follicles deep within the dermis provide a source for re-epithelialization, second-degree wounds typically heal spontaneously in 2 to 3 weeks.

Third-degree burns can be white, dark, tan, or charred in appearance and often have a rubbery or leathery texture. These burns are relatively insensate and will not heal by re-epithelialization. Wound closure is accomplished either by autolysis of necrotic tissue followed by contraction and closure by secondary intention or by surgical removal of the eschar and autologous skin grafting.

Can you now calculate the estimated fluid volume for Mr. Folino?

4 mL × 70 kg body weight × 63% = 17,640 mL

If he arrived in the emergency room 1 hour after being injured, 8820 mL is to be given over the next 7 hours with another 8820 mL administered over the following 16 hours.

Now that you have calculated the estimated fluid requirements for Mr. Folino, does it matter?

No, not really. The formula only gives you a general guideline as to what would be an expected volume of fluid needed for adequate resuscitation. Renal perfusion is an important gauge for the adequacy of perfusion for the rest of the body. If urine output is low, then, regardless of the fluid volume advocated by the formula, more fluid is needed. Thus, a physician gives fluids to maintain urine output of at least a 0.5 mL per kg per hour. If there is concern that either cardiac or renal failure combined with excessive fluid administration may precipitate pulmonary edema and hypoxemia, monitoring of cardiac filling pressures such as central venous pressure may be helpful.

For Mr. Folino, fluid administration was initiated at 1.3 L per hr using Ringer's lactate. Urine output for the first hour was 42 mL. However, his pulse oximetry decreased to 82% despite adjustment of the fraction of inspired oxygen (FIO_2) on the ventilator to 100%. He has palpable pulses in all extremities, his blood pressure is 130/60 mm Hg, and his heart rate is 110 beats per minute.

What are some likely explanations for the poor oxygenation?

There are several possible explanations for Mr. Folino's hypoxemia. In addition to a myriad of underlying medical problems, such as chronic obstructive pulmonary disease (COPD) or heart failure, one possibility may be that Mr. Folino is suffering from carbon monoxide poisoning (7). Carbon monoxide binds very strongly to the hemoglobin molecule and displaces oxygen, thereby impairing oxygen delivery. Pulse oximetry measures the oxygen saturation of hemoglobin and thus monitors the delivery of oxygen. In contrast, blood gas measurements quantify the partial pressure of oxygen (PO_2). This value may be deceptively high in patients affected by carbon monoxide. Other signs and symptoms of carbon monoxide poisoning include bright red skin, mental obtundation, and metabolic acidosis, all findings related to inadequate availability of oxygen. To combat carbon monoxide poisoning, high concentrations of oxygen are given. Over time, carbon monoxide concentrations decrease as it is expired through ventilation.

Another possible explanation for the hypoxemia is smoke inhalation. Inhalation of toxic fumes is common in burn patients trapped in a closed space, such as a house or a car, and especially common in patients with impaired mentation. In such victims, smoke enters the airway, damaging the bronchial endothelium. Necrotic tissue combined with the infiltration of inflammatory cells creates a thick tenacious coagulum, which clogs the airways, instigates bronchospasm, and impairs ventilation. Unventilated segments of lung incite pulmonary artery vasoconstriction, potentially leading to cor pulmonale and right-sided heart failure. The diagnosis is most readily verified by bronchoscopy. This maneuver is also considered therapeutic because some of the large debris can be cleared from the airway and ventilation restored. Frequent use of bronchodilators is also helpful in improving airflow and ventilation. Oxygen need also be administered to inhibit the pulmonary artery vasoconstriction and minimize hypoxemia.

Pneumonia is a very common sequela with smoke inhalation, thus frequent assessment of microbial colonization of the lungs and airway is important. Prophylactic antibiotics are not generally considered beneficial in that they do not appear to reduce the frequency of pneumonia yet promote the proliferation of organisms resistant to the administered antibiotics. Thus, antibiotics and antifungals should be reserved for those patients with symptoms of pneumonia.

How can you tell if there is damage to the eyes?

Corneal damage is fairly common in patients with burns to the face and head. It is important to examine the eyes soon after the injury because periorbital edema may quickly preclude subsequent inspection. Fluorescein dye and examination using blue light provides a facile manner for detecting corneal damage. If damage is present, an antibiotic ointment is recommended.

Bronchoscopy identified smoke inhalation. With bronchial lavage and bronchodilators, Mr. Folino's oxygenation slowly improved, his hemodynamics remained good, and his urine output was adequate. His body temperature is 37.8°C.

What is the best way to address Mr. Folino's wounds?

Once the patient is warm with good hemodynamics, you can address the wounds. Most burn units are equipped with large whirlpool baths, which allow for partially submerging patients in warm water. Blisters are débrided and the thick eschar washed to remove as soon as possible any residual dirt and debris. Once cleaned, antibiotic ointments are routinely placed over the wounds to impede bacterial contamination. Silver sulfadiazine (Silvadene) is popular because of its soothing sensation on application and because it has a very low incidence of adverse reactions; neutropenia is the only rare side effect. Another commonly used antibiotic ointment is sodium mafenide acetate (Sulfamylon). This antibiotic penetrates into the eschar, and it is efficient not only as a barrier to wound colonization but also as a possible aid in clearing infection from burned eschar. Side effects from sodium mafenide acetate include metabolic acidosis and pain on application.

What is the best way to feed this severely injured, intubated patient?

Enteral feedings are an essential component in the care of severely burned patients (8). Placement of tube past the pylorus and into the small intestine allows feeding on a continuous basis, while an accompanying nasogastric tube helps ensure gastric decompression. Enteral feedings should begin as soon as feasible.

How many calories and how much protein should be given to Mr. Folino?

Severely injured patients, especially those with burn injury, respond with increased resting energy expenditure, extensive catabolism of muscle, and resistance to the action of insulin on peripheral tissues accompanied by increased hepatic glucose production. Resting energy expenditure often increases to 40% or 50% above baseline, thereby implying the need for greater than normal caloric support. However, recent information suggests that "excessive" caloric supplementation may be very detrimental because it promotes fat deposition in the liver and engenders hepatic dysfunction (9). Frequent use of indirect calorimetry may be helpful in guiding the appropriate amount of calories given.

Large amounts of protein are given, yet the loss of lean body mass is pervasive regardless of the amount of calories or protein administered. The metabolic consequence of peripheral insulin resistance along with increased gluconeogenesis is hyperglycemia. Recent evidence strongly suggests that hyperglycemia has a detrimental influence by promoting infection, retarding wound healing, and adversely affecting survival of burn patients. Thus, aggressive correction to normalize the plasma glucose concentration is imperative. This is most appropriately accomplished with the graded administration of insulin. Enteral nutrition is also said to be important in its ability to maintain the integrity of the gut and thereby lower the frequency and severity of a septic complication, presumably by reducing the translocation of bacteria and/or endotoxin from the gut lumen.

With ongoing fluid resuscitation, Mr. Folino's hemodynamics and urine output remain good, yet over the next 3 hours, the pulses at the wrist are absent for the right arm and greatly diminished at the left wrist.

What can be done to improve blood flow to the hands?

Escharotomies (10). Frequently, deep third-degree burns create a thick nonelastic eschar. The underlining tissue edema then increases the pressure within the arm as confined by the noncompliant burn eschar. This increasing pressure can eventually impede blood flow to the extremity. The proper management is to cut the eschar (*escharotomy*), and thus allow the underlining tissue edema to expand, thereby reestablishing extremity blood flow. Pulse oximetry monitoring of all burned extremities is useful for early detection of this scenario.

Suspecting a high probability of infection from Mr. Folino's inhalation injury and deep burns, should antibiotics be started now?

No, prophylactic antibiotics do not appear to reduce the subsequent incidence of infection, yet they do foster proliferation of pathogens resistant to the given antibiotics. Therefore, prophylactic antibiotics are not indicated. Aggressive surveillance for infection is appropriate, and once infection does appear to have set in, antibiotics directed specifically to the infecting organism are appropriate. The high incidence of resistant *Pseudomonas*, methicillin-resistant *Staphylococcus aureus*, and fungus in burn units is a vivid consequence of this common, prior practice of excessive antibiotic use.

Now that Mr. Folino has completed successful resuscitation and is doing well with supportive care, is there any utility in surgical management?

Over the last 20 plus years, there has been an increasing propensity toward earlier and more complete excision of deep burn eschar. Now, many burn surgeons excise the burn eschar to 20% and 30% of the total body surface area within the first several days after burn injury and place autologous skin grafts over the débrided open wounds. When skin graft donor sites are limited, cadaveric or porcine skin is placed over the débrided wounds. This provides a temporary wound cover until donor sites heal and can be reharvested, usually every 7 to 10 days. Traditionally, burn eschar excisions are limited after 20% to 30% body surface area débridement because of the extensive blood loss.

Following resuscitation and a period of stability, patients are brought back to the operating room to complete the débridement of any residual burn eschar, usually on a 2- to 3-day cycle. Studies assessing this manner of early aggressive surgical débridement of deep second- and third-degree burns followed by prompt skin grafting note a quicker time for healing, reduced rates of infection, and improved cosmetic and functional recovery.

What can be done to minimize Mr. Folino's scarring and deformity once the skin grafts have healed?

Having the patient wear tight-fitting, elastic garments and encouraging early mobilization with extensive involvement from occupational and physical therapists are considered important to the cosmetic and functional recovery of burn patients (11). Although the mechanism of action is unknown, many burn specialists place sheets of silicone over the scar and claim it reduces scarring and improves skin compliance.

REFERENCES

1. Yowler CJ, Fratianne RB. Current status of burn resuscitation. Clin Plast Surg. 2000;27:1–10.
2. Ramzy PI, Barret JP, Herndon DN. Thermal injury. Crit Care Clin. 1999;15:333–352.
3. Danks RR. Burn management: a comprehensive review of the epidemiology and treatment of burn victims. J Emerg Med Serv. 2003;28:118–141.
4. Sheridan RL. Burn care: results of technical and organizational progress. JAMA. 2003;290:719–722.
5. Monafo WW. Initial management of burns. N Eng J Med. 1996;335:1581–1586.
6. Sheridan RL. Comprehensive treatment of burns. Curr Probl Surg. 2001;38:657–756.
7. Sheridan RL. Burns. Crit Care Med. 2002;30:S500–S514.
8. Cioffi WG. What's new in burns and metabolism. J Am Coll Surg. 2001;192:241–254.
9. Dickerson RN. Estimating energy and protein requirements of thermally injured patients: art or science? Nutrition. 2002;18:439–442.
10. Wong L, Spence RJ. Escharotomy and fasciotomy of the burned upper extremity. Hand Clin. 2000;16:165–174.
11. Young A. Rehabilitation of burn injuries. Phys Med Rehabil Clin N Am. 2002;13:85–108.

CHAPTER

30

TRAUMA

Michel B. Aboutanos

John Smith is a 30-year-old man brought in by the emergency medical team (EMT) after a high-speed motor vehicle collision (MVC). He is unconscious and does not respond to verbal or physical stimuli.

What information should be elicited from the prehospital EMTs?

EMT can provide valuable information regarding (a) mechanism of injury, (b) vital signs, and (c) level of consciousness.

Why is mechanism of injury important?

Mechanism correlates with the type, severity, and patterns of injury. For MVCs, important information includes use of restraints (seat belt, air bags), steering wheel deformation, direction of impact (front, lateral, rear), extent of damage to the vehicle, rollover of the vehicle, and ejection of the passenger. A patient is 25 times more likely to be injured if thrown from a car than from being belted in place.

Why are prehospital vital signs and level of consciousness important?

Prehospital vital signs and the level of consciousness are the first steps in the triage of the patient. If vital signs are abnormal at the scene, serious injury should be suspected. Evidence of depressed level of consciousness immediately after the accident indicates either a decreased cerebral oxygenation/perfusion or a possible closed head injury (CHI). Patients with a loss of consciousness (LOC) lasting more than 5 minutes have an increased likelihood of significant head injury even if they are mentating normally on admission (1).

At the scene, Mr. Smith's blood pressure was 170/90 mm Hg and his heart rate was 110 beats per minute. His Glasgow Coma Scale (GCS) score was 3 (Table 30.1). He lost a significant quantity of blood from a head laceration. He had an obvious deformity of the right thigh.

TABLE 30.1.

GLASGOW COMA SCALE

Indicator	Score
Eye opening	
Spontaneous	4
To voice	3
To pain	2
None	1
Verbal response	
Oriented	5
Confused	4
Inappropriate words	3
Incomprehensible words	2
None	1
Motor response	
Obeys command	6
Purposeful movement (pain)	5
Withdraw (pain)	4
Flexion (pain)	3
Extension (pain)	2
None	1
Total GCS points	3–15

From Michael DB, Wilson RF. Head injuries. In: Wilson RF, Walt AJ, eds. Management of Trauma: Pitfalls and Practice. Baltimore, Md: Williams & Wilkins; 1996:173–202, with permission.

What is the GCS, and what is its significance in evaluation of trauma patients?

GCS is a simple objective neurologic evaluation that has prognostic value at the time of admission (2). It correlates with the severity of the head injury and its predictive outcome. The components of GCS include motor, verbal, and eye-opening responses. Motor response is most predictive of patient outcome. The normal (and maximum) score is 15; the minimum score is 3. A GCS of 8 or less indicates coma. GCS is also used to classify brain injury. A GCS score of 13 to 15 is designated as mild, 9 to 12 as moderate, and 3 to 8 as severe brain injury (3,4).

What initial monitoring procedures are appropriate for all patients with major trauma?

Baseline monitoring consists of cardiac rate and rhythm measurement, noninvasive blood pressure measurement, pulse oximetry, and capnography if the patient is intubated. The pulse oximeter measures the oxygen saturation and pulse amplitude via the toes, fingers, or earlobes. Capnography measures the carbon dioxide tension in expired air. A sudden decrease in the tension may suggest mechanical problems in the airway or hypoventilation. Note that the blood pressure is a poor measure of actual tissue perfusion.

What initial therapeutic interventions are appropriate for all patients with major trauma?

All patients with major trauma receive high-flow oxygen, two large-bore intravenous (IV) cannulas placed in peripheral veins, and resuscitation fluid composed of either lactated Ringer's (LR) solution or normal saline (NS). LR is preferred over NS because of the high chloride content in NS (154 mEq), which can lead to metabolic acidosis. Patients are also immobilized on a backboard with a cervical collar until injuries to the axial skeleton are ruled out. All obvious fractures or deformities of the extremities are immobilized, usually via a splint.

In the trauma bay, Mr. Smith is connected to cardiac and blood pressure monitors. His initial blood pressure is 120/90 mm Hg, with a heart rate of 120 beats per minute. The arterial oxygen saturation is 98% on 100% oxygen via facemask.

How should the initial assessment of this patient be carried out?

All trauma patients are assessed in a systematic manner, addressing the most life-threatening injuries first. The primary survey follows an ABCDE sequential protocol and addresses the immediate life-threatening problems. The secondary survey is a head-to-toe evaluation that begins after the primary survey is complete and the resuscitative efforts are established (4). The primary survey consists of the following:

Airway is always addressed first regardless of the type or severity of injuries. A common mistake is to be distracted by a grossly deformed, non–life-threatening, peripheral injury such as a mangled extremity. By definition, a patient who can talk has a patent airway. An unconscious patient is presumed incapable of maintaining his or her airway integrity, and a definitive airway via tracheal intubation must be established. Signs of possible airway obstruction include agitation, stridor, decreased breath sounds, and evidence of increased airway resistance such as respiratory retractions and the use of accessory muscles. Continuous protection of the cervical spine via either a cervical collar or an inline manual stabilization is an essential part of the airway assessment and management.

Breathing is assessed by visual inspection, auscultation, palpation, and percussion. The respiratory rate and depth are determined. Pay attention to the presence of bruising, deformity, paradoxical chest wall motion, chest wall tenderness, crepitus, and diminished breath sounds. In a hemodynamically stable patient with oxygen saturation above 98%, it is reasonable to wait for a chest radiograph to verify the presence of a suspected thoracic injury. In unstable and hypotensive patients with diminished breath sounds and low pulse oximeter readings, early intervention before radiograph is life saving. Conditions that may impair breathing include tension pneumothorax, flail chest, pulmonary contusion, and hemothorax.

Circulation is best assessed by level of consciousness, pulse, and skin color. Hypotension in a multitrauma patient is considered hypovolemic in origin until proven otherwise. Decreased cerebral perfusion secondary to decreased circulating blood volume (BV) leads to a depressed level of consciousness. A person with brisk capillary refill and pink skin is rarely critically hypovolemic. An ashen, gray color characterizes hemorrhage. Full, slow, and regular pulses indicate normovolemia. Rapid, thready pulses usually indicate hypovolemia. Normal pulses can be present with severe hypovolemia in the elderly trauma patient on beta-adrenergic-blocking agents. Absent central pulses usually indicate severe BV depletion with impending death. Hemorrhage control is achieved in the primary survey.

Disability is determined by a baseline neurologic evaluation by means of GCS scoring and pupillary response. Patient's pupillary size and reaction and the ability to move all extremities is quickly assessed. Drugs and alcohol can affect a patient's level of consciousness. Until proven otherwise, a head injury is suspected in a multitrauma patient who has a depressed level of consciousness and shows no evidence of hypovolemia or hypoxia.

Exposing the entire patient by removing all clothing is important for complete examination and assessment. This is accomplished with minimal movement of the patient by cutting off all garments. The patient is covered with warm blankets or an external warming device is used (e.g., Bair-Hugger) to prevent hypothermia. IV fluid is warmed before infusion.

Mr. Smith's arterial oxygen saturation is 98%.

How should his airway be managed?

Any patient with a GCS of 8 or less is at risk for respiratory failure and should have a definitive airway, regardless of the adequacy of the pulmonary function. A flaccid tongue may obstruct the airway, and progression of intracranial injury may cause the patient to stop breathing. Definitive airways include orotracheal intubation, nasotracheal intubation, and surgical airway (cricothyroidotomy or tracheostomy).

The preferred intubation method is via the orotracheal route following rapid-sequence anesthesia and inline cervical spine immobilization. Nasotracheal intubation is contraindicated in the apneic patient. Other relative contraindications to nasotracheal intubation include facial fractures, frontal sinus fractures, basilar skull fractures, and cribriform plate fracture. All of these fractures may result in a nasotracheal tube being misguided into the cranial vault. Initially, an oral airway is placed and the patient is ventilated with oxygen-enriched air via a bag-valve-mask unit. Jaw-thrust chin-lift maneuver are used to expose the airway and to avoid hyperextension of the neck. If intubation is unsuccessful, surgical cricothyroidotomy through the cricothyroid membrane is indicated (4).

Mr. Smith is successfully intubated with an endotracheal tube and placed on a ventilator. He suddenly becomes tachycardic (heart rate, 120 beats per minute) and hypotensive (blood pressure, 90/40 mm Hg). His oxygen saturation decreases to 89% with increasing airway pressures. Diminished breath sounds are noted upon repeat auscultation of the right chest.

What are the possible causes of hypotension in a patient in the trauma bay? What is the most likely cause of Mr. Smith's hypotension?
The causes of hypotension in a trauma patient should be divided into hypovolemic and non-hypovolemic causes.

Non-hypovolemic causes of hypotension in a trauma patient

1. Blunt cardiac injury leading to cardiogenic shock
2. Spinal cord injury leading to neurogenic shock.

Note that septic shock is rarely a cause of hypotension in the trauma bay.

Hypovolemic causes of hypotension in a trauma patient

1. Cardiac compressive shock resulting from tension pneumothorax and pericardial tamponade
2. Hemorrhagic shock caused by external or internal blood loss

It is important to note that head trauma is not a cause of hypotension, except in the terminal events of brainstem herniation. Although blood loss is the most common cause of hypotension in trauma patients, the most likely cause of Mr. Smith's hypotension is tension pneumothorax.

How is tension pneumothorax diagnosed and treated?
Tension pneumothorax results from an injury to the lung that causes a one-way valve air leak into the pleural space upon inspiration. This leads to elevated intrapleural pressures that displace the mediastinum to the opposite side and results in decreased venous return and cardiac output, causing hypotension. It is a life-threatening condition that necessitates immediate action.

There is no time and no need for a chest radiograph to confirm the diagnosis. The diagnosis is made clinically by the unilateral absence of breath sounds and the presence of distended neck veins, tracheal deviation, hyperresonance on percussion, respiratory distress, arterial desaturation, and signs of hypoperfusion such as tachycardia and late cyanosis. The sudden decompensation of Mr. Smith shortly after intubation is the result of a sudden increase in positive pressure leading to the conversion of simple pneumothorax into a tension pneumothorax. Not all of these signs may be present.

If tension pneumothorax is suspected, a large-bore (14- or 16-gauge) IV catheter is inserted into the thorax through the second intercostal space in the midclavicular line to decompress the tension and alleviate the cardiac compromise. After needle decompression, a tube thoracostomy is placed in the lateral fifth intercostal space to treat the remaining simple pneumothorax.

What other thoracic etiology has the same pathophysiology as tension pneumothorax with similar clinical manifestation?

Cardiac tamponade has the same pathophysiology as tension pneumothorax except that the increased pressure is in the pericardium, rather than the pleural space. It results from the accumulation of blood in the inelastic pericardial sac leading to increased pressure in the pericardium that exceeds the central venous pressure (CVP) and prevents venous return and cardiac filling. Arterial hypotension, muffled heart sounds, and distended neck veins (*Beck's triad*) are the classic manifestation of cardiac tamponade (5,6). Beck's triad may be falsely positive or falsely negative in up to one third of patients (7).

Other clinical manifestations of cardiac tamponade include *pulsus paradoxus* (a decrease of systolic blood pressure of more than 10 mm Hg on inspiration) and *Kussmaul's sign* (an increase in CVP with inspiration during spontaneous breathing). Any of these findings, however, may also be absent and are rarely detected in acute trauma.

Mr. Smith's tension pneumothorax was treated with needle thoracentesis followed by tube thoracostomy with rapid normalization of his blood pressure. During assessment of the circulation, brisk arterial bleeding is noted from a deep laceration on his right forearm.

How can this bleeding be controlled?

External hemorrhage is controlled with direct manual pressure. Tourniquets only impede venous drainage; therefore, they should not be used except in the field in cases in which a traumatic amputation has occurred. Probing deep wounds with a hemostat is also contraindicated. It is unproductive, time-consuming, and may cause injury to adjacent vital structures such as nerves and veins.

What are the different classes of hemorrhage (Table 30.2)?

A grading scale from I to IV assesses the clinical degrees of hemorrhage (4).

Class I hemorrhage: classified as the loss of 750 mL or 15% of BV. Physical findings are very subtle at this stage: slight delay in capillary refill and mild tachycardia to less than 100 beats per minute. Blood pressure, pulse pressure, and urine output remain unchanged. Resuscitation begins with a balanced crystalloid solution (LR).

Class II hemorrhage: loss of 15% to 30% of BV (750 to 1500 mL). There is mild delay in capillary refill time and unchanged or minimally decreased pulse pressure and urine output. A mild tachycardia greater than 100 beats per minute along with tachypnea is noted. Most patients require crystalloid and blood transfusion at this stage.

Classes III and IV hemorrhage: marked by the presence of hypotension. Class III is the loss of 30% to 40% of BV. Class IV is the loss of more than 40% of BV. Life-threatening signs are clearly apparent. Patients are

TABLE 30.2.

ESTIMATED FLUID BLOOD LOSSES BASED ON PATIENT'S INITIAL PRESENTATION

	Degree of Hemorrhage			
Parameter	**Class I**	**Class II**	**Class III**	**Class IV**
Blood loss (mL)	Up to 750	750–500	1500–2000	>2000
Blood loss (% blood)	Up to 15%	15%–30%	30%–40%	>40% volume)
Pulse rate (beats/min)	<100	>100	>120	>140
Blood pressure	Normal	Normal	Low	Low
Pulse pressure	Normal	Low	Low	Low or high
Respiratory rate (breaths/min)	14–20	20–30	30–40	>35
Urine output (mL/hr)	>30	20–30	5–15	Negligible
CNS, mental status	Slightly anxious	Mildly anxious	Anxious and confused	Confused and lethargic
Fluid replacement (3:1 rule)	Crystalloid and blood	Crystalloid and blood	Crystalloid	Crystalloid

CNS, central nervous system.

From American College of Surgeons (ACS). Advanced Trauma Life Support Program for Physicians: Instructor Manual. Chicago, Ill: American College of Surgeons; 1993:21, with permission.

anxious, confused, cold, constricted, and tachycardic. All patients require blood transfusion (type-specific blood or universal donor blood) to avoid delays in cross-matching.

Mr. Smith is initially resuscitated with 2 liters of LR. His heart rate decreases to 90 beats per minute, and the primary survey is continued. The neurologic assessment (disability) reveals that he can move all four extremities and that his response to painful stimuli is purposeful, but he does not follow commands. His eye-opening response is negative and he does not attempt to speak. His GCS is 7. The laceration of the right forearm has stopped bleeding actively. After the removal of his clothes (exposure), angulation of his right lower leg is noted. His pulses are absent in the right foot, which is slightly pale. He is covered with warm blankets to prevent the rapid development of hypothermia.

What are the major presumptive diagnoses at this time?

The persistent alteration in mentation suggests a CHI. CHIs can be focal (subdural and epidural hematomas) or diffuse processes (brain contusions and diffuse axonal or shear injury). Diffuse processes are usually caused by the sudden deceleration encountered in motor vehicle crashes or falls. The deformity of the right lower leg with absent foot pulses points to a likely fracture of the tibia and fibula with associated vascular injury.

What therapy is indicated for patients with blunt trauma and suspected head injury?

Brain injury is the leading cause of morbidity and death in patients with blunt trauma (2). A noninjured brain maintains normal cerebral perfusion in the face of low or high pressure. The injured brain loses this *autoregulation,* or the ability to maintain a normal cerebral blood flow, leading to variations in cerebral perfusion. Increased pressure in the cranial vault from mass lesions or diffuse edema may contribute to decreased perfusion (8–10).

The only treatment for primary head injury is prevention. The main task in the medical management of head injury is to prevent and treat secondary brain injury by scrupulous maintenance of cerebral perfusion. Hypotension and hypoxia are the principle causes of secondary brain injury. Therefore, it is important to maintain euvolemia and treat hypotension aggressively. Mild hyperventilation to a partial carbon dioxide pressure of 30 to 35 mm Hg or end-tidal carbon dioxide pressure of 25 to 30 mm Hg should be maintained; this induces intracerebral alkalosis and mild vasoconstriction and may offer benefit by decreasing intracranial pressure (ICP) (1). Other medical therapies used to reduce ICP include mannitol and furosemide (Lasix). Steroids have not been shown to reduce ICP or improve outcome in severe head injury patients. As soon as the patient is stable, computed tomography (CT) of the head is obtained. Laboratory tests are performed to rule out other causes of altered mentation, such as hypoglycemia and substance intoxication. Dextrose (50% water) and naloxone may be administered empirically.

What initial interventions and diagnostic procedures are performed at this time?

1. A Foley catheter is inserted after the rectal examination. Gastric decompression, nasally or orally, is performed to reduce the risk of aspiration, especially in a suspected CHI. Nasogastric tube is avoided in suspected facial fractures and midface instability where fracture of the cribriform plate may lead to cranial penetration (4).
2. A basic radiologic assessment is performed in cases of blunt trauma, including radiographs of the chest and pelvis. A lateral cervical spine radiograph is indicated if there are signs or symptoms of cervical spine injury or if the patient has altered mentation, has distracting injuries, or has received analgesia (4).

What are the contraindications for passing a urethral catheter in a trauma patient?

A rectal examination is performed before placement of a urinary catheter in men. A high-riding prostate gland felt during the rectal examination, blood at the urethral meatus, or a penile or periscrotal hematoma may indicate urethral rupture. If any of these findings are present, a urethrogram should be performed before a urinary catheter is placed. This is followed by a cystogram to assess the integrity of the bladder after the catheter is placed. In unstable patients, a suprapubic catheter may be placed in the bladder by percutaneous techniques, and genitourinary evaluation is delayed.

How and when should Mr. Smith's right leg fracture be treated?

Fractures may cause long-term disability if not properly treated, but they are not life-threatening injuries. They are addressed during the secondary survey. Fractures are placed in a splint or on traction, as appropriate, for later definitive treatment. Adequate analgesia should be used for fracture reduction. Vascular compromise with long-bone fractures may be due to kinking of the blood supply, direct vascular injury, or compartment syndrome.

What is compartment syndrome?

Compartment syndrome is compression of the nerve or blood supply within fascial compartments because of either accumulation of blood or edema within a limited space. This leads to decreased capillary perfusion and potential muscle necrosis and loss of limb. With most closed fractures, pulses that were absent return after the fracture is reduced. If this is the case, at many centers further evaluation for vascular injury is deferred with good results.

Measurement of ankle [illegible] an also be performed. If t[illegible]ed by angiography. Mea[illegible] an assess compartment syndrome, or fasciotomy can be performed on a presumptive basis. Remember that correction of life-threatening injuries in the trauma patient with multiple injuries takes precedence over treatment of a threatened extremity.

The fracture is manually reduced, and this leads to return of pulses and improvement in color and warmth of the foot. A posterior splint is placed.

What are the components of the secondary survey?

Components of the secondary survey include a complete history and a full head to toe physical examination, including a rectal examination, and for women, a pelvic examination. It begins after life-threatening injuries are dealt with in the primary survey.

Basic trauma radiographs consisting of a lateral cervical spine, a chest radiograph, and pelvic radiograph were obtained. The chest radiograph reveals multiple left-sided rib fractures and a well-positioned thoracostomy tube. The mediastinal silhouette is abnormally wide.

What is the significance of a wide mediastinum on chest radiographs in patients with blunt trauma?

A wide mediastinum is the most common radiographic indicator of aortic rupture. Other signs that may be present include the following:

1. Obliteration of the aortic knob
2. Deviation of the trachea to the right
3. Pleural cap (an indication of extrapleural hematoma)
4. Elevation and shift to the right of the right main stem bronchus
5. Depression of the left main stem bronchus
6. Deviation of the esophagus (nasogastric tube) to the right
7. Obliteration of the aortopulmonary window

A normal radiograph does not rule out a transected aorta. Helical (spiral) CT of the thorax is currently the most used modality for the diagnosis of aortic injury (11–13). Transesophageal echocardiography may be used for rapid diagnosis in the operating room or intensive care unit. The gold standard for diagnosis of aortic transection is still aortography.

The radiograph of the pelvis reveals an open-book type of pelvic fracture with a widened pubic symphysis and sacroiliac joints. The cervical spine radiograph is normal. A comminuted fracture of the tibia and fibula is

revealed from a radiograph of the right femur. Mr. Smith remains stable for about 15 minutes before his systolic blood pressure drops again to 80 mm Hg, and the diastolic blood pressure is not audible. His heart rate is 120 beats per minute. There is no arterial desaturation and he is easy to ventilate. The initial assessment is rapidly repeated. The tube thoracostomy is in good position and there are bilateral breath sounds. There is a small air leak, as expected. The neck veins are collapsed and the trachea is in midline position. Crystalloid infusion is given, but the response is only partial.

What is the cause of the recurrent hypotension? What is the significance of a partial response to resuscitation?

With other causes ruled out, the most likely cause of recurrent hypotension in this patient is hypovolemic shock consequent to ongoing hidden blood loss. The partial response to crystalloid resuscitation indicates profound hypovolemia or loss of red cell mass. Failure to respond to crystalloid infusion or recurrent hypotension indicates continuing blood loss at a significant rate and is a definite indication to transfuse type-specific or universal donor blood immediately (4) (Table 30.3).

What is shock?

Shock is inadequate tissue perfusion and oxygen delivery. It manifests as peripheral vasoconstriction and tachycardia as the earliest findings, a narrowed pulse pressure, altered sensorium, oliguria, and metabolic acidosis. Hypotension is a late finding in shock because homeostatic mechanisms maintain blood pressure until volume loss is greater than 30%. Any trauma patient who has vasoconstriction and tachycardia should be considered to be in shock until proven otherwise (4).

What are the types of shock commonly identified in trauma patients?

1. *Hypovolemic or hemorrhagic shock:* the most common form of shock seen in trauma (14)
2. *Cardiac compressive shock:* is consequent to pericardial tamponade or tension pneumothorax
3. *Neurogenic shock:* occurs after spinal cord injury and is caused by bradycardia and pooling of blood consequent to sympathetic denervation
4. *Septic shock:* is secondary to infection and often complicates the later hospital course after major injury but is rarely seen immediately after the injury
5. *Cardiogenic shock:* is rare in acute trauma but may occur as a consequence of ischemic myocardial injury due to prolonged hypovolemia, hypoxia, or preexisting coronary artery disease (14).

TABLE 30.3.

RESPONSES TO INITIAL FLUID RESUSCITATION

Tests	Rapid Response	Transient Response	No Response
Vital signs	Return to normal	Transient improvement; recurrence of drop in blood pressure, rise in heart rate	Remain abnormal
Estimated blood loss	Minimal (10%–20%)	Moderate, ongoing (20–40%)	Severe (>40%)
Need for more crystalloid	Low	High	High
Need for blood	Low	Moderate to high	Immediate
Blood preparation	Type and cross-match	Type-specific release	Emergency
Need for surgery	Possible	Likely	Highly likely
Surgical consultation	Yes	Yes	Yes

Fluid resuscitation consists of 2 L Ringer's lactate in adults, 20 mL/kg Ringer's lactate in children, over 10–15 min.

From American College of Surgeons. Advanced Trauma Life Support Program for Physicians: Instructor Manual. Chicago, Ill: American College of Surgeons; 1993;3:75–94, with permission.

What are the possible sites of blood loss in trauma patients?

The trauma patient can bleed in five compartments. Each must be ruled out in a systematic manner:

1. Chest—one or both pleural spaces
2. Peritoneal cavity—solid organ injuries (liver and spleen) or mesenteric tear
3. Retroperitoneum—pelvic fracture or other retroperitoneal injuries causing a retroperitoneal hematoma
4. Muscle compartments—severe contusion to muscular and subcutaneous tissues or long bone fractures, particularly a fracture of the femur, in which 1.0 to 1.5 L of blood may accumulate in each thigh
5. The street—missed external injuries with underestimated losses into linens, into dressings, and onto the floor

How is the site of bleeding determined?

All of the possible sites must be assessed. Hemothorax should be checked for with a repeated chest radiograph. The patient should be quickly reexamined for external bleeding and expanding hematoma of the lower extremities or soft tissues. This process of elimination points to the abdomen (peritoneal cavity) and fractured pelvis (retroperitoneum) as the likely sites of bleeding in Mr. Smith.

What are the options for evaluating abdominal injuries? Which modality is most appropriate for this patient?

Patients with evidence of blood loss who show signs of peritoneal irritation (e.g., rebound tenderness) are taken promptly to the operating room for laparotomy without further diagnostic tests. Barring any evidence of peritonitis, or in situations in which the physical examination is unreliable (depressed or altered mental status from CHI or drugs and alcohol), the different modalities for evaluating the abdomen depend on the hemodynamic stability of the patient and the available resources. If the patient is stable, ultrasonography (US) and CT can be used. CT scan is the most sensitive and the most specific modality.

Unstable patients with episodes of persistent or recurrent hypotension are evaluated with US or diagnostic peritoneal lavage (DPL). Focused abdominal sonographic examination for trauma (FAST), performed by surgeons trained in it, has supplanted DPL in most centers because it is similarly accurate and is noninvasive (15). DPL is more sensitive than US and requires minimal equipment, but it is invasive, nonspecific, and nondiagnostic for retroperitoneal injuries, and it can lead to many nontherapeutic laparotomies. It involves passing a catheter through a small incision in the abdomen, followed by aspirating fluid and irrigating with saline solution. The presence of gross blood or an irrigation return containing more than 100,000 red blood cells per cubic millimeter indicates significant shed blood in the abdomen.

Unstable patients with positive results from US should undergo prompt laparotomy. Unstable patients with equivocal US results may be further assessed with DPL. Stable patients with positive US results may safely have further evaluation by CT, which is more specific than US and may assist in the nonoperative management of certain solid organ (liver, spleen, kidney) injuries (15). A patient such as Mr. Smith, whose condition is unstable, should be evaluated in the trauma room by US or by DPL.

What is the role of laparoscopy in the evaluation and management of abdominal trauma?

The use of laparoscopy as a primary diagnostic tool in blunt abdominal trauma is still very limited. It can be used as an adjunct to CT scan, especially in the presence of peritoneal fluid and the absence of solid organ injuries. The greatest challenge in abdominal trauma is the optimal management of penetrating abdominal injuries in a stable patient with doubtful intraperitoneal trajectory (tangential abdominal and lower thoracic wounds). Since the mid-1990s, laparoscopy has established its role in the evaluation and management of penetrating abdominal trauma in stable patients. It minimizes unnecessary laparotomies while avoiding missed injuries and safely manages these injuries in a cost-effective manner without significant complications. However, mandatory celiotomy is still the treatment of choice where advanced skills in laparoscopy are lacking. Laparoscopy has no role in the unstable patient (16–18).

Mr. Smith undergoes US, and a large amount of fluid is revealed in Morrison's pouch. He continues to be borderline hypotensive, with a blood pressure of 95/40 mm Hg despite the ongoing blood transfusion. It is now known that the sites of blood loss are the abdomen and most likely the retroperitoneum as a result of his pelvic fracture.

How should a patient such as Mr. Smith be treated next?

An exploratory laparotomy is performed to control abdominal bleeding. The presumed pelvic fracture bleeding is treated concurrently. Pelvic fractures, such as Mr. Smith's, bleed from torn sacral veins at the sacroiliac joints and from arterial branches of the hypogastric arteries. Treatment usually entails placement of an external orthopedic fixator device in the operating room. By compressing the pelvis, the external fixator reduces the fracture and decreases bleeding from the sacral veins. At many centers, iliac angiography is performed to embolize bleeding branches of the hypogastric arteries with coils, synthetic gel, or autologous clot.

Mr. Smith is taken to the operating room and was found to be bleeding from a shattered spleen. Splenectomy is performed. A pelvic external fixator was placed by the orthopedic service.

What are the options for managing splenic injury?

Splenic injury ranges from grade I to grade V (19), with *grade I* being a small subcapsular hematoma and *grade V* being a shattered spleen or a hilar injury with complete devascularization of the spleen. CT is needed to grade splenic injuries.

At present, 40% to 60% of splenic injuries can be managed nonoperatively (20,21). The major requirement is that the patient be hemodynamically stable without evidence of major ongoing blood loss, as monitored by hematocrit, vital signs, and physical examination. Detection of a blush on CT is an indication for angiographic embolization in the stable patient. An ongoing decrease in the hematocrit value or a worsening examination indicates unsuccessful nonoperative management, and immediate surgery is dictated. To protect against overwhelming postsplenectomy sepsis from encapsulated gram-negative bacteria, Mr. Smith needs vaccination against pneumococcal and *Haemophilus influenzae* infection before hospital discharge.

On the second postoperative day, Mr. Smith's fluid requirement to maintain blood pressure increases, and his urine output decreases. A meticulous search for bleeding sites is unproductive. A pulmonary artery catheter is passed to assess volume and cardiac function; the results reveal high cardiac output, normal pulmonary capillary wedge pressure, and low systemic vascular resistance. The arterial oxygenation level decreases, and the chest radiograph shows patchy infiltrates indicating acute respiratory distress syndrome (ARDS). The urinary sediment is compatible with a diagnosis of acute tubular necrosis. Liver enzymes are mildly elevated, and prothrombin time is prolonged. The platelet count decreases to 75,000 per mm^3.

What do these findings indicate?

These findings indicate multisystem organ failure (MSOF), the cause of which is poorly understood but probably multifactorial. The major contributors may be direct ischemic injury to organs and the systemic inflammatory response syndrome (SIRS).

What is SIRS?

Formerly called *sepsis syndrome, SIRS* is now known to be initiated by stresses that do not involve infectious agents. These include ischemic insult, pancreatitis, burns, and trauma. Inflammatory mediators, such as cytokines and kinins, released from damaged tissues may cause the organ injury and the high-output hemodynamics of SIRS. These substances include tumor necrosis factor (TNF), interleukins, and interferons (Table 30.4). They regulate immune, cardiovascular, and metabolic responses to injury in a complicated cascade that amplifies the response to injury for an extended period after the initial insult (22). Exaggerated production of or response to cytokines may produce both the hemodynamic manifestations of septic shock and the refractory catabolic state and tissue wasting seen in severe injury and infection.

What is the treatment for SIRS and MSOF?

The alleviation of persisting causes, such as infection, ischemia, shock, and any necrotic tissue, offers the best hope for treating MSOF. Beyond this, the treatment for SIRS is supportive care only. Organ function is supported by mechanical ventilation, inotropic agents, dialysis, correction of coagulopathy, and nutritional support. Inhibitors and antibodies to various cytokines may have a clinical role in limiting SIRS and preventing death from MSOF in trauma. In the past, however, despite numerous clinical trials using novel pharmacological agents (anti-endotoxin antibodies, antibodies to TNF, interleukin-1 [IL-1] receptor antagonist) placebo-controlled trials have failed to demonstrate convincing clinical benefit. The only Food and Drug Administration–approved agent with proven

TABLE 30.4.

BIOLOGIC ACTIVITIES OF SELECT CYTOKINES

	Tumor Necrosis Factor	Interleukin-1	Interleukin-2	Interleukin-6
Immune system				
Neutrophils	↑ Bone marrow release ↑ Margination ↑ Transendothelial passage ↑ Activation	↑ Bone marrow release ↑ Influx to site of injury ↑ Transendothelial passage	Leukocytosis	
Monocytes	↑ Blood monocyte differentiation ↑ Activation ↑ Cytotoxicity	↑ Blood monocyte differentiation ↑ Activation		
Lymphocytes	↑ Lymphokine production	↑ T-cell activation ↑ Lymphokine production	↑ T-cell proliferation ↑ Cytotoxicity ↑ Lymphokine synthesis	↑ Differentiation ↑ B-cell proliferation ↑ Cytotoxicity
Eosinophils	Activation of eosinophils		Eosinophilia Organ infiltration	
Cardiovascular system	Hypotension Shock ↑ Vascular leak	? Hypotension	↑ Vascular leak ? Hypotension	
Metabolic effects	Anorexia Weight loss Fever	Anorexia Weight loss Fever	? Fever	Fever

continued

TABLE 30.4.

BIOLOGIC ACTIVITIES OF SELECT CYTOKINES—*Continued*

	Tumor Necrosis Factor	Interleukin-1	Interleukin-2	Interleukin-6
Hepatic	↑ Lipogenesis ↑ Amino acid uptake ↑ Acute-phase protein synthesis ↓ Albumin synthesis	↑ Acute-phase protein synthesis ↓ Albumin synthesis		↑ Acute-phase protein synthesis
Skeletal muscle	↓ Resting membrane potential ↑ Amino acid loss ↑ Myofibrillar protein mRNA ↑ Hexose transporters ↓ Cellular glycogen ↑ Lactate production	↑ Nitrogen loss ↓ Myofibrillar protein mRNA		
Lipid	Inhibition of lipoprotein lipase ↓ Free fatty acid synthesis ↑ Lipolysis	Inhibition of lipoprotein lipase		

From Fong Y, Lowry S. Trauma: cytokines and cellular response to injury and infection. In: Wilmore DW, Brennan MF, Harken AH, et al., eds. ACS Care of the Surgical Patient. New York, NY: Scientific American; 1996;4:1–25, with permission.

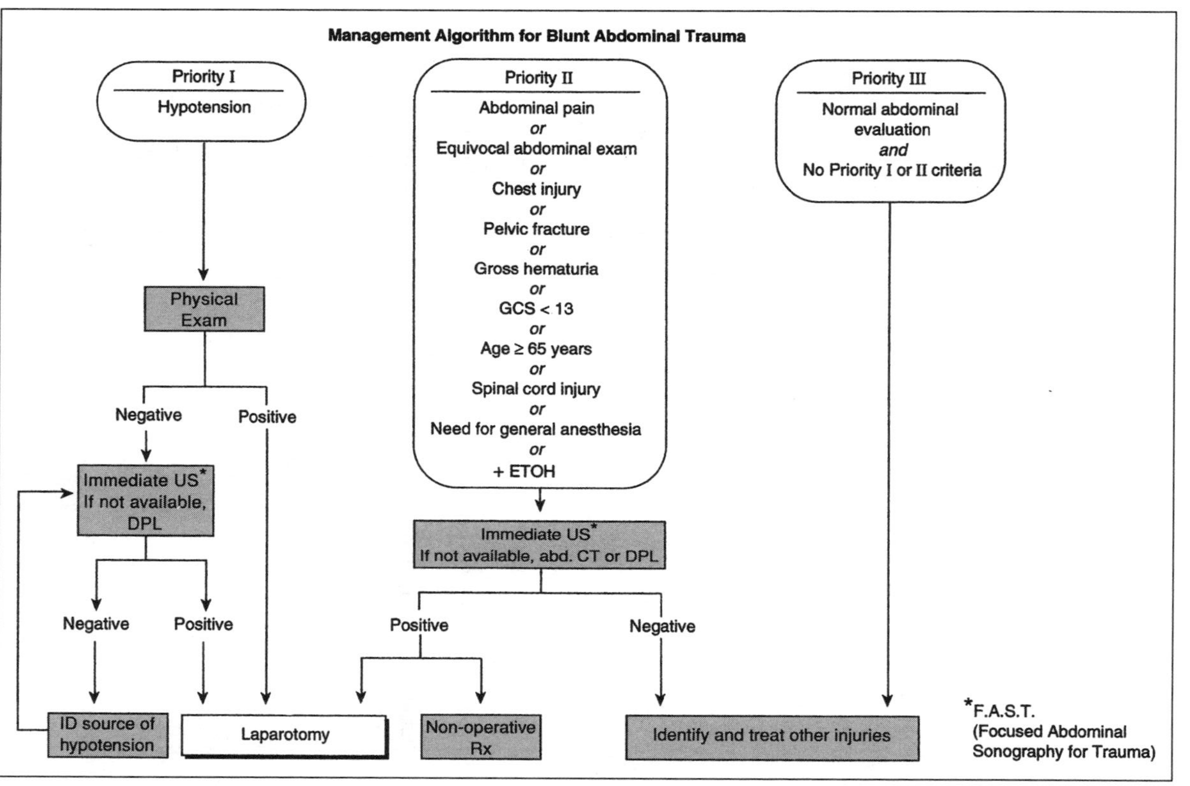

Algorithm 30.1.

reduction in mortality in patients with severe sepsis is the human recombinant form of activated protein C (Xigris, or Drotrecogin Alpha [Activated]) (23,24).

REFERENCES

1. Miller SM. Management of central nervous system injuries. In: Capan LM, Miller SM, Turndorf H, eds. Trauma: Anesthesia and Intensive Care. Philadelphia, Pa: WB Saunders; 1985:207.
2. Michael DB, Wilson RF. Head injuries. In: Wilson RF, Walt AJ, eds. Management of Trauma: Pitfalls and Practice. Baltimore, Md: Williams & Wilkins; 1996:173–202.
3. Teasdale G, Jennett B. Assessment of coma and impaired consciousness. A practical scale. Lancet. 1974;2:81–84.
4. American College of Surgeons Committee on Trauma. Advanced Trauma Life Support for Doctors. Instructor Course Manual, 1997. Chicago, Ill: American College of Surgeons; 2002.
5. Demetriades D, Vander Veen PW. Penetrating injuries of the heart: experience over two years in South America. J Trauma. 1983;23:1034.
6. Arom KV, Richardson JD, Webb G, et al. Subxiphoid pericardial window in patients with suspected traumatic pericardial tamponade. Ann Thorac Surg. 1977;23:545–549.
7. Wilson RF, Basset JS. Penetrating wounds of the pericardium or its contents. JAMA. 1966;195:513.
8. Maull KI. Alcohol abuse: its implications in trauma care. South Med J. 1982;75:794.
9. Walls RM. Rapid-sequence intubation in head trauma. Ann Emerg Med. 1993;22:1008.
10. Woster PS, LeBlanc KL. Management of elevated intracranial pressure. Clin Pharm. 1990;9:762.
11. Hunink MG, Bos JJ. Triage of patients to angiography for detection of aortic rupture after blunt chest trauma: cost-effectiveness analysis of using CT. AJR Am J Roentgenol. 1995;165(1):27–36.
12. Gavant ML, Menke PG, Fabian T, et al. Blunt traumatic aortic rupture: detection with helical CT of the chest. Radiology. 1995;197(1):125–133.
13. Gavant ML, Flick P, Menke P, et al. CT aortography of thoracic aortic rupture. Am J Roentgenol AJR. 1996;166(4):955–961.
14. Holcroft JW. Shock. In: Willmore DW, Brennan MF, Harken AH, et al., eds. Care of the Surgical Patient. New York, NY: Scientific American; 1989:1–12.
15. McElveen TS, Collin GR. The role of ultrasonography in blunt abdominal trauma: a prospective study. Am Surg. 1997;63:184–188.
16. Ivatury R, Zantut L, Yelon J. Trauma care in the new millennium. Laparoscopy in the new century. Surg Clin North Am. 1999;79:1291–1295.
17. Mazuski J, Shaoiro M, Kaminski D. Diagnostic laparoscopy for evaluation of penetrating abdominal trauma. J Trauma. 1997;42:163.
18. Townsend M, Flauncbaum L, Choban P, et al. Diagnostic laparoscopy as an adjunct to selective conservative management of solid organ injuries after blunt abdominal trauma. J Trauma. 1993;35:647.

19. Moore EE, Shackford SR, Pachter HL, et al. Organ injury scaling: spleen, liver, kidney. J Trauma. 1989;29:1664–1666.
20. Cogbill TH, Moore EE, Jurkovich GJ, et al. Nonoperative management of blunt splenic trauma: a multicenter experience. J Trauma. 1989;29:1312–1317.
21. Pachter HL, Guth AA, Hofstetter SR. Changing patterns in the management of splenic trauma: the impact of nonoperative management. Ann Surg. 1997;227:708.
22. Fong Y, Lowry S. Trauma: cytokines and cellular response to injury and infection. In: Wilmore DW, Brennan MF, Harken AH, et al., eds. ACS Care of the Surgical Patient. New York, NY: Scientific American; 1996:1–25.
23. Vincent J-L, Angus DC, Artigas A, et al. Effects of drotrecogin alfa (activated) on organ dysfunction in the PROWESS trial. Crit Care Med. 2003;31:834–840.
24. Matthay M. Severe sepsis: A new treatment with both anticoagulant and anti-inflammatory properties. N Engl J Med. 2001;344:759–762.

CHAPTER

31

COMMON POSTOPERATIVE COMPLICATIONS: OLIGURIA, DYSPNEA, FEVER, AND HYPOTENSION

Bruce Simon

OLIGURIA

Mrs. Jones is a 70-year-old woman without previous known medical history who had not seen a physician in many years. She presented to the emergency department of your hospital complaining of 3 days of nausea, vomiting, and abdominal pain. Although her vital signs were stable on admission, she required fluid resuscitation in the emergency department for low urine output. At surgery, strangulation obstruction of the small bowel was found and a resection of some necrotic bowel and primary anastomosis was performed. Mrs. Jones remained stable throughout surgery and was admitted to the surgical intermediate care unit postoperatively.

Why was Mrs. Jones admitted to an intermediate care unit after surgery?
Mrs. Jones is at risk for developing significant complications, even though her surgery went uneventfully. Although some complications may result from intraoperative events, others are related to pre-existing medical conditions, the clinical situation, and the urgency of operation. Mrs. Jones has no known medical history; however, occult cardiovascular disease is certainly possible. She was dehydrated at presentation with evidence of organ malperfusion and is at significant risk for infectious complications from her necrotic bowel.

Six hours postoperatively the nurse calls you because Mrs. Jones' urine output has been 15 mL per hour for 2 hours and she has produced no urine output for the last hour. Vital signs are stable but she is slightly

TABLE 31.1.

COMMON ETIOLOGIES OF OLIGURIA IN THE SURGICAL PATIENT LISTED BY PHYSIOLOGIC CATEGORY

Prerenal	Renal	Postrenal
Hypovolemia	Acute tubular necrosis	Outflow obstruction
Congestive heart failure		Blocked urinary catheter
Nonhypovolemic shock states (i.e. cardiogenic)		

tachycardic at a rate of 110 beats per minute. Mrs. Jones's problem must be evaluated.

What is normal urine output?

Normal urine output is usually thought to be greater than 0.5 mL per kg per hour. It is an important estimate of the adequacy of end-organ (in this case, the kidney) perfusion, and it is important to focus on organ perfusion rather than the strict number of milliliters of urine. When urine output is low, it is useful to consider prerenal, renal, and postrenal causes (Table 31.1) (1).

Prerenal oliguria is caused by inadequate glomerular perfusion or renal ischemia; hypovolemia is a classic example and is the most common cause of oliguria in the postoperative patient. Low cardiac output syndromes and congestive heart failure can also cause prerenal azotemia.

Renal causes of oliguria include injury to the renal tubules from toxins, antibiotics, intravenous (IV) contrast, and other direct insults. They may progress to acute renal failure.

Postrenal causes of oliguria are those factors distal to the renal tubules that obstruct the drainage of urine. Eventually, this back-pressure leads to renal injury. The most common and easily correctable example of a postrenal process is obstruction of the urinary catheter by clot or debris. Obstruction of the ureter by hematoma can occur as a complication of certain abdominal procedures, but bilateral obstruction would be required to impair urine output.

While you are considering the etiology of oliguria in the postoperative setting, the nurse asks you what you want to do.

How do you proceed?

First, confirm the patency of the indwelling bladder catheter. This is particularly crucial when it is reported that urine output has suddenly dropped to zero.

Once this is done, assess the patient for signs and symptoms of hypovolemia or hypervolemia. The fluid balance since surgery and the dilutional state of the urine may provide further useful information. A urine specific gravity equal to or greater than 1.020 is concentrated and supports the assessment of hypovolemia. An increased hematocrit, sodium, or urea-to-creatinine ratio further strengthens this impression. A chest radiograph may complete the assessment of the patient's volume status if it remains otherwise unclear.

Patients who are hypovolemic receive one or two fluid boluses of crystalloid or colloid solution; 500 mL of lactated Ringer's solution or one unit of albumin constitute reasonable fluid boluses. Those patients who appear hypervolemic may receive a trial dose of an IV loop diuretic such as furosemide.

If there is no response to these diagnostic challenges or if the picture remains unclear, consider assessing the intravascular volume status with central venous pressure (CVP) monitoring. CVP roughly correlates with intravascular volume (2), although the normal CVP may range between 0 and 8 mm Hg. A low or equivocal CVP may justify further fluid resuscitation and monitoring of urine output. An elevated CVP indicates a need for more aggressive diuresis. It is particularly useful to follow the trends in CVP as therapeutic interventions are made.

When should pulmonary artery catheterization be considered and how does it work?

Failure to obtain urine output with therapy directed by CVP may be an indication for placement of a flow-directed pulmonary artery catheter (3,4). The pulmonary artery catheter has a balloon at its tip. Inflation of this balloon causes the catheter to float across the tricuspid valve, into the right ventricle, and across the pulmonic valve. The catheter and tip rest in the proximal pulmonary artery of either the right or the left lung.

When the balloon is inflated, the catheter wedges in the pulmonary artery. The pressure sensor at the tip of the catheter reads the pressure downstream, called the *pulmonary capillary wedge pressure* (PCWP). Because there are no valves between the left atrium and the pulmonary arteries, the PCWP closely approximates left atrial pressure and is an excellent barometer of left ventricular preload. A low PCWP indicates hypovolemia and prompts further fluid loading. If the PCWP is normal (10 to 14 mmHg), intravascular volume is adequate and a search for other causes of oliguria is necessary. Persistent oliguria in the face of a high PCWP raises the possibility of renal failure or postrenal obstruction.

When reviewing Mrs. Jones's flowsheet you note that she received only 2 L of fluid during her surgery. Although her recorded operative fluid loss was minimal, you are aware that she probably had the small-bowel obstruction for several days and had come to surgery with a considerable pre-existing deficit. Vital signs are normal. Examination shows

clear lungs and dry mucus membranes. Urine specific gravity is 1.025. Hematocrit is elevated at 46% and blood urea nitrogen (BUN) elevated at 21 mg/dL. You are confident that Mrs. Jones is hypovolemic and order two 500-mL fluid boluses of normal saline (NS). An hour later, the urine output has not picked up. A central venous line is inserted and the CVP is 4 mmHg. Another liter of NS is given, raising the CVP to 7 mm Hg. The urine output improves significantly.

RESPIRATORY INSUFFICIENCY

Mrs. Jones remains well with normal vitals signs until the middle of postoperative day 1. She has previously been resting comfortably but now the nurse calls to inform you she is complaining of dyspnea or shortness of breath. You are told that her respiratory rate is 34 breaths per minute and she is tachycardic to 105 breaths per minute. Her oxygen saturation is 94% on 2-L nasal cannula. Her blood pressure is normal.

Mrs. Jones's arterial saturations are adequate; should you be concerned?

Yes. When assessing patients with respiratory complaints, it is necessary to differentiate those with subjective dyspnea who are well compensated, those with true but mild insufficiency, and those with impending respiratory failure (5,6). Patients in acute respiratory distress requiring intubation will need ventilatory support before determination of the exact cause of the problem. Arterial oxygen desaturation on pulse oximetry may provide a clue, but arterial desaturation is a late event, particularly if supplemental oxygen is being provided. A rapid, shallow respiratory pattern (rate greater than 40 breaths per minute), the use of accessory muscles of respiration, or paradoxical motion of the diaphragm may indicate respiratory muscle fatigue and impending mechanical ventilatory failure. Confusion, anxiety, or cyanosis are signs of inadequate oxygen delivery and should prompt inhalation of ventilatory support.

When you arrive in the intermediate care unit, you note that Mrs. Jones is slightly tachypneic as claimed. Her heart rate is 90 beats per minute. She is not breathing with accessory muscles, is pink, and is easily able to talk. Intubation does not seem necessary at this time. On examination, Mrs. Jones has decreased breath sounds at the bases and is taking shallow breaths at a slightly increased rate of 30 breaths per minute. Her incentive spirometry is only 4 mL per kg (greater than 10 mL per kg acceptable), and she volunteers that deep breathing is painful.

A chest radiograph obtained by the nurse shows only decreased lung volumes and increased density at the bases. Oxygen saturation improves

to 98% on 4 L. Your presumptive diagnosis is atelectasis and you order increased analgesia and aggressive physiotherapy and encourage spirometry. On a follow-up visit later that evening, Mrs. Jones is much improved and appreciative of your help.

Why did you choose this course of action?

When respiratory failure is not impending, increasing supplemental oxygen may improve arterial blood saturation and improve symptoms but may not address the primary problem. Assessment of events surrounding the patient's symptoms may be helpful. For example, sudden onset of dyspnea may occur due to mucus plugging in a sedentary patient. Pulmonary embolism may present suddenly in a patient recently mobile. Gradual worsening of breathing may be more indicative of atelectasis or a developing pneumonia (7). Sudden shortness of breath while eating may indicate aspiration.

The physical examination is particularly important and can suggest a diagnosis, as in patients with bronchospasm, congestive heart failure, or a pneumothorax. A chest radiograph should routinely be obtained and can make the diagnosis. Arterial blood gases are helpful to define worsening oxygenation and hypercapnia.

Finally, cardiovascular complications such as acute myocardial infarction can manifest with respiratory distress. The diagnostic features and major treatments for the most common causes of postoperative respiratory insufficiency are outlined in Table 31.2 (8–10).

FEVER

Mrs. Jones continues to do well into postoperative day 3 when the nurse notifies you that she has recorded a temperature spike of 101.2°F. Other than the temperature, Mrs. Jones is reportedly well and without symptoms. You tell the nurse you will come down shortly to see Mrs. Jones.

Is the timing of her fever important? What is atelectasis?

The most common causes of postoperative fever, their usual time frames for occurrence, and risk factors are outlined in Table 31.3. The most common cause of fever in the early postoperative period is atelectasis, for which fever may be the only clinical sign. *Atelectasis* is characterized by alveolar collapse due to poor inspiratory effort. Patients may complain of pain on deep breathing and have decreased breath sounds at the lung bases. Most notably, atelectasis is characterized by its low-grade temperature of less than 101.5°F and mild leukocytosis of less than 12,000 per mm^3; higher values lead to suspicion of another diagnosis. Although atelectasis may progress to pneumonia, it is not a bacterial process (11,12) and consequently, blood cultures are generally not useful (13,14).

TABLE 31.2.

DIAGNOSTIC FEATURES AND MAJOR TREATMENTS FOR THE MOST COMMON CAUSES OF POSTOPERATIVE RESPIRATORY INSUFFICIENCY

	Risk Factors	Lung Exam	Chest Radiography	Other Factors	Treatment
Atelectasis	Abdominal/thoracic incision	Decreased: Breath sounds Respiratory excursions	Decreased volume Hazy diaphragms	Poor spirometry, good response to O_2	Analgesia, spirometry, chest physiotherapy, encouragement, Mucolytics, Occasional bronchoscopy
Aspiration of Gastric Contents	Emergency operation; tube feeding	Localized rales	Lobar infiltrate; often RLL	Increased secretions +/− temp, WBC	Physiotherapy, spirometry, sputum culture, +/− antibiotics
Congestive Heart Failure/Pulmonary Edema	Cardiac history + fluid balance	Rales, wheezes, JVD	Pulmonary vascular congestion; alveolar infiltrates	High CVP	Diuresis, digitalization preload reduction (nitrates)
Pneumothorax	COPD, positive pressure ventilation, central venous catheter	Unilateral absent breath sounds; hypertympany	No lung markings		Tube thoracostomy
Pulmonary Embolism	Obesity, malignancy, immobility, DVT, previous PE	Normal	Clear	Sudden onset Hypoxia fails to improve with O2; confirmatory study	Anticoagulation, vena cava filter
Bronchospasm	Asthma, COPD, blood transfusion	Wheezes or minimal air movement	Clear		Bronchodilators, steroids
Myocardial Infarction	Coronary artery disease	+/− rales, +/− JVD	Usually clear; Occasional congested	Tachycardia +/− cyanosis, ECG, CPK, troponin	Nitrates, beta-blockers, Heparin, inotropic agents if shock

COPD, chronic obstructive pulmonary disease; CPK, creatine phosphokinase; DVT, deep venous thrombosis; JVD, jugular venous distension; PE, pulmonary edema; WBC, white blood cell; ECG, electrocardiogram.

TABLE 31.3.

MOST COMMON CAUSES OF POSTOPERATIVE FEVER, ASSOCIATED TIME FRAMES, AND RISK FACTORS

	Time Frame	Risk Factors
Atelectasis	1–2 days	Abdominal incision
Urinary infection	3 days with catheter	Catheter
Wound infection	5–7 days	Malnutrition, diabetes, cancer, immune suppression, contaminated surgery
Abdominal Abscess	5–7 days	As above Peritonitis, contamination, bowel anastomosis Emergency surgery
Pneumonia	Anytime	Altered mentation, lung disease, tube feedings, prolonged mechanical ventilation
***C. difficile* colitis**	During/after antibiotics	Prolonged broad spectrum antibiotics (cephalosporins)
Deep venous thrombosis	Anytime	Obesity, immobility, cancer, smoking, oral contraceptive, previous deep venous thrombosis or pulmonary embolism
Transfusion reaction	Transfusion within 2 hrs	Previous transfusion reaction

Pneumonia can occur at any time. In general, malnutrition, cancer, and emergent surgery all create subtle immune compromise and increase the risk for infectious complications (15). Bacterial pneumonia may secondarily affect atelectatic lungs or may be associated with aspiration. Colonization of the trachea and proximal tracheobronchial tree is common in patients with endotracheal tubes on ventilatory support. The postoperative patient with pneumonia usually complains of shortness of breath but may not produce sputum. There may be any combination of purulent sputum, cough, rales, and an infiltrate on radiograph. Treatment is based on appropriate antibiotics and pulmonary physiotherapy.

Mrs. Jones is breathing without difficulty. You notice that her Foley catheter is still in place. She asks you not to remove it because she has trouble walking to the bathroom and does not want to use a bedpan.

Urinary tract infection (UTI) may occur anytime after bladder catheter insertion, either from colonization after prolonged use or earlier, from inadvertent contamination during insertion. UTIs may also occur in patients with urinary retention and stasis after catheter removal. Symptoms of frequency, urgency, and dysuria may not be present with an indwelling catheter. The urine may be cloudy, and a positive test for leukocyte esterase in the urine may provide further evidence of infection. Diagnosis is easily made with a urinalysis and culture. The mainstay of diagnosis is the presence of bacteria and white blood cells in the urine. The main pathogens are gram-negative enteric organisms, particularly *Escherichia coli*, and the treatment is by appropriate antibiotic therapy based on cultures. The catheter should be removed or changed if possible. Alternatively, intermittent catheterization may allow resolution of the infection.

Mrs. Jones has her catheter removed and she is encouraged to increase her ambulation. Two days later, she tells the medical student she is having more pain at the site of her incision. The medical student reminds her to take her pain medication and dismisses it, thinking that all patients have pain after surgery.

Is this of concern?

Yes. Abdominal wound infections generally occur from 5 to 7 days after surgery. They are characterized by a spiking fever curve, increased wound pain, and tenderness. Eventually, increased wound erythema and warmth develop. Early signs of a wound infection may be subtle, and the only symptom may be a change in the pain pattern. Regular, serial examination of the wound is critical. Probing the wound with a cotton sw will often reveal purulent drainage.

The mainstay of treatment involves wide opening of the infected subcutaneous layer and removal of all infected material. The incision is then treated as an open wound in a variety of ways and may or may not be closed later. Antibiotics are a secondary component of treatment. The offending organisms are usually skin *Staphylococcus* and *Streptococcus* but may involve gram-negative rods and anaerobes when intestine has been opened during the operative procedure.

A critical exception to the principles of postoperative wound infection is that of necrotizing fasciitis. This virulent polymicrobial infection is commonly seen after contaminated trauma cases but may also be seen with general surgical and gynecologic procedures. It is especially important as it may manifest within several hours of surgery with severe wound pain and tenderness extending far beyond the wound. Serous drainage from the wound may occur, although gross purulence is minimal. Severe systemic toxicity occurs. Wound infection is discussed in greater detail elsewhere in this text and the reader is also referred to the additional references within this chapter (16).

Abdominal abscess is another infectious complication of abdominal surgery. An abdominal abscess is more likely to occur when there is pre-existing peritoneal contamination or peritonitis such as might follow emergent surgery for a colon perforation or for necrotic bowel. It is also more likely when an intestinal anastomosis is performed in the presence of malnutrition, shock, or compromised perfusion. As with wound infection, abdominal abscess is associated with a spiking temperature and a high leukocytosis. There may or may not be abdominal complaints based on the location of the abscess, and abdominal examination may be normal. Suspicion is based on the surgical history and diagnosis is usually made by CT scanning. Treatment involves antibiotics and drainage, either by radiologically guided catheter or by open surgery.

What is pseudomembranous colitis?

Clostridia difficile colitis or pseudomembranous colitis is traditionally associated with the prolonged use of broad-spectrum antibiotics, most commonly cephalosporins, but has been documented with short courses of other agents. The condition is manifest by non-bloody diarrhea, abdominal pain, tenderness, and leukocytosis. Varying degrees of toxicity may occur and diagnosis is usually made by assay for toxin in the stool. Treatment involves cessation of the offending antibiotic and institution of oral metronidazole or vancomycin.

Mrs. Jones does not have a UTI, her wound is pristine, the abdominal CT is negative, and her chest radiograph is clear. Yet she still has intermittent fevers.

Should you start empiric antibiotics?

Fever of unknown origin in the surgical patient usually means the physician has not looked hard enough for the diagnosis. Treatment of fever of unknown etiology with antibiotics in the postoperative patient remains controversial. Untreated sepsis is certainly to be avoided and early therapy can be life-saving; however, injudicious use of broadspectrum antibiotics has been associated with fatal fungal infection and antibiotic-associated colitis (17,18), as well as development of antibiotic-resistant organisms.

What else could it be?

Two less common causes of postoperative fever are deep venous thrombosis (DVT) and transfusion reaction. DVT is characterized by a low-grade fever and minimal leukocytosis. Thrombus may occur in the iliac, femoral, or calf veins. There may or may not be leg edema tenderness, a palpable cord, or a positive Homan's sign. Diagnosis is best made by duplex ultrasound of the femoral veins. Febrile transfusion reactions are usually heralded with temperatures lower than 101.5°F within 2 hours of transfusion. They are caused by pyrogens in the blood or by recipient antibodies to donor white cells. Temperature usually resolves within 2 hours. There may be a mild urticaria but none of the severe symptoms associated with hemolytic transfusion reactions. It may not be necessary to terminate transfusion.

POSTOPERATIVE HYPOTENSION

Mrs. Jones is doing well without further fever or respiratory problems. It is now postoperative day 5. She still manifests an intestinal ileus, has a nasogastric tube in place, and is receiving total parenteral nutrition. That evening, the nurse calls you because Mrs. Jones is hypotensive to a systolic pressure of 85 mmHg. Her diastolic pressure is not detectable.

Is she in shock?

Maybe. The most important consideration in the evaluation of hypotension in the postoperative setting is the potential for shock. Because shock is a state of impaired organ perfusion, not all patients with mild hypotension of short duration are in shock (19). Signs of perfusion such as mental status, skin color and temperature, capillary refill, and pulse strength are assessed. Mild hypotension in response to narcotic administration may indicate hypovolemia.

Why is her ileus important?

The most common cause of postoperative hypotension in general surgery patients is hypovolemia, especially in patients with an ileus who are receiving IV alimentation (19). Because hypovolemia responds at least transiently to fluid loading, a fluid challenge is usually the first therapeutic maneuver in response to hypotension. This fluid infusion may be made with a crystalloid IV fluid, a colloid- or protein-containing fluid, or blood if the patient's hematocrit is low (20).

While the fluid challenge is being administered, a search for the etiology of the hypotension should be made. Low urine output for the previous few hours may point toward hypovolemia. Coincident fever or leukocytosis may indicate infection and sepsis. An electrocardiogram (ECG) is obtained for evidence of myocardial ischemia, as postoperative myocardial infarction occurs most commonly days after the operation. Medications are reviewed for the presence of narcotics or sedatives.

If the patient responds well to one or two fluid challenges, no further action may be necessary. Vital signs and urine output should be monitored. If hypotension continues, more aggressive and invasive monitoring is needed with either a CVP or pulmonary artery catheter. Although the use of pulmonary artery catheters is somewhat controversial and it has been difficult to show that their use improves outcomes, advocates say the information these catheters provide is important for clinical decision-making. Measurement of mixed venous pH or serum lactate may

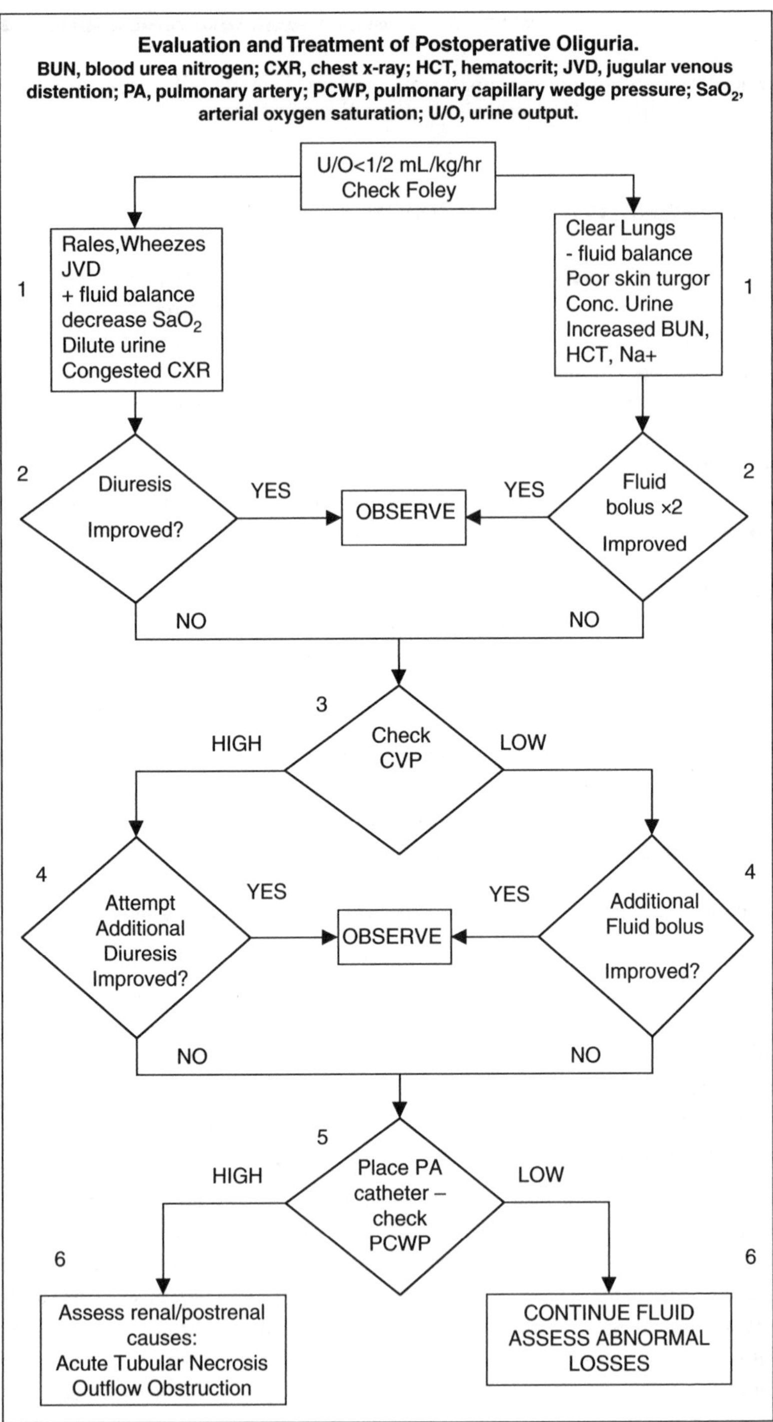

Evaluation and Treatment of Postoperative Oliguria.
BUN, blood urea nitrogen; CXR, chest x-ray; HCT, hematocrit; JVD, jugular venous distention; PA, pulmonary artery; PCWP, pulmonary capillary wedge pressure; SaO_2, arterial oxygen saturation; U/O, urine output.
U/O<1/2 mL/kg/hr
Check Foley
1
Rales, Wheezes
JVD
+ fluid balance
decrease SaO_2
Dilute urine
Congested CXR
1
Clear Lungs
- fluid balance
Poor skin turgor
Conc. Urine
Increased BUN,
HCT, Na+
2
Diuresis
Improved?
YES
OBSERVE
YES
2
Fluid
bolus ×2
Improved
NO
NO
3
Check
CVP
HIGH
LOW
4
Attempt
Additional
Diuresis
Improved?
YES
OBSERVE
YES
4
Additional
Fluid bolus
Improved?
NO
NO
5
Place PA
catheter –
check
PCWP
HIGH
LOW
6
Assess renal/postrenal
causes:
Acute Tubular Necrosis
Outflow Obstruction
6
CONTINUE FLUID
ASSESS ABNORMAL
LOSSES

Algorithm 31.1.

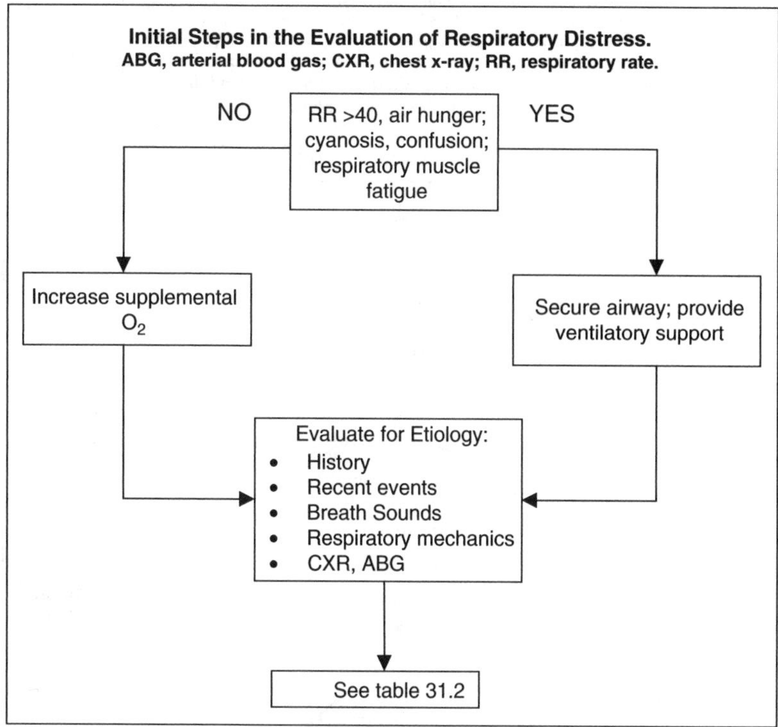

Algorithm 31.2.

indicate the severity of hypoperfusion (21). The use of inotropic or alpha-agonist pressor agents without invasive monitoring is discouraged.

Mrs. Jones appears pale with a rapid but regular pulse. Her systolic blood pressure remains in the 80s and fails to respond to several boluses of lactated Ringer's solution. She is transferred to the intensive care unit. A recent hematocrit is normal and the nurse says that Ms. Jones's urine output had been acceptable until just an hour ago, when her pressure began to drop. She has no fever or leukocytosis. A recent arterial blood gas shows a significant metabolic acidosis. A pulmonary artery catheter is placed; her PCWP is high and the cardiac output normal. A 12-lead ECG demonstrates ST depression in the inferior leads, and Mrs. Jones subsequently is diagnosed with myocardial infarction. Cardiac catheterization demonstrates a significant right coronary artery stenosis, which is successfully treated percutaneously. Her ileus resolves and the rest of her recovery is uneventful.

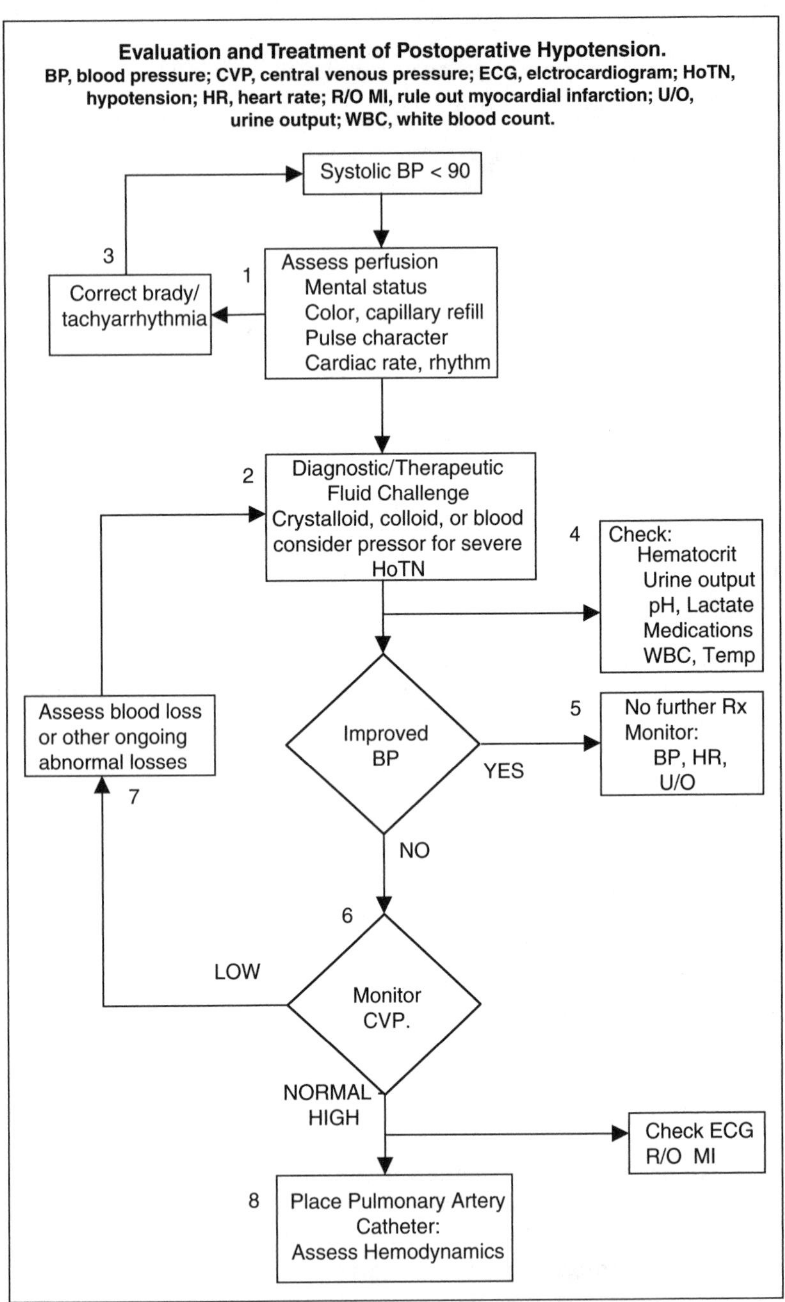

Algorithm 31.3.

REFERENCES

1. Espinel CH, Gregory AA. Differential diagnosis of acute renal failure. Clin Nephrol. 1980;13:73.
2. Varon AJ. Arterial, central venous and pulmonary artery catheters. In: Civetta JW, Taylor RW, Kirby RR, eds. Critical Care. 3rd ed. Philadelphia, Pa: JB Lippincott Co; 1999:852–853.
3. Varon AJ. Arterial, central venous and pulmonary artery catheters. In Civetta JW, Taylor RW, Kirby RR, eds. Critical Care. 3rd ed. Philadelphia, Pa: JB Lippincott Co; 1999:853–863.
4. Shah KB, Rao TLK, Laughin S, et al. A review of pulmonary artery catheterization in 6,245 patients. Anesthesiology. 1984;61:271.
5. Doherty GM, Mulvihill SJ, Pellegrini CA. Postoperative complications. In: Way LW, Doherty GM, eds. Current Surgical Diagnosis and Treatment. 11th ed. New York, NY: Lange Medical Books/McGraw-Hill; 2003:25–27.
6. Roukema JA, Caval EJ, Prins JG. The prevention of pulmonary complications after upper abdominal surgery in patients with non-compromised pulmonary status. Arch Surg. 1988;123:30.
7. Duncan SR. Atelectasis during anesthesia and in the postoperative period. Acta Anesthesiol Scand. 1986;30:54.
8. Cvitanic O, Marino PL. Improved use of arterial blood gas analysis in suspected pulmonary embolism. Chest. 1989;95:48–51.
9. PIOPED Investigators. Results of the prospective investigation of pulmonary embolism diagnosis. JAMA. 1990;263:2753.
10. Silver D, Sabiston DC Jr. The role of vena cava interruption in the management of pulmonary embolism. JAMA. 1990;263:2759.
11. Garibaldi RA, Brodine S, Matsumiya S. Evidence for the non-infectious etiology of early postoperative fever. Infect Control. 1985;6:487.
12. Freischlag J, Busutil RW. The value of postoperative fever evaluation. Surgery. 1983;94:358.
13. Howard RJ. Finding the cause of postoperative fever. Postgraduate Med. 1988;85: 223.
14. Galicier C, Richard H. A prospective study of postoperative fever in a general surgery department. Infect Control. 1985;6:487.
15. Tchervenkov JI, Meakins JL. Altered Host Defense Mechanisms in Septic Patients. 19–34.
16. Nichols RL. Bacterial infectious disease considerations in the surgical patient. In Civetta JW, Taylor RW, Kirby RR, eds. Critical Care. 2nd ed. Philadelphia, Pa: JB Lippincott Co; 1992:793–797.
17. Solomkin JS, Anaissie E. Candida infections and candidemia. In: Fry DE, ed. Surgical Infections. Boston, Mass: Little Brown and Company; 1995:579–581.
18. Demarest GB. *Clostridium difficile* enterocolitis. In: Fry DE, ed. Surgical Infections. Boston, Mass: Little Brown and Company; 1995:635–639.
19. Barber A, Shires GT 3rd, Shires GT. Shock. In: Schwartz SI, Shires GT, Spencer FC, et al., eds. Principles of Surgery. New York, NY: McGraw-Hill; 1999:101–120.
20. Lyon AJ, Bernards WC, Kirby RR. Fluids and electrolytes in the critically ill. In: Civetta JM, Taylor RW, Kirby RR, eds. Critical Care. Philadelphia, Pa: JB Lippincott Co; 1992:477.
21. Jiminez E. Shock. In: Civetta JW, Taylor RW, Kirby RR, eds. Critical Care. 3rd ed. Philadelphia, Pa: JB Lippincott Co; 1999:359–362.

CHAPTER

32

PEDIATRIC SURGERY

Daniel A Saltzman, Sean J. Barnett, Nathan Kreykes, and Robert D. Acton

Author's Note: Pediatric surgery is an encompassing field that covers many aspects of the surgical diseases of infants and children. In this chapter, we have used five cases to illustrate the more common problems encountered in pediatric surgery. If you want more information, we encourage you to examine the numerous comprehensive texts that are available that cover the realm of pediatric surgery (see Suggested Readings).

A 2-day-old term infant boy was admitted to the neonatal intensive care unit (NICU) for feeding intolerance, progressive abdominal distention, and bilious emesis. His prenatal course has been unremarkable and he has been alert and active since birth. On examination, the baby appears well. His vital signs are normal and his abdomen is moderately distended. Rectal examination reveals an anatomically normal anus and there is no meconium in the rectal vault. A complete blood count (CBC) and serum electrolytes are normal. An abdominal radiograph reveals a distal gastrointestinal obstruction.

What is the differential diagnosis for this infant's abdominal problem and how would you proceed with a workup?

Differential diagnosis for a distal gastrointestinal obstruction includes the following:

- Jejunal-ileal atresia
- Neonatal small left colon syndrome
- Meconium plug syndrome
- Meconium ileus
- Hirschsprung's disease
- Malrotation
- Colonic atresia

The workup begins with a detailed history specifically looking for a diabetic mother, family history of jejunal–ileal atresias, or family history of Hirschsprung's disease. Infants with neonatal small left colon syndrome have a diabetic mother.

Next, an abdominal radiograph is obtained. The air–gas pattern obtained on this simple test can point you to the right diagnosis. The absence of colonic gas may indicate a more proximal atresia, Hirschsprung's disease, or neonatal small left colon syndrome. A nonspecific gas pattern may indicate a malrotation, whereas "soap bubbles" in the right lower quadrant may indicate a meconium ileus. If you suspect malrotation or a midgut volvulus, you must exclude these diagnoses.

What do you do next?

In this case, abdominal radiograph revealed absent colonic gas with more proximal intestinal distention. If suspected, a limited upper gastrointestinal (UGI) series should be obtained to exclude a malrotation. A contrast enema with isotonic water-soluble contrast is indicated. This study demonstrated a *microcolon,* that is, unused colon, indicative of a jejunal–ileal atresia (Fig. 32.1).

- In *meconium plug syndrome,* intraluminal colonic masses would have been visualized.
- A transition zone may be seen with *Hirschsprung's disease.*
- A small sigmoid and left colon with a normal caliber transverse colon is generally observed with *neonatal small left colon syndrome.*
- A complete bowel obstruction secondary to malrotation is from the development of a *volvulus.* These patients are tender and appear septic and do not look generally healthy, in contrast to the way this patient presented.

Operative exploration is now indicated and no further studies are necessary.

What is the pathophysiology of jejunal–ileal atresias?

Unlike duodenal atresia, which is thought to be a failure of recanalization, jejunal–ileal atresias are thought to arise from an intrauterine vascular accident with subsequent ischemic necrosis. Pathologically, one can see a spectrum of defects with intestinal atresias that range from a stenosis to multiple atretic segments throughout the intestine.

How are jejuno–ileal atresias treated?

The operative procedure performed is dependent on the pathologic findings. Generally, a limited resection of the proximal dilated and hypertrophied bowel with a primary end-to-end anastomosis with or without tapering is commonly performed.

A 16-month-old girl had a cough and cold for approximately 5 days when she developed intermittent abdominal pain associated with dark and

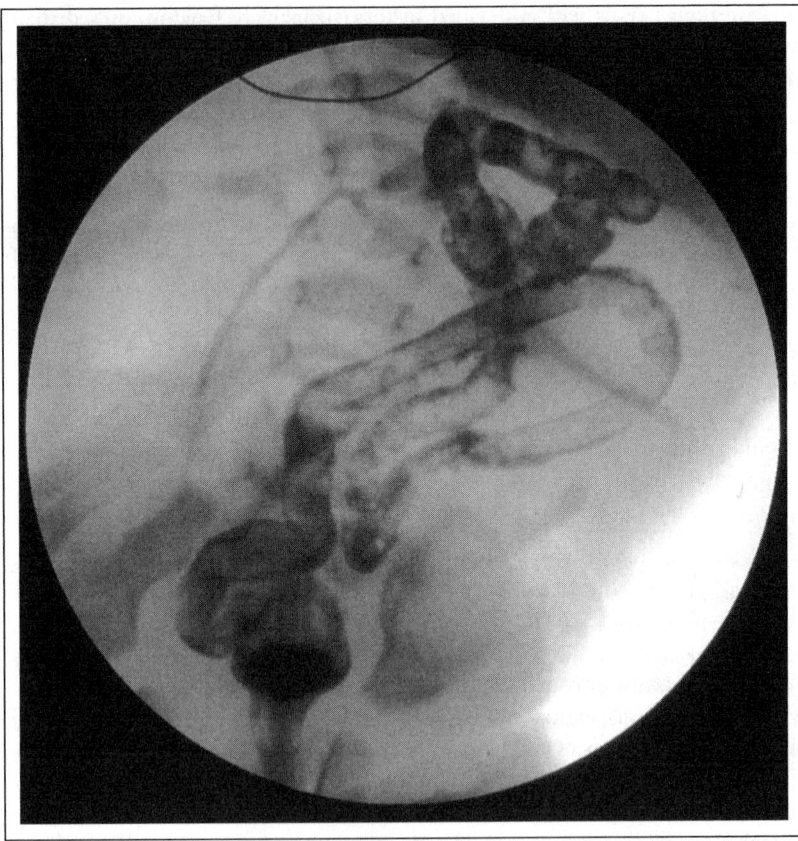

Figure 32.1. Contrast enema in newborn with jejunal-ileal atresia demonstrating a microcolon or unused colon.

bloody stools and presents to your emergency department. On examination, her vital signs are normal and she is lying comfortably on the examination table. During her examination she begins to cry and draw up her legs. Significant findings during her examination include abdominal tenderness and a mass in the right lower quadrant with heme-positive stools. An abdominal radiograph performed the night before in an urgent care center revealed proximal intestinal dilation.

What is your working diagnosis?
Intussusception, appendicitis, or Meckel's diverticulitis.

An abdominal ultrasound (US) is ordered and confirms an ilio-colic intussusception. After establishing intravenous (IV) access, volume

resuscitating the child, and starting IV antibiotics, a prompt air-contrast enema is obtained. The intussusception cannot be reduced. The child then undergoes an emergent operative reduction. She has an uneventful postoperative course and is discharged home on postoperative day 3.

How successful are radiologic reductions of intussusceptions and what is their etiology?

Intussusception is the telescoping of one portion of the intestine into another. Most are ilio-colic and the lead point is the resultant hypertrophy of the lymphoid tissue at the terminal ileum from a nonspecific viral syndrome. Nonoperative radiologic reductions of intussusceptions are successful 50% to 95% of the time. Success is dependent on the skill of the radiologist, the technique used, and the delay from onset of symptoms.

A 2-year-old boy is noted by his parents to have a right inguinal bulge that becomes more prominent with crying. He has no pain associated with this and his parents report that it occasionally goes away. On examination, you determine an easily reducible right inguinal hernia and a normal left inguinal canal. Both testicles are descended bilaterally and there is no evidence of testicular atrophy.

What is the pathophysiologic basis for groin hernias in children?

A patent processus vaginalis is the pathophysiologic basis for an indirect hernia in the child. The processus vaginalis is a peritoneal diverticulum that is present in the developing fetus by the 12th week. As the intraabdominal testicles descend into the scrotum by the 7th or 8th month of gestation, a portion of the processus attaches to the descending testis. The portion of the processus that envelops the testis becomes the tunica vaginalis and the remaining processus in the inguinal canal eventually obliterates. It is the persistence of this processus that establishes a communication between the peritoneal cavity and the inguinal canal that defines the pediatric indirect hernia.

What is the incidence of inguinal hernias in children?

It is estimated that 1% to 5% of all children have developed an inguinal hernia. The incidence in premature infants has been reported to be as high as 30%. Direct or femoral hernias in children are exceedingly rare and are considered to be an acquired condition.

What is a hydrocele?

A *hernia* is defined as a persistent processus vaginalis that contains an intraabdominal structure (e.g., bowel, ovary), whereas a *hydrocele* contains only peritoneal fluid. Hydroceles can be divided into two types: communicating and noncommunicating. *Communicating hydroceles* indicate a communication with the peritoneal cavity and should be treated as an inguinal hernia. A *noncommunicating hydrocele* is trapped fluid within the inguinal canal and is usually self-limiting. Most surgeons advocate repair at age 1 year if the noncommunicating hydrocele persists.

What is the essence of repair of the pediatric inguinal hernia?
High ligation of the sac.

A previously healthy 3-year-old girl was noted by her parents to have an asymptomatic mass of the left hemiabdomen during a recent bath. In her pediatrician's office, she had no complaints. On examination, she was found to be hypertensive at 135/88 mm Hg and a 7 × 8 cm mass was palpated beneath the left costal margin. Laboratory evaluation revealed a normal CBC and electrolytes; however, a urinalysis demonstrated hematuria.

What is the differential diagnosis for this asymptomatic mass and how would you proceed with the workup?
Usually, only two tumor types come to mind: Wilms' tumor and neuroblastoma. An US is a good first step to establish the origin of the tumor and assess the patency of the inferior vena cava to determine if there is caval extension of disease. Chest radiograph is important to screen for metastatic disease. A computed tomography scan of the head, chest, and abdomen will allow determination of extent of renal extension and presence of local and metastatic disease (Fig 32.2).

Wilms' tumor, also called *nephroblastoma,* is the most common renal malignancy seen in childhood. Boys and girls are nearly equally affected, and the average age at presentation is between 3 and 4 years. There is an increase in association of Wilms' tumor in children with aniridia, hemihypertrophy, genitourinary anomalies, and the Beckwith–Wiedemann syndrome.

Neuroblastoma arises from neuroblasts of the sympathetic nervous system and consequently can arise in the ganglia of the sympathetic chain, preaortic ganglia, and most commonly, in the adrenal medulla. Approximately 80% of neuroblastomas arise in children younger than 4 years of age, and staging is based on the extent of localized or distant disease. A *unique stage (4S)* is defined as a localized primary tumor with dissemination limited to the skin, liver, and bone marrow in children younger than 1 year of age. Neuroblastoma commonly presents with vague symptoms of abdominal pain, weight loss, fever, and malaise. Initial diagnostic workup includes a determination of urinary catecholamines (vanillylmandelic acid and homovanillic acid), which are usually elevated in cases of neuroblastoma. Treatment involves a multidisciplinary approach, and the goal of operative therapy is gross total resection. Radiation and chemotherapy are usually administered as well. Overall survival from neuroblastoma is approximately 60%, whereas survival of those with advanced stages is considerably less. One

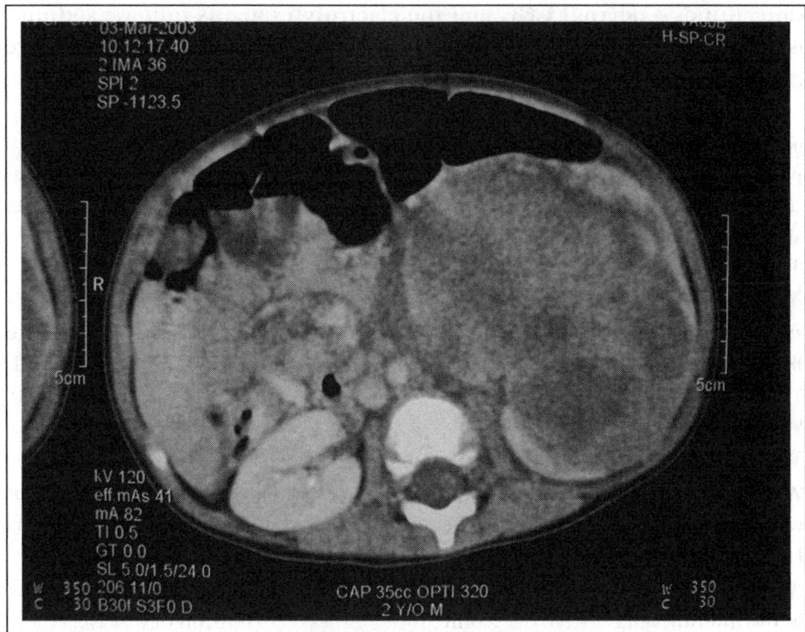

Figure 32.2. CT scan of abdomen demonstrating a large left Wilms' tumor.

exception is Stage 4S. Survival rates for Stage 4S have approached 90%, and spontaneous regression of the tumor has been reported.

This 3-year-old girl's preoperative workup did not reveal any metastatic disease, and she successfully underwent a radical left nephrectomy and later followed with chemotherapy for a Stage I Wilms' tumor.

What is this child's prognosis?

Histopathology is the most important prognostic factor in these children. Specific pathologic characteristics define these tumor types into two broad categories: favorable and unfavorable histology. Overall survival of patients with favorable histology exceeds 90%, whereas survival of those with unfavorable pathologic subtypes is 20% to 80%.

A 6-week-old boy presents to his local emergency department with a 2-day history of persistent vomiting after feedings. His mother describes the emesis as nonbilious and projectile. On examination, you find an irritable infant with normal vital signs. On abdominal examination, an "olive" is palpated in the right upper quadrant. Laboratory evaluation

determines a normal CBC and the electrolytes are as follows: sodium, 141 mEq/L; potassium 2.9 mEq/L; chloride 90 mEq/L; and bicarbonate 35 mEq/L.

What is your working diagnosis?

Most likely diagnosis is hypertrophic pyloric stenosis (HPS); the differential diagnosis for nonbilious emesis also includes gastroesophageal reflux disease, salt-wasting adrenogenital syndrome, and elevated intracranial pressure.

You admit the child to the general care ward and begin your fluid resuscitation. His electrolytes reveal a hypochloremic, hypokalemic metabolic alkalosis. Over the next 24 hours, his metabolic abnormality is corrected.

What is your next step?

With a palpable olive in your initial examination, the diagnosis is pyloric stenosis. If you are unable to palpate an olive, an US of the pylorus is extremely helpful in establishing a diagnosis. After correction of the metabolic alkalosis, the child is ready for the operating room. The standard procedure is a Ramstedt pyloromyotomy; in this procedure, the serosa and muscularis are split to allow the mucosa to bulge out.

Six hours postoperatively the child was slowly advanced to his regular diet. He was discharged home on postoperative day 1.

SUGGESTED READINGS

1. Ashcraft KW, ed. Pediatric Surgery. 3rd ed. Philadelphia, Pa: WB Saunders; 2000.
2. O'Neill JA Jr, Grosfeld JL, Fonkaslrud EW, et al., eds. Principles of Pediatric Surgery. 2nd ed. St. Louis, Mo: Mosby; 2004.
3. Blakely ML, Ritchey ML. Controversies in the management of Wilms' tumors. Semin Pediatr Surg. 2001;10:127–131.
4. La Quaglia MP. Surgical management of neuroblastoma. Semin Pediatr Surg. 2001;10:132–139.
5. Moss RL, Skarsgard ED, Kosloske AM, et al. Case Studies in Pediatric Surgery. New York, NY: McGraw-Hill; 2000.

CHAPTER

33

PERIPHERAL ARTERIAL OCCLUSIVE DISEASE

W. Charles Sternbergh III

David Brown is a 68-year-old retired carpenter who for the past 2 years has had cramps and aching in the right calf after walking. The discomfort has been gradually worsening and is now reproducible after he walks approximately two blocks; it subsides within 5 minutes of resting but reappears when he walks another two blocks. He denies having any pain in the left leg while walking or in the right calf or foot at rest, nor does he have any history of trauma to the extremities. He smokes two packs of cigarettes a day.

Mr. Brown's medical history is significant for coronary artery disease (CAD), for which he underwent coronary artery bypass grafting (CABG) 3 years ago. Since the CABG, he has had no angina, dyspnea on exertion, or orthopnea. He has no history of stroke, transient ischemic attacks, or hypercholesterolemia. He has mild chronic obstructive pulmonary disease because of smoking. His only medications are diltiazem and aspirin.

A physical examination indicates that Mr. Brown is normotensive and in sinus rhythm; findings of the neck, chest, abdominal, and neurologic examinations are normal. Evaluation of his peripheral pulse reveals a 2+ carotid pulse bilaterally without bruits, 2+ radial pulses, and 2+ femoral pulses without bruits. Mr. Brown is bilaterally pulseless in the popliteal, posterior tibial, and dorsalis pedis arteries, but these vessels produce a monophasic signal when evaluated with a Doppler study. The right leg has a well-healed longitudinal scar from the excision of the saphenous vein for the CABG. There is no muscle atrophy, ulceration, or any other sign of tissue loss in either leg; capillary refill in the toes is good.

What is claudication?

Claudication is exercise-induced intermittent discomfort in a particular muscle group that subsides within 1 to 5 minutes after the exercise is stopped. This discomfort may be described by the patient as pain, cramping, burning, or weariness. In the lower extremities, the calves, thighs, and buttocks are most frequently affected. Because the pain is reproducible by the same degree of exertion, claudication is typically quantified by the distance a patient can walk before its onset (e.g., two-block claudication).

What causes claudication?

Claudication occurs when a particular muscle group becomes hypoxic because the increased metabolic demands for oxygen during exercise cannot be met. Normal arteries can increase flow 5- to 10-fold when regional metabolic demands rise; however, stenosed or occluded vessels have limited capacity to augment flow during exercise. The stenosis or occlusion is usually caused by progressive atherosclerosis.

What is the differential diagnosis for lower extremity pain?

Claudication is a characteristic symptom in patients with significant chronic arterial occlusive disease. Because of the reproducibility of hypoxic muscle pain after exercise, a history and physical examination should be sufficient to rule out most other causes. The differential diagnosis for lower extremity pain includes the following:

Chronic peripheral arterial occlusive disease (PAOD): pain or weariness of the calf (most common), thigh or buttock that occurs with exercise but not at rest. The distance required to induce the discomfort should be fairly constant. The discomfort should be promptly relieved (1 to 5 min) by standing still.

Acute arterial embolism: the precipitous reduction of blood flow that results from acute arterial embolism can cause an acute onset of diffuse lower extremity pain at rest in a patient with no history of arterial occlusive disease.

Acute aortic dissection: dissection of the thoracic aorta can extend into an iliac artery, acutely compromising arterial flow and thus presenting like an acute embolus. Many patients will also complain of a "tearing" chest or back pain.

Neurologic disorders: lumbar disc herniation or spinal stenosis may cause characteristic shooting pain or extremity weakness that is sometimes quite distinct from claudication. However, other patients can have extremity complaints that are similar to that caused by PAOD. Patients who develop leg pain with standing only and those who must sit or lie down to relieve the discomfort after exercise typically have a neurologic etiology to their leg symptoms.

Diabetic neuropathy: many patients with long-standing diabetes develop significant burning pain in the feet at rest, which may be easily confused with pain caused by critical arterial ischemia.

Chronic venous disease: venous valve incompetence and the resulting relative stasis can cause chronic swelling, hyperpigmentation, and ulcers at or proximal to the malleoli.

Deep vein thrombosis: characterized by swelling in the extremities or vague pain, deep vein thrombosis cannot be accurately diagnosed from the history and physical examination.

Musculoskeletal disorders: patients with musculoskeletal disorders have a history of recent trauma or of pain associated with movement of a joint.

Infection: local erythema and tenderness that are not exacerbated by exercise are present.

What are some significant risk factors for arterial occlusive disease?

Hypercholesterolemia, tobacco use, hypertension, diabetes mellitus, male gender, age, and hereditary influences are all significant risk factors (1).

What are the signs of significant arterial occlusive disease?

These signs may be observed during a physical examination:

1. Lack of distal pulses
2. Pallor of the extremity on elevation and rubor on dependency
3. Trophic changes such as thinning of the skin, loss of hair, and thickening of the nails
4. Muscle atrophy
5. Tissue loss (e.g., ulcers distal to the malleolus or gangrene). Ulcers proximal to the malleolus are almost never primarily caused by arterial ischemia.

What is the natural course of lower extremity claudication?

Symptomatic arterial occlusive disease has a surprisingly benign course; 75% to 80% of patients have stable or diminished claudication with conservative management (2). Reported amputation rates for all patients with claudication who are managed without surgery range from 1.6% to 7% after a 6- to 8-year follow-up (3,4). Approximately 20% of patients with claudication ultimately require invasive intervention for limb salvage.

What is an appropriate initial treatment for claudication?

Because of the relatively benign natural course of this disease, an initial conservative approach is generally warranted. This includes the following measures:

Cessation of smoking. Tobacco use is clearly associated with a significant exacerbation of vascular occlusive disease. Smoking doubles an elderly patient's risk of claudication (5). Most smokers with claudication show a significant improvement in exercise tolerance after quitting (6).

Exercise. A graded exercise program stimulates formation of collateral vessels. The resulting increase in blood flow can increase the walking distances by 80% to 120%. Unfortunately, these beneficial effects are sometimes difficult to achieve without a supervised and highly structured exercise program.

Aggressive modification of risk factors. PAOD is a strong marker for generalized atherosclerotic disease. As such, patients with PAOD, even if clinically asymptomatic, should be assessed for elevated cholesterol and triglycerides. Younger patients should be checked for elevations in homocysteine and perhaps LP(a). Appropriate dietary modifications and possibly drug therapy should be instituted.

Medications for claudication. Cilostazol (Pletal) has been available in the Unites States for the treatment of claudication since 1999. It significantly increases walking distance in approximately 50% of patients who take the medication. Pentoxifylline (Trental) is a less effective medication for claudication and is now rarely prescribed.

Mr. Brown's physician instructs him to stop smoking and begin a graded exercise program, but his interest and participation in exercise are limited, and he does not stop smoking. He does not go to scheduled follow-up visits. Over the next 2 years, his walking distance before onset of the characteristic right calf pain gradually shortens. He also begins to have pain in his right foot at rest, especially at night; the discomfort is relieved by dangling the foot off the bed. The intensity and duration of the pain gradually increase, and after 3 weeks, he seeks help.

What is rest pain, and what causes it?

Rest pain is caused by inadequate delivery of oxygen to the tissues during rest. This hypoperfusion inevitably manifests as ischemic pain in the foot at rest. The lower extremity muscles that are prone to claudication (the calf, thigh, and buttock muscles) *rarely* if ever exhibit rest pain because they are not at the end of the arterial tree. Conversely, the foot does not claudicate because it has relatively little muscle mass that is susceptible to exercise-induced hypoxia. By definition, the pain caused by claudication is intermittent, whereas rest pain can be continuous. Rest pain is characteristically worst at night, when the patient is supine, because the arterial flow to the foot is not aided by gravity. The pain is relieved by dangling the foot off the bed, walking a few paces, or sleeping in a chair.

What is the natural history of rest pain?

In contrast to claudication, true ischemic rest pain ultimately progresses to limb loss in most untreated patients. An aggressive treatment regimen is therefore warranted in the absence of prohibitive comorbid medical conditions.

What are the indications for treatment of arterial occlusive disease?

1. **Rest pain.**
2. **Tissue loss.** This may be a nonhealing inframalleolar ulcer, nonhealing distal amputation, or gangrenous changes in the toes.
3. **Disabling claudication.** The availability of minimally invasive endovascular treatments has resulted in a more liberal policy for interventional treatment of claudication in many centers.

How is arterial occlusive disease evaluated?

A thorough history and physical examination are essential, and any comorbid medical conditions must be addressed. Segmental arterial Doppler studies and an ankle-brachial index (ABI) are obtained.

What does an arterial Doppler study measure? What is the ABI? What are pulse volume recordings (PVRs)?

Segmental arterial Doppler studies measure the systolic pressure at several locations on the extremity. A pressure difference greater than 20 mm Hg between levels suggests significant occlusive disease. The ABI (obtained by dividing the ankle pressure by the highest brachial pressure) provides a value indicating distal perfusion. A *normal ABI* is 0.9 to 1.1; an ABI of 0.5 to 0.7 is typical of *claudication;* and an ABI of less than 0.5 may accompany *rest pain* or *tissue loss.* The ABI is only a relative number, and many patients with an ABI of 0.5 have no symptoms.

Because diabetic patients sometimes have heavily calcified arteries that are poorly compressible, their ABI may be misleadingly high. That is one reason PVRs should also be routinely obtained with the ABI. PVRs are arterial waveforms that give subjective but important information about arterial blood flow. Normal PVRs have a triphasic waveform whereas patients with significant PAOD will have a sigmoidal waveform. Patients with very severe PAOD may have a flat line PVR with no pulsatility whatsoever.

At what point does arterial stenosis become hemodynamically significant?

The cutoff point is a 75% reduction of the cross-sectional area, which is equivalent to a 50% reduction of the diameter. At this level of stenosis, poststenotic pressure and blood flow are maintained at 90% to 95% of normal values; however, any further stenosis causes a precipitous fall in distal perfusion.

Mr. Brown's physician orders a lower extremity segmental arterial Doppler study. It reveals a reference right brachial pressure of 130 mm Hg, high thigh pressure of 140 mm Hg, above-knee pressure of 73 mm Hg, below-knee pressure of 60 mm Hg, ankle pressure of 51 mm Hg, and toe pressure of 45 mm Hg. The ABI is calculated to be 0.39. The contralateral leg has fairly similar pressures and an ABI of 0.5.

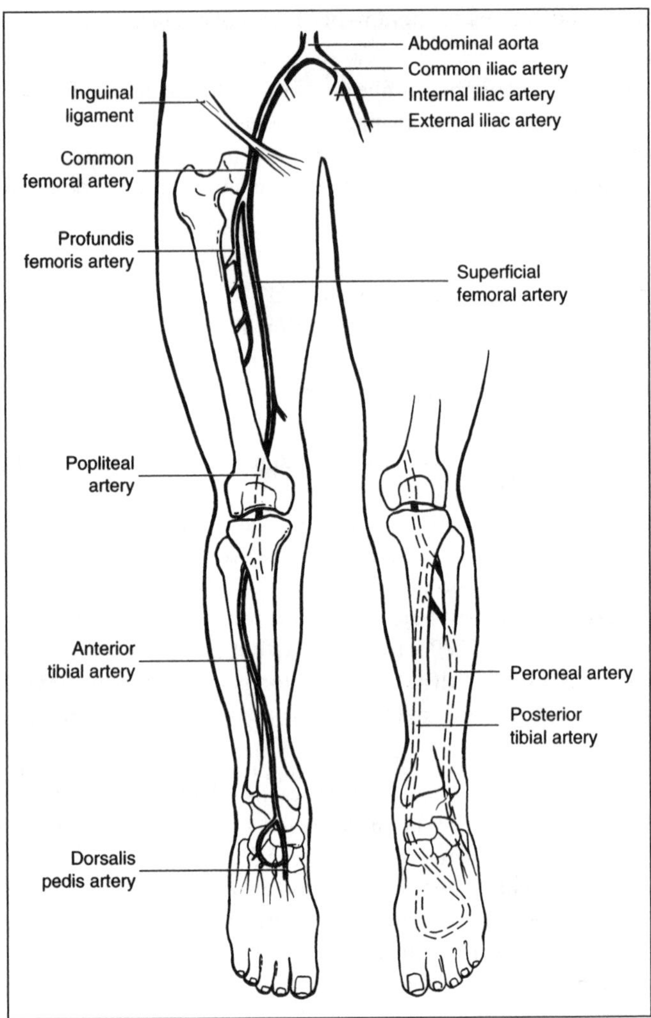

Figure 33.1. Anatomy of the lower extremity arterial tree.

What is the anatomy of the vascular tree in the lower extremities?

The vascular anatomy of the lower extremity is shown in Figure 33.1.

How does the location of the pain suggest the probable area of stenosis or occlusion?

In 60% to 70% of patients, the arterial lesion is one level above the claudicating muscle group. Calf claudication, as in Mr. Brown's case, therefore suggests superficial femoral artery (SFA) or popliteal artery disease, whereas thigh or buttock claudication indicates more proximal aortoiliac occlusive disease. However, up to 40% of patients with aortoiliac disease may have calf claudication without thigh or buttock symptoms.

What is Leriche's syndrome?

In 1940, Leriche described a group of patients with distal aortic occlusion resulting from progressive atherosclerotic disease. These patients exhibited characteristic signs and symptoms: impotence, symmetric lower extremity muscle wasting, pallor of the legs and feet, and easy fatigability. Impotence is caused by the greatly decreased flow to the hypogastric arteries. Because of the extensive formation of collateral vessels, these patients can remain asymptomatic for as long as 5 to 10 years, but many ultimately need surgery.

What is the most likely location of Mr. Brown's lesion?

Both the Doppler studies, which reveal a large decrease in pressure between the high and the low thigh, and the patient's initial symptom (right calf claudication) suggest an occlusion of the SFA. The most common site of occlusion in the lower extremities is the distal SFA as it passes through the adductor canal.

The patient is referred to a vascular specialist for further evaluation and definitive treatment. Further imaging of the PAOD is needed before treatment.

What types of imaging studies are available for PAOD?

1. **Angiography.** This has been the gold standard for vascular imaging and is still used routinely in most practices. A small catheter is percutaneously placed in the aorta via the femoral or brachial artery, and contrast material is injected. Excellent imaging of the arterial vascular anatomy should be obtained. However, newer noninvasive imaging modalities continue to improve and are being used at an exponential rate.
2. **Computed tomography angiography (CTA).** Very fast spiral CT scanners obtain thin-cut axial slices while giving contrast material via a peripheral intravenous (IV) line. Reconstructed 3D vascular images are then available. The advantages of CTA are its noninvasiveness (no arterial puncture) and ability to manipulate and rotate the reconstructed images in any orientation. Limitations include difficulty in accurately imaging occlusive lesions in smaller (less than 3 to 5 mm) vessels, potential artifact caused by heavily calcified vessels, and the need for the same amount of contrast dye as with conventional arteriography.
3. **Magnetic resonance arteriography (MRA).** MRA is similar to CTA, except non-nephrotoxic gadolinium is given via IV rather than standard contrast material. Advantages of MRA include its noninvasiveness, no radiation

exposure, and lack of need for standard contrast material. This is most helpful in patients with advanced chronic renal insufficiency who are at greatly increased risk of nephrotoxicity with administration of contrast material. Limitations include inability to image vessel flow inside a previously placed stent, making the image always appear that a segmental occlusion exists when it may not (stent artefact). In vessels smaller than 6 mm, MRA may have difficulty discriminating between a high-grade stenosis (greater than 70%) and an occlusion (a signal drop-out). The small vessel imaging of both MRA and CTA will undoubtedly continue to improve, ultimately making these the primary modalities for diagnostic vascular imaging in the future.

4. **Duplex ultrasound (US).** Scattered centers have significant experience with the use of highly detailed duplex US mapping of the iliac, femoral, popliteal, and tibial arterial system. Its main advantage is its complete noninvasiveness (no IV, no contrast of any kind). Disadvantages include its great technician dependence and variability and the length of examination (usually longer than 1 hr). As such, it is unlikely that duplex US will become the definitive diagnostic vascular imaging in most practices.

What are the indications for arteriography?

Arteriography is performed only if the patient is to undergo invasive intervention. It should not be used as a screening tool. Arterial Doppler studies are a good noninvasive tool for screening.

What are the risks of arteriography, and how can they be minimized?

The risk of a life-threatening reaction to the contrast medium is 1 in 14,000. The reported incidence of renal dysfunction from contrast toxicity ranges from 0 to 10% in low-risk patients. Minimizing contrast medium–induced renal dysfunction is done by the use of iso-osmolar non-iodinated contrast material (such as Visipaque) and judicious use of IV hydration, both before and after the study. Oral acetylcysteine (Mucomyst) given the day before and day of contrast administration to patients with pre-existing renal insufficiency has been demonstrated to reduce the incidence of further renal dysfunction.

Mr. Brown's arteriogram reveals mild to moderate atherosclerotic changes in the distal aorta and common iliac arteries in the absence of hemodynamically significant stenoses. The right extremity has a patent profunda femoris, but the SFA and proximal popliteal are completely occluded, with reconstitution at the distal popliteal artery below the knee. There is one vessel runoff (anterior tibial artery). The left extremity has diffuse mild to moderate occlusive changes; there is a 3-cm occlusion at the distal SFA, with popliteal reconstitution.

If an arteriogram reveals significant occlusive disease in both extremities but the patient has symptoms on only one side, should both extremities undergo invasive treatment?

Only symptomatic lesions should be treated.

What type of cardiac evaluation before surgery is appropriate for a patient who has had a myocardial infarction (MI)?

Perioperative MI is the most common cause of postoperative death in patients operated on for PAOD. The prevalence of severe CAD in this patient population is high; 34% of patients with clinically suspected coronary disease have severe correctable CAD, as do 14% of patients with no history of CAD (7). It is therefore important to identify patients at risk for a perioperative cardiac event. Any history of CAD, angina, or congestive heart failure necessitates further study. An abnormal electrocardiogram in the absence of clinical symptoms should also prompt further investigation. Frequently used cardiac stress tests include the dobutamine-stressed echocardiogram and the dipyridamole (Persantine)-stressed thallium (radionuclide) scan. If a significant portion of myocardium is found to be at risk for ischemia, cardiac catheterization is indicated.

When in the perioperative period is a MI most likely?

A MI is most likely to occur 3 to 5 days postoperatively. Although reasons for this temporal relation are not completely understood, a major contributing factor may be the mobilization of third-space fluid that accumulates intraoperatively. This internal fluid challenge may overwhelm a marginally vascularized heart and cause ischemia and infarction.

What is the mortality from an acute MI in the perioperative period in a patient undergoing noncardiac surgery?

Mortality associated with an MI in the perioperative period is 20% to 50%, in contrast to 8% to 14% mortality after acute MI in nonsurgical patients. These statistics underscore the importance of aggressive preoperative cardiac risk assessment.

Mr. Brown has a standard electrocardiogram that reveals a normal sinus rhythm of 80, Q waves in leads II, III, and aVF, but no other Q waves or ST segment abnormalities. Because of his history of CAD, he undergoes a dipyridamole-thallium cardiac stress test that reveals no redistribution and thus indicates that the risk of perioperative MI is low.

What is the treatment for severe symptomatic occlusive peripheral vascular disease?

Revascularization of the limb at risk for ischemia is essential. This may be accomplished by the surgical placement of a conduit that bypasses the area of disease or by percutaneous endovascular techniques that use balloon angioplasty and stents. Endovascular treatment is inherently attractive to the patient and physicians because of its minimally invasive nature. These procedures can usually be performed in an outpatient setting and have reduced morbidity, mortality, and cost of treatment compared with conventional surgery.

What is the role of balloon angioplasty in the treatment of PAOD?

Percutaneous interventional techniques have become very common and important procedures in a vascular surgical practice. Most progressive vascular surgeons now perform both percutaneous endovascular treatments and conventional bypass surgery. Many occlusive lesions that were treated with bypass surgery in the past can now be effectively managed with an outpatient percutaneous procedure.

Although the durability of endovascular treatment has generally been inferior to surgical revascularization, the differences in outcome between the two treatments have narrowed significantly in some areas. The ideal lesion for successful primary angioplasty is a proximal lesion less than 5 cm long with no significant distal occlusive disease.

After successful angioplasty of an isolated common iliac stenosis, the 5-year patency rate is 80% to 85%. Angioplasty may also be useful as a secondary procedure, such as dilating a discrete stenosis in a failing bypass graft. A vessel with an occluded segment longer than 10 cm, a more distal location, and multilevel disease all impede the initial and long-term success of angioplasty.

What are stents? Do they improve the patency rate after angioplasty?

Stents are metal scaffolds made of nitinol or stainless steel that are either self-expanding or balloon-expandable. Balloon-expandable stents have the greatest radial strength and are easiest to precisely position; they are routinely employed with aorto-ostial lesions. Self-expanding stents are more flexible and cannot be externally crushed; they are used in more tortuous vessels and those such as the femoral artery that might be subject to external compression.

Percutaneous treatment of both aorto-ostial stenotic lesions (iliac, renal, brachiocephalic) and vessel occlusions are generally improved with the routine use of stents (primary stenting). Stent use also improves results when used after an initial angioplasty that leads to a suboptimal technical result (provisional stenting). Although many physicians routinely stent all iliac arterial occlusive lesions, the data to support improved patency are mixed in this location. Multiple randomized studies have demonstrated that primary stenting of femoral occlusive lesions does not improve patency rates. However, drug-eluting stents for these vessels are now in clinical trials, and these have the potential to improve long-term patency results by reducing in-stent restenosis caused by intimal hyperplasia.

How does balloon angioplasty affect an atheromatous plaque?

An increase in the cross-sectional diameter of the vessel occurs primarily through disruption or cracking of the plaque. Extrusion of the plaque contents contributes 6% to 12% to this increase, whereas compression of the plaque, which earlier was considered to be the primary mechanism, is now believed to contribute only about 1%.

What factors determine successful revascularization?

Three elements are essential for a durable revascularization: inflow of blood, a conduit for the blood, and an outflow tract. A bypass of an SFA occlusion from the common femoral to the popliteal artery is destined for early thrombosis if there is a significant iliac stenosis (inflow problem). The same bypass will also fail early if there is extensive occlusive disease in the tibioperoneal trunk (outflow problem). Clearly, the vasculature of the entire limb must be studied to plan an effective and long-lasting revascularization.

What are the types of conduits used for peripheral bypass procedures, and how durable are they?

The choice of conduit is based on the long-term patency of the grafts. Grafts for revascularization in decreasing order of preference are listed:

Autogenous vein. The greater saphenous vein is preferred to the basilic, cephalic, and lesser saphenous veins because of its superior patency.

Synthetic material (polytetrafluoroethylene [PTFE] or polyester [Dacron]). PTFE conduits also have good patency rates in bypasses from the common femoral to the popliteal artery above the knee. After 2 years, reversed saphenous vein and PTFE bypasses have a similar patency rate, approximately 80%; however, after 4 years, the patency of PTFE decreases to 54%, whereas the patency of the reversed vein graft is still 76% (8). Arterial reconstruction to the tibial vessels with PTFE leads to very low patency rates—12% with PTFE versus 49% to 75% with vein—at 4 years (8) and should be avoided. A composite graft consisting of a proximal PTFE graft sewn to a distal vein may be used for a bypass to the tibial vessels when an available vein is insufficient.

Cryopreserved or glutaraldehyde-preserved umbilical vein. Cryopreserved veins are a poor choice for a conduit because of their uniformly low patency rate.

What is the difference between a reversed saphenous vein bypass graft and an in situ graft?

For a reversed saphenous vein bypass, the vein is removed from the leg, the branches are ligated, and the vessel is reversed so that the distal end of the vein is used as the proximal origin of the bypass conduit. The vein is reversed so that arterial flow is not impeded by its numerous valves. For in situ saphenous vein grafts, the greater portion of the vein is left in situ; only the most proximal and distal aspects are dissected free for the arterial anastomoses. The valves are excised with special instruments. These valve cutters, or valvulotomes, are inserted through a side branch or through the distal end of the vein. Finally, all of the branches of the vein are ligated, with minimum dissection in surrounding areas.

What are the advantages of the in situ technique?

Most of the advantages of the in situ technique are predicated on the concept of endothelial cell preservation. The endothelium has remarkable antithrombotic properties that are easily compromised by ischemia and reperfusion. Therefore, avoiding the ischemic damage caused by surgical excision of the vein segment has great theoretic appeal. The vasa vasorum, which supply the media and adventitia with blood, are minimally injured. Manipulation-induced spasm and the resulting need for hydrostatic dilation, which may lead to additional damage, are avoided. Also, a smaller-caliber vein may be used.

Do in situ techniques give better long-term patencies than standard reversed bypasses?

Although some proponents of in situ techniques claim better patency rates (9), the emerging consensus is that with precise attention to detail, the two techniques produce equivalent results. Controlled trials have shown no differences in long-term patency between them (10).

What are the types of vascular procedures for lower extremity occlusive disease? What is the usual choice of conduit? What are their approximate 5-year patency rates?

The various procedures, together with the conduits and duration, are listed in Table 33.1. The indicated patency rates are only average rates. Thus, bypasses performed for claudication have a higher patency rate than those done for rest pain or tissue loss. Finally, limb salvage rates are higher than the 5-year patency rates.

Mr. Brown undergoes surgery, during which the left greater saphenous vein is harvested, reversed, and anastomosed to the common femoral artery proximally and to the popliteal artery below the knee distally. An arteriogram obtained after completion of surgery reveals no technical defects and excellent runoff. The right dorsalis pedis artery has a palpable pulse.

What is the role of intraoperative arteriography or duplex US?

Both modalities can be used to assess the technical adequacy of a bypass. Duplex US may be more sensitive than arteriography to technical problems with the graft, particularly with the in situ technique (11,12). Sometimes, the preoperative

TABLE 33.1.

RELATION OF LOCATION OF ARTERIAL BYPASS TO LONG-TERM PATENCY

	Conduit Type	5-Year Patency Arterial Bypass Type (%)
Aortobifemoral or aortoiliac	Polyester or PTFE	85–95
Axillary-femoral	PTFE or polyester	35–35
Femoral-bifemoral	PTFE or polyester	50–70
Femoral-femoral	PTFE or polyester	50–80
Femoral-popliteal	Vein	60–80
	PTFE	45–60
		35–60
Femoral-tibial or femoral-peroneal	Vein	50–70
	PTFE	<20

PTFE, polytetrafluoroethylene (Gore-Tex).

angiogram does not provide sufficient detail of the distal vasculature. In these cases, an intraoperative arteriogram, directed specifically to the area of interest, may guide the arterial reconstruction.

What are some important considerations in the postoperative management of a patient who has had vascular surgery?

Careful management of coexisting medical problems. As a group, patients who have undergone vascular surgery have a higher prevalence of coexisting diseases than does any other subset of surgical patients. Accordingly, meticulous attention should be directed to cardiac, pulmonary, and renal disease.

Frequent assessment of graft patency. The functioning bypass should produce a palpable pulse or a strong Doppler signal in the distal vessels. This pulse should be checked hourly for the first 12 hours and then several times a day for the next few days. A baseline ABI should also be recorded at the bedside. Any sign of graft thrombosis demands an imaging study (duplex study or angiography) and immediate surgical reexploration.

Use of anticoagulation. Routine perioperative anticoagulation with dextran or heparin is usually not indicated. Exceptions are patients with high-risk grafts from technical difficulties, marginal conduit, or poor runoff; patients with grafts that are prone to thrombosis; and patients with hypercoagulable conditions. These patients may be treated with heparin postoperatively, and they can be maintained on warfarin indefinitely. Those patients with intermediate risk may be maintained on long-term clopidogrel (Plavix), a potent platelet inhibitor.

Administration of antibiotics. Patients undergoing vascular surgery are typically treated with a single preoperative and one to three postoperative IV doses of a first-generation cephalosporin (e.g., cefazolin). If a prosthetic graft is used, many surgeons prolong the postoperative coverage to 5 days. If the patient has an infected foot or ulcer, the antibiotic therapy is prolonged and the coverage is widened.

Walking. Most patients should be encouraged to begin walking a day or two after surgery.

Mr. Brown's right ABI increases from 0.39 preoperatively to 0.8, and he maintains a good right dorsalis pedis pulse. His rest pain is gone. He begins limited walking the day after the operation and is discharged on the fifth day with continued good distal pulse.

What is the 5-year survival for patients such as Mr. Brown, who have had surgery for PAOD?

The 5-year survival rate for patients after peripheral arterial reconstruction ranges from 22% to 85% (Table 33.2). Survival of individual patients depends on the severity of any CAD, status of the CABG, gender, and any diabetes mellitus. Stratification of the patients according to gender and diabetes reveals that nondiabetic men gain the greatest benefit from CABG. This subgroup has 81% 5-year survival after CABG, compared with 58% in women and diabetic patients (13). Thus, Mr. Brown, who is not diabetic and who has undergone CABG, has approximately a 70% to 80% chance of surviving 5 years.

TABLE 33.2.

EFFECT OF CORONARY ARTERY DISEASE ON SURVIVAL AFTER PERIPHERAL ARTERIAL RECONSTRUCTION

Status of CAD	5-Year Survival (%)
No significant CAD	85
Severe CAD with CABG	72
Advanced compensated CAD (no CABG)	64
Severe CAD without CABG	43
Severe inoperable CAD	22

CABG, coronary artery bypass grafting; CAD, coronary artery disease.

From Hertzer NR. The natural history of peripheral vascular disease: implications for its management. Circulation. 1991;83(Suppl):12–19, with permission.

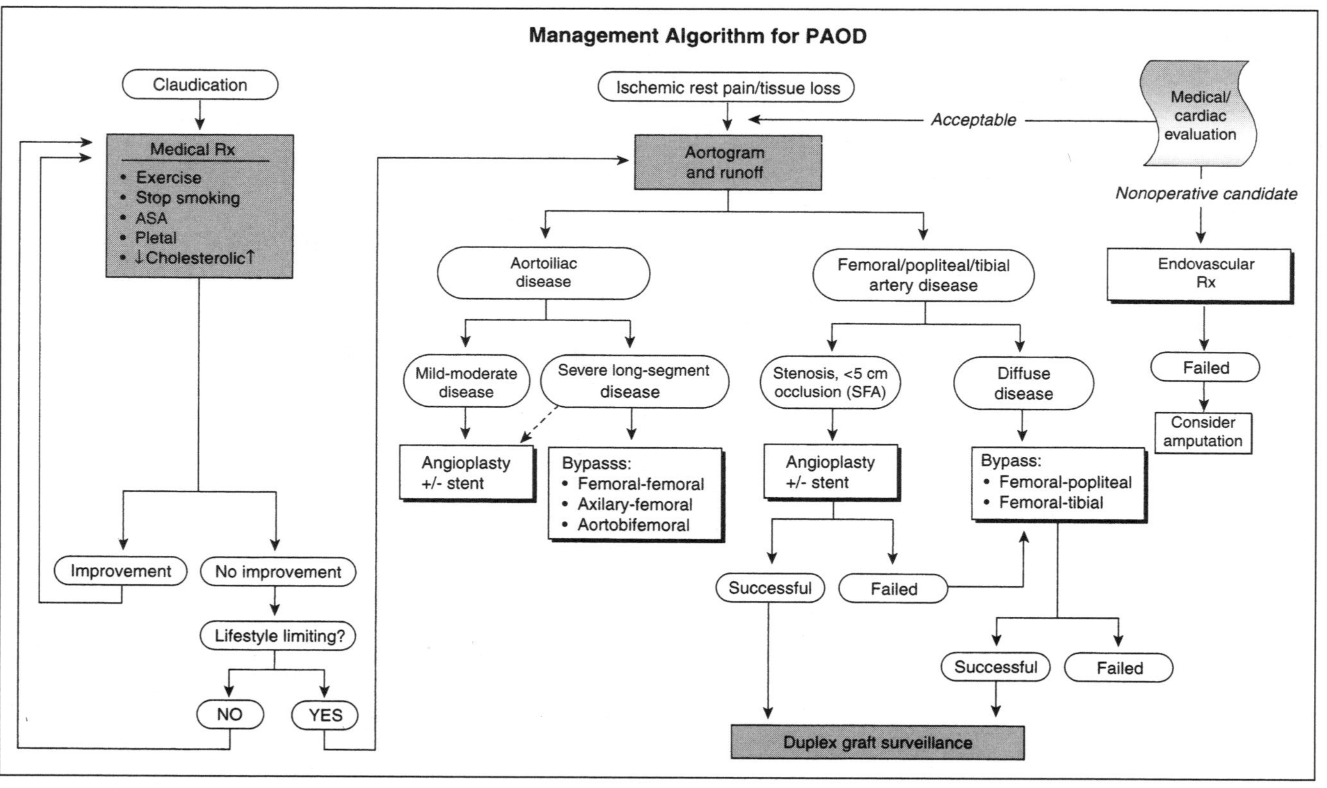

Algorithm 33.1.

Why is it important to maintain long-term surveillance for a failing graft?

The patency rates for grafts that are threatened and revised before thrombosis sets in are 15% to 25% higher than patency rates for grafts that are revised after thrombosis (14,15). A discrete area of stenosis may be treated with balloon angioplasty, open patch angioplasty, or a short jump graft. After total occlusion and thrombosis, the revision is more difficult and the outcome less favorable.

What causes bypass graft failure?

Technical problems with the graft. Most graft thromboses within the first 30 days of surgery are due to technical problems such as a kinked graft, an inadequate venous conduit, or an unrecognized intimal flap. Prompt surgical revision is indicated.

Intimal hyperplasia at the anastomosis. For reasons that are not well understood, significant stenosis caused by intimal hyperplasia may occur at the distal anastomosis. The pathogenesis may be related to shear stress, operative handling of the anastomosis, and the degree of compliance mismatch between the conduit and recipient artery. Intimal hyperplasia is the most frequent cause of graft failure 2 to 24 months after a bypass operation.

Progression of arterial disease. Atherosclerotic disease may progress proximal or distal to the bypass, compromising its inflow, outflow, or both. Progression of atherosclerotic disease is the most common cause of graft occlusion after 3 to 4 years.

Degenerative changes in the graft. The body of the graft can also be affected by intimal thickening, atherosclerotic changes, and fibrosis, especially at the old valve sites. These degenerative changes may appear within months or many years after surgery.

How is a failing graft detected?

Patients with significant graft stenoses may have recurring rest pain, claudication, or tissue loss; however, many patients have no symptoms. Although examination of the strength and character of the pulses is important for monitoring a patient after peripheral vascular reconstruction, variation between examinations and the difficulty in comparing pulses over time may make the physical examination unreliable. Duplex US is therefore important in surveillance of these patients. Changes in pulse volume or Doppler velocity usually precede a drop in the ABI. Any suspicion of impending graft failure should be cause for prompt arteriography and any necessary correction for the best long-term results.

REFERENCES

1. Dawber TR. The Framingham Study: The Epidemiology of Atherosclerotic Disease. Cambridge, Mass: Harvard University Press; 1980:105–110.

2. Imparato AM, Kim GE, Davidson T, et al. Intermittent claudication: its natural course. Surgery. 1975;78:795–799.
3. Kannel WB, Skinner JJ, Schwartz MJ, et al. Intermittent claudication: incidence in the Framingham study. Circulation. 1970;41:875–883.
4. Mcallister FF. The fate of patients with intermittent claudication managed nonoperatively. Am J Surg. 1976;132:593–595.
5. Kannel WB, Shurtleff D. Cigarettes and the development of intermittent claudication. Geriatrics. 1973;28:61–65.
6. Quick CRG, Cotton LT. The measured effect of stopping smoking on intermittent claudication. Br J Surg. 1982;69:S24–S26.
7. Hertzer NR, Bever EG, Young JR, et al. Coronary artery disease in peripheral vascular patients: a classification of 1000 coronary angiograms and results of surgical management. Ann Surg. 1984;199:223–233.
8. Keith FJ, Gupta SK, Ascer E, et al. Six-year prospective multicenter randomized comparison of autologous saphenous vein and expanded polytetrafluoroethylene grafts in infrainguinal arterial reconstruction. J Vasc Surg. 1986;3:104–114.
9. Leather RP, Veith FJ. In situ vein bypass. In: Haimovici H, ed. Vascular Surgery. Norwark, Conn: Appleton & Lange; 1989:524–526.
10. Wengerter KR, Veith FJ, Gupta SK, et al. Prospective randomized multicenter comparison of in situ and reversed vein infrapopliteal bypasses. J Vasc Surg. 1991;13:189–199.
11. Papanicolaou G, Aziz I, Yellin AE, et al. Intraoperative color duplex scanning for infrainguinal vein grafts. Ann Vasc Surg. 1996;10:347–355.
12. Bandyk DF, Johnson BL, Gupta AK, et al. Nature and management of duplex abnormalities encountered during infrainguinal vein bypass grafting. J Vasc Surg. 1996;24:430–438.
13. Hertzer NR. The natural history of peripheral vascular disease: implications for its management. Circulation. 1991;83(Suppl 1):I-12–I-19.
14. Berkowitz HD, Greenstein SM. Improved patency in reversed femoral infrapopliteal autogenous vein grafts by early detection and treatment of the failing graft. J Vasc Surg. 1987;5:755–761.
15. Caps MT, Cantwell-Gab K, Bergelin RO, et al. Vein graft lesions: time of onset and rate of progression. J Vasc Surg. 1995;22:466–475.

APPENDIX

BASICS OF MECHANICAL VENTILATION

Edgar Rodas and Michael B. Aboutanos

The number one reason for intensive care unit (ICU) admission is the need for mechanical ventilation (MV). Therefore, it is essential that the clinician be well versed on when to initiate MV, how to provide patients this specialized treatment modality safely, how to monitor ventilated patients to diagnose and prevent potential complications, and when to discontinue MV.

What is MV?

MV is a means to provide full or partial respiratory support to patients who otherwise cannot adequately sustain their requirements for oxygenation and/or ventilation secondary to a disease process, trauma, or surgical procedure.

Why do we need to provide ventilatory support?

Patients require ventilatory support to overcome an imbalance between the supply and demand of oxygen created by a pathologic process that alters the patient's capacity to perform the work of breathing, alters their muscle strength, or inhibits the efficiency of breathing and results in respiratory distress or inability to protect the airway. Whatever the disease process—neurogenic (stroke), pulmonary (acute lung injury, acute respiratory distress syndrome (ARDS), atelectasis, bronchospasm), cardiogenic (myocardial infarction, impending cardiopulmonary arrest) nephrogenic (uremia), metabolic (severe diabetic ketoacidosis, intoxications), infectious (pneumonia, sepsis), traumatic (closed head injury, thoracic trauma), or mechanical (aspiration pneumonitis, inhalation injury)—the ultimate goal of MV is to restore balance between supply and demand, improving gas exchange until the underlying cause is corrected and the patient can support him- or herself.

What are the indications for MV?

Although unique to each clinical situation, the indications for MV in general are as follows:

- *Failure to oxygenate:* partial pressure of oxygen (PO_2) less than 50 mm Hg on high oxygen delivery content, resulting in tachypnea or respiratory distress.
- *Failure to ventilate leading to progressive hypercapnia:* PO_2 less than 50 mm Hg, associated with moderate to severe acidosis, pH less than 7.3, and acute mental status changes.
- *Compromised airway control with impending hypoventilation or apnea:* For example, compromise found in closed head injury or stroke.

How is MV provided?

MV can be provided by either negative pressure or positive pressure. Only positive pressure ventilation is covered here, in view of the fact that negative pressure ventilators are no longer used in today's ICUs.

In general, MV is an invasive therapy because it requires endotracheal intubation or tracheostomy tube placement to deliver it. There are noninvasive forms of MV that can provide continuous positive airway pressure delivered through a facemask. Its use has been shown to be effective for improving gas exchange in patients with acute exacerbation of chronic obstructive lung disease and risk of respiratory failure, thus avoiding complications associated with endotracheal intubation (1,2).

What are the types of ventilation modes?

Volume control. The amount of ventilation is preset by tidal volume, thus regardless of the state of the patient's pulmonary mechanics, a known volume of air is delivered into the patient's lungs. Depending on the lung compliance, the inspiratory pressure may vary. In normal lungs, large tidal volumes result in normal peak inspiratory pressure. However, in stiff lungs (e.g., in patients with ARDS), a small tidal volume may result in a high peak inspiratory pressure, resulting in barotrauma or pneumothorax.

Pressure control. This is also known as volume-variable mode. The inspiratory pressure is preset, and volume is delivered into the lungs until the set pressure is met, at which point the MV ceases to deliver air. The actual tidal volume depends on lung compliance and the preset inspiratory pressure. The tidal volume is variable, but the advantage is that dangerously high inspiratory pressures can be avoided in patients with stiff lungs.

High frequency. This mode is effective in patients with bronchopleural fistula. High-frequency jet ventilation may provide adequate ventilatory support for a short time while maintaining a relatively low mean airway pressure. This mode also has been used with variable results in the treatment of patients with severe ARDS or refractory respiratory failure whose need for pressure-controlled ventilation has been pushed to the limit.

What are the ventilator settings?

Ventilator settings are parameters needed to provide adequate support to patients during the respiratory cycle and decrease their work of breathing. These settings are rate or mode, FIO_2, tidal volume, pressure, and inspiration-expiration ratio.

Rate or Mode

In *intermittent mandatory ventilation* (IMV), the patient receives a mandatory preset rate of MV in addition to what the patient breathes on his or her own. The mandatory MV and the patient's spontaneous breathing are not synchronized. The initial setting is usually 10 breaths per minute.

In *synchronized intermittent mandatory ventilation* (SIMV), a preset rate of ventilation is delivered in synchrony with the patient's own breathing pattern. A preset rate of 10 delivers only 10 breaths per minute in synchrony with the patient's own breathing, even if the patient is taking 30 breaths per minute. (Compare with assisted control ventilation, next.)

In *assisted control ventilation* (ACV), each breath initiated by the patient triggers the MV to deliver the tidal volume. A preset rate of 10 delivers at least 10 ventilatory breaths per minute if the patient is breathing at less than that rate. However, if the patient is breathing at 30 breaths per minute, ACV provides 30 assisted breaths per minute.

In *pressure support ventilation* (PSV), each breath initiated by the patient triggers the MV to deliver a variable flow of air into the lungs until the inspiratory pressure reaches a preset value. The actual assisted volume provided by the respirator depends on the preset pressure, the lung compliance, and the patient's inspiratory efforts. This mode has been designed to diminish the work required by the patient to breathe and is useful for patients with weaning difficulties.

FIO_2

The FIO_2 is the fraction of inspired oxygen in the air delivered to the patient, commonly expressed as a percentage of oxygen. Avoiding long periods of time at a 100% setting is recommended to prevent oxygen toxicity and nitrogen washout. The threshold concentration for preventing this toxicity is 0.6 FIO_2 (3).

Volume Parameter

Minute ventilation is the *tidal volume* (TV) multiplied by the respiratory rate per minute. TV is usually calculated as 6 to 8 mL per kg per breath. This lower tidal volume was determined to be safer than the traditional 10 mL per kg in a clinical trial after demonstrating its role in protection against barotrauma and decreasing mortality in patients with acute lung injury and ARDS (4).

Pressure Parameters

Peak inspiratory pressure (PIP) is the peak pressure achieved in the respirator-lung circuit during inspiration. When tidal volume is preset, PIP depends on lung compliance. In stiff lungs, even a small tidal volume may result in high PIP. A PIP greater than 50 cm H_2O is associated with barotraumatic pneumothorax.

Peak negative inspiratory pressure is the peak negative pressure generated by the patient's own breathing. It is used as an index of the patient's ability to breathe on his or her own following extubation.

Positive end-expiratory pressure (PEEP) is the pressure in the respirator-lung circuit at end expiration. Increased PEEP raises functional residual capacity by distending small patent alveoli and recruiting collapsed alveoli (those with more than 10 cm H_2O). Alveolar oxygen exchange improves, and Po_2 increases. PEEP is generally used in cases of suboptimal oxygenation (e.g., ARDS; pulmonary edema; severe pneumonitis, as in AIDS-related *Pneumocystis pneumonia;* and severe COPD). As a disadvantage, the cardiac output is known to fall with increasing PEEP because of decreased venous return, right ventricular dysfunction, and decreased left ventricular distensibility. Barotraumatic pneumothorax is also a known complication of PEEP therapy.

Continuous positive airway pressure (CPAP) keeps the inspiratory airway pressure above atmospheric pressure without increasing the work of breathing, whereas PEEP is applied to the patient's spontaneous breathing. CPAP maintains improved functional residual capacity, improved lung compliance, and a subjective sensation of breathing better. CPAP is therefore helpful in weaning patients who have been chronically dependent on a respirator.

Inspiration-Expiration Ratio

The inspiration-expiration (I:E) ratio is the ratio of the inspiratory time to expiratory time of each ventilatory cycle. The physiologic I:E ratio is 1:2. By increasing the inspiratory time, one can improve oxygenation by recruiting alveoli.

What are strategies for improving oxygenation and recruitment of alveoli?
Generally, the fractional concentration of oxygen in inspired gas (Fio_2) and PEEP effect changes in Po_2. In patients with ARDS, PEEP has been shown to improve oxygenation by decreasing intrapulmonary shunting (5).

Other unconventional means of recruiting alveoli are noted in the following paragraphs.

Inversing the I:E ratio improves oxygenation by increasing the mean airway pressure (6). This leads to improved oxygenation while allowing for arise in the Pco_2.

Permissive hypercapnia is thus employed, allowing for improved oxygenation while sacrificing ventilation and accepting a respiratory acidosis (7); however, there are no current controlled randomized trials that support this.

Changing patients into the prone position intermittently has also been shown to recruit collapsed lung tissue (8). Prone positioning improves oxygenation, reduces pulmonary shunt, and leads to improved lung volumes and uniformity of perfusion.

Use of selective pulmonary vasodilators such as inhaled nitric oxide in conjunction with other strategies has produced an additive short-term improvement in oxygenation in ARDS (9); however, no level I evidence exists to show any improvement in survival. Other agents such as prostaglandins are also under investigation and could yield promising results.

High-frequency ventilation (HFV) modes are new forms of MV for treatment of refractory hypoxemia. HFV uses low tidal volumes at remarkably high rates to produce gas exchange at lower airway pressure than conventional ventilation and to maintain the alveoli recruited throughout the respiratory cycle (10,11). There are three types of HFV: (a) high-frequency jet ventilation (HFJV), (b) high-frequency percussive ventilation (HFPV), and (c) high-frequency oscillatory ventilation (HFOV).

What are strategies for improving ventilation?

The parameters that alter minute ventilation (e.g., tidal volume, rate, and pressure support ventilation) effect changes in the partial pressure of carbon dioxide (P_{CO_2}), thus by manipulating any of these parameters alone or in conjunction one can alter ventilation.

How can you monitor patients on MV?

Patients on MV need to be assessed periodically to ensure their safety. Six main parameters have been described to monitor ventilated patients (12): (a) bedside findings, (b) oxygenation, (c) ventilation, (d) hemodynamics, (e) pulmonary mechanics, and (f) ventilator function.

What are the complications of MV?

Complications can be related to the endotracheal tube or tracheostomy tube and include (a) injuries from direct contact during tube placement or after prolonged intubation with development of tracheal stenosis or tracheo-innominate fistula; (b) infectious complications such as ventilator-associated pneumonia and sinusitis; (c) barotrauma and tension pneumothorax; (d) complications from alterations in the hemodynamics due to increased pressure causing a variety of alterations such as reduced cardiac output from decreased venous return; and (e) decreased renal and hepatic function (12).

What are the new ventilator modalities, and how do they differ from conventional ventilation?

The new ventilator modalities strive to limit lung injury associated with MV. The two most recent modalities are BiLevel and airway pressure release ventilation (APRV). They differ from conventional ventilation by allowing the patient to spontaneously breath throughout the entire ventilatory cycle with decreased sedation use and without neuromuscular blockade. They simultaneously maintain lower airway pressures, lower minute ventilation, and minimal adverse effect on the cardiocirculatory function (13).

What is BiLevel mode?

BiLevel means two levels of PEEP generated in a pressure-controlled–like ventilation mode; however, the patient is able to breathe spontaneously at either the high or the low PEEP. This mode of ventilation is beneficial because it decreases the need for paralytics and sedatives and their side effects. It can be applied clinically in patients with ARDS as well as during the weaning process when patients need less support.

What is APRV?

APRV is CPAP with regular, brief releases in airway pressure. It begins at an elevated baseline pressure. Releasing volume from this high baseline pressure to zero pressure in order to augment ventilation distinguishes APRV from other types of ventilation. Spontaneous breathing is also allowed in the upper pressure level, allowing additional ventilation (13).

How does BiLevel differ from APRV?

BiLevel is biphasic positive airway pressure (high PEEP, low PEEP). It differs from APRV only in the timing of the upper and lower pressures. In APRV, the lower pressure is set at zero for a brief duration (i.e., 0.8 second).

What is ventilator weaning?

Ventilator weaning is the process of gradually decreasing ventilatory support, allowing the patient to regain full control of the work of breathing and facilitate separation of the ventilator successfully. It is important to discontinue MV when resolution or correction of the primary cause that led to intubation and the need for respiratory support have been achieved (14). It is imperative that the physician understand how to assess and interpret the different weaning parameters.

How is a patient weaned from MV?

There is no standarized way to wean patients from MV. The three most popular modes are T-piece, PSV, and SIMV. There are no randomized, controlled trials to determine which is the best mode of weaning (15). How the technique of weaning is applied is as important as the mode of weaning. Protocol-directed weaning has been shown to decrease weaning time independent from the mode used (16,17). Ventilator management protocol was associated with decreased incidence of ventilator-associated pneumonia in trauma patients (18).

What are weaning parameters?

When the patient's ventilatory status nears that of extubation, a set of weaning parameters is obtained to assess the patient's likelihood of successful extubation (19); these parameters and their threshold values follow:

$\dot{V}_E$ (minute ventilation) = 10 to 15 L per min
NIF (negative inspiratory force) = −20 to −30 cm H_2O
PImax (maximal inspiratory pressure) = −15 to −30 cm H_2O
$P_{0.1}$/ PImax (mouth occlusion 0.1 sec after onset of inspiratory effort) = 0.30
CROP score (index including compliance, rate, oxygenation, and pressure) = 13
RR (respiratory rate) = 30 to 38 beats per minute
V_T(tidal volume) = 4 to 6 mL per kg
F:V_T ratio (respiratory rate/tidal volume) = 60 to 105 per L

The decision to wean and extubate a patient is primarily based on clinical judgment. No predetermined set of criteria may suffice to replace individual consideration.

GUIDELINES FOR WEANING AND DISCONTINUING MECHANICAL VENTILATORY SUPPORT

The following recomendations were made by a collective task force facilitated by the American College of Chest Physicians, the American Association of Respiratory Care, and the American College of Critical Care Medicine (20) in addition to guidelines used in our ICU.

1. Search for causes that may contribute to ventilatory dependency in all patients requiring MV for more than 24 hours. These can be neurologic, pulmonary, mechanical, cardiovascular, infectious, metabolic, nutritional, or psychological.
2. Assess the following criteria before considering the patient to be ready for MV weaning:
   - Reversal of underlying cause of respiratory failure
   - Hemodynamic stability, without pressors or low dose vasopressor (i.e., dopamine or dobutamine less than 5 μg per kg per min)
   - Adequate oxygenation: P:F ratio greater than 150 to 200, PEEP 5 to 8, F_{IO_2} 0.4 to 0.5, pH greater than or equl to 7.25
   - PSV of 15 cm or less

- Adequate mentation and ability to initiate inspiratory effort
- Able to handle secretions and intact cough reflex

3. If the patient meets all the criteria just listed, obtain a rapid shallow breathing index (RSBI). This consists of the respiratory rate:tidal volume ratio (F:VT) in liters in 1 minute. The number obtained should be less than 105.
4. Initiate a spontaneous breathing trial (SBT). SBTs are used to assess the patient's ability to breathe on his or her own on a subjective comfortable level, with a normal respiratory pattern, maintaining adequate gas exchange and hemodynamic stability. SBT should last between 30 and 120 minutes.
5. In order to discontinue MV, the patient's airway must be patent and the patient should be able to protect the airway. Before removal of the endotracheal tube, deflate the cuff to ensure the clear passage of air around the lumen of the endotracheal tube. This is a very simple test that can prevent early respiratory distress secondary to obstruction due to airway edema or extrinsic compression.
6. When patients fail a SBT, they are placed back on ventilatory support and allowed to rest. A search for the cause of failing is initiated and, if all steps are once again cleared, another attempt is carried out in 24 hours.
7. Use adequate analgesia and sedation strategies.
8. Use of protocol-directed weaning will hasten the extubation process.
9. Consider tracheostomy when it is apparent that the patient will require prolongued MV.

REFERENCES

1. Abou-Shala N, Meduri GU. Noninasive mechanical ventilation in patients with acute respiratory failure. Crit Care Med. 1996;24:705–715.
2. Antonelli M, ContiG, Rocco M, et al. A comparison of noninvasive positive-pressure ventilation and conventional mechanical ventilation in patients with acute respiratory failure. N Engl J Med. 1998;339:429–435.
3. Lodato RF. Oxygen toxicity. Crit Care Clin. 1990;6:749–765.
4. The Acute Respiratory Distress Syndrome Network. Ventilation with lower tidal volumes as compared with traditional tidal volumes for acute lung injury and the acute respiratory distress syndrome. N Engl J Med. 2000;342:1301–1308.
5. Dantzker DR, Brook CJ, Dehart P, et al. Ventilation-perfusion distributions in the adult respiratory distress syndrome. Am Rev Respir Dis. 1979;6:749–765.
6. Yanos J, Watling SM, Verhey J. The physiologic effects of inverse ratio ventilation. Chest. 1998;114:834–838.
7. Bidani A, Tzouanakis AE, Cardenas VJ, et al. Permissive hypercapnea in acute respiratory failure. JAMA. 1994;272:957–962.
8. Voggenreiter G, Neudeck F, Aufmkolk M, et al. Intermittent prone positioning in the treatment of severe and moderate posttraumatic lung injury. Crit Care Med. 1999;27:2375–2382.
9. Kaisers U, Busch T, Deja M, et al. Selective pulmonary vasodilation in acute respiratory distress syndrome. Crit Care Med. 2003;31:S337–S342.

10. Hynes-Gay P, MacDonald R. Using high-frequency oscillatory ventilation to treat adults with acute respiratory distress syndrome. Crit Care Nurse. 2001;21(5):38–47.
11. Bohn D. The history of high-frequency ventilation. Respir Care Clin N Am. 2001;7:535–548.
12. Brown BR. Understanding mechanical ventilation: patient monitoring, complications, and weaning. J Okla State Med Assoc. 1994;87:411–418.
13. Frawley PM, Habashi NM. Airway pressure release ventilation: theory and practice. AACN Clinical Issues. 2001;12(2):234–246.
14. Esteban A, Alía I, Ibañez J, et al. Modes of mechanical ventilation and weaning: a national survey of Spanish hospitals. Chest. 1994;106:1188–1193.
15. Butler R, Keenan S, Inman KJ, et al. Is there a preferred technique for weaning the difficult-to-wean patient? A systematic review of the literature. Crit Care Med. 1999;27:2331–2336.
16. Kollef MH, Shapiro SD, Siver P, et al. A randomized controlled trial of protocol-directed versus physician-directed weaning from mechanical ventilation. Crit Care Med. 1997;25:567–574.
17. Brilli RJ, Spevetz A, Branson RD, et al. Critical care delivery in the intensive care unit: defining clinical roles and best practice model. Crit Care Med. 2001;29:2007–2019.
18. Marelich GP, Murin S, Battestella F, et al. Protocol weaning of mechanical ventilation in medical and surgical patients by respiratory care practitioners and nurses: effect on weaning time and incidence of ventilator associated pneumonia. Chest. 2000;118:459–467.
19. Cook D, Meade M, Guyatt G, et al. Evidence report on criteria for weaning from mechanical ventilation. Rockville, Md: Agency for Health Care Policy and Research; 1999.
20. Cook DJ, Ely EW, Epstein SK, et al. Evidence-based guidelines for weaning and discontinuing mechanical ventilatory support. A collective task force facilitated by the American College of Chest Physicians, the American Association of Respiratory Care, and the American College of Critical Care Medicine. Chest. 2001;120:375S–395S.

APPENDIX

HEMOSTASIS AND COAGULATION DISORDERS

Cornelius Dyke

OVERVIEW OF HEMOSTASIS AND FIBRINOLYSIS

The body's intrinsic control of hemorrhage necessitates a complex interplay between clot formation and lysis. Clot formation is essential to maintain hemostasis when vessel injury occurs, yet uncontrolled clot formation results in thrombosis and its ischemic complications.

Hemostasis may be considered to occur in three steps: (a) blood vessel vasoconstriction, (b) platelet activation and aggregation, and (c) formation of the insoluble fibrin clot. These three manifestations of the hemostatic response occur in unison to arrest bleeding. When a blood vessel is injured, local factors produced by platelets and endothelial cells result in an intense vasoconstrictive response that effectively reduces the rate of ongoing blood loss.

The disruption of the endothelial barrier also exposes underlying tissue factor in the vessel wall, resulting in potent platelet activation and aggregation as well as activation of the extrinsic pathway of the coagulation system (Fig. A2.1). The net result is the conversion of fibrinogen, a soluble plasma protein, into fibrin, an insoluble protein, which, when cross-linked, results in a stable clot. Simultaneously with clot formation, the fibrinolytic system is geared up to control and limit this process, preventing disseminated clot formation (Fig. A2.1).

Antithrombin III and the protein C and S system are the two dominant anticoagulant systems that prevent uncontrolled thrombosis. Antithrombin III binds to thrombin and activated factor X, inhibiting their procoagulant functions. (This reaction is powerfully potentiated by heparin, which makes it an effective anticoagulant.) Proteins C and S work together as cofactors to inhibit activated factors V and VIII, limiting thrombin formation.

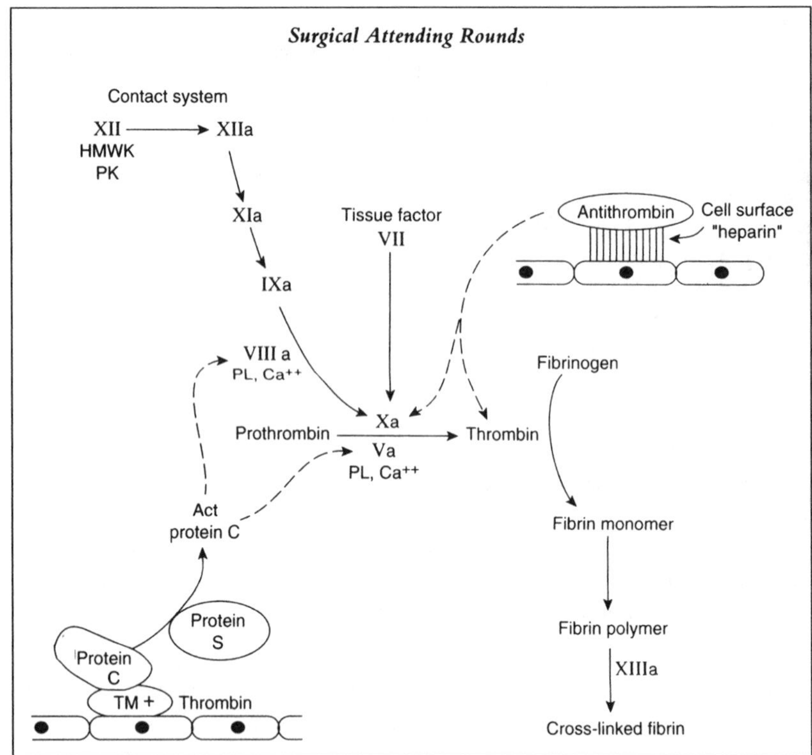

Figure A2.1 The coagulation cascade illustrates how soluble proteins interact when triggered to form an insoluble clot.

NORMAL PLATELET FUNCTION

Platelets are the first, middle, and last lines of defense against hemorrhage, and they contribute to every aspect of hemostasis and blood vessel repair after injury. Platelets from the initial platelet plug spread over the area of vessel injury and attract and promote migration of other platelets and inflammatory cells. In doing so, they create a dynamic scaffold for fibrin cross-linking and clot stabilization, and they modulate the remodeling process of the vessel wall. Thrombin is an especially potent stimulant for platelet activation, causing a change in platelet glycoprotein (GP) receptors that up-regulates their adhesiveness.

Two platelet membrane GP receptor complexes—the GP Iv–factor IX-V complex and the GP IIb/IIIa complex—are important for platelet adhesion and aggregation. The GP Ib complex, which is constitutively expressed on the platelet membrane, mediates initial adhesion of the platelet to the injured vessel wall via its interaction with von Willebrand factor, a protein associated with the subendothelial matrix. The importance of the GP I receptor to platelet adhesion is illustrated in Bernard-Soulier syndrome, a rare genetic disorder resulting in a dysfunctional GP I receptor on the platelet plasma membrane. Patients with Bernard-Soulier syndrome have platelets that respond normally to platelet agonists and activation but not to thrombin. These patients have significantly impaired platelet adhesion.

After initial platelet contact with subendothelial proteins (e.g., tissue factor) and subsequent activation, the platelet releases granules containing serotonin, epinephrine, thrombin, adenosine diphosphate, and thromboxane. These substances cause local vasocontriction, increase capillary permeability, and are potent chemoattractants, causing cellular migration of inflammatory cells and other platelets. The initial platelet plug is stabilized through interactions between another platelet GP complex expressed on the plasma membrane, that is, the GP IIb/IIIa receptor, causing high-affinity binding with fibrin, von Willebrand factor, and other platelet receptors. This results in a firm, sticky, solid clot of platelets and coagulation proteins covering the site of vessel injury.

Without activation of the GP IIb/IIIa complex, mature clot formation does not occur. This is remarkably demonstrated in patients with Glanzmann's thrombasthenia, a condition caused by a point mutation that results in a congenitally defective GP IIb/IIIa receptor. People with this disorder have a normal platelet count and normal initial adhesion; however, platelet aggregation is completely impaired, resulting in a clinically significant bleeding disorder.

Current Clinical Anticoagulants

For nearly 100 years, the mainstays of anticoagulation therapy have consisted of heparin, warfarin, and aspirin. Only recently, within the past 10 to 15 years, have other anticoagulants come to market and become widely used. Although heparin, warfarin, and aspirin are effective and remain commonplace, each has undesirable characteristics that have led to the development of newer agents.

Currently, clinicians are faced with an abundance of choices for their patients who require anticoagulation. The following summary of anticoagulant medications is meant to offer a convenient list of currently available drugs, recognizing that this field is rapidly evolving and additions to the market are expected. Additionally, as the choice of anticoagulants has increased, indications for their use continue to evolve.

Antiplatelet Agents

Cyclooxygenase Inhibitors

Aspirin. The first antiplatelet agent created, aspirin remains a critical component of the treatment and prevention of atherosclerotic heart disease and stroke. The usual dose is between 81 and 325 mg per day. Aspirin inhibits platelet activation by inhibiting the cyclooxygenase pathway, preventing the production of prostaglandin and thromboxane A_2 (an important activator of the platelet GP IIb/IIIa receptor). Aspirin's effects last for the lifetime of the platelet.

Adenosine Phosphate Antagonists

Clopidogrel (Plavix). Clopidogrel and ticlopidine are thienopyridines, potent noncompetitive inhibitors of the low-affinity platelet adenosine diphosphate (ADP) receptor. Clopidogrel and ticlopidine are metabolized in the liver, and the active metabolite binds irreversibly to the receptor, inhibiting platelet aggregation for the lifetime of the platelet. Because the ADP pathway is only one of several pathways for platelet activation, inhibition of aggregation is approximately 40% normal when patients are given a full dose. Clopidogrel and ticlopidine are usually used in conjunction with aspirin for the treatment and prevention of myocardial infarction and stroke.

Ticlopidine (Ticlid). Although both clopidogrel and ticlopidine have side effects, the incidence of bone marrow suppression and neutropenia is more common with ticlopidine than clopidogrel. This severely curtails its use in the United States.

Phosphodiesterase Inhibitors

Cilostazol (Pletal). Cilostazol is an oral, mild phosphodiesterase inhibitor that weakly inhibits platelet activation. Its vasodilatory effects are useful for the symptomatic relief of claudication in patients with peripheral vascular disease. It is not used to prevent cardiovascular events or stroke.

Glycoprotein IIb/IIIa Inhibitors

The GP IIb/IIIa receptor on the platelet is the final pathway for platelet activation and aggregation. The active GP IIb/IIIa receptor allows cross-linking with fibrinogen and subsequent clot stabilization. Inhibition of the GP IIb/IIIa receptor results in potent inhibition of platelet aggregation (>80%). Two of the GP IIb/IIIa inhibitors (Integrelin and Aggrastat) bind noncompetitively to the receptor, whereas the third GP IIb/IIIa inhibitor (ReoPro) is a chimeric monoclonal antibody that irreversibly binds to the receptor. These drugs are given intravenously to patients with acute coronary syndromes and to patients undergoing percutaneous coronary interventions. Although oral GP IIb/IIIa inhibitors have been developed, enthusiasm for their use has been erased by several negative clinical trials and there are none on the market.

Adenosine Reuptake Inhibitor

Dipyridamole (Aggrenox). Usually used in combination with aspirin, dipyridamole is a weak platelet inhibitor used most commonly for the prevention of stroke in at-risk patients. Dipyridamole stimulates prostacyclin synthesis and inhibits phosphodiesterase. It has no role in the prevention or treatment of cardiac events.

Antithrombin Agents

Heparin. *Unfractionated heparin* is an indirect thrombin inhibitor that asserts its effect by potentiating naturally circulating antithrombin III. Heparin should be thought of as a group of long polysaccharides whose action is mediated by a small segment of the molecule that binds and activates antithrombin III. The rest of the molecule has no anticoagulant activity.

Commercial preparations of heparin are derived from either pork intestine or beef lung and are a mixture of molecules with molecular weights from 3000 to 30,000 daltons. As the level of anticoagulant activity varies with each preparation, monitoring of the anticoagulant effect is critical. Classically, heparin monitoring is done by measuring the activated partial thromboplastin time (aPTT), although measurement of anti-Xa activity is becoming common. Heparin is given intravenously and has a half-life between 1 and 2 hours. Antibody formation to heparin preparations is common and can result in life-threatening complications. Heparin is reversed by protamine sulfate (a foreign protein isolated from fish sperm), which binds and inactivates it.

Low Molecular Weight Heparin. Another indirect thrombin inhibitor, fractionated or low molecular weight (LMW) heparins (Lovenox, Fragmin) are preparations that have been fractionated to contain molecules of heparin below 10,000 daltons. LMW heparins bind to antithrombin III and inhibit factor Xa. LMW heparin does not significantly affect the aPTT and the level of anti-Xa activity is consistent, eliminating the need for monitoring for its effect. LMW heparins are given through subcutaneous injection and are dosed on a weight-based regimen every 12 hours. LMW heparins have been shown to be effective for patients with acute coronary syndromes and for the prevention of venous thrombosis. They are not reversible with protamine sulfate.

Direct Thrombin Inhibitors. Hirudin, lepirudin, argatroban, and bivalirudin directly inhibit thrombin. They do not rely on adequate circulating amounts of antithrombin and do not bind to plasma proteins; as a consequence, their effect is very predictable and potent. Additionally, and unlike indirect thrombin inhibitors, they bind to clot-bound thrombin as well as circulating, fluid-phase thrombin. These direct thrombin inhibitors are given intravenously and are not reversible, although the short half-life of bivalirudin eliminates the need for a reversal agent and increases its clinical utility.

Bivalirudin binds to thrombin bivalently and is auto-cleaving, such that its antithrombin effects are gone in approximately 25 minutes. It has been approved for use in patients with acute coronary syndromes undergoing percutaneous coronary angioplasty.

Ximelagatran is an oral direct thrombin inhibitor derived from the saliva of the vampire bat. It has been shown in large clinical trials to be as effective as warfarin for the prevention of stroke in patients with atrial fibrillation, but unlike warfarin, it does not require monitoring of its anticoagulant effect. It is also being intensively studied for the prevention of deep venous thrombosis (DVT) and other clinical scenarios in which warfarin is classically indicated. Although not approved for use in the United States as of early 2004, its approval is expected.

Factor Xa Inhibitors. A new class of anticoagulant, the selective factor Xa inhibitor fondaparinux (Arixtra) is indicated for the prevention of DVT in patients at high risk for DVT after orthopedic surgery. It has a long half-life (15 hours) and is given as a daily subcutaneous injection dosed according to patient weight.

Vitamin K Antagonists. The anticoagulant effect of warfarin was first described in the veterinary literature in the 1920s after an outbreak of hemorrhagic disease in cattle. Warfarin inhibits the synthesis of the vitamin K–dependent factors VII, IX, X, and proteins C and S in the liver. It has a long half-life (approximately 40 hours). Because its anticoagulant effect is dependent upon inhibition of the synthesis of coagulation factors and because it does not affect circulating coagulation factors, the anticoagulation effect takes time to achieve. Careful monitoring with the prothrombin time is essential as diet, drug interactions, drug absorption, and liver function all affect the level of inhibition of factor synthesis in the liver. Warfarin is not readily reversible. Rapid reversal requires infusion of coagulation factors, and the effect of vitamin K supplementation takes time.

The Future

The dramatic increase in the number of drugs that affect coagulation in the past decade is a direct result of our improved understanding of the science of blood clotting. As our understanding of the intricate biology of hemostasis and thrombosis continues to accelerate, increasingly sophisticated manipulation of the coagulation and fibrinolytic systems will become possible. The tools for anticoagulation will continue to becoming increasingly delicate, improving efficacy and increasing safety for our patients.

PREOPERATIVE EVALUATION OF THE COAGULATION SYSTEM

The preoperative hemostatic assessment of the surgical patient raises three questions:

1. Are there any preexisting coagulation abnormalities?
2. What corrections should be made?

3. What are the intraoperative and postoperative transfusion requirements likely to be?

A careful history and physical examination are the most important components of the preoperative assessment of the coagulation system in the surgical patient; they are more important than a routine battery of coagulation tests. A congenital bleeding diathesis is elicited by careful questioning about bruising ability, prolonged bleeding from minor cuts or shaving, frequent nosebleeds, or arthralgias. The physical examination is important in confirming these findings. A medication history is particulary important because many medications affect the coagulation system.

Routine laboratory testing ("coag screen") is not cost-effective and adds little information about patients who have no evidence of coagulation defects on history or physical examination and who are undergoing surgery in which blood loss is expected to be minimal. Laboratory testing is useful in patients who may have a coagulation defect or whose potential for intraoperative bleeding is high.

ORDERING BLOOD PRODUCTS

Blood typing and screening are usually performed for patients who may, but are unlikely to, need transfusion (e.g., before a routine colectomy). When antibodies in the patient's blood sample are detected, donor blood lacking those antibodies is identified in case it is needed. Although antigens may be present in the blood that is set aside, they usually do not cause a serious hemolytic reaction.

A type-and-cross-match order completely cross-matches donor and recipient blood and makes available compatible blood cells.

Partially cross-matched blood transfusions use blood that is ABO-type specific, Rh matched, and tested for acute phase reactants without cross-matching lesser antigens. These transfusions are used in emergencies and are slightly safer than type-specific blood only.

The last choice for emergency transfusion (limited to exsanguination) is the use of type O Rh-negative blood. Hemolytic reactions from antibodies in the plasma may occur (a form of graft-versus-host disease) when non–cross-matched O-negative blood is used.

AUTOLOGOUS BLOOD TRANSFUSION

Selected patients electively scheduled for surgery may donate their own blood preoperatively for planned transfusion during the operation. Self (autologous) blood donation is frequently used by patients undergoing elective operations

TABLE A2.1.

ESTIMATED RISK OF BLOOD TRANSFUSION PER UNIT

Reaction or Adverse Event	Incidence
Minor allergic reaction	1:100
Fatal hemolytic reaction	1:600,000
Viral hepatitis (A, B, C, or D)	1:50,000
HIV infection	1:500,000

who have a high risk of bleeding, including those undergoing prostatic resection and major orthopedic surgery. The obvious benefit is the elimination of the infectious complications of donor blood transfusion (Table A2.1). Candidates for predonation of blood are patients without significant cardiopulmonary or neurologic disease who have a hemoglobin level greater than 11 g per dL. Patients may donate 2 to 3 units of blood in the weeks preceding surgery, with the last donation no later than 3 days before the operation. Patients take supplemental iron to enhance red blood cell production in the bone marrow. The use of erythropoietin to stimulate red blood cell production and allow more voluminous blood donation has been described, but it is not necessary in patients who are stockpiling only 2 or 3 units.

TRANSFUSING BLOOD PRODUCTS

Before transfusing blood or blood products, careful identification of the patient is mandatory. Human clerical error is the most common cause of blood transfusion reactions. Although there are infectious complications of blood transfusion, careful and universal testing has ensured a safe blood supply in the United States (Table A2.1). Normal saline is used with packed red blood cells to decrease the viscosity of the transfused blood. Calcium-containing solutions are not appropriate because they may induce clotting; hypoosmolar solutions are not used because they may induce cell lysis. Blood is filtered through a 170-μm filter to remove aggregates and cellular debris. Smaller filters may be used to remove white blood cells and thereby reduce febrile reactions that may occur with transfusion; however, the cost utility of this has been questioned. Blood should be warmed before transfusion in the operating room or when large quantities are needed.

Major signs of a transfusion reaction include flushing, hypotension, urticaria, hemoglobinuria, back pain, pruritis, chills, and fever. Obviously, in the anesthetized patient, these signs and symptoms are not apparent. Excessive bleeding and coagulopathy are a common sign of a transfusion reaction intraoperatively.

INTRAOPERATIVE BLOOD SALVAGE

When significant amounts of intraoperative bleeding occurs, blood may be scavenged from the operative field with suckers, washed, and the red blood cells returned to the patient. The hematocrit of this washed red blood cell volume is approximately half that of a unit of blood from the blood bank. However, it does have the advantage of being autologous. Intraoperative blood salvage is not appropriate in all patients. Patients with active infections or sepsis and those with cancer undergoing localized resection are not candidates for intraoperative blood scavenging because of the risk of spread of infection or tumor. Similarly, patients in whom significant bleeding and blood transfusion is unlikely do not justify the additional cost of the equipment to scavenge, wash, and retransfuse red blood cells "just in case."

ADJUNCTS TO HEMOSTASIS

Electrocautery (the Bovie) is ubiquitous in surgical practice today. Developed by William Bovie, a physicist, and Harvey Cushing at Johns Hopkins University, electrocautery dessicates tissue and locally destroys body proteins, creating an intense stimulus for thrombosis and heat-welding small blood vessels. Normal coagulation is needed for effective use.

Thrombin and collagen may be used topically on raw surfaces to stimulate coagulation and platelet adherence and activation. When used in sheets or pads, local tamponade may also contribute to hemostasis. Numerous commercial varieties are available.

Gelatin foam is also used as a local hemostatic agent. Although it has no procoagulant effect, gelatin foam soaks up blood and plasma increasing in size. This causes the gelatin foam to exert a local tamponade effect and to concentrate plasma proteins at the site of bleeding.

Fibrin glue may be used to create an instant clot at a specific site. Fibrin glue is created by putting fibrinogen in one syringe and calcium and thrombin in another. These ingredients must be kept separate until used because a fibrin clot is formed instantly when these ingredients are mixed.

BioGlue is another topical sealant with quick action. Composed of albumin and glutaraldehyde (separately), it is applied in liquid form. Within minutes, it forms a rigid and adherent seal when applied to a dry surface. Most commonly used during vascular procedures (especially large vessel and aortic surgery), it is especially useful to seal needle holes in prosthetic material.

None of the surgical adjuncts to hemostasis replaces meticulous surgical technique.

APPENDIX

SURGICAL NUTRITION

Jeannie F. Savas

The nutritional status of a patient may be poor because of inadequate food intake, poor absorption, or an increased metabolic state, such as is seen with sepsis or recent surgery. The nutritional assessment begins with the history and physical examination.

Has there been weight loss, diarrhea, vomiting, dysphagia, anorexia, or steatorrhea?

Has the patient had surgery or a medical condition that is associated with malabsorption or malnutrition?

Many surgical patients are unable to eat because of recent abdominal surgery, bowel obstruction, ileus, pancreatitis, or alteration of mental status. All of these factors should be considered in determining whether a patient is at risk for malnutrition. The physical examination may reveal cachexia, abdominal distention, jaundice, poor skin turgor, edema, or dermatitis. Calculations such as the Harris-Benedict equation estimate the nutritional needs.

Nonspecific laboratory tests that may be clues to malnutrition include serum albumin, transferrin, total protein, liver function tests, total lymphocyte count, and prealbumin. A 24-hour urine specimen for nitrogen can evaluate whether a patient is in positive or negative nitrogen balance. The respiratory quotient (R/Q) is an accurate means of determining the adequacy of and proper balance of protein, carbohydrate, and fat calories in the diet. However, this test is difficult to perform unless the patient is on a ventilator.

Indications for supplementation include the following:

- No intake for more than 5 days
- Inadequate intake
- Inadequate absorption
- Hypermetabolic state that renders the patient in negative nitrogen balance

The route of supplementation should then be decided. Enteral nutrition, if possible, is preferred. This may be accomplished orally or via nasogastric or nasojejunal tube. If long-term supplementation is expected, a gastric or jejunal tube should be placed either endoscopically or surgically. Oral or gastric routes should be used only for patients not at high risk for aspiration. Common complications of enteral feeding are tube dislodgment or dysfunction, abdominal distension, and diarrhea. The latter two can usually be avoided by beginning with a diluted formula and advancing the amount slowly as tolerated. Sometimes the addition of kaolin pectin or antimotility agents is necessary once infection is excluded. Enteral nutrition is beneficial to maintain mucosal integrity and prevent bacterial translocation even if parenteral supplementation is also required to meet the patient's nutritional needs. Special formulas are available for patients with diabetes, renal failure, hepatic failure, and ileus or malabsorptive states.

If enteral nutrition is not an option (e.g., bowel obstruction, severe ileus, bowel ischemia, or malabsorptive state) parenteral nutrition is instituted. If short-term or partial supplementation is necessary, it may be achieved via a peripheral venous catheter. If long-term or complete supplementation is needed, the patient must have a central venous catheter despite the risks of sepsis, glucose intolerance, and catheter-related complications. There are special formulations for patients with renal or hepatic failure. All patients need to be monitored for glucose intolerance, electrolyte imbalances, hypophosphatemia, and cholestasis.

The amount and type of supplementation a patient requires should be periodically assessed with routine laboratory tests, measurement of nitrogen balance, and/or the R/Q. As a guideline, the nonstressed person needs 25 kcal per kg per day. Stresses such as sepsis, tumor, trauma, burns, multiple illnesses, and/or recent surgery may increase these needs by 50% to 400%. Underfeeding a patient produces a catabolic state and an inability to heal or fight infection. Overfeeding a patient may result in carbon dioxide retention and ventilator dependence.

Occasionally, a patient who is nutritionally depleted needs surgery, such as for cancer. If possible, supplementation should be given until the patient is in positive nitrogen balance in order to diminish the perioperative morbidity and mortality. This is particularly important if the serum albumin is less than 2.0 mg per dL. Studies have shown that severely hypoalbuminemic patients experience a greater incidence of complications and death following surgery.

Surgical patients are often at risk for malnutrition. Start feeding and/or supplementing patients at risk as soon as possible, and frequently reassess the adequacy of nutrition. Feed enterally whenever possible, even if parenteral nutrition is also required to meet the patient's needs. Consider placing a feeding tube at the time of surgery in patients at risk. Remember that stress, such as experienced during trauma, surgery, or sepsis, greatly increases the metabolic needs of the patient.

INDEX

Page numbers in italics denote figures; those followed by a t denote tables.